The Women's Book: Volume 1

A Guide to Nutrition, Fat Loss, and Muscle Gain

by Lyle McDonald

ISBN: 978-0-9671456-9-3

For information contact:
Lyle McDonald Publishing
1200 Hatteras Drive
Austin, Tx 78753
Email: support@bodyrecomposition.com

A portion of the sale of this book will benefit the Women's Sports Foundation, a 501c3 charity founded by Billie Jean King and dedicated to creating leaders by ensuring all girls access to sports.

Acknowledgements

A number of people contributed to the completion of this book that I want to acknowledge. Several including Keith Caskey, Adam Rafalowsky, J Fred Muggs and others helped me to get some of the research papers that I needed.   Lisa Vickers suggested a title change and the book is better for it.

Finally, I want to thank the many, many women online who made me aware of female specific issues that I would likely not have thought to address if they hadn't.

Preface

Preface

Having been in the fitness field for nearly 20 years, it's been clear to me for quite some time that women face issues that men simply don't. They have more overall trouble with fat loss, seem to gain weight and fat more easily along with endless other differences. And while I had made observations regarding this over the years, I had never really examined it in any sort of of enormous detail. But this lack of attention to the issue came to a head in 2007 which is when I can say that this book really started. I had a female trainee who I simply could not figure out. Her performance was all over the place in the gym with her coordination, strength and mood changing seemingly weekly. She'd hit personal bests one week and be unable to lift 60% of her best in others with smaller variations in other weeks. Her mood shifted constantly and she suffered from fairly debilitating PMS along with the typical female body fat issues.

One day, in the midst of a tangentially (and unfinished) related project, I decided to finally get this worked out and to "solve PMS". I spent the day reading endless research papers and, without exaggerating, was done in about a day. At least in regards to her training, a basic model of what needed to be done fell right into place. While that should have been the start of the project it wasn't. I'd write my Stubborn Fat Solution (addressing women's bodyfat issues) shortly thereafter and essentially retire for about 8 years.

In 2015, after a few years of craziness, I finally got back to work. About February of that year, I found out that one of my earlier books, A Guide to Flexible Dieting (written in 2004), had been plagiarized by someone claiming to have pioneered the concept. It wasn't even the first time I'd been plagiarized but this made me angry. Very angry. For little to no reason other than spite, I decided to rewrite that book. A lot of my thoughts had changed and, being 11 years old, it was a little rough around the edges.

As I started that project, I realized that I needed to add a section and add a section and all of a sudden it had turned into a completely different book, one on general fat loss. I'd needed to write that kind of book for a while so that's what I began doing. I pulled information from my other books, from my website and suddenly what started as a basic rewrite had spiraled into a 400 page tome. My purpose, ignoring dealing with my anger, became to write the be-all, end-all book on the topic of fat loss. If it wasn't discussed in my book, it didn't matter or the concept didn't yet exist. As a secondary, and also anger driven goal, I wanted to give people in the field something to plagiarize for the next decade. They were going to do it anyway so I figured I might as well give them a comprehensive (and correct) resource to rip off.

Women's Issues

Which brings me in a very roundabout way to the book you hold in your hands. I had reached a point where I was about 90% done with the mega fat loss book, at least in its initial form when I realized there was one last topic I needed to discuss. A topic that I had promised a book on years previously but had avoided (consciously or unconsciously) as I knew the difficulty it would entail. Of course that topic was women's issues as they pertained to diet, fat loss and training. As trite as it sounds, it was clear that women are "not just little men" even if they are often treated as such by coaches, physiologists and the medical establishment alike. There are physiological, anatomical, neurological and psychological differences to begin with and that's just as a baseline. During the course of the menstrual cycle, changes in a woman's hormone levels cause large-scale shifts in a woman's physiology. Her insulin sensitivity, whether she uses fat or carbohydrates for fuel, her metabolic rate, hunger, propensity to store fat along with her strength, endurance, coordination, injury risk and almost any other topic you could think of all change. In contrast, men are basically the same every day.

Originally I figured I could cover the topic in maybe a chapter or so. Hahahahaha. Not only would it have been totally unfair to relegate women's issues to one short chapter, it became rapidly clear that it was impossible. Women make up ~51% of the population and a single chapter wouldn't do even if I could do the topic justice in that few pages. I figured I'd expand it to the length of the other sections in that book, that I might get it done in 40-50 pages. How wrong I was. As I started writing that section and was putting up excerpts on my Facebook wall or in my group, women on both started going kind of nuts and clamoring for that information. They didn't want to wait for the tome to be finished and wanted it earlier rather than later. Given the general lack of information that was out there, and knowing my generally obsessive approach to projects, they knew anything that I wrote would cover the topic in a way that only I seem able to. Make no mistake, some of it already existed (I had personally read an older book by two Australian sports scientists/coaches on the topic that I am fairly sure nobody else has seen) and was on the web and I Googled what was out there myself to see what had been written. What I was found was either vague, incomplete or, in some cases, incorrect.

And it then dawned on me that, while information on women would be included in the mega-project to one degree or another, the topic truly needed its own stand-alone book. I'd have to pull some information from the big book since I couldn't say "Refer to Chapter 17" from a book that hasn't been release but that was fine. And I started writing and researching and writing and researching. As I got deeper into the topic, the complexity would multiply seemingly exponentially. The menstrual cycle alone introduced complications in women's physiology that simply don't occur in men. Even here, there is an added complexity. The "normal" menstrual cycle really isn't with a great deal of variability. Any two women may have different cycle lengths and even the same woman may have her cycle length change from month to month. Women also show differences in terms of how their mood, hunger, etc. change with almost no two women having the same exact pattern.

The cycle can also be disrupted. In oligomenorrhea, menstruation occurs infrequently. In amenorrhea (altogether too common in dieters and athletes), the cycle may be lost completely. Even that was only the tip of the iceberg due to the presence of what I call hormonal modifiers. Birth control (which is supremely complicated) is one of the most common but Poly-Cystic Ovary Syndrome (PCOS) along with the changes that occur around menopause are all important issues. There are endless other situations, disease states (some of which women are more susceptible to than men), that change the system but they are far beyond the scope of this book. But each of the above situations are subtly or not so subtly different from the others. The hormonal profile may change (or not) with a given reproductive hormone being relatively more dominant in terms of impacting or changing a woman's physiology. In contrast, a man's primary hormone is effectively a flat line that changes only minimally day to day and goes down gradually with age. Certainly levels of that hormone vary between men which may have implications for fat loss and training but these are really slight variations on a theme rather than being distinctly different physiologies entirely. Comparatively speaking, men are profoundly simple from a physiological (and some might say other) standpoint.

The Writing

While I was writing this book, I joked repeatedly that I had been putting it off for a decade and that's not really untrue. As I mentioned above, while I had recognized some of the issues purely from experience, I knew that delving into the topic thoroughly would be exhausting and I wasn't wrong. Covering even the general physiological differences would have been difficult enough but by the time the hormonal modifiers were added, addressing the topic in any degree of detail was overwhelming. A project that I thought I'd get done quickly and easily would rapidly spiral out of control. While I originally intended to talk about fat loss and training in the one book, I would end up having to split the information into two volumes (as I write this preface in September of 2017, the training book is only partially written).

None of this was made any easier by the fact that I was basically starting completely from scratch in terms of even the terminology that is used. I was a man writing about a topic that I have no fundamental (and certainly not personal) familiarity with studying information that doesn't resonate with me on any sort of intuitive level. I don't have a menstrual cycle and the entire concept is fundamentally foreign to me beyond my observations of female trainees. I would find that many women don't really understand the menstrual cycle so what chance, as a man did I have? Over the next 2.5 years, I would manage to wrap my head around the topic although I would be lying if I didn't say it was exhausting. In podcasts I would describe it as soul crushing with no negative intention meant. The topic is simply overwhelming. At the same time writing this book has been immensely gratifying (finishing it perhaps moreso) Not only did it allow me to expand my knowledge base, both on women and physiology in general by an enormous amount, but I also knew that I was ultimately contributing positively to the field, in a way that had never really been done before with this book.

This Book

This book is a book about women's physiology, diet, nutrition and fat loss. As I mentioned above, originally it was meant to cover training issues but doing those justice will require a second volume. In it I will look at what may seem like an endless number of topics. This will include a woman's general physiology, focusing on the menstrual cycle itself and what changes are occurring throughout it. Since they are so common, the hormonal modifiers will be discussed in some detail in terms of how they impact on or alter a woman's physiology. For background I'll look briefly at exercise types and some of the common goals a woman might seek

To ensure that readers are clear on certain concepts, I will look at some fairly general topics such as body composition (what it is, tracking it and altering it) along with the issue of energy balance and metabolic adaptation. The next sections of the book will look in detail at how women utilize different nutrients, store and mobilize fat along with the potential differences in fat gain and fat loss. Since it is such a critical issue, I will address the topic of menstrual cycle dysfunction in some detail along with a large chapter on stress (a place where women and men differ drastically). This will lead into a chapter where I look at how to fix the various issues women face.

The remainder of the book will be aimed at providing practical recommendations on a number of topics with a primary focus being on dieting and fat loss as that is such a prevalent goal for women (it is also a place where there is simply a staggering amount of either incorrect or outright damaging information present). This includes setting and adjusting calorie levels, determining nutrient requirements along with nutrient sources, fluid intake and others. I will discuss the concept of flexible eating strategies (originally discussed in the 2004 book that indirectly led to this one), around workout nutrition, meal frequency and patterning and finally supplements (including phase or hormonal specific supplement recommendations). I will also talk about estimating dieting times, identifying and breaking the inevitable dieting plateaus and adjusting the diet over time. Since training is a critical part of fat loss, I will address it in brief, once again a full discussion of women's training issues will have to wait for Volume 2 of this series. Finally I will provide hormonal templates for each of the potential situations a woman might find herself in along with diet templates for women of different starting body fat. Since lean females have the most issues, they will get their own chapter along with an examination of what should happen when and if they develop amenorrhea. Since recovery from amenorrhea is absolutely critical, I will spend a chapter discussing how that is optimally done.

In many places in this book, I will be addressing some of the mistaken ideas that exist for women in terms of dieting and fat loss. There is simply a tremendously large amount of mistaken beliefs and information on the topic. And the recommendations, which as often as not come from men (especially in the athletic realm) are either ineffective or damaging to a woman's health. And while I will, as often as not, compare a woman's physiology to a man's (primarily to differentiate women), the fact is that this is a women's book. Others have been written (and I've read them all) but they tend to be either clinical and aimed at researchers or, frankly, simply aren't that good. Many are incomplete and it's not uncommon to find flatly incorrect information in them (based on the research available). While this book may have started out as part of another book before becoming what was meant to be a relatively small side-project, it morphed over 2.5 years into something completely unique. It's not just a general guide to women's physiology as books of that nature exist. Rather it exists as a comprehensive guide to not only women's unique physiology but what implications that uniqueness has in terms of optimizing her nutrition, diet, health, etc. Finally, the book I promised years ago is here. Well, Volume 1 anyway.

An Important Note About This Book

While I have tried to make this comprehensive regarding women in different types of hormonal situations, there are several topics that I have chosen not to cover. The first are any medically based pathophysiologies. There are far too many of them to address in any type of detail, it is an area far outside of my expertise and which should be treated by a health practitioner or OB/GYN in any case. I will mention the occasional issue in brief but, beyond that, the topic will not be addressed.

While I will address some of the changes that occur throughout a woman's lifespan (especially the menopausal transition), I will not explicitly address girls between puberty and the age of 18. Certainly much of the information in this book applies in terms of good nutrition, improving bone mineral density and the consequences of things such as amenorrhea (Common in young female athletes) but there are too many issues involved with the growing female that I have neither the expertise nor ability to cover.

Similarly, I will not be covering the issue of pregnancy or breast feeding. Women's hormones go through enormous changes at this time with some of their effects effectively reversing in some ways and addressing that in detail would be impossible. Of more importance, I am both unqualified and unwilling to provide dietary advice on either situation. The developing fetus and newborn are too sensitive to changes in a mother's food intake and the idea of giving suggestions that might cause harm fills me with dread (I will mention pregnancy in one or two places, however). There are already numerous books on the topic, written by people far more qualified than I available and I would recommend that women interested in the topic use them as a resource.

Finally is the topic of eating disorders (ED's). While absolutely relevant to the topic of women, diet and fat loss, it is another topic that requires professional help and intervention rather than advice from a book (no matter how well researched). As with pregnancy, I will mention it once or twice in this book, primarily as it pertains to other topics, but I will not address treatment or recovery.

A Few Qualifications

In the modern world, discussions of sex or gender can be problematic for any number of reasons and I want to make some qualifications about the language and concepts that I'm going to discuss first. This section may seem excessive or pedantic but I want to make absolutely sure that none of what I will write throughout this book will be misconstrued.

First and foremost, in terms of their specific meaning sex and gender are not identical concepts. Sex refers to an individual's biology in terms of their genetics and which reproductive organs are present. In contrast, gender refers more to the roles an individual plays in society or how they self identify. Someone with female reproductive organs (female by sex) might identify as a male (male by gender) or perform what are traditionally referred to as a male gender role. The opposite can hold true and there are many more possibilities than just those two (my choice of that example is not meant to be exclusionary).

That said, in the scientific literature, and certainly among a majority of the lay-public, sex and gender are used interchangeably, with scientific researchers showing no real tendency towards one or the other. This is especially true in physiological research which is what most of this book focuses on. While acknowledging that it is technically incorrect, I will do the same throughout this book using the terms sex and gender or sex differences and gender differences synonymously. In most cases, I am likely talking about sex differences since my focus is on physiology and biological differences but I will still use both at varying times. I just want to make it clear that I am in no way dismissing or denying the differences.

In a similar fashion, I may occasionally refer to female-like or male-like characteristics or personality traits. With no intent to imply or maintain traditional gender roles, this is simply a descriptive shorthand that I will be using since I expect readers to be familiar with what the terms have traditionally represented. Clearly, women can show what are traditionally thought of as male-like characteristics (in terms of behavior or personality) and vice versa and there is a tremendous range of behaviors that might be seen between any given extreme. Again, it's nothing more than a descriptive shorthand since most know what the terms refer to and I use it only for convenience.

About the Title

This book has gone through a number of title changes. My first working title was "50 Shades of Hormones" which became "More than Just Little Men" but I was thankfully convinced that neither were appropriate. While I frequently compare women and men's physiology throughout this book, my primary goal was simply to point out those differences and nothing more. To compare women to men in the title misses the point of what this book is. That is, this is a book about women and the differences and situations that they face. Hence the change to simply "The Women's Book" which describes exactly what it is.

Chapter 1: Introduction to Women's Physiology

While this is meant to be a book about women's specific physiology and how that impacts on diet, nutrition and fat loss, to at least some degree it will be a book about the differences between women and men. This is a topic that is sometimes dangerous to discuss as, to many in the modern world, it smacks of inherent sexism to even consider that there are any differences between women and men. Certainly in the past, the idea that there were gender differences got co-opted into the idea that one gender was superior or inferior to the other. Since it was usually men who were writing about this, and since they tended to assume that they were the default setting, the idea that women were different from men came to mean that women were inferior to men. Many seem to feel that to discuss or even suggest gender differences is to tie into what some see as inherent male-dominant (or androcentric) sexism. I think this confuses issues.

In my mind, the concept of a difference is no way implies an inherent inferiority or superiority even if many interpret it that way. Even in the case where women and men are different, there are clear places where women show a greater response than men and others where they show a lesser response. In most sports, at the elite level, women's performance is about 8-10% below men. However, in ultra-endurance running and cold water swimming, women's performance is generally superior. Women also show better endurance an tolerate heat better than men. While they often lose fat more slowly, they also lose less muscle than men. Regardless of whether the response is better or worse, I will simply consider them to be differences going forwards and nothing more. Honestly, the only reason to address them as differences (rather than simply focusing on women's physiology) is that so much of the information is based on men with the flawed idea that it automatically applies to women. But even this raises the question of why it took so long to even recognize that there were differences between the two.

Scientific Research: Part 1

For quite some time, it was basically assumed that research on men, and this cut across most disciplines including general physiology, exercise, fat loss, etc. would apply directly to women. It just wasn't really questioned on any level. In the realm of sports performance, it wasn't until about the mid 80's that any amount of comparative studies on women and men started to be done (1). But even from the earliest research, it became clear that there were significant differences.

A singular example will hopefully make the point. Endurance athletes such as runners or cyclists will often use a dietary strategy referred to as carbohydrate loading where they combine intense exercise with a drastically increased amount of carbohydrate in their diet. The goal of this is to increase the store of carbohydrate in the body (muscle and liver) to improve performance. Early studies showed that this worked well for men. They increased the storage of carbohydrate in their bodies and their performance improved. But in women it didn't seem to have the same effect. In one comparative study, while men increased their muscle carbohydrate stores when fed a 70% carbohydrate diet, women did not. For fairly logical reasons, biological differences were assumed to be the case since, as often as not, it does explain the differences that are seen. But this was at least partially wrong.

It turned out that part of the reason the female subjects didn't carb-load as well as the men was due to the fact that the same 70% carbohydrate diet provided much smaller amounts of total carbohydrate due to the women being smaller and having a lower energy expenditure. That is, a woman burning 2000 calories per day and eating 70% carbohydrate is getting 350 grams of carbohydrate while a man burning 3000 calories per day and eating 70% carbohydrate is getting 525 grams. The percentage is identical but the total amounts aren't. When women were fed equivalent amounts as the men, most of the differences went away

When both women and men were given even larger amounts, there was no gender difference in carbohydrate loading. It had purely to do with the total amount of carbohydrate. But this raised another problem, it created an impossible diet for the women. To get enough total carbohydrate meant eating too many total calories. Their smaller size and energy expenditure basically made it impossible to achieve what men could without eating too much food. There was another issue. Many females are restricting their food intake to one degree or another for various reasons. If they need or want to lose fat, they have to eat less than they burn and that may not leave enough total food to support their training. There are solutions to this, what some call nutritional periodization (alternating time periods of restricting food intake with increasing it) and I'll talk about them in a variety of contexts later in this book.

But even this singular example brings up one of the key problems that often shows up which is that dietary approaches that work for men (or are used by male coaches) don't work or prove impossible for women to implement. There will be more examples of this throughout this book.

Scientific Research: Part 2

So why did it take so long to include women in research, especially in sports science and exercise research? Some it probably represented pure chauvinism: the majority of scientists were male and they tend to bring a male-oriented mentality to things. But perhaps a bigger part of it was that for the first half of the 20th century, and even into the 70's, women simply weren't as involved in sport as men.

In certain sports, it was long thought that women were incapable of performing them or that they would do physical damage to themselves. Up through the 70's, for example, women were barred from even competing in marathons (there is a famous picture of referees trying to pull a woman off of the course). Some of this mentality persists today as many sports still maintain shorter distances or slightly different events for women versus men. A lot of it was sociocultural as well; there was a lot of social pressure against women entering sports. It was seen as being unfeminine (or outright masculine) and simply remained mostly a male domain. This started to change in America in the 70's with the passing of Title IX which required similar sporting availability for women. And as they started to enter sport, gradual changes started to occur. I'd note that this wasn't true in many other countries. Due to the status for winning at the world and Olympic level, females were both allowed and encouraged to compete. In the 80's, for example, the German Democratic Republic (GDR) women were absolutely dominant in swimming and track.

But the point is that most research in sports science was done on men because men represented the majority of people involved in sport at the time. There wasn't much reason to study women since they didn't make up a large proportion of athletes. Even when research was done either on women or to compare women to men, early research was poorly done and the results were questionable at best. The reason for that has to do with the incredible complexity of women compared to men which due to the menstrual cycle. This is the roughly 28 day cycle a woman goes through monthly during which her hormonal status and physiology can change in subtle or not so subtle ways. The cycle is typically divided evenly into two phases called the follicular (from menstruation to ovulation) and the luteal phase (from ovulation through PMS) and each is distinct from another. There are even shifts that occur in the early- and late- phases of each and some even divide each phase into an early-, mid- and late- phase. During this cycle, a woman's primary reproductive hormones (estrogen and progesterone) show complex overlap.

This makes studying women incredibly difficult. Researchers have to control for the phase of the cycle itself and even this can be difficult as determining where in her a cycle a woman is isn't always easy (recent studies will use ultrasound and blood work to determine this but this is not easy or cheap). Add to that that no two women have an identical menstrual cycle and even an individual female's cycle may vary from month-to-month. A woman who starts menstruating a day early might have to wait a month to be retested. To begin to compare women to men, you must control for the phase of the cycle. But when you study her may change what conclusion you reach. In one phase a woman's response may be identical to a man's; in the other it may be different or even the compete opposite. As a singular example, women's metabolism of caffeine is similar to men's during the first half of her cycle but different in the second half. If you don't study all of those conditions, you can draw incorrect conclusions and early studies didn't even pay attention to where in her cycle a woman was. She'd come to the lab to be measured and that was it. The results were meaningless. In contrast men have one primary reproductive hormone which changes very little day-to-day. So long as you control a few simple variables like time of day and whether or not the eaten, you can test them any day of the month. Ultimately, it's just simpler to study men.

An Amusing Exception

There is an amusing exception to the above that I only mention for completeness, a place where by and large there is relatively more research on women compared to men and that is in the realm of diet studies. Here, women tend to be drastically over-represented, making up the majority of subjects. This is primarily reflective of the fact that women are far more likely to be dieting than men. Hence they are more likely to enter the studies. For example, there is a database of successful weight losers called the National Weight Control Registry (NWCR) and it is composed of roughly 80% women. In the same way males represented the majority of athletes in the 70's, women continue to represent the majority of the dieting population now. While I mention it only as a point of trivia, the reality is that a great many weight loss approaches, studies, etc. are either done exclusively or predominantly on women and there has been some recent question whether or not this information applies equally to men. Dieting, diet groups, etc. are often seen as a "woman's domain" and men may be less likely to pursue either for a variety of reasons. To address this, researchers have been working on more "male oriented" weight loss programs including male humor (which I take as fart and poop jokes) and sports team affiliation (2).

2

Gender Differences: Introduction

Regardless of all of the above, it's abundantly clear that there are distinct differences between men and women and they cut across nearly all domains including those covered in this book such as diet, nutrition and fat loss (exercise and training being covered in Volume 2). Let me state up front that the differences I will be discussing, especially many of the physical differences represent no more than averages. Usually researchers study a huge number of subjects and look at the average response. But an average response says nothing about any given individual and it's trivial to find an exception to just about any topic I will discuss. For example, despite the fact that women are, on average, shorter than men, clearly you can find a woman who is taller than a man. Despite the fact that the average woman typically has narrower shoulders and wider hips than a man, you can find a woman with narrower hips and wider shoulders. As frequently as not the variation within a gender is actually greater than the difference between genders (3). And at least in some area, women may show even more variability than men.

Throughout most of this book when I address gender differences I will put it in terms of "Women show such and such of a difference compared to men." and I want to address my choice of that phrasing. A recent book about the Chinese female Olympic Lifting team makes a fairly impassioned point that using men as the baseline for sports performance represents not only the history of the idea of men being inherent superior but an androcentric (male) viewpoint overall (4). That is, typically speaking, women are compared to men in terms of their physiology, biomechanics, response to training, etc. instead of the other way around. And strictly speaking it would make just as much sense to reverse it. For example, women tend to handle heat better than men (at least during some phases of the menstrual cycle) and it would be just as accurate to state that "Men handle heat worse than woman" as "Women handle heat better than men." That said, when examining gender differences I will still discuss them in terms of a woman's response relative to a man's. There are three reasons for my choice in this.

The first is that is a book about women's issues related to nutrition and fat loss. To describe differences in physiology in terms of men's responses relative to women would make little sense since it is the woman's response that is important The second is that, with one odd exception discussed above regarding dieting studies, staggeringly more research has been done on men relative women (even now research on men is done at about a 4:1 ratio to that on women). It's only been fairly recently that women's response, or explicit gender difference studies have become more common place. And since there is far more research on men, comparing women's responses to men's makes logical sense to me here.

Finally, and perhaps most importantly from a practical sense, the fact is that a majority of ideas about nutrition and fat loss that are applied to women typically come out of either research or practice on men. Since most athletes have traditionally been male, most coaches have as well. This is changing in modern times and there are more and more female coaches (usually coaching women) but many of the ideas and approaches to training, exercise, dieting and fat loss come out of male-oriented approaches which may not only be ineffective but damaging. Addressing that means comparing women to men to some degree.

A Snapshot of Gender Differences

In no particular order of importance, here is a brief look at a a few of the (again, average) differences between women and men. On average, women are lighter, with less lean body mass and more body-fat than men. They also carry their fat differently with a more lower-body fat patterning. Their bodies utilize protein, carbohydrates and fats differently than men both at rest, after a meal and during exercise. They regulate what is called energy homeostasis differently than men (ultimately sparing the loss of body fat).

Physically, women's wider hips alter their knee biomechanics (predisposing them to certain kinds of injuries). Women tend to be more flexible with relatively more mobile tendons and joints. And while women's muscles are physiologically identical to male's for the most part, there are differences in how they generate force or fatigue in response to exercise. As I mentioned above, on average female athletes perform at a level roughly 10% below that of men in most sports (with two exceptions). While women typically start out with lower levels of fitness than men, they respond similarly if not identically in terms of the relative improvements that they make in response to training.

Perhaps the most major difference between women and men has to do with hormones, especially the existence of the menstrual cycle. Discussed in detail later in this book, this represents the roughly monthly cycle of hormonal variations that a woman undergoes (in contrast, a man's hormones are relatively stable across the month). This changes her physiology at a fundamental level and introduces a complexity that simply isn't seen in men. This can also be modified in a stunning number of ways with what I will call hormonal modifiers changing a woman's physiology subtly or not so subtly.

The Cause of The Differences

This raises the next important question which is what the genesis of these differences is. Of some interest is the fact that most parts of a woman and man's bodies are actually identical in a physical sense. Under a microscope, a woman's bone is the same as a man's bone in terms of it's cellular structure, it's just not as dense. A woman's muscle is almost identical to a man's in terms of it's cellular structure, it's just typically smaller (there are other small differences I won't get into here). A woman's heart, lungs, etc. are all identical in cellular structure (albeit smaller) with the largest physical difference arguably being in the genitalia. Of course there are clearly differences that appear in terms of the relative amounts of fat, muscle, etc. So if the underlying structures are more or less identical, why are these differences seen?

Whenever a fairly large scale difference between women and men shows up, it's been traditional to assume that it is due to underlying genetic/chromosomal or hormonal differences. In recent years, the idea that all physical differences between women and men, especially the differences in strength or sports performance, are culturally generated is being more commonly heard. As usual, the truth lies between the two extremes. Certainly it would be absurd to dismiss the role of environment or society and culture on women's, or for that matter anyone's, overall nature. But it's equally absurd to dismiss the differences between the sexes in terms of biology. And since this isn't a book about society or culture, it is the biology that I will *primarily* focus on. Because not only are those changes significant, it's actually the case that many of them are set in place before birth, before any social or cultural influences are present.

A woman and a man's genetic code differs, readers may remember that woman have XX and men XY chromosomes which are a huge part of what "tells" the body how to develop (especially in terms of the reproductive organs). Related to this, in recent years there have been issues concerning women in sport and biological sex testing. As this topic has more to do with emotion and political agendas rather than biology or physiology at this point, I am not going to begin to touch it in this book.

The Role of Hormones

Other than genetics and the difference in genitalia, arguably the largest biological difference between women and men is in the relative amounts of the primary reproductive hormones. In women, these are estrogen and progesterone and in men it is testosterone. Both sexes make all three hormones but the relatively amounts in adults differ significantly. On average women having roughly 1/10th to 1/30th the testosterone levels of men; men have similarly low levels of estrogen and progesterone. It would be patently absurd to pretend that this isn't impacting on the physiology of a woman versus a man directly in addition to any interaction with aspects of her genetic programming.

A singular example is that women's bodies genetically form more of what are called pre-adipocytes (think of these as baby fat cells) in their lower bodies. These pre-adipocytes are stimulated to become fully formed fat cells and this occurs under the impact of hormones estrogen and progesterone with estrogen specifically impacting on the development of lower body fat cells in women (5). Even that doesn't occur until what might be described as one of the most profound times of life for both girls and boys occurs which is puberty. Prior to that, little girls and boys are more or less physically and physiologically identical. When there are differences they tend to be small and are generally in the same direction I mentioned above (i.e. girls are still slightly shorter or carry slightly more fat).

But it is at puberty, when the reproductive organs become active and hormonal levels diverge enormously that the primary physical and physiological differences between the sexes appear . A woman's specific physiology develops under the effects of estrogen and progesterone as does a male's under the influence of testosterone. Women develop their traditional body fat patterns, increasing not only total body fat but lower body fat specifically while men develop more muscle mass while losing fat. Effectively puberty is when the typical feminine and masculine physiologies develop and let me reiterate (for those who skipped the preface) that I am using these terms only as descriptive shorthand with no implication about whether or not one is a relatively more or less appropriate or superior gender role than the other. We all know what these terms refer to and it's just easier writing it this way.

This is further shown by the fact that even small changes in hormones can have a profound impact. Even small changes in the levels of testosterone in women can drastically impact on her physiology, effectively masculinizing her in many ways (the effect is even more pronounced in women who use anabolic steroids, derivatives of testosterone).. I'll talk about specific examples of this in later chapters and other factors that change or modify a woman's overall hormonal profile drastically impact her physiology. Menopause is one of the most profound of those as through the process peri-menopause through the menopausal transition itself, her hormones drop from their youthful levels to nearly zero.

None of the above is meant to in any way dismiss the role of culture and environment in this. Clearly it plays a role and to ignore it is a mistake. When I talk about training and injury risk in Volume 2, I'll talk about a very specific place where culture/environment (specifically women's typically lower involvement in sport at a young age) interact with her biology in a profoundly negative way. For now I want to briefly discuss a topic I said I wasn't going to talk about much in the preface.

Eating Disorders

Perhaps no more clear an example of the above lies in an issue of enormous importance for women that I said I wouldn't discuss in this book but should at least address and that is the topic of eating disorders (EDs) such as anorexia, bulimia and others. Because, depending on what statistics you see, women may be anywhere from 3-9 times more likely to have a true ED as a man. Unbelievably, some studies indicate that 95% of true ED's are seen in women which is simply enormous (6). Quite in fact, for some time it was actually thought that ED's occurred only in women. We now know that this is false as relatively more men are developing some form of ED in the modern world. Presumably this due to increasing pressure for men to meet the same type of physical ideal that women have faced for far longer (8).

Even here there can be a gender difference. Women's ED's tend to revolve around the quest for extreme thinness while men's are often focused on increased muscle mass, although extreme leanness can also be a goal. Similarly pathological behaviors are often seen here as well. The idea of bigorexia or body dysmorphia is being used to describe males who, despite objectively being muscular and large, still see themselves as small, unmuscled and weak. This is fundamentally no different than the anorexic who still sees themselves as fat despite objective evidence to the contrary. It's just working in the opposite direction.

But focusing on women, there is absolutely no doubt that environmental and cultural issue that play into this with factors such as a mother with an ED, early dieting practices, stressful environments, being teased about body weight, media images or being involved in traditionally female sports such as gymnastics, ballet and ice skating that stress thinness and low body weights that are present (9). But most overt ED's occur in women under the age of 24 and tend to develop at puberty which suggests a biological factor. And that biological factor, simply, is estrogen more specifically the increase in estrogen that occurs at puberty which is when the majority of true ED's develop (10). It's clearly the interaction of a woman's biology along with a certain environment causing one of the most potentially damaging effects and one that is seen nearly exclusively in women. But the hormonal effects are simply incontrovertible and the changes that occur at puberty are what lead to the physiological, physical and other changes that are seen.

Prenatal Hormone Exposure

But it actually goes even deeper than the above. A great deal of a person's biology is actually set in place during fetal development. A pregnant woman's diet, environment and other factors can drastically and permanently impact the risk of disease including obesity, diabetes and even brain development in the developing fetus (10,11). There is a lot of recent concern in this regard over environmental compounds (such as environmental estrogens) and the impact they may be having on biology and I'll actually talk one specific issue relative to dietary supplements later in the book that is important here.

The above is not strictly a gender difference since it can occur in both women and men. However, there is an effect of reproductive hormones, in this case the relative levels of testosterone and estrogen that the fetus is exposed to that not only plays an enormous role in the final physiology seen but can act to have a relative masculinizing or feminizing effect that is seen later in life. Prenatal hormone exposure expresses itself externally in what is called second to fourth (2:4) digit ratio: the ratio of length between the index (second) and ring (fourth) finger. When exposed to high levels of testosterone, the index finger is typically shorter than the ring finger (a male-like pattern). When exposed to lower levels of testosterone, the index finger is equal or longer than the ring finger (a female-like pattern). And while this ratio doesn't seem to show any relationship to adult hormone levels, it is clearly related to prenatal hormone exposure (11).

A female exposed to relatively more testosterone may undergo different biological "programming" than a female exposed to less, developing relatively more "masculine" characteristics physiologically. The same occurs in reverse in men; men exposed to less testosterone may develop a more "feminine" physiology, body structure and set of behavior patterns. This ratio ends up being predictive of many factors such as bodyweight, waist to hip ratio (here there are common female and male patterns) and health risk (12). But there is also a strong relationship between the male-like finger pattern (again indicative of relatively more testosterone exposure in the womb) and traditionally masculine behaviors. Hopefully a few examples will suffice (and there is fairly endless research on this).

In general, the more male-like digit ratio correlates strongly with the typically seen differences between women and men in behavior, being related to such behaviors as aggression, thrill seeking and attention seeking (13).   A male-like digit ratio is associated with better athletic performance in at least some sports, presumably those requiring higher levels of aggression and other masculine characteristics (14).   Both men and women with a male-like digit ratio have more masculine faces in men this is associated with attractiveness in women (15,16).   In contrast women with a more male-like digit ratio are rated as less desirable and less faithful than those with the female-like digit ratio (17). It's interesting to note that in at least one high-level sport, coaches specifically select female athletes by looking for a more male-like facial structure, smaller breasts and less triceps fat as they feel this corresponds with higher testosterone levels and better chance of sporting success (18).

As well, and this is relevant to training issue that I will discuss in Volume 2, digit ratio may predict what adult preferences are shown (19). Women exposed to higher pre-natal testosterone show different preferences in terms of activities, toys, etc. that they are drawn to (20,21).   Digit ratio also interacts with adult hormone levels. Women injected with testosterone show increased levels of aggression and decreased empathy (both traditionally masculine behaviors) but only if they have the more male-like digit ratio to begin with (23).   In this case, the effects of pre-natal hormone exposure and programming determine how a woman's biology will be impacted by changes in her hormones later in life. Returning to the topic of eating disorders, Binge Eating Disorder (BED) which is far more prevalent in women is thought to be related to the combination of a relative lack of androgen exposure during fetal development that puts a woman at higher risk for developing BED at puberty when estrogen levels increase (24).

All of this sets up an enormously interactive situation. Prenatal hormone exposure may have a relatively masculinizing or feminizing effect on women in terms of biology, body structure and personality which leads them to prefer certain types of activities, which they are then prepared to succeed in. But it's the interaction of factors with my only point being that there are clear and enormous impacts of not only the differences in reproductive hormones between women and men but that exposure to those hormones has an impact on all aspects of woman's physiology before birth or puberty.

In this vein and to get back to the topic of this chapter a relatively informal piece of Russian research found a strong correlation between a relatively crude measure of personality called the Bem Sex Role inventory in terms of ratings of femininity, androgyny and masculinity in terms of what types of sports they were found in (25). Women with higher ratings of masculinity were more likely to be found in sports requiring more strength, power and aggression while higher ratings of femininity predicted the opposite effect. Women who rated for androgyny were in the middle. The more masculine women could be trained more like men due to their prenatal biological programming and adult hormone levels for this reason. As well, they were less likely to be impacted by the changes that typically occur with the menstrual cycle. Because, as I mentioned, in addition to genetics, hormonal changes at puberty, and clear cultural influences, there is still the presence of the menstrual cycle.

Scientific Research: Part 3

In addition to the different levels of hormones seen between women and men, there is another factor that makes the study of women so much more complicated which is the presence of the menstrual cycle. Because, in addition to making observations, about what the differences may be from phase to phase or to men, researchers usually want to know what is causing those changes.   And here the incredible swings that occur in the menstrual cycle in estrogen and progesterone can make determining what is causing what to occur very complicated. Both hormones rise, fall, overlap and interact. When looking at any given response, is it the increase in one, the decrease in the other, the combination of the two changing or the ratio of the two? It can be excruciatingly different to determine this.

Frequently researchers use animal models where it's easier to control their hormone levels but this raises issues of whether or not they make a good model for humans. Usually they do not and in some cases the effect of one or the other hormones in animals is the opposite of what is seen in humans. Another interesting approach is to inject a woman's hormone (usually estrogen) into a male to see if the same effect is seen. Often it is. But sometimes the effects are different are reversed (for example, increasing testosterone levels in women often has the opposite effects as what is seen in men). Usually what is done is to first shut down a woman's hormone production completely. Then either estrogen, progesterone or some combination of the two is put back in to study the effects under isolated or at least controlled situations. And while there were endless questions as to which hormone or what hormonal interaction was causing what effect in women, in recent years, the picture has become far more clear.

Adding even to that, women have a number of what I will call hormonal modifiers that change the picture further. The normal cycle can be disrupted either becoming longer than normal (called oligomenorrhea) or being lost entirely (amenorrhea). Many women use birth control (BC), either a combination of synthetic estrogen and progesterone (or just progesterone) of which there are a staggering number of forms and types all of which may act slightly differently. Many women suffer from Poly-Cystic Ovary Syndrome (PCOS) which is typically marked by higher than normal testosterone levels and there is a subclinical hyperandrogenism where a woman's normally low testosterone levels are higher than normal and both change her physiology drastically.

A woman's physiology also changes throughout the lifespan around menopause where her reproductive organs start to shut down. First there is a peri-menopause (with an early- and late-stage) and menopause itself. That is modified by whether or not a woman chooses to go on Hormone Replacement Therapy (HRT), synthetic estrogen and progesterone. There is also a specific estrogen only HRT used in women who have had a partial hysterectomy. All of these situations in women are subtly or no so subtly different physiologically. To study women completely on any given topic means to study each of these situations separately. In some cases it's to see what the changes are from aging; pre-menopausal and post-menopausal women may be compared. In some cases, a normally cycling female may be compared to a woman using BC or one who is amenorrheic. Different types of BC may be compared. The possibilities are nearly endless.

In contrast, males may have slightly lower or higher testosterone although some men produce more estrogen than others. Men with very low testosterone (hypogonadal) do need to be studied but even with age, a man's testosterone only goes down. It doesn't drop to near zero as occurs in menopause. Getting very off topic, this is why I think the concept of andropause, means to be equivalent to menopause is incorrectly named. In menopause, a woman's reproductive hormones go effectively to zero. In the supposed andropause, a man's testosterone is simply going down with aging. They are simply not the same.

Implications for this Book

It's a bit of a running joke that nobody understands women and there is much truth to this. As I have worked on this project and posted a great deal about it online, it's become clear to me that many women aren't familiar with the terms I used above, the phases of their menstrual cycle or how their hormones (much less their) physiology changes. Outside of the ob/gyn, neither are their health care providers and there the focus is primarily medical rather than being applied in terms of how it impacts on diet, nutrition, fat loss or training. It should be clear that if females don't understand the topic, men, whether coach, athlete, or significant other has no chance of understanding it. There are a few implications of this.

The first is that, fairly obviously, a woman has to be treated at least somewhat differentially than a man when it comes to both her diet, training and fat loss. Make no mistake, the same generalities will always hold here. While I'll talk about training in detail in Volume 2, I'll I'd mention that improving fitness, strength, power or performance requires certain general aspects of training. It's the specifics of how those aspects are specifically applied that may differ in a woman than in a man. Women face issues that men simply never will, for example some women experience changes in their performance, coordination, etc. throughout the month. This means that their training may have to be adjusted to better synchronize with those changes. This will never apply to men. There are other examples and this is a problem as, in the same way males dominated athletes for a long period of time, most coaches have traditionally been males. They know what they did as a (male) athlete and usually know how to coach male athletes.

Keeping with the topic of this book, one place this perennially shows up is when it comes to dieting and fat loss. Due to the differences in all aspects of their biology, some of the approaches that are effective for men are either ineffective or outright damaging to women (this is especially true in the physique subculture where strategies to diet down to the lowest extremes of body fat were originally developed on and for men). Additionally, since they are typically larger, men have more food and calories to "work with". This allows them to use strategies that end up being inappropriate for women or at least to avoid certain problems that female athletes run into (i.e. not having enough calories in their diet to get sufficient protein and fat and still have enough carbohydrate to sustain training). This fact typically goes completely ignored by most.

Some writers and coaches (generally male) have at least paid lip service to the potential differences between female and male trainees but often they reach completely opposite conclusions. Some feel that training should or can be modified across the menstrual cycle (early Russian training literature even talked about this) while others argue that women should be trained effectively the same as men with the variations being more about the individual athlete than being based on gender at all. Sometimes high-level coaches change from one stance to another but this tends to go along with the use of anabolics in sport. With high enough doses of testosterone in women, the menstrual cycle usually disappears and women can be trained just like men. Even without drugs, women with relatively higher levels of testosterone (often seen in PCOS but also in other situations) can often be trained relatively more like men and, as I'll discuss later in the book, tend to show superior performance.

Quite in fact, one of the dirty little secrets in women's physique sports such as bodybuilding, physique or figure is that there is often some degree of low-level drug use occurring. This might include anabolic steroids (to increase muscle size or hardness) and various fat burners that help the athletes to get into contest shape while avoiding the problems that natural women face. Since they are successful, much of the idea about how dieting and training should be done comes from them which leaves women who are not using those compounds with a very poor idea about how they should approach their diet or training.

All of the above is made further complex by the variation between women. Certainly two men may show differential responses to diet, fat loss and training but, in the aggregate, it's more a matter of degrees than anything else. Two women may show differences from one another and any given woman may vary from month to month. Looking at training and considering only the menstrual cycle, one woman may see her performance vary enormously while another has no such change. Changes in mood during the final week of the cycle (i.e. when PMS typically occurs) are monstrous. One woman may have no issues while a second might have severe mood swings or fatigue and a third may be completely physically debilitated and suffer from clinical depression. The patterns of mood swings can vary as can any other aspect of a woman's physiology. While some of the hormonal modifiers actually work to stabilize this, they still change a woman's physiology to some degree and add another level of complexity. And one that no male or coach training a male will ever have to face or deal with.

And that is really the crux and goal of this book. I want to not only look at the differences in physiology between women and men and to identify places where a woman's response differs in some fundamental way which may make an approach that is effective for men be less so for women. More importantly, I want to address those differences in terms of what changes a woman should (or should not) make in how she approaches reaching her goals. To help readers not only understand how the physiology of women and men differ but how a woman's approach to diet, nutrition, fat loss or training (again, in Volume 2) should differ because of that. And to begin to understand that means starting with a discussion of arguably the primary factor that differentiate women from men. That is not only the differences in the primary female reproductive hormones from that of men's but in how they change across the monthly menstrual cycle.

Chapter 2: The Normal Menstrual Cycle

In the last chapter, I not only looked at some of the problems that have plagued both studying women and comparing them to men but looked, in brief, at some of the clear gender differences that have been found to exist in aspects of their physiology. While there are other reasons that I will discuss later in the book, a great deal of those differences are due to the relative levels of hormones, primarily the reproductive hormones, present in women and men. This is further complicated by the changes in those hormones that occur on a roughly monthly basis which act to change her physiology. And while hormonal modifiers exist that further complicate this system, understanding any of them means first understanding cycle itself.

In this chapter, I want to sketch out the normal menstrual cycle from start to finish, primarily focusing on the changes that occur in estrogen, progesterone and testosterone in terms of levels and how they impact on her physiology. I will also look at several other hormones that vary to one degree or another in women and men and which are important to various aspects of this book. One hormone that I will not discuss in this chapter is cortisol, a stress hormone that is so crucial to understanding many of the issues that women's face that it will be discussed in a separate chapter.

A note on terminology: Strictly speaking there is no "normal" menstrual cycle It varies in duration between women and even the same woman can differ from month to month. In using the term "normal", I in no way mean to imply that any other pattern is abnormal. It's just a descriptive shorthand for the typical cycle of hormonal changes that occurs under standard situations. It's modified enormously by other situations but it's just easier to call it "normal" for writing purposes.

An Overview of the Menstrual Cycle

The menstrual cycle derives from the Latin word for month and refers to the roughly one month (28 day cycle) that a woman goes through from the time she enters puberty until she loses her cycle at menopause. While I will treat the menstrual cycle as if it were exactly 28 days, a normal menstrual cycle may be anywhere from 24-32 days in duration (quite in fact, while most women report a 28 day cycle, few actually have a 28 day cycle). The primary purpose of the menstrual cycle is to prepare for the potential of pregnancy and most of the hormonal changes and their effects are aimed at this goal. When the menstrual cycle is functioning normally, this is called eumenorrhea ("eu" means well or good). By convention, Day 1 of the cycle occurs at the onset of menstruation (i.e. her period), the bleeding that occurs as the uterine lining (thickened in preparation for implantation of the egg) is expelled. This typically lasts 3-5 days. From this point, the remainder of the cycle is divided into two distinct phases, described next.

The Follicular Phase

The first half of the cycle is termed the follicular phase and within a 28 day cycle will typically last 14 days. Strictly speaking this can be divided up into an early, mid-, and late follicular phase of roughly 3-5 days each but I'll only use early- and late follicular in this book with the split happening halfway through (i.e. day 7). In research, women are frequently measured during the mid-follicular phase to get a more or less average indication of what is going on physiologically. Under certain conditions, the follicular phase can lengthen as well. During this phase, the follicle (hence the name) develops due to the effects of Follicle Stimulating Hormone (FSH). Technically, multiple follicles develop but only one releases an egg.

Hormonally, progesterone remains very low during the follicular phase. Estrogen starts at a low level, shows a gradual increase leading up to a large surge in the final few days of the cycle. This surge causes a follicle to burst open, releasing an egg from the ovaries which then implants itself into the lining of the uterus (thickened to provide nutrients in the case of pregnancy). The surge in estrogen also causes a thickening of vaginal mucus, which makes the vagina less acidic and more hospitable to sperm. Women have often used this thickening as an indication of their fertility.

The Luteal Phase

The release of the egg on day 14 (the halfway point of the cycle) is termed ovulation and this marks both the middle of the menstrual cycle along with the end of the follicular phase (testosterone spikes briefly at this stage as well). At this point, a woman enters the luteal phase which can again be subdivided into early-, mid- and late phases. As with the follicular phase, I'll only use early- and late luteal phase in this book. As in the follicular phase, researchers often measure women in the mid-luteal phase for consistency and to obtain an average response in terms of physiology.

During this phase, the follicle which released the egg develops into a structure called the corpus luteum (hence the name luteal phase) which starts to produce the hormone progesterone. Over the first half of the luteal phase both progesterone and estrogen increase gradually reaching a peak at mid-cycle. Progesterone levels are higher than those of estrogen, which only reaches about half of the level seen during the peak of the follicular phase. Body temperature also increases slightly (about 0.2°C or 0.4°F) after ovulation and basal body temperature (BBT) can be used not only to tell when ovulation has occurred when pregnancy is the goal but is can also be used to tell when the follicular phase has ended and the luteal phase has begun. Along with this increase in body temperature is a slight increase in metabolic rate which I will discuss in more detail later in the chapter..

Late Luteal Phase

In the late luteal phase, progesterone and estrogen start to drop again and this is the when Pre-Menstrual Syndrome (PMS), if present, typically occurs. PMS can be marked by an enormous number of symptoms including cramping (as a woman's body prepares to shed the uterine lining) mood swings, low energy, depression, breast tenderness and others (this is called dysmenorrhea). In extreme cases, women may experience debilitating pain from cramps, depression, anxiety or suicidal thoughts (often requiring medication) and this is referred to as Pre-Menstrual Dysphoric Disorder (PMDD).

Depending on the source in question, PMS is reported to occur in roughly 30-40% of women with clinical relevant PMS occurring in 20% and PMDD occurring in 5-10% of women. Cramps per se are reported in 45-95% of women with 3-33% of women being physically incapacitated due to them (1a). While cramping is often thought to occur primarily during the late luteal phase, it is common for it to continue through menstruation as the uterine lining is shed.

Summarizing the Cycle

I've drawn an essentially idealized menstrual cycle in the graphic below, just showing the relative changes that occur in estrogen (black line), progesterone (gray line), testosterone (bottom black line) and body temperature (at the very top). I've also shown when menstruation, ovulation and PMS generally occur and how the different phases are named and divided.

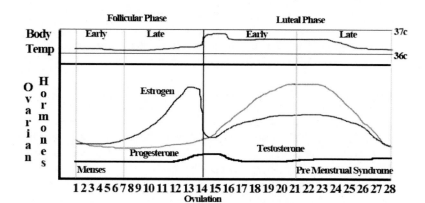

As I will be focusing primarily on the effects of estrogen and progesterone in this book, I have deliberately left out two fairly important hormones which are Follicle Stimulating Hormone (FSH) and Leutinizing Hormone (LH). FSH is primarily involved with the development of the follicle itself while LH controls estrogen production, ovulation, implantation of the egg and development of the corpus luteum. I mention them here as the disruption of LH release patterns can occur under a variety of stressful conditions and this is what fundamentally leads to the menstrual cycle becoming disrupted (discussed in Chapter 12). Interested readers can find more complete graphics online.

In any case, you can see how the dynamics of the cycle change which I will summarize. Menstruation occurs from roughly day 1 to 5 before estrogen starts to climb slowly during the follicular phase of the cycle, surging in the final few days before dropping rapidly when ovulation occurs. Into the luteal phase, both estrogen and progesterone show a slow increase during the luteal phase hitting a peak at the middle of the cycle before gradually decreasing over the second half. If occurs at all, PMS or PMDD will occur in the last 4-7 days (roughly) before menstruation occurs and the cycle starts over.

As I discussed in the previous chapter, the above dynamics should help to illustrate just how much more complex women are compared to men. Women have two primary hormones that are increasing, decreasing and criss-crossing and, as you'll see, interacting in complex and fascinating way. In contrast, a man's hormonal profile would be a more or less straight line for testosterone across every day of the month with not much else changing significantly. Those gender differences are present even before considering the hormonal modifiers that I will discuss in the next chapter.

Individual Variability in the Menstrual Cycle

While the above graphic and description represents a sort of idealized menstrual cycle, there are enormous variations that can occur both between women or in the same woman from month to month (when women first start menstruating their cycles may be extremely variable although this decreases with age). Technically a normal menstrual cycle can last anywhere from 24-32 days with 28 simply being an average or assumed length and any two women might easily have different cycle lengths. While some women are extremely consistent in their cycle lengths, others show more variability where the length of the cycle varies from month to month. A woman might have a 30 day cycle one month and a 23 day cycle the next or what have you. While not a variation per se, a large number of factors including diet, exercise and stress can change or disrupt the cycle. One of these is a shortening of the luteal phase where the time from ovulation to menstruation is less than normal. Here cycle length may actually remain the same which means that while the luteal phase is shortened, the follicular phase is lengthened.

Other variations may be present as well After ovulation, there can be variations in how much of a temperature increase is seen with women experiencing relatively smaller or larger increases. There is also significant variation in how much or how little metabolic rate increases. Even with an apparently normal cycle length, there are times when an egg is not released (termed an anovulatory cycle). This is common when women first start menstruating but can also occur due to diet, exercise and stress.

While PMS lasts 5-7 days on average there is enormous variability in this with many patterns having been observed. Some women show shorter or longer phases of PMS and some women may experience PMS symptoms at other times of the luteal phase. So she might have a day or two of symptoms early in the luteal phase that then end along with several more days of PMS in the late luteal phase. As I've mentioned, there are also huge differences in how much of an effect PMS has on any given woman. This can be true in terms of the number of symptoms present, their severity and many other factors.

While an average menstruation may last 3-5 days,this too can vary with women having shorter or longer durations of bleeding. The level of bleeding can vary a well. Some may only spot lightly (and it's not uncommon for women to spot briefly and then stop before experiencing true menstruation a few days later), others will bleed lightly and others have what is referred to as heavy flow (I'll mention this again when I talk about iron requirements in women). In extreme cases, women will expel what they usually call "chunky bits", clots of blood and tissue from endometrial buildup that is being expelled.

I won't look into the details of these variations but they most likely relate to the relative levels of estrogen, progesterone (or other hormones) that are present along with how any given woman's body responds to them. Women's health care providers often refer to women as being relatively estrogen or progesterone dominant, meaning that they have higher than expected levels of a given hormone during a given phase of the cycle, and this can impact on every aspect of a woman's physiology including her menstrual cycle. There is also assuredly a genetic component.

The existence of this degree of variation is why I said at the outset that there is really no truly normal menstrual cycle. Certainly there is no consistent one. Yes, the general pattern is the same between women but the specifics of hormone levels, durations of the phases, bleeding, presence of absence of PMS/PMDD all vary enormously. As stated, two women can show completely different responses and any individual woman may vary from month to month. I bring this up as I can't cover every possible eventuality and will be working, in a practical sense, from the idealized 28-day menstrual cycle throughout this book. Any given reader of this book will have their own pattern (or patterns) and, within the context of this book (and perhaps moreso Volume 2), women or their coaches will have to be their own best scientist. Regular tracking of factors such as energy, hunger, mood, etc. will help illustrate a given woman's individual patterns and used to adapt how diet or training is applied or utilized.

But with those general patterns and changed sketched out, let me now look at how a woman's reproductive hormones impact on her physiology since that will provide a picture of how her physiology is changing across the cycle. To do so, I need to provide a bit of background information.

Hormones

A hormone is any compound in the body that exerts a biological effect somewhere else in the body (it's technically a little more complex than this but this is good enough). That effect occurs when a hormone binds to its receptor and causes something to happen. The standard analogy here is that the hormone is a key and the receptor is a lock and only the right key can open the right lock. For the most part, every hormone has a specific receptor that it can bind to. Estrogen binds to the estrogen receptor, progesterone binds to the progesterone receptor, etc. This isn't universal as I'll discuss below and sometimes a given hormone can kind of bind to a receptor. As well, there can be different receptor subtypes, estrogen has an alpha and beta subtype for example, found in different parts of the body. This simply allows a single hormone to have different effects in the body depending on which receptor subtype is present. Estrogen might have one impact on fat cells and a different effect on muscle or breast tissue.

So a hormone (key) binds to its receptor (lock) and this causes something to happen and some signal to be sent in the body. How much of an actual signal is sent by a given hormone is related to three primary factors. The first is the level of the hormone itself. Simplistically, the more of a hormone present, the more of an effect that is seen. The second is something referred to as affinity, that is how well or poorly a given hormone binds to the receptor. A hormone with high receptor affinity binds very tightly, generally sending more of a signal, while one with low receptor affinity binds poorly and sends less of a signal.

The third has to do with the sensitivity of the receptor to that hormone. When a receptor is very sensitive, that means that any given level of a hormone will send a larger signal. When a receptor is insensitive or is said to be resistant, either a given level of hormone will send less of a signal or more will be required to send the same signal. Readers maybe familiar with the concept of insulin resistance (or insensitivity) which occurs when the insulin receptor no longer responds well to the hormone insulin. This means that insulin can't send its signal as well as it otherwise would which causes a number of effects in the body. One is that hormone levels may increase in an attempt to overcome the resistance. In the opposite situation, someone with good insulin sensitivity doesn't need much insulin to send a strong signal.

Sometimes a given hormone can sort of bind to another hormone's receptor, called cross reactivity. When this occurs, the cross reacting hormone prevents the hormone that would normally bind from sending its signal (the lock is literally blocked). Usually this means that less of a signal is sent than otherwise would be. As one example, cortisol (a stress hormone) can partially bind to what is called the mineralocorticoid receptor (MR), which normally binds a hormone that causes water to be retained in the body. While cortisol sends less of a signal at the receptor, when enough of it is present, it can still cause water retention. Progesterone is notable in this regard as it can bind to four different receptors in the body.

Finally, a hormone can also act as an antagonist at a receptor meaning that it binds and directly prevents the normal signal from being sent. So a hormone acting as an androgen receptor antagonist will prevent the androgens from sending their normal signal. Additionally, since most tissues in the body have receptors for more than one hormone, with those hormones often having different or even opposite effects, there can be complex interactions. In some cases, the effects of the hormones compliment one another, in others one hormone can effectively block the effects of another. As I'll discuss below, progesterone not only has effectively opposite effects of estrogen but blocks the effects estrogen would normally cause. And this is all mostly relevant as variations in all of the above, hormone levels, hormone ratios, receptor affinity, sensitivity, etc. are probably what are contributing primarily to some of the variability seen in women.

The system can get even more complicated but the above should give readers at least a general picture. The main take away message is that specific hormones have specific effects and they do so through their specific receptor. But that there are endless ways that the system is modified, some of which are critical understanding the changes in a woman's physiology during her cycle. It's probably fair to say that there are differences in the levels (or effects) of many, if not, most hormones in a woman's body compared to a man's but I don't intend to detail all of them here. While I will look at other hormones at the end of the chapter I will focus on the reproductive hormones, testosterone, estrogen and progesterone in terms of their effects on fat gain or fat loss.

Androgens/Testosterone

While estrogen and progesterone are the primary women's reproductive hormones, I want to start by looking at the androgens/testosterone. The term androgen is a general one, referring to any hormone with masculinizing or androgenic effect, and includes a variety of hormones. Testosterone is probably the most well known and is produced primarily in a woman's ovaries. However other androgens such as androstenedione, DHEA, DHEA-sulfate (DHEA-S) which are produced in the adrenal gland, are extremely important to women as they represent a large portion of a woman's overall androgen output. After menopause, especially, when the ovaries are no longer production testosterone, the adrenal androgens become that much more important. DHEA is especially critical in terms of a woman's exercise performance and I will discuss it more in Volume 2. That said, in this book I will primarily focus on testosterone as it tends to generally represent the effects of this type of hormone.

Testosterone is a steroid hormone which simply means that it is produced from cholesterol. Estrogen, cortisol and progesterone are steroid hormones as well. While often thought of as a "male" hormone, women do produce relatively small amounts of testosterone (in the same way men produce small amounts of estrogen and progesterone). On average, women have testosterone levels about 1/15th (ranging from 1/10th to 1/30th) the levels of testosterone as men. An average testosterone level for men might be 545 ng/dL (this varies from 300-900 ng/dL) while women might have levels of 25-35 ng/dL.

As mentioned, women release testosterone and other androgens from their ovaries and adrenal cortex but androgens can also be produced via chemical reaction in other parts of the body. Testosterone can also be converted to dihydrotestosterone (DHT, a hormone involved in hair loss) and estrogen (fat cells convert testosterone to estrogen, via an enzyme called aromatase, in both women and men). As I mentioned above, the receptor for testosterone, DHT and other androgens is called the androgen receptor or AR.

Testosterone has a number of effects in the body which are typically subdivided into anabolic (tissue building) and androgenic (masculinizing). Anabolic effects include increasing protein synthesis and muscle mass. Testosterone also increases blood cell number and women generally have a lower hematocrit (the ratio of red blood cells to plasma) than men due to their reduced levels of testosterone. Androgenic effects can be thought of as other secondary male sexual characteristics such as increased body hair, a deepened voice, oily skin, acne, hair loss and others (the increase in testosterone at puberty is what causes these changes in boys). As mentioned, elevated testosterone also contributes to hair loss due to it's conversion to DHT in the scalp. Testosterone has a pronounced effect on tissues such as skeletal muscle and bone where it increases the size and strength of both.

For the most part, the effects of testosterone in women are similar to that of men but there are exceptions. For example, in women elevated levels of testosterone impairs insulin sensitivity and causes insulin resistance while, in (hypogonadal) men, it generally improves it. Testosterone also directly impacts on both body weight and body fat levels but in a gender specific way. Elevated testosterone in women, for example, increases bodyweight and body fat (and specifically fat around the midsection) while those same elevations in testosterone (especially if low levels are being corrected) tend to reduce both in men. Overall, women's lower levels of testosterone decrease both the anabolic and androgenic effects. Women have less muscle mass and bone density, carry more total body fat with a different distribution and, unless testosterone levels are elevated, don't show the typical male secondary sexual characteristics.

At the same time, even small increases in testosterone have more profound effects in women due to their higher sensitivity to it. Women with slightly or significantly elevated levels of testosterone may have increased body hair, oily skin, acne or experience hair loss. They store larger amounts of fat around the midsection and often show increased levels of muscle mass or improved athletic performance. This occurs in women who use anabolic steroids (synthetic derivatives of testosterone) and I will describe two biological causes of elevated testosterone levels in women in the next chapter. There are endless other effects of testosterone in both the female and male body but to detail them all would be impossible. They can involve behavior, with at least some linkage between testosterone and overall aggressive behavior, psychology and others and the differences between women and men are at least partially due to the differences in hormone levels (along with the potential for genetic and biological programming from prenatal hormone exposure as I discussed in Chapter 1).

Testosterone levels do impact health on a number of ways and are a large part of why men are at a greater risk for certain diseases such as cardiovascular disease than women. This is primarily related to body fat patterning with a woman's lower body fat pattern being more protective than a man's more central body fat pattern (2). For women, it's actually a little bit more complicated as her relatively lower risk is due as much to having lower testosterone levels (which reduces risk) as having elevated estrogen levels (which are protective). Women who have elevated levels of testosterone and who have a more male-like body fat pattern are at an increased risk due to the elevated testosterone levels. At menopause, when women's estrogen and progesterone levels drop, there is also an increase in cardiovascular disease risk (and changes to a more male fat patterning). It is the balance of and combination of effects of the two hormones that are at work here and, overall, women who have a relatively higher levels of estrogen and testosterone are relatively healthier than the reverse (3).

As a piece of trivia, women live, on average, about 7 years more than men and at least part of this is due to differences in testosterone levels with men's higher testosterone levels being responsible for their earlier deaths. Studies of modern day eunuchs, men who have had their testicles removed and who produce no testosterone live 14-19 years longer than the average male (4). At the same time, men with only lower testosterone (rather than producing none) are at a higher health risk and lower testosterone levels in men tend to cause the same problems as elevated levels in women (5).

But ultimately most of the effects of testosterone in women are fairly small, due to the lower levels that are typically present. As well, outside of the small burst right around ovulation, testosterone levels stay relatively stable across the menstrual cycle meaning that it's effects will be relatively stable. As the primary reproductive hormones, estrogen and progesterone play by far the greater role.

Estrogen and Progesterone: Introduction

The two primary female sex hormones are estrogen and progesterone and you've seen above how they change across the menstrual cycle. In the same way that women have roughly 1/15th the testosterone levels of men, men have about 1/10th (or so) the levels of estrogen and progesterone (as men's physiology is not the topic of this book I will not discuss it further). I mentioned in Chapter 1 that determining the effects of estrogen and progesterone on a woman's physiology was very difficult for researchers for quite some time. Was it the increase in one hormone, the decrease in another, the combination, the ratio? After decades of research, the effects of each hormone is fairly well established.

The follicular phase is actually fairly simple in that progesterone is very low and has very little effect overall with estrogen being the primary determinant of what is occurring physiologically. The surge of estrogen in the late follicular phase has a number of effects but the overall picture there is fairly simple. Things become more difficult in the luteal phase where estrogen first drops (this drop causing one set of effects) before both estrogen and progesterone increase and then fall again, causing different effects still. While I will discuss each hormone individually below, the simplest way of looking at this issue is that estrogen and progesterone have effectively opposite effects on a woman's physiology. Importantly, when progesterone is high during the luteal phase, its effects dominate as it blocks/opposes estrogen's effects.

Even here there is a further complication as estrogen sensitizes the progesterone receptor so that progesterone will have a larger impact during the luteal phase. In that sense, at least some of progesterone's overall effects are can be indirectly attributed to estrogen. Regardless, once I've looked at the effects of both estrogen and progesterone and consider the interactions (along with the spike of estrogen before ovulation), the overall structure of the menstrual cycle should make some logical sense in how it is trying to prepare a woman's body for the potentiality and eventuality of pregnancy.

Estrogen

There are actually three primary estrogens which are estrone (E1), estradiol (17 beta-estradiol or E2) and estriol (E3) which have slightly different effects. Each tends to predominate at different times in a woman's life with estrone most relevant during pregnancy and estriol most relevant after menopause. Since I am discussing the normal menstrual cycle here, I will exclusively focus on estradiol or simply use the term estrogen generally. Estrogen is produced primarily by a woman's ovaries although it can be produced elsewhere, generally by the conversion of other hormones such as testosterone via aromatase.

As I mentioned above, estrogen has its own specific receptor and there are two subtypes called estrogen receptor alpha and estrogen receptor beta. These are found in varying levels in different tissues in the body which not only explains how estrogen can have differential effects in different places but also why certain drugs that target specific receptors can be used to treat such diseases as breast cancer. In this case, it is estrogen receptor alpha that is primarily at play and drugs that specifically block that receptor allow estrogen to work in other tissues that express estrogen receptor beta while still treating the disease itself.

In the same way that testosterone is responsible for the development of male secondary sexual characteristics, estrogen has a primary effect on the development of female secondary sex characteristics. Estrogen is critically involved in the deposition of breast fat and contributes both to women's increwased overall body fat levels and her lower body fat patterning. In men estrogen can have the same effect, for example and some males develop gynecomastia, the development breast tissue, under some conditions such as puberty or testosterone abuse. High levels of estrogen can also cause water retention.

Estrogen causes the growth plates of bones to close and this is part of why women are typically shorter than men; at puberty their bones fuse and stop lengthening. Critically, estrogen is a major player in increasing bone density although it is not the only factor here. Estrogen also plays a role in cognition and mental function and there are endless other effects that I won't detail here (6). Since is is the primary topic of this book, I will focus primarily on the impact of estrogen on processes related to fat loss and fat gain with a brief mention of some of its effects on exercise, training and muscle growth (discussed in detail in Volume 2). Recall again that estrogen dominates during the follicular phase (first half of the cycle), starting at a low level and gradually increasing to a surge prior to ovulation. It then drops before rising gradually during the luteal phase, reaching a level about half of that of the peak during the follicular phase.

Since estrogen has typically been blamed for a woman's issues with body fat, let me start with its effects in this regard. It turns out that estrogen has both positive and negative impact on fat metabolism, fat cells and fat loss although, in the aggregate most of its effects are positive (this may come as a surprise to many readers). I should mention that one very confusing issue regarding the role of estrogen and body fat in women is that it has different effects in different parts of the body. This is a large contributor to the typical fat patterns in women. I'll talk about some of the implications of this later in the book.

Discussed more below, estrogen can impact negatively on thyroid levels which can have an indirect effect on body fat by lowering metabolic rate; estrogen also has a number of other potential negative effects on body fat. I haven't talked about how fat stores or mobilizes fat yet but estrogen does increase the levels of a specific receptor in fat cells (the alpha-2 receptor) that inhibits the release of fat from fat cells by decreasing the fat mobilizing effect of hormones released during exercise (7). These receptors are found to a greater degree in women's lower body and this is one way that estrogen may at least indirectly impact on body fat levels in the lower body. In contrast, estrogen does not impact on the levels of the alpha-2 receptor in the upper body and increases the fat cell's sensitivity to fat mobilizing hormones (8).

Estrogen thickens the connective tissue in the skin and fat matrix in the lower body and this is the primary cause of cellulite (9). What is happening is that excess body fat pushes through the connective tissue and you can think of it as a holiday ham pushing through the mesh it comes wrapped in. Cellulite is not a different type of fat and it doesn't respond to nearly any of the supposed treatments for it short of some invasive almost surgical treatments (fat loss generally improves its appearance). The presence or absence of cellulite seems to be partially genetic (perhaps due to elevated estrogen levels

Beyond that, most of estrogen's other effects are relatively positive in terms of body weight and body fat levels. First, there is an enzyme in fat cells called lipoprotein lipase (LPL) which breaks fatty acids off of what are called chylomicrons (produced after fat is eaten) for storage. Unless levels are very low, estrogen inhibit the activity of LPL in lower body fat cells inhibiting fat storage in that area (9a). Estrogen also inhibits the storage of visceral fat which is at least part of why it is protective against heart disease.

While LPL was long-considered the singularly important enzyme for fat storage, there is a second, far more important enzyme responsible for fat storage in fat cells called acylation stimulating protein (ASP) that plays a far larger role. While progesterone (discussed next) affects ASP, estrogen does not. Estrogen also increases LPL activity in muscle cells which causes fat to be stored there as Intramuscular Triglyceride (IMTG). These provide a quick source of energy during certain types of exercise and women's higher levels of estrogen cause them to store more IMTG than men (10). Estrogen also increases the level of fat-burning enzymes in skeletal muscle along with activating a compound (called AMPk) which enhances the use of fat for fuel.

Although many of estrogen's effects clearly limit fat gain in women, there is no doubt that many aspects of its metabolism clearly function to increase lower body fat. This fat exists primarily to provide energy during pregnancy and breastfeeding and given the large calorie requirements of both, it makes logical evolutionary sense to store calories there (11). Demonstrating this is an oddity of female metabolism where, during pregnancy, normal fat storage and mobilization patterns effectively reverse. The normally easy to store and difficult to mobilize hip and thigh fat becomes the easiest to mobilize as it is being used to provide energy for pregnancy and breastfeeding.

Despite it's potentially negative effect on body fat, and especially lower body fat, estrogen also has a number of significant positive effects helping to regulate appetite, body weight and body fat levels (12). Demonstrating this is the fact that postmenopausal women who do not go on Hormone Replacement Therapy (HRT) gain significant amounts of weight and body fat (with a shift in distribution) and this is prevented if estrogen levels are maintained with HRT. And at least some of this is mediated by the interaction of estrogen with the hormone leptin (discussed briefly below and in much greater detail later in the book) which acts to regulate appetite, body weight and body fat. Among its many other effects, leptin acts to improve the brain's response to other hormones that help to regulate appetite and body weight. Simply, when leptin is low (as occurs during dieting), these signals don't work as well and this is part of the overall adaptation to dieting that I will discuss in detail in Chapter 9.

Not only does estrogen increase leptin production from fat cells, it also increases leptin sensitivity in the brain causing leptin to send an even stronger signal. Estrogen also sends it's own leptin-like signal in the brain further increasing the effect (13). The end result of this is that estrogen helps to control hunger, with the largest effect occurring during the follicular phase and hunger being lowest in the 4 days or so before ovulation when estrogen surges. As well, falling levels of estrogen after ovulation contribute to the increase in hunger and cravings that are seen during the luteal phase (14). At least one way that estrogen does this is through it's effects on the brain chemicals (effectively hormones in the brain) serotonin and dopamine. Serotonin is involved in overall mood and appetite (especially carbohydrate cravings) and low levels can contribute to depression. Dopamine is part of the reward system and low levels can drive cravings for high-calorie/high-sugar foods. When estrogen is high during the follicular phase/before ovulation, serotonin and dopamine levels will be higher; when estrogen levels decrease, the levels of both serotonin and dopamine will as well, increasing hunger and cravings.

Estrogen has many other positive effects on metabolism. One is that it increases insulin sensitivity. This means that, when estrogen is the dominant hormone, the body will burn more carbohydrates for fuel and this has implications for both diet and exercise. Insulin also inhibits fat release from fat cells and this change is yet another way that estrogen can impact on body fat levels. Finally, the surge in estrogen during the second half of the follicular phase causes a woman's body to retain more sodium; on a high-salt diet this will cause her body to retain water. While training will be discussed in detail in Volume 2, let me briegly address estrogen's overall positive effects here. Estrogen prevents inflammation, limits free radical damage, may limit muscle damage itself (reducing soreness) and acts to help remodel and rebuild skeletal muscle (15). At the same time, estrogen may negatively impact on tendon strength and this has enormous implications for the risk of knee injury in women that I will discuss in Volume 2 (16).

While estrogen is most commonly blamed for all aspects of woman's body fat (and especially lower body fat problems), it's clear that the picture is more complicated than that. Certainly estrogen has some effects in fat cells, especially in the lower body. that can be considered negative. At the same time, estrogen also has a number of positive effects on fat metabolism, body weight regulation and appetite control. In the aggregate, estrogen probably has a more overall positive than negative effects in this regard. I'd add that the impact of estrogen on any aspect of fat gain or fat loss interacts with the diet. Many of estrogen's negative effects are primarily seen when combined with a high dietary fat intake. Regardless, while estrogen receives much of the blame, the fact is that progesterone causes far more problems.

Progesterone

Progesterone is the second primary reproductive hormone in women and is released from the corpus luteum that develops after release of the egg at ovulation. While it has a tremendous number of roles in the body most of them aren't that relevant to this book and I will once again focus on fat loss, fat gain while briefly addressing training. As a steroid hormone, progesterone has a structure similar to many other hormones in the body and can actually be converted to aldosterone (involved in water balance), cortisol (a stress hormone), and the androgens. Due to that structural similarity, progesterone can bind to four different receptors. The first is the progesterone receptor itself where a normal signal will be sent. At the cortisol receptor, progesterone only sends a weak signal, weaker than cortisol itself. Progesterone is also an antagonist at the androgen and aldosterone receptor, not only blocking the effects of the hormones that would normally bind there but sending an actual negative signal. This cross reactivity not only explains many of progesterone's effects but is critical for the discussion of birth control in Chapter 3.

As I described above, progesterone remains low during the follicular phase of the menstrual cycle and has little to no effects at that time. During the luteal phase, following ovulation, progesterone starts to increase gradually, reaching a peak halfway through the cycle before decreasing again prior to menstruation. And as I'll describe, as much as estrogen tends to get the blame for so many aspects of women's fat loss issue, progesterone is of far more importance. Not only does it have its own profoundly negative direct effects, it also acts to cancel out estrogen's many positive effects, essentially doubling its negative effects in this regard.

Before discussing progesterone's negative effects, let me examine its one potential benefit in terms of fat loss. I mentioned above that the increase in progesterone is the cause of an increase in women's body temperature after ovulation and that Basal Body Temperature (BBT) has long been used to indicate when ovulation has occurred. Along with changes in vaginal mucus (due to estrogen), this can be used to determine a woman's peak fertility. Along with this increase in body temperature comes an increase in energy expenditure and resting metabolic rate. This is another effect that is variable between women with increases ranging from 2.5-10% over normal which might amount to roughly 100-300 extra calories per day burned. In premise this should benefit weight and fat loss.

This is counteracted by the fact that, during this time, both hunger and cravings are increased, adding to the fact that women are more prone to food cravings already (16a). Women also show an increased attention/notice of tasty, high-calorie foods (16b). This can make controlling food intake more difficult and, on average, women's calorie intake increases more than their metabolic rate. The increase in hunger during the luteal phase occurs for several reasons. As I mentioned above, a primary one is the drop in estrogen from before ovulation which causes both serotonin and dopamine levels to go down. While progesterone by itself does not appear to increase hunger, it does so in the presence of estrogen, which describes is the hormonal profile at this time (17). Progesterone causes some degree of insulin resistance (described below) and one consequence of this is that blood sugar may become unstable. This can cause blood sugar levels to fall, also stimulating hunger. Finally, although leptin levels go up during the luteal phase (which should help to control hunger), leptin resistance also develops so that this effect is blunted.

Overall, the above effects result in increased hunger and cravings, especially for high-sugar/high-fat foods (chocolate is the most commonly reported craving although other foods are often craved). When diet is uncontrolled, an increase in food intake of 90-500 calories has been observed during the luteal phase and this can readily exceed any small increase in metabolic rate that occurs. There are supplements that can potentially help to avoid this that I will discuss in Chapter 23. In premise, so long as food intake can be controlled during this time, the increase in metabolic rate during the luteal phase can be used to enhance fat loss. If a woman is able to avoid an increase in calorie intake, the 100-300 calorie/day increase in metabolic rate with an average duration of 10 of the 14 days of the luteal phase would burn ~1000-3000 extra calories. This amounts to somewhere between 1/3rd to just under one pound of extra fat lost. Alternately, food intake could be increased slightly during this phase which could increase diet adherence for those women seeking fat loss (I will discuss this again in Chapter 19).

I mentioned above that progesterone can bind to the aldosterone receptor, which is involved in water retention in the body. Since it blocks aldosterone from binding and causing water retention, progesterone causes women to be less likely to retain water during the first half of the luteal phase. As progesterone drops during the late luteal phase/PMS week, there is a rebound effect which can cause water retention. As with the surge in estrogen before ovulation, this drop in progesterone changes how the body handles sodium and women on a high-sodium diet during this time may show extreme amounts of water retention. Dietary strategies to limit this will be discussed later in the book.

The above are the potentially good effects of progesterone on a woman's body weight and body fat levels. Now let me look at the large number of bad effects. Like estrogen, progesterone increases LPL activity in women's lower body fat, breaking fatty acids off of chylomicrons for storage (17a). This is compounded by the fact that progesterone also activates ASP (mentioned above) which is not only one of the key enzymes in storing body fat but has been described as the most potent enzyme for the fat storage process. ASP is found preferentially in subcutaneous fat (which women have more of to begin with) and, for all these reasons, one researcher has called ASP "A female fat storing factor" (18). All of which is important as, unlike estrogen, progesterone potently activates ASP (ensuring storage of the fatty acids made available by its effects on LPL). Within the context of the menstrual cycle this sets up a sequence of events where the surge in estrogen before ovulation not only sensitizes the progesterone receptor but also increases the number of the fat loss inhibiting alpha-2 receptors. Increasing progesterone levels then activates LPL and ASP ensuring that excess calorie intake (driven by increased hunger) is stored as body fat.

As well, progesterone opposes estrogen in that it impairs insulin sensitivity meaning that the body doesn't utilize carbohydrates as well. This can be good or bad depending on the situation. In the context of a high-carbohydrate, low-fat diet, insulin resistance is not a good thing as there will be an overproduction of insulin. In contrast, insulin resistance can be beneficial on a lowered or low-carbohydrate diet (19). The practical implications of this, discussed in Chapter 19, is that a higher carbohydrate/lower fat diet will be superior in the follicular phase while a lowered carbohydrate/higher fat diet will be superior in the luteal phase. As mentioned above, this insulin resistance also causes blood glucose levels to become more unstable, affecting energy levels, mood and potentially hunger. Perhaps confusingly, the insulin resistance that develops during the luteal phase causes a decrease in carbohydrate use and an increase in fat utilization both at rest and during aerobic exercise. While this sounds beneficial, most of the additional fat being burned is from the IMTG stored within the muscle so this does not impact the visible subcutaneous fat stores directly (I will discuss this in detail in Chapter 10). The combined effect is that progesterone increases the storage of fat in a woman's fat cells while increasing the use of fat stored in her muscles.

Taken as a whole, the effects of progesterone are to ensure and enhance not only general fat storage but fat storage specifically in a woman's lower body. Following ovulation, in preparation for pregnancy, the increase in progesterone will not only block estrogen's beneficial effects but will cause her to store more fat in her fat cells while burning more in her muscles. Although metabolic rate may be up slightly, hunger and cravings will increase and this tends to increase calorie intake far above the small increase in metabolic rate. If calorie and fat intake is too high during this phase, there will be increased fat storage. In contrast, if calories can be controlled, the changes in metabolic rate can be harnessed to potentially increase fat loss.

Looking briefly at training, progesterone's overall effects are quite negative. First and foremost, progesterone binds to the androgen receptor which would normally bind testosterone. This not only prevents testosterone from binding and having a positive effect on muscle but progesterone acts as a receptor antagonist, inhibiting any effect that might be seen. Due to this, progesterone tends to decrease tendon strength and decrease the ability to build muscle (recall that estrogen directly improves a woman's muscular remodeling and growth). For endurance athletes primarily, the increase in body temperature during the luteal phase can cause problems with thermoregulation during exercise in hot or humid conditions. High-intensity endurance performance may also be impaired as the use of carbs for fuel is lowered because of the insulin resistance that develops.

An Overview of Menstrual Cycle Changes

With the above discussed, let me summarize the changes that are occurring.

Early and Late Follicular Phase

After menstruation, during the early follicular phase, estrogen and progesterone are both fairly low although estrogen will start to increase and have the dominant effect overall. Insulin sensitivity will be high with a woman's body using more carbohydrate for fuel at rest. Appetite and hunger will be stable and controlled, especially in comparison to the previous luteal phase. Blood glucose levels will remain stable as well. Her metabolic rate will be normal and fat storage will be normal and/or lowered at least relative to the luteal phase. Estrogen will be exerting anti-inflammatory effects and have a positive effect on muscular remodeling from training. Early in the follicular phase, water retention will be low after any retention from the previous late-luteal phase has disappeared and this is when women will show their lowest bodyweight. For the most part all of the above will hold in both the early and late follicular phase with one or two exceptions. Due to the surge in estrogen, appetite will be reduced significantly in the 3-4 days prior to ovulation. This same surge can cause water retention, especially if a woman is on a high sodium diet.

Early Luteal Phase

During the early luteal phase, most of the above reverses or at least starts to reverse. Body temperature increases slightly and with this will come a small increase in metabolic rate. Hunger and cravings will tend to go up both due to the fall in estrogen after ovulation along with increasing progesterone levels. This can cause an increase in food intake that can easily overwhelm the small increase in metabolic rate. Due to the impact of progesterone on both LPL and ASP, fat storage will be higher than in the follicular phase and this is compounded by estrogen's effects both on anti-fat mobilizing receptors and it's sensitizing of the progesterone receptor. Since progesterone causes insulin resistance, a woman's body will use more fat for fuel (and less carbohydrates) both at rest and during exercise but the fat comes from within the muscle. Blood sugar becomes unstable and this can cause energy and mood swings along with hunger. Binding of progesterone to the aldosterone receptor will cause a loss of body water and there tends to be little water retention during this phase. Due to the negative impact of progesterone on muscle along with it's blocking of the androgen receptor, muscle growth and remodeling are negatively impacted. The increase in body temperature may harm endurance performance especially in the heat.

Late Luteal Phase/PMS/PMDD

Moving into the late luteal phase, estrogen and progesterone continue to drop and this has a large number of effects on a woman's body. Blood sugar levels often become even more unstable during this time period and this can cause women to experience low blood sugar (hypoglycemia) negatively affecting energy, mood and hunger. Just as with earlier in the luteal phase, cravings for high-fat and high-sugar foods are usually high here, related both to the drop in serotonin and dopamine levels. Falling dopamine levels also cause levels of the hormone prolactin to increase, causing breast tenderness. The same basic pattern of fat storage and fuel utilization seen in the early luteal phase will be maintained. As progesterone drops, there is a rebound effect with water retention typically being the worst at this time with the effect being increased for women on a high-sodium diet.

While not frequently mentioned, sleep is often interrupted during the late luteal phase as well. Melatonin, a hormone predominantly involved in sleep, is more inhibited by the impact of even small amounts of light, and this can prevent women from sleeping well (20). There are a number of strategies including avoiding light late at night, sleeping in a dark and cool room that can help with this. A sleep mask may also be useful and I will discuss specific sleep supplements in Chapter 23 that can be used.

Finally, in that proportion of women that experience it at all, the late luteal phase is also when Pre-menstrual syndrome (PMS) or Pre-Menstrual Dysphoric Disorder (PMDD) will typically occur (21). Again, there are different patterns here with some women experiencing symptoms in the early luteal phase or having those same symptoms continue through the first days of menstruation. Women may suffer from headaches, joint or muscle ache, digestive problems, issues with coordination and many others. Exhaustion, irritability, anger, problems with concentration and mood swings are common as well (as I mentioned, in PMDD, this may reach the extreme of depression, anxiety or suicidal thoughts). Anti-depressants have shown a benefit for PMS and PMDD which further suggests that serotonin levels are involved with some of the typical PMS symptoms As well, due to low estrogen levels, a large percentage of women suffer from hot flashes, identical to what is seen after menopause (21a). As mentioned, some women experience none of the traditional effects whatsoever.

Treating the symptoms of PMS have always been of great interest (for what should be obvious reasons) and many approaches have been tried or shown to be beneficial with an equal number of often claimed remedies having zero effect. Regular exercise appears to reduce the symptoms of PMS but this may be problematic if the presence of PMS or PMDD makes it difficult for women to maintain an exercise program (21b). A number of dietary supplements, including specific vitamins and minerals along with others may help to alleviate many of the typical PMS symptoms as well and I will provide recommendations in Chapter 23.

Finally, in preparation for shedding the uterine lining and the start of menstruation, cramps are common here and these may continue into the early stages of menstruation as bleeding starts. Related to falling levels of progesterone, the cause of the cramping are prostaglandins, short lived chemical messengers, that cause the uterus to contract. This can generally be treated with Non-Steroidal Anti-Inflammatories such as aspirin, Naproxen Sodium, Ibuprofen and others. Although the reason is unclear, approximately 18% of women are resistant to their effects and may require medical treatment (22). As the late luteal phase ends, menstruation and the next cycle begins.

Summary of the Menstrual cycle

I've summarized the primary general changes that occur in a woman's physiology that occur across the menstrual cycle and this chart, or a variation on it, will appear multiple times throughout this book. As you can see clearly, there are changed in fuel utilization, fat storage, hunger, appetite, water retention and others that occur due to the impact of either estrogen, progesterone with estrogen and progesterone typically having roughly opposite effects in the body. From a fat loss perspective, both estrogen and progesterone have positive and negative effects although it's arguable that the late luteal phase when progesterone is dominant is truly the problem time.

Day	1	2	3	4	5	6	7	8	9	10	11	12	13	14	15	16	17	18	19	20	21	22	23	24	25	26	27	28
Phase	Early Follicular							Early Follicular							Early Luteal							Late Luteal						
Note	Menses (3-5 days)							Ovulation														PMS (4-7 days)						
Dominant Hormone	Estrogen							Estrogen							Progesterone							Progesterone						
Insulin Sensitivity	High							High							Lowered							Lowered						
Fuel at Rest	Carbs							Carbs							Fat							Fat						
Fuel During Exercise	Fat							Fat							Fat (increased)							Fat (increased)						
Fat Storage	Lowered							Lowered							Increased							Increased						
Metabolic Rate	Normal							Normal							Increased							Increased						
Hunger	Lowered							Lowered							Increased							Increased						
Blood Glucose	Stable							Stable							Unstable							Unstable						
Water retention	Lowered							Increased							Lowered							Increased (highest)						
Muscle Growth	Increased							Increased							Decreased							Decreased						

Hopefully the above chart makes it clear just how much more complicated a woman's physiology is compared to a man's. There are major changes occurring at least every 2 weeks and in some cases even more frequently than that. These changes interact, overlap and often reverse completely (in contrast, men are basically the same daily). Addressing women's needs for diet or fat loss means taking those changes into account, taking advantage of the positives while minimizing the negatives.

Other Hormones

While I have focused on the differences in the reproductive hormones in this chapter in order to describe the menstrual cycle, there are other differences between women and men's hormones that are important or worth addressing at least briefly and I'll round out the chapter by looking at a few of them. One hormone that will not be discussed here is cortisol as it will be discussed in detail in Chapter 13.

Growth Hormone (GH)

Growth hormone is involved in many processes in the body but a primary one in adults is the mobilization of fat. Women show higher levels of GH than men along with an larger increase in response to exercise. This is probably part of why women use more fat for fuel under some conditions.

Insulin

The hormone insulin is one about which there is a great deal of confusion and mistaken information. While all too frequently blamed for being the cause of fat gain it's better to think of insulin as a general storage hormone. It impacts on fat metabolism, stimulating fat storage and inhibiting fat mobilization and burning but it also increases the storage of carbohydrate in skeletal muscle and liver and is involved in skeletal muscle growth. In general, women have lower levels of insulin along with better insulin sensitivity than men. This is more pronounced during the follicular phase when estrogen increases insulin sensitivity and is decreased in the luteal phase when progesterone causes some degree of insulin resistance.

Thyroid

I would imagine that almost all readers are familiar with thyroid hormone although, like so many things, there is a lot of confusion and misinformation about it. Among it's other effects in the body, thyroid hormones are a primary controller of metabolic rate, interacting with other hormones (such as the catecholamines discussed below). Thyroid also impacts on fat cell metabolism (helping to mobilize fat out of the cells) and skeletal muscle.

There are two primary types of thyroid hormone called T4 (thyroxine) and T3 (triiodothyronine) which are released from the thyroid gland in a ratio of about 80% T4 to 20% T3. T4 is primarily a storage hormone which is converted to the more active T3 in other tissues in the body, especially the liver. The conversion of T4 to T3 is important as this process goes down while dieting, leading to lower levels of T3 and a lowered metabolic rate; I'll talk about this more later in the book. Reproductive hormones interact with T3, estrogen decreases levels of active thyroid hormone while progesterone increases them. This may be part of the metabolic rate increase during the luteal phase. T3 can also be converted inside of tissues to T2 which has it's own metabolic effects there (23).

Women are significantly more likely to be hypothyroidal (meaning that their thyroid gland releases insufficient levels of thyroid hormones) having more issues when iodine intake is insufficient. They are also three times as likely to suffer from thyroid cancer as men and this is probably related to the direct effect of estrogen on thyroid hormone metabolism (24). Women are also more likely to suffer from depression and, while far from the only cause, low thyroid levels are an often undiagnosed cause. While beyond the scope of this book, Hashimoto's thyroiditis, an autoimmune condition, is far more common in women than men (women are more likely to suffer autoimmune disease in general). In the case of Hashimoto's the immune system attacks the thyroid gland and can cause swings from low to high thyroid.

All medical cases of hypothyroid are treated with thyroid hormone to replace the hormone that is not being produced normally. Either T4 or a combination of T4 and T3 are typically given and some women report better results from a type of thyroid called Armour (25). Determination of hypothyroid of any sort must be made through blood tests and medication should be used under the care of a health practitioner. Of more relevance to this book, in addition to their already generally lower levels of thyroid hormones, women's levels can be impacted significantly by certain diet and training practices, this effect being both large and rapid. Women's overall dietary choices can also negatively impact on thyroid hormone levels (and by extension their metabolic rate) and I will discuss these later in the book.

The Catecholamines

    The catecholamine hormones are refers to adrenaline and noradrenaline in America and epinephrine and norepinephrine everywhere else in the world   Adrenaline (epinephrine), as it's name suggests is released from the adrenal gland into the bloodstream and has effects throughout the body. In contrast, noradrenaline (norepinephrine) is released from nerve terminals and only has effects very locally where it is released.   Many readers may have heard these hormones referred to as the fight or flight hormones although, as I'll discuss in Chapter 13, they appear to have slightly different effects in women.

    Released in response to a variety of stressors, the catecholamines raise heart rate, blood pressure, mobilize fuel for energy and have many other functions.   In general women show lower levels of the catecholamines at rest along with a generally lower response to exercise compared to men. While women initially increase levels during exercise to the same degree as men, they rapidly adapt to exercise and no longer match men's levels.   As with the differences in GH described above, these differences are probably part of why women's overall nutrient utilization patterns at rest and during exercise are what they are.

    The catecholamines also interact with thyroid hormone in controlling metabolic rate along with fat mobilization. Thyroid hormones sensitizes the catecholamine receptors (meaning that the hormones send a more potent signal) while the catecholamines stimulate conversion of T4 to T3 in the liver. Like thyroid, levels of the catecholamines drop during dieting and these two factors are a large part of the overall decrease in metabolic rate.

Leptin

    I mentioned leptin briefly above want to examine it equally briefly here (I will discuss its effect in detail in later chapters). Leptin is a hormone released primarily from fat cells and it's discovery in 1994 changed the field of obesity research forever. Not only did it indicate that fat cells were far more than just an inert storage space but would lead to the realization that they produced numerous hormones involved in regulating the body's metabolism (26).   Relative to body weight and body fat specifically leptin helped to fill in a number of gaps in previous research in terms of how body fat and body weight were regulated. Early research had suggested that there was some way that the body or brain could "know" how much fat an animal was carrying or how much it weighed so that metabolism and food intake could be adjusted. Although the system is much more complicated, leptin provided a mechanism for how this could occur.

    Leptin levels turn out to be related to two primary factors. The first is the amount of body fat someone is carrying with higher levels of body fat leading to higher leptin levels. The second is the amount someone is eating over several days with leptin levels rapidly changing in response to alterations in food (especially carbohydrate intake). In the early days of leptin research, it was thought that leptin acted to prevent obesity but this is now known to be false. Rather, leptin acts primarily as an anti-starvation signal with decreasing levels (in response to food restriction or fat loss) signaling the body to lower metabolic rate, increase hunger/appetite along with other effects. (this will be discussed in detail in Chapter 9). Decreasing leptin levels is also involved in menstrual cycle dysfunction, discussed in Chapter 12.

    Perhaps surprisingly, women turn out to have higher levels of leptin than men. While some of this is simply due to having more total body fat, women's fat cells also produce more leptin than men's due to the effect of estrogen. While estrogen acts to generally sensitize the brain to leptin as I mentioned above, women do tend to show relatively more leptin resistance than men overall, meaning that it cannot send as potent of a signal. As well, although leptin levels increase during the luteal phase (possibly in response to the surge of estrogen right before ovulation), leptin resistance increases further. Finally, in response to dieting and exercise, women's bodies show a different response than men's and it looks like woman's brains may respond differently to changing leptin levels than men's. All of this adds to a woman's general physiological tendency to store and hold onto body fat as it means that women's bodies may fight back harder and adapt more quickly to dieting or exercise, slowing fat loss to a greater degree than would be seen in men. I will discuss this in detail in Chapter 9.

Chapter 3: Hormonal Modifiers

Having examined the normal menstrual cycle in detail in the last chapter in terms of the major hormonal changes that occur and how it affects a women's physiology, I want to next look at some commonly experienced situations that will change a woman's physiology from that of the normal menstrual cycle (this will not include explicit disease states which are outside of the scope of this book). I will refer to these as hormonal modifiers throughout this book and each will alter a woman's physiology in a very specific and often dramatic way with implications for her nutritional or fat loss guidelines. While each hormonal modifier is distinct in its own way, there are commonalities and this will allow me to group them somewhat going forwards.

Effective Hormonal States

In the previous chapter, I discussed the three primary hormones which impact on a woman's overall physiology which are estrogen, progesterone and testosterone. Each has its own distinct effects and, when one or the other is relatively dominant in a woman's body, it generally results in a fairly similar physiology. So regardless of the specific hormonal modifier present, two women with an estrogen-like, progesterone-like or androgen-like physiology will be considered to have a similar physiology in terms of the nutritional and other recommendations I will make later in this book. Each effective hormonal state will be related to the menstrual cycle itself meaning that I will consider the estrogen-like physiology to be the equivalent of the follicular phase physiology described in the last chapter and a progesterone-like physiology to be the equivalent of the luteal phase physiology. The androgen-like physiology is slightly more complicated in that it may generate an estrogen-like or progesterone-like physiology depending on other factors.

Amenorrhea/Oligomenorrhea

While there is no truly "normal' menstrual cycle, in that the variation between two women (or within the same woman) can be extremely large, it is still possible for the cycle to become extremely disrupted. While there are less severe disruptions I will mainly focus on amenorrhea and oligomenorrhea here. As both will be discussed in some detail in Chapter 12, I will only look at each briefly here. Amenorrhea refers to the absence of a menstrual cycle and is defined clinically as a lack of menstruation for 90 days or more with less than three total cycles in a year (some women will not menstruate for extended lengths of time). Strictly speaking, amenorrhea can occur under many different situations. This can include a woman who has begun to menstruate at all (called primary amenorrhea), pregnancy (where menstruation stops due to not being needed) and birth control (which deliberately shuts off the normal cycle although some bleeding may still occur). There can be numerous medical causes for amenorrhea but none of these represent the type of amenorrhea that I will discus in this book.

Rather, I will focus only on Functional Hypothalamic Amenorrhea (FHA). As the name suggests, FHA originates in the hypothalamus (a structure in the brain I will discus later) which will shut down the menstrual cycle under certain circumstances. Within the context of this book, these tend to be stress related including the stress of dieting, the stress of exercise, mental stress or some combination of the three. Physiologically, in amenorrhea, estrogen drops to about 33% of normal levels and progesterone drops to roughly 10% of normal. The normal cyclical changes are also lost and hormonal levels of both are effectively a flat line. The release of LH and FSH, which I described briefly in the last chapter, also disappears such that the follicle never matures or implants, the corpus luteum doesn't develop and there is no uterine lining to shed (hence the lack of bleeding). When amenorrhea develops, a woman's physiology changes enormously and I will discuss those changes in detail in Chapter 12.

Oligomenorrhea refers to an infrequent or delayed menstrual cycle and is defined clinically as a cycle that only occurs every 35-90 days (recall that the normal menstrual cycle occurs within 24-32 days). In contrast to amenorrhea where a woman's primary hormones drop to low levels and show no cyclical changes, in oligomenorrhea those hormones are lowered but are still changing. On some days hormone levels may be identical to the normal menstrual cycle but on others their levels will be random. Like amenorrhea, oligomenorrhea can occur for many reasons. This includes some types of birth control (where light bleeding may occur) and a variety of medical conditions (including PCOS, discussed next).

There are two types of oligomenorrhea that I will consider in this book. The first is part of the continuum of adaptations to dieting that can lead to amenorrhea that I will discuss in Chapter 12. While all women were originally thought to have this type of oligomenorrhea although it's now known that there is a subgroup of women who are oligomenorrheic due to elevated androgen/testosterone levels.

Hyperandrogenism

In the last chapter, I mentioned that the term androgen is sort of a catch-all for a variety of hormones that are produced in the body including testosterone, DHEA, DHEA-sulfate and a few others but I'll continue to use the term androgen or testosterone generally throughout this book. When those levels are elevated above normal, this is referred to as hyperandrogenism. Here I am combining two slightly different hormonal situations which are absolute and relative hyperandrogenism. Absolute hyperandrogenism will refer to any situation where a woman's testosterone levels are elevated above normal. Relative hyperandrogenism will refer to a situation where testosterone levels are not elevated above normal but estrogen and progesterone levels have decreased so that androgens are relatively higher.

In this section, I only want to look absolute hyperandrogenism, when a woman's testosterone levels are elevated above their normally low level along with the implications that has. Given the effects of testosterone, overall the effect of absolutely hyperandrogenism is some degree of masculinization or virilization of a woman's body with an increased prevalence of male secondary sexual characteristics along with other potentially negative effects. This includes increased body and facial hair, oily skin, acne and an increased risk of hair loss. Hyperandrogenic women often have a more "male" like body in that they have narrower hips and tend to carry relatively more of their body fat around their midsection. Relevant to this book, women with elevated testosterone levels often show an increased amount of muscle mass along with potentially improved sports performance and an ability to respond to training. I'll come back to this below and discuss it in detail in Volume 2.

Probably the most common cause of elevated testosterone in women, and the one I suspect most readers are at least passingly familiar with, is Poly-Cystic Ovary Syndrome or PCOS. PCOS has been found in somewhere between 6-20% of women and one of the most common effects is either oligomenorrhea, amenorrhea or infertility (due to a lack of an egg being released). In fact, roughly 15-20% of women who are infertile are diagnosed as having PCOS. PCOS is often associated with weight gain (I'll look at the reasons why in a later chapter) and obesity with more fat being carried around the midsection. Here even small amounts of weight loss (5-10% of current body weight) drastically improve health markers and fertility (1). Interestingly, while PCOS women often report having trouble losing weight, research shows no difference in weight loss between PCOS and non-PCOS women, at least within tightly controlled research (1a). In Chapter 23, I'll discuss a number of supplements specifically for PCOS symptoms.

PCOS is clinically diagnosed according to the Rotterdam criteria and requires that two of the following three symptoms be present: multiple cysts on the ovaries, clinical or biochemical signs of hyperandrogenism, and either oligomenorrhea or anovulation (an egg is not released). Practically this means that there are four distinct types of PCOS. A woman could have all three symptoms or any combination of two symptoms (i.e. cysts+hyperandrogenism, cysts+oligomenorrhea/anovulation, or hyperandrogenism+oligomenorrhea/anovulation). When hyperandrogenism is present (and this will usually manifest with oily skin, acne, central fat distribution or hair loss), the PCOS woman's testosterone levels may be 2.5-3 times a woman's normal levels. While this is still well below even the low normal range in males, women's greater sensitivity to androgens means that this will have a profound effect on her overall physiology. PCOS women also have lower levels of Sex-hormone Binding Globulin (SHBG) which results in more free testosterone (the biologically active type) being available.

Perhaps the most commonly seen metabolic dysfunction in PCOS is insulin resistance, an inability of the body to properly respond to insulin. Not only does this have numerous health consequences, it acts to maintain elevated androgen levels as elevated levels of insulin affect adrenal metabolism so that it produces even more androgens. This is even more true if excessive amounts of refined carbohydrates are being consumed but this turns into a vicious cycle where the elevated androgens cause insulin resistance which increases the insulin response which increases androgen levels.

Insulin resistance is extremely prevalent in PCOS and is estimated to occur in 60-80% of women with PCOS. This may increase to 95% if obesity (especially fat around the midsection, called central obesity) is present. The impact of obesity appears to be significant as lean women (defined later in this book) women with PCOS show relatively normal insulin sensitivity along with other physiological differences (1b,1c). Regular activity in overweight women also improves insulin sensitivity although it is still impaired compared to lean/normal weight PCOS women (1d). While I don't intend to cover every possible medical situation a woman might encounter, I do want to mention that women with PCOS are also 3 times more likely to suffer from thyroid disease (especially Hashimoto's thyroiditis, mentioned last chapter) than non-PCOS women (2). This adds up to a particularly problematic condition although, as I will discuss briefly below, it tends to aid athletic performance.

This second situation where a woman might show elevated testosterone levels is currently referred to as subclinical hyperandrogenism, representing a situation where testosterone levels are 20-30% above normal. While smaller than in PCOS, this is enough to have physiological effects without the clinical health issues of PCOS. Finally is an extreme rare condition (occurring in 1 in 12,000-18,000 people) called congenital adrenal hyperplasia (CAH, which can also occur in males). For complicated reasons, individuals with CAH produce adrenal androgens at an enormously elevated level. In both females and males, this causes an early puberty, extreme masculinization (including an enlarged clitoris or penis) and infertility. Since it is so rare, I won't discuss it further in this book and only mention it for completeness.

Even when oligomenorrhea was thought to be related to amenorrhea, it was often found that the oligomenorrhea seen in female athletes was accompanied by elevated testosterone levels. This was assumed to be a consequence of the changes in estrogen and progesterone but this is actually reversed and it is the elevated testosterone levels causing both oligomenorrhea and the changes in hormones such as estrogen and progesterone that occur (2a). In athletes, the elevated testosterone seen in this type of oligomenorrhea appears to be directly for the improvement in performance that is seen (3). The effects of testosterone such as increased muscle mass, bone density, the ability to respond to training and even aggressiveness can be beneficial for many sports which would explain its high prevalence. Subclinical hyperandrogenism was first identified in swimming, a sport requiring strength and power with less of an emphasis on leanness, although up to 30% of female runners have been found to have elevated testosterone levels as well. Women with this type of testosterone caused oligomenorrhea are likely to show an enhanced response to training regardless of sport. Supporting this is the fact that both PCOS and hyperandrogenism (along with menstrual cycle dysfunction) is found in female Olympic athletes (4).

As I mentioned above, it's not uncommon to see women with elevated testosterone levels, to have a different body structure than women without elevated testosterone levels. Narrower hips, what researchers call a linear body type (meaning less curves), are one example and these types of changes can make women relatively more or less suited to succeed at certain types of sports. This is in addition to any other benefits that even slightly elevated testosterone levels have in terms of trainability mentioned above. You might recall my comments in Chapter 1 about Chinese coaches looking for girls with certain physical characteristics as they tend to indicate elevated testosterone levels which will improve performance.

In all three cases of elevated testosterone in women, there is a continuum of effects in terms of the masculinization/virilization and other effects which may occur. CAH is the most profound with PCOS related hyperandrogenism the next and subclinical hyperandrogenism the least. In both PCOS and subclinical hyperandrogenism, it's common to find some degree of increased male sexual characteristics (i.e. the sub-clinically hyperandrogenic woman may carry relative more fat on her stomach) and this is often the first indication that androgens are elevated relative to normal. Oligomenorrhea or outright amenorrhea may be present but, distinguishing it from FHA, this will have been present from a fairly early point in a woman's life as it is related to her baseline level of testosterone in the first place.

For women interested in sports performance, hyperandrogenism can have enormous benefits, improving the ability to build muscle mass, strength, power and endurance. But this frequently comes with the consequence of increased body hair, acne, etc. along with the potential of infertility (important to those women who want to become pregnant). For inactive or relatively fatter women (defined later), the androgen-like physiology and the insulin resistance it tends to cause will generate a luteal phase physiology. For lean hyperandrogenic females who are highly active, insulin sensitivity should be relatively normal and an effective follicular phase physiology can be assumed to be present.

Since women with PCOS/hyperandrogenism may have distinctly different goals (i.e. performance vs. improved health/fertility), I will discuss them somewhat separately when I talk about diet and supplement recommendations. I'd note again that even small amounts of weight/fat loss can drastically improve health in women with overt PCOS. At the extremes, this may be insufficient and more pharmaceutical strategies may be required. Many approaches are used here with Metformin being a primary one. Hormonal birth control, which doesn't improve fertility but does improve many health parameters, is also commonly used and is discussed in detail in the next section.

Hormonal Birth Control

Formerly referred to as oral contraception (OC, a term no longer accurate due to other modes of application), hormonal birth control (BC) is used by a large percentage of women and is likely to represent the most common hormonal modifier readers may encounter. As they have no effect on a woman's physiology, I will not include barrier methods of birth control in this discussion. When I use the abbreviation BC it should be taken to only refer to hormonal forms. As the name suggests, a primary use BC is for its intended purpose which is to prevent unwanted pregnancy but there are other situations where BC is used. One is simply to control or regulate the menstrual cycle. This may be necessary to treat endometriosis, regulate irregular cycles (as in oligomenorrhea), to control heavy bleeding or excessive acne, or in cases of severe PMS/PMDD. For reasons I will explain below, BC is often used to treat PCOS as well. Finally, BC is often used by female athletes to regulate the timing of their cycle. Many women experience changes in performance across the menstrual cycle and it can be disastrous if an important competition falls during the part of a woman's cycle when her performance is decreased. By using BC, this can be avoided by either controlling or eliminating the changes in her physiology that would be occurring. While a potential benefit, there are also drawbacks to BC for athletes; this will be discussed in Volume 2.

Of all the hormonal modifiers I will discuss in this book, the discussion of BC is likely to be the most complicated along with being somewhat incomplete. The difficulty here is that there is no single type of BC. There are multiple general categories of BC but they may differ in the types of hormones present, how they are applied and the ultimate effects that they have on metabolism. New forms and combinations of BC are constantly being developed and there is simply little to no data on their specific effects in most cases. To try and keep the individual variance to a minimum, I will be dividing the different types of BC into distinct categories in terms of their general metabolic effects and will focus only on the issues that might be relevant in terms of diet and fat loss.

Types of BC

Since their introduction, all forms of BC have been based around synthetic versions of estrogen and progesterone. And regardless of how it is taken or used, in the most general sense, BC can be divided into combination BC (containing synthetic estrogen and progesterone) and progestin only BC (containing only synthetic progesterone). The synthetic estrogen ethinyl estradiol (EE) has been used almost exclusively in BC for decades. In early forms of the pill, doses were very high with 150 micrograms of EE. Newer forms of BC typically have 15-30 micrograms of EE on average with the reduction improving safety and reducing side effects (higher doses of EE are only used for emergency contraception). In contrast, there are at least 8 different types of progestins (synthetic progesterones) with newer types being developed.

While both EE and the progestins act very similarly to estrogen and progesterone in the body they are not identical to the hormones that a woman naturally produces. EE is significantly more potent than a woman's natural estrogen in many ways and can impact on a woman's physiology depending on how it is taken (i.e. orally vs. any other method). Progestins are even more complicated and differ in how well or poorly they bind to the progesterone, androgen, cortisol and mineralocorticoid receptor and this has an enormous impact on their overall effect in the body. The progestins are generally grouped into one of four generations based on when they were developed. They may also be distinguished by their chemical structure and what hormone they are synthesized from but the details of this are unimportant here. The development of newer types of progestins was driven by the desire to improve menstrual cycle control while reducing the side effects that were commonly seen with earlier progestins (5).

The first three generation progestins were all derived from testosterone due to the similarity in chemical structure and their effects were often very different from natural progesterone. For example, while natural progesterone is anti-androgenic, blocking the normal signal at the androgen receptor, testosterone derived progestins are androgenic, sending a positive signal. The androgenic effects of synthetic progestins the cause of many of the observed side effects such as oily skin, acne and body hair in addition to other effects described below. While sending an androgenic signal, synthetic progestins do not send the same anabolic (tissue/muscle building) signal and some forms of BC will impair gains in strength and muscle mass (this will be discussed in Volume 2). Within the context of this book, the progestins with the most androgenic effects tend to have the worst metabolic effects overall.

First generation progestins had significant androgenic effects although this was addressed by simply lowering the doses being used. Second generation progestins are the most androgenic and the third generation progestins have the least androgenic effects. A fourth generation progestin called drospirenone (found in products such as Yaz/Yasmine) is not derived from testosterone and shows effects nearly identical to a woman's normal progesterone including blocking any effect at the androgen receptor along with preventing water retention due to binding at the mineralocorticoid receptor. Like a woman's natural progesterone, drospirenone actually has anti-androgenic effects causing it to reduce body hair, acne and oily skin. There are also multiple new progestins, some of which are in use and some of which are still in development, that seem to act in broadly similar ways to drospirenone in terms of their overall effects (including the anti-androgenic effects).   Given the differences in how synthetic estrogen and progesterones work in a woman's body, there has been some recent interest in the use of bio-identical hormones instead. Some recent forms of BC such as Qlaira and Zoely contain a bio-identical form of 17-beta estradiol and I will touch on this when I talk about hormone replacement below. A new form of synthetic progestin called 19-nor-progesterone, which lacks most of the negatives of other progestins has recently been developed but it is not active orally.

Forms of BC

BC can come in many forms and this adds to the complexity of the situation as there are often subtle differences in the physiological effects that are seen. The original form of hormonal BC, still in use, is a pill taken daily. Most commonly the pill is taken for 21 days with a 7-day withdrawal period when an inert pill or nothing is taken. A woman's normal hormone levels will be suppressed during the 21-days of use with a rebound of estrogen during the washout period where light bleeding and other side effects may occur. At least two forms of the pill (Zoely and Yaz/Yasmine) use a 24 day on/4 day off schedule and 26 day on/2 day off pills also exist. The reduced withdrawal period limits the hormonal swings that would normally occur during the withdrawal period. In recent years, using BC for 3 months straight before a month off has become more common. There is also a progestin only mini-pill, taken daily.

For reasons related primarily to convenience and adherence, non pill based BC was developed. The patch is applied once per week for three weeks with a one week withdrawal period. The vaginal ring is placed within the vagina and provides a continuous release of hormone for 21 days and may be used with or without a withdrawal period (used without there is no bleeding). Depo-provera is a progestin only based shot given into the muscle or under the skin which provides constant birth control for three months. Nexplanon (an updated form of Implanon) is a small rod implant places in the arm which releases hormone for 3 years. Mirena, a hormonal intrauterine device (IUD), provides 3+ years of birth control.

Combination pill and patch forms of BC can come in what are termed monophasic, diphasic, triphasic and quadraphasic forms which refers to the pattern of hormone levels over the course of the month. For all practical purposes, all of these keep the dose of EE stable with only the level of the progestin changing on a weekly basis. Monophasic keep levels of both hormones stable through the cycle while diphasic increases progestin levels for the last 11 days of use. As diphasic BC seem to offer no benefit over monophasic it isn't used frequently. Triphasic raises levels of the progestin twice during the 21-day cycle in an attempt to more closely mimic the menstrual cycle while quadraphasic raises levels of the progestin four times (there is only one quadraphasic compound as of this book's writing and little is known about it).

Hopefully readers can begin to see why the topic of hormonal BC is so complex. There are multiple forms of BC taken on different schedules, some of which contain both EE and a progestin, some of which are progestin only with 8+ progestins in four different generations which may have different effects.   The combinations become almost endless although there are some combinations which aren't seen. Only the pill, patch and vaginal ring use a combination of synthetic estrogen and progesterone while the mini-pill, shot, implant and intrauterine methods are progestin only. Basically, all continuous forms of BC are progestin only while the intermittent use forms contain both both synthetic estrogen and a progestin.

The Physiological Effects of BC

With the above background, I want to look at the general physiological and hormonal effects of BC in terms of how it modifies or alter's a woman's physiology from what would be seen during the normal menstrual cycle. Some of the effects are common to all forms of BC while others can be attributed to either the EE component (which at least remains constant across different forms of BC for the most part) or the progestin component. As seen during the normal menstrual cycle, EE and the progestin interact and tend to have opposing effects with the side effects due to the EE component being offset/reduced by the progestin or vice versa. Progestin only BC lacks this interaction along with any EE based effects.

With one exception, the most general effect of hormonal BC a suppression of a woman's normal hormone levels and menstrual cycle to prevent pregnancy. Fundamentally, they do this by inhibiting the release of FSH and LH, the two hormones that underlie the development and release of the follicle, cyclical hormonal changes, etc. This causes a woman's natural estrogen and progesterone levels to drop although BC with a withdrawal week allow estrogen to rebound to roughly mid-follicular levels during that week. The decrease in LH and FSH also reduces a woman's testosterone levels which can have direct consequences for training. The exception to the above is the hormonal IUD which only has a local effect in the uterus and does not impact on LH/FSH or other hormones at all.

The EE component of BC has a number of specific metabolic effects. Due to being stronger than a woman's normal estrogen, EE impacts on how a woman's body handles sodium (recall from the previous chapter that the surge in estrogen at ovulation causes water retention for this reason) and may cause more water retention than a woman would otherwise experience. This will be especially true if her sodium intake is high. This effect can be offset by the progestin component although this depends on the specific type and its effect. Newer progestins tend to offset the EE the most, helping to eliminate water retention and the fourth generation progestins often cause water loss to occur.

Specific only to oral forms of birth control is that EE causes the liver to increase production of what are called binding proteins which bind hormones and make them inactive. The two of importance here are thyroid binding globulin (TBG), which bind to thyroid hormones, and sex hormone binding globulin (SHBG) which binds to hormones such as testosterone. Both are increased with oral EE although the increase in TBG doesn't seem to be that important as the body simply increases its production of thyroid hormones to compensate witht free (active) thyroid levels remaining normal.

However, this is not true for SHBG with BC lowering a woman's testosterone levels through several mechanisms. The first is that testosterone production in the ovaries is reduced due to the reduction in LH/FSH levels (adrenal androgen production is unaffected). The increase in SHBG also means that there will be less free (i.e. unbound) testosterone. The practical effect of this is that oral BC can reduce both total and free testosterone by up to 50% (6). This not only has implications for athletes but is probably part of the reduction in sex drive that occurs in some women on hormonal BC. Interestingly, oral BC containing bio-identical estrogen does not cause the same increase in SHBG or reduction in testosterone (6a). While progestin only BC does not increase SHBG, testosterone levels still drop to a similar degree due to the changes in LH/FSH and reduction in testosterone production in the ovaries.

I mentioned above that BC is often used to treat PCOS (primarily the hyperandrogenic type) and it is this 50% reduction in testosterone that makes it effective. BC containing one of the newer progestins which have anti-androgenic qualities (such as drospirenone) have an even greater impact here as the anti-androgenic effects further reduce some of the effects of PCOS such as body hair, acne, oily skin and others. While this is a benefit to women suffering from PCOS related effects, and may not matter to many women either way, this is of potentially huge concern for female athletes. Even a woman's relatively low testosterone levels are important to her ability to gain muscle, strength or improve performance and a 50% decrease will impact on that ability enormously. Again, this will be discussed in detail in Volume 2.

Looking next at the progestins, an early observation was that some degree of insulin resistance along with increases in blood glucose often occurred which raised questions about long-term health effects. This is primarily seen with the first and second generation progestins while the third and fourth seem to lack this effect, at least in women who don't have insulin resistance in the first place (7). I would expect newer progestins to have no effect here. Practically this means that women using BC containing a first or second generation progestin will be in a progesterone-like state with an effectively luteal phase physiology. If a one-week withdrawal phase is present, that week will be an estrogen-like/effectively follicular phase physiology. Any woman on BC with a third or fourth generation progestin, whether continuous or not will be in an estrogen-like hormonal state with an effectively follicular phase physiology.

BC and Weight/Fat Gain

Perhaps one of the largest concerns regarding birth control is its potential impact on body weight, body fat or body composition (the relative proportions of fat and muscle, discussed later in the book). There is a pervasive idea that BC causes weight gain and even a brief online search will find women reporting significant weight gain while using BC. Weight gain is also one of the most commonly given reasons for the discontinuation of BC. With a few caveats, research has not generally supported this idea with a 2014 review of all papers available at the time finding at most a small effect of combined BC on body weight although the effect depends on the specific type of BC being discussed (8). Monophasic oral BC may cause a 3-4 lb water weight gain while triphasic BC has been found to cause a small increase in body fat after three months of use, probably due to the high-dose progestin during the third week. In contrast, a recent study found that a new form of combined BC (using one of the newer anti-androgenic progestins) caused a slight fat loss after 6 months of continued use (9).

The same general pattern has been found to occur for progestin only BC with an average weight gain of 3-4 pounds over 12 months typically occurring (10). The primary exception to this is Depo-Provera, a long-acting high-dose first generation progestin shot that is fairly notorious for causing weight gain and making weight loss very difficult. In one study an average weight gain of 11 pounds with a fat gain of 9 pounds over 3 years was seen; the shot also doubled the risk of becoming obese (11). This is actually somewhat surprising as Depo-Provera has been shown to increase metabolic rate, especially if it is started during the luteal phase of the cycle (12). This suggests that any impact on weight is due to increased food intake and Depo has been shown to increase women's attention to highly tasty foods which might cause her to eat more (12a). I'd note that other forms of BC have no generally been found to increase appetite unless a high-dose and/or high-potency progestin is present. The progestin component of BC raises metabolic rate similar to what is seen during the luteal phase although the effect is only 60 calories per day (12b).

I should note that changes in body weight alone are not all that is relevant and changes in body composition are far more important overall. Body weight can remain unchanged but if fat is gained and lean body mass (i.e. muscle) is lost, appearance, health and body composition can worsen. And while most studies only look at body weight, some have examined body composition and found that BC may cause a preferential gain in fat and loss of lean mass. In the Depo-Provera study cited above, a group of women using a combined BC (with a third generation progestin) gained about half as much weight as the Depo group but they also gained fat while losing lean body mass.

Another study compared a progestin only intrauterine implant (Mirena) with a copper IUD over 12 months of use (12c). The progestin group gained nearly 6 pounds while increasing body fat and losing lean body mass while the copper IUD group gained just over 3 pounds while losing a small amount of fat and gaining an equally small amount of lean body mass. While the weight gain in the hormonal BC was not enormously higher, the overall impact on body composition was. Other studies have found no difference in the body composition changes over time between hormonal and non-hormonal BC users and this may depend on the specific BC being used (12d).

With the exception of Depo-Provera, there seems to be a disconnect between the public perception (or anecdotal reports) and research into the effect of BC on weight gain and I want to look at a few reasons why this might be the case. A very real possibility is that women differ in their propensity to gain weight in response to the use of hormonal BC. Some clinicians report that one in four women are more prone to weight or fat gain with BC. Women tend to report different physical, emotional and other side effects from different types of BC and it would seem reasonable to assume that the metabolic effects could also differ. There is some indication that women already carrying more body fat are more likely to gain fat from BC so there may be an interaction here with either the pre-existing physiology or lifestyle factors such as diet or activity. While beyond the scope of this book, black women are more prone to weight gain with BC.

In this vein, I want to point out that while studies may only find a relatively small weight gain overall, this is an average of all women in the study. Averages may mask individual changes but some studies have looked not not only at average weight gain but at individual gains and losses. In one study women, using triphasic BC for 4 months had zero average weight gain but this ranged from a 32 pound loss to a 15 pound gain (12e). In another, women using one of three types of progestin only BC (Mirena, Implanon or Depo Provera) or a non-hormonal copper IUD were followed for 12 months (12f). While the average body weight change in the groups was fairly small (ranging from no increase for the copper IUD to an increase of 2-5 pounds in the other groups), the individual variability was huge. The minimum and maximum changes in body weight ranged from a loss of 36 lbs (16.3 kg) to a gain of an incredible 72 lbs (32 kg) in the Implanon group for example. Similar results were seen for Mirena (-35 lbs/16 kg to + 42 lbs/19kg), and Depo Provera (-16 lbs/7.7 kg to + 48 lbs 21.7 kg). And while this suggests that any given BC might be relatively worse or better for any given woman, the copper IUD group had changes in body weight ranging from a loss of 36 lbs (16.3 kg) to a gain of 36 gain lbs (16.3 kg). This suggests that other factors such as age or lifestyle are responsible more than the form of BC itself.

Clearly overall lifestyle factors such as diet and activity are key here but one worth serious consideration is simply time and the normal aging process. Generally with age there is a gain in body weight and some studies find that the weight gain that occurs with hormonal BC is about the same as what is seen in women using non-hormonal BC or nothing at all. Due to the fact that earlier forms of BC which used high dose estrogens and progestins did generally cause weight gain, this is now part of the lore of BC and it's been suggested that the weight gain from BC is due primarily to expectation and belief (12g). That is, hormonal BC may be getting blamed for what is primarily nothing more than age or lifestyle related weight gain. I say primarily as the difference in body composition change that have been found to occur can't be ignored. Obviously hormonal BC has profound hormonal effects in a woman's body and hunger, appetite, body weight and body composition can all be affected. Even in the absence of true or even significant weight gain a worsening of body composition is never good and I'll only conclude by saying that, on average, the overall effect of most forms of BC on body weight appears to be mild at best.

Birth Control and Fat Loss

Related to the above issue is whether or not the use of hormonal BC will impair fat loss while dieting. Certainly there have been anecdotal reports of this with Depo-Provera being one of the worst offenders but other women report that hormonal BC has little to no effect on their ability to lose fat and weight so long as their diet and activity are well controlled. There is shockingly little research into this topic although a paper I will discuss later in the book found that female physique competitors were able to reach the lower limits of female body fat despite the majority of them using BC. A recent study found that BC did not limit women's abilities to lose weight after pregnancy (13). Just as with weight gain, it may also be that BC impacts women differently in terms of their ability to lose weight.

Birth Control and Bone Health

Since it is so critical to women's long-term health (especially with age), I want to briefly discuss the impact of BC on bone mineral density or BMD. Although it interacts enormously with other hormones, dietary factors and activity, estrogen is a key player in bone health (both amenorrhea and menopause is associated with a reduction in estrogen with bone loss being a common consequence). This raises the question of whether or not synthetic EE has the same effects as estrogen in terms of bone health.

Looking first at healthy young (pre-menopausal women), the data is mixed with most studies showing no major effect and a small number showing a positive effect. Of some concern, 7 studies showing that BC might negatively impact on BMD (13a). While the mechanism by which this might occur is unknown, it is potentially problematic. Several studies found that BC might also prevent exercise from having it's normal benefit on BMD although this may be due to inadequate calcium, other hormonal effects or negative effects of the synthetic progestin. BC has not been shown to have any benefit on BMD in women suffering from anorexia and the data on it's effects in women with menstrual cycle dysfunction is mixed with some studies showing a benefit and some not. Related to this, the use of BC may increase fracture risk slightly with Depo-Provera having the largest negative impact (13b).

Summarizing BC

I said above that this section would likely be the most complicated of all of the hormonal modifiers and I imagine readers now see why. Differences in hormones, dosing, potencies (primarily of the progestins), methods and types of application make the potential number of combinations of BC immense. Not all combinations are seen in practice but most of what is available have no data available on them yet. At best it's clear that early forms of progestins (typically with higher androgenic effects) have distinctly different effects than the newer forms. I have used those differences to draw conclusions about the effective hormonal situation a given BC will generate below.

First and second generation progestins are known to cause most of the metabolic effects that have been noted and the one I'm focusing on here is the change in insulin sensitivity and resistance. Their tendency to cause insulin resistance will cause progesterone-like hormonal status and a luteal phase physiology (where progesterone induces insulin resistance). Third and fourth generation progestins do not impair insulin resistance and generate an estrogen-like hormonal status and effective follicular-phase physiology. I would expect any newer progestins that are developed to be identical to the third and fourth generation progestins.

This is true whether the progestin is found in a combination form of BC or as a progestin only and even this is complicated by the fact that any form of BC with a withdrawal period will have the fourth week as an effectively follicular/estrogen dominant phase regardless of what progestin is present. I've attempted to summarize this in the chart below, listing the typical first through fourth generation progestins that are currently in common use.

Generation	Progestin	Androgenic Effects	Hormonal State	Effective Phase
First	Norethindrone*, etnyodiol diacetate, medroxyprogesterone*	Medium	Progesterone	Luteal
Second	Levonorgestrel, norgestrel	High	Progesterone	Luteal
Third	Desogestrel*, norgestimate, gestodene	Low	Estrogen	Follicular
Fourth	Drospirenone	Anti-androgenic	Estrogen	Follicular

All of the above types progestins are found in varying amounts in combination BC while the forms with an * after them are found in progestin only BC. Norethindrone is found in the mini-pill, medroxyprogesterone is found in the Depo-Provera shot and etonogestrel (the active form of desogestrel) is found in the Nexplanon implant.

Obesity

The next hormonal modifier I want to address is obesity, focusing here on the negative hormonal changes that occur as body fat levels increase. It's important to realize that, in some cases, the presence of the hormonal modifier may be causing a woman's predisposition to obesity. PCOS is a common one and it's overall effects on a woman's physiology, especially combined with the modern diet and lifestyle, put woman at risk for fat gain to begin with and this becomes a vicious cycle where PCOS causes insulin resistance which causes the PCOS to worsen, worsening the insulin resistance, etc. But even when PCOS or another hormonal modifier is not present, as women begin to gain excessive amounts of fat, there are a variety of hormonal changes that start to occur and much of this is due to the development of insulin resistance. Both progesterone and estrogen levels may go up and the production of androgens may increase as well creating a state of elevated testosterone/androgen levels, causing a PCOS-like state.

Obesity, like PCOS, is also associated with infertility and other pregnancy related problems. Ovulation may be impaired, the risk of miscarriage is increased and this is all fundamentally related to the hormonal changes that occur, and primarily the insulin resistance that tends to develop. For women wanting to become pregnant, this presents a problem but, as with PCOS, the loss of even moderate amounts of weight/fat drastically improves the situation. There are also supplements which can help to both improve the health issues along with fertility itself and I will discuss these in Chapter 24.

Overall, increasing levels of body fat create an androgen-like physiology and the insulin resistance that will usually be present will create an effective luteal phase physiology. As with other forms of hyperandrogenism, female athletes in certain types of sports, this effect might actually be seen as a benefit although the health risks need to be managed. For women wanting to improve health or fertility, these effects are clearly a negative. But for all practical purposes, I will treat women with a certain level of body fat as being hyperandrogenic for all practical purposes since the resulting physiology is the same.

Age Related Changes in Women's Physiology

In addition to the above modifiers, which can occur at any age in women, there are also a number of age-related changes that occur in a woman's physiology over her lifespan. Here I am only focusing on those changes that occur later in life such as peri-menopause and menopause itself. At peri-menopause, a woman's reproductive function begins to decrease, a process referred to as the climacteric. Effectively, a woman runs out of potential follicles/eggs to fertilize and this signals the reproductive system to shut down at which point her estrogen and progesterone production is nearly eliminated. This is yet another place where women and men differ significantly. As I discussed earlier in this book, with increasing age a man's testosterone levels are reduced (which some are calling andropause to liken it to menopause) but at no point does it drop to zero. In contrast, at menopause, a woman's reproductive hormone production essentially stops.

Regardless, the menopausal transition that a woman undergoes has a profound impact on her overall physiology although this is another area of some complexity as there are four different situations that have to be considered. These include peri-menopause, the time before true menopause occurs which has both an early and late phase along with menopause itself. After menopause, women who go on Hormone Replacement Therapy (HRT) show a different physiology than those women who do not. I should mention that in addition to the profound changes that are occurring in a woman's hormones at this time, there are other changes that are simply age-related that also contribute to the changes in physiology.

Peri-Menopause

Peri-menopause literally means near menopause and refers to the changes that occur as a woman begins the transition into menopause itself. While peri-menopause is typically thought to occur in the 50's, it is possible for some women to enter peri-menopause in their 40's or even 30's. The entire peri-menopausal period can last anywhere from 12 months up to four years and is divided into an early- and late-phase depending on the specific hormonal profile which is seen. Unfortunately, only blood work to determine the actual levels of estrogen and progesterone can pinpoint exactly where a woman is at this time. During peri-menopause, cycles may become infrequent or change in length and some cycles will be anovulatory with no egg being released.

If there is a perceived "benefit" to peri-menopause it's that falling estrogen may decreases PMS symptoms (15). At the same time, other symptoms, similar to what is seen postmenopausally often appear. Hot flashes, sleep problems, mood changes, a decline in sexual interest and function and a loss of bone density may all occur (full lists of symptoms can be found online). The occurrence of these symptoms, especially the easily observable ones, can actually act as an indicator that peri-menopause has started; blood work would support or confirm this. There are supplements, discussed in Chapter 24 that may help with some of the side effects and I will discuss hormone replacement therapy below.

In early peri-menopause estrogen levels can start to shift up and down but there is typically a decrease in progesterone without much change in estrogen levels. For that reason, I will consider early peri-menopause to be an estrogen-like situation, creating an effectively follicular-phase physiology. In late perimenopause, estrogen starts to drop along with the drop in progesterone and this will create a state of relative hyperandrogenism. Androgen levels are not elevated above normal but their effects become relatively dominant unless hormone replacement is begun.

Late peri-menopause is often accompanied by the beginnings of a change in body weight, body fat and fat distribution and this is due to the drop in estrogen levels. Muscle loss often accelerates and with this metabolic rate can begin to slow down. Fat gain may start to occur with a shift in body fat from the lower body to around the midsection and this is typically accompanied by the development of insulin resistance. For this reason I will consider the late peri-menopausal woman to to have a hyperandrogenic/progesterone-like hormonal state with an effective luteal phase physiology. This will be altered if Hormone Replacement Therapy (HRT) is begun.

Menopause

Once a woman has not had a menstrual cycle for 12 months after entering peri-menopause, she is considered to have entered menopause and to be postmenopausal Here, the same side effects that may have started in peri-menopause can be come more pronounced . This includes hot flashes, mood swings, depression, vaginal dryness, cloudy thinking and many others. Her reproductive system has effectively shut off completely and her hormone production drops significantly. Her estrogen levels will continue to drop from the peri-menopausal level and can be as low as 95% below her pre-menopausal levels (16). Her progesterone levels will already have dropped since there are no longer follicles being released or implanting with no development of the corpus luteum.

After menopause, testosterone levels may be slightly higher than average and this can happen for a few reasons. Some women will have had PCOS to begin with but there can be reasons such as testosterone secreting tumors which are present. Even without those medical conditions being present, postmenopausal women often see a slight increase in testosterone levels after menopause before levels fall gradually over the next five years. The consequence of the above is that the immediate postmenopausal women will develop the same type of hyperandrogenic state I described previously (17, 18). This will put the postmenopausal woman in an effectively luteal-phase physiology.

This includes the development of insulin resistance along with a shift from the typical female lower body fat pattern to a more male-like central body fat pattern. Along with this comes an increase in heart disease risk. In addition to this shift in body fat patterning, there is often an increase in body weight and total body fat levels as well with a reduction in energy expenditure and metabolic rate (19). The lack of estrogen also causes an accelerated rate of bone loss increasing a woman's risk of developing osteopenia or osteoporosis. A majority of these effects are reversed by the use of hormone replacement therapy (HRT) which I will discuss below. Once again, all of this is occurring along with or in addition to the many age-related changes that are occurring.

Hysterectomy

Before finishing up the chapter with a brief discussion of HRT, I want to address one other potentially major hormonal modifier that women might encounter (outside of the myriad medical conditions) and that is a hysterectomy. Usually done for medical reasons, a hysterectomy refers to a surgery where part or all of a woman's reproductive organs are removed. In a full hysterectomy, the ovaries, uterus and cervix are all removed and this brings on a state identical to menopause described above (it may be referred to as surgical menopause). But there is also a partial hysterectomy where only the uterus is removed, leaving the cervix and ovaries intact. This decreases levels of both estrogen and progesterone which necessitates estrogen-only Hormone Replacement Therapy (HRT). While often thought to occur later in life, hysterectomies may be required at any time during a woman's reproductive life.

Hormone Replacement Therapy (HRT)

As women approach and enter the menopausal transition, the issue of whether or not to begin hormone replacement therapy (HRT) arises. Like hormonal BC, HRT has typically contained a synthetic form of estrogen, typically conjugated equine estrogen (CEE), along with the same progestin found in the Depo-Provera shot. The goal here is to reduce or eliminate the many negative effects that often occur at menopause due to the reduction/near elimination of a woman's estrogen and progesterone production. There is also some interest in androgen replacement for postmenopausal women, discussed below.

The topic of HRT is one filled with some controversy and I want to look at some of the arguments both in favor of and against the use of HRT after menopause. In favor or HRT is the fact that it can reverse or at least attenuate many of the negative effects that occur at menopause in terms of body weight, body fat, increased heart disease risk, etc. I'd note that this is only true if HRT is started fairly early after menopause occurs (20). Just as with BC, HRT does not appear to cause any weight gain outside of what typically occurs with age (20a). At the same time, there is a long-standing concern with the potential of HRT to increase the risk of breast cancer.

Much of this concern comes from one of the earliest study on long-term HRT use, the Women's Health Initiative (WHI) study which was actually terminated due to an increase in breast cancer risk among the study subjects. These results caused a drastic decrease in the use of HRT which has been accompanied by decreased incidence of breast cancer (21). However, re-analysis of the WHI and other studies suggest that the benefits outweigh the risks so long as HRT is begun shortly after menopause occurs with the health risks only increasing substantially in women over 60-70 years of age (22-24).

Without meaning to trivialize breast cancer in any way, there is the fact that heart disease is a far more common cause of death after menopause than breast cancer. Since I have no intention of giving recommendations as to whether any woman should or should not use HRT, I only mention this as it may impact on the choice of any individual woman's choice of whether or not to use HRT. A woman with a familial history or genetic risk (i.e. BRCA mutation) for breast cancer might make a very different choice regarding HRT than one without that risk or with a family history of heart disease, for example. With time, there may be the potential to identify who is or is not not a good candidate for HRT based on this and other factors (25). As with the newer forms of BC that include low- or ultra-low dose estrogens and different types of progestins, newer forms of HRT are in development and these seem to show similar benefits to the older forms with fewer side-effects (26,27).

I'd note that, in addition to estrogen and progesterone based HRT, there is interest in the use of low-dose androgen replacement postmenopausally. This has typically been used to improve sexual function but may provide other benefits (28,29). Of some interest is that androgens can be converted to estrogen within specific tissues such as fat cells and skeletal muscle via an enzyme called aromatase. As aromatase is not present in breast tissue, by providing androgens replacement, a woman's body could make estrogen where it is needed without raising levels in the bloodstream or in breast tissue, avoiding any increased risk of breast cancer. Like BC, HRT can come in a number of forms including pills, patches, nasal spray, skin gels, vaginal cream and a vaginal ring and each can have slightly different effects that I can't realistically describe (30,31). Overall, most forms of HRT seem to improve or at least maintain insulin sensitivity and practically I will consider postmenopausal women on HRT to be in an estrogen-like hormonal state with an effective follicular-phase physiology (32,33).

Following hysterectomy, HRT seems to be universally given, probably due to the fact that it can occur earlier in life. While there is some interest in the use of androgens or progesterone following a hysterectomy, only estrogen replacement is considered required (34). In this case, the female on estrogen only HRT following a partial hysterectomy will be considered to be in a permanent estrogen-like state with a follicular-phase physiology.

Bio-identical Hormones

Although I won't go into detail on the topic, I want to briefly address the topic of bio-identical hormones. For most of the time they have been in use, the traditional forms of estrogen and progesterone in both BC and HRT have been synthetically derived chemicals that don't always act in exactly the same way as a woman's normal hormones. And in some cases, it's fairly clear that the synthetic forms have distinctly different effects than the natural hormones have. Fairly recently, there has been some interest in the use of bio-identical hormones. While this term lacks specific definition at this point, it basically refers to chemical compounds that are structurally identical to a woman's own hormones. These includes 17-beta estradiol (which I mentioned is found in some new forms of BC) estriol, estrone and a micronized progesterone all of which are chemically identical to the hormones a woman's body naturally produces.

While many claims have been made for the superiority of bio-identical hormones, the science on the topic is not so clear and is only now developing. At worst, bio-identical hormones appear to be no worse than the synthetic forms and limited research suggest that they may minimize some of the risks and negatives that have been associated with the synthetic forms of the hormones (35-38). The ideal combination of bio-identical hormones is also unknown although it has recently been suggested that the combination of transdermal estradiol combined with micronized progesterone may be optimal although this requires further research (39). Specifically related to BC, a small amounts of research suggests those containing the bio-identical forms of estrogen may provide twice the contraceptive effectiveness with half of the potential negatives (40).

Summarizing Hormonal Modifiers

I covered a lot of different information in this chapter in terms of the major hormonal modifiers that women might encounter, how they might change her physiology relative to the normal menstrual cycle and touched on what overall hormonal situation it might put her in. I want to summarize that information below, looking at each of the different modifiers and what effective hormonal state it will put her in. I'll also indicate which of the two normal menstrual cycle phases, follicular or luteal, a given situation effectively puts a woman in in terms of overall physiology. To a great degree, my focus here is on the degree of insulin sensitivity or resistance as this impacts all aspects of nutrient utilization and what diet may or may not be ideal.

The chart below will appear again later in this book since it's relevant to both diet set up and the actual diet and training templates so don't worry about memorizing it.

Hormonal Status	Hormonal State	Effective Phase	Insulin Sensitivity
PCOS/Hyperandrogenism Lean and/or active	Testosterone	Follicular	Improved/Normal
PCOS/Hyperandrogenism Obese and or/inactive	Testosterone	Luteal	Lowered
Birth Control (1st,2nd gen.)* Progestin only BC	Progesterone	Luteal	Lowered
Birth Control (3rd,4th gen.)*	Estrogen	Follicular	Unaffected/Good
Amenorrhea	None	N/A	Increased
Obesity	Testosterone	Luteal	Lowered
Early Peri-Menopause	Estrogen	Follicular	Decreasing
Late Peri-Menopause	Testosterone	Luteal	Lowered
Menopause (no HRT)	Testosterone	Luteal	Lowered
Menopause (HRT)	Estrogen	Follicular	Unaffected/Good
Partial Hysterectomy w/HRT	Estrogen	Follicular	Unaffected/Good

*Birth control with a withdrawal period show a rebound week
where estrogen increases, creating a single follicular phase week.

With the normal menstrual cycle and various hormonal modifiers having been discussed, I want to present some background information that will be important for many later chapters of this book.

Chapter 4: Types of Exercise and Goals

Although I don't expect all readers of this book to be on an exercise program (and exercise will be discussed in far more detail in Volume 2), I want to define some terms and concepts first as they will be used many later chapters and I want to make sure everyone understand the terminology I'll be using. First I want to look at the general categories of exercise that are most commonly seen or used. In addition, I want to categorize some of the major different training or diet goals that readers might be pursuing. This interacts with the different types of training since different combinations of exercise may (or may not) be used depending on those goals.

Types of Exercise

Although they can overlap to a slight degree and are frequently combined, I want to first look at the primary different types of exercise that might be done. For each I'll look at what they are, their goals or the types of adaptations that they generate along with any other issues that are specific to women, especially the issue of bone mineral density (BMD).

Stretching

Stretching refers generally to any type of activity done that is meant to improve flexibility. There are multiple types of stretching that can be done including static stretching (simply holding the muscle at an increased length), dynamic stretching (movements that gradually take body parts through increasing ranges of motion) or something called PNF stretching (a type of stretching that alternates contracting and relaxing a muscle). Typically stretching is done as part of a workout (generally before and/or after) but there are pure stretching classes that can be found. Yoga classes often have a focus on flexibility but it's not unheard of for gyms to offer pure stretching classes. Athletes whose sport requires extreme amounts of flexibility such as gymnastics often perform additional stretching outside of their normal training.

A huge number of benefits has been attributed to stretching such as injury prevention, decreased muscle soreness and others but for the most part none of these are true (1,2). Being flexible in and of itself doesn't prevent injuries; quite in fact both too little and too much flexibility can increase the risk of injury. In general, women are already more flexible than men which is probably why they tend to enjoy stretching (men often dislike stretching since they aren't very good at it). Arguably Yoga classes are taken more by women than men as well. But outside of the sports that require it, excessive flexibility might actually increase their injury risk as it can destabilize their joints (women's injury risks are discussed in Volume 2).

This isn't to say that stretching has no place in women's training. Light stretching as part of a warm-up may be useful (although is often unneeded by women) or as a cool-down. Yoga can be good for relaxation and light stretching before bed often help with sleeps. With age there is often a loss of flexibility which means that peri- and postmenopausal women are more likely to need stretching as part of their overall exercise program (3). Since it is low intensity, stretching can be done as frequently as desired. Simply keep in mind that more flexibility is not automatically better. Stretching has no impact on BMD.

Aerobic, Cardiovascular or Aerobic Training

Aerobic, cardiovascular or endurance training refers to any type of exercise involving the larger muscle of the body in a continuous and rhythmic (usually repetitive fashion) that lasts a minimum of 20 minutes (some athletes may perform aerobic work for multiple hours). This includes such activities as walking, running, cycling, swimming, rowing, cross country skiing along with exercise machines such as Ellipticals, stairclimbers, rowing machines and group aerobics classes. Certain types of weight training (discussed below) can have an aerobic-like effect.

The adaptations to aerobic training include strengthening the heart and lungs, improving endurance, and increasing the levels of enzymes that help burn fat in skeletal muscle. For endurance athletes, there is an increase in blood volume and overall oxygen carrying capacity. Aerobic work also improves the body's ability to buffer acid which is a cause of fatigue during high intensity activities. When high-intensity exercise such as intervals or sprints are being done, a higher level of aerobic fitness improves recovery. Except in complete beginners, aerobic exercise isn't good for building muscle and generally doesn't have an enormous impact on improving BMD. Some forms of aerobic activity can actually harm BMD.

Aerobic exercise can be subdivided into different intensities typically based on heart rate (I will provide a better method in Chapter 28). Low-intensity aerobic exercise refers to anything done at a heart rate of roughly 130 or lower, medium intensity aerobic exercise at a heart rate of 130-150 or so and high-intensity aerobic exercise between 160-180 heart rate (or up to maximum). As the intensity of workouts increase, the length of aerobic workouts must come down. Low intensity exercise can be done almost indefinitely while high-intensity aerobic work might be limited to no more than an hour. It is always possible to perform shorter workouts at a lower intensity. Runners or cyclists often do easy recovery workouts for 30-60 minutes at low intensities.

It's safe to say that aerobic exercise has been the singularly most common recommended form of exercise for health, fitness and fat loss for decades. While it has its place, women tend to not only gravitate to aerobic exercise but often do far too much, frequently with poor results. Certainly aerobic exercise burns calories and some amount of fat but the effect tends to be fairly small for realistic amounts of exercise. Excessive amounts, especially if done without a progressive build up can cause a number of negative effects in women. This is discussed in Chapter 12 and 13.

High-Intensity Interval Training (HIIT)

Somewhat related to aerobic training is high-intensity interval training (HIIT) or simply interval training. Unlike aerobic exercise which can be continued for extended periods, interval training is done at such a high intensity that only a short period of time can be sustained at once. The high-intensity or "interval" portions are alternated with short periods at a lower intensity for recovery. This might mean alternating 30-60 seconds of near maximal intensity work alternated with 30-60 seconds (or longer) at a much lower intensity and this alternation might be done 5-10 total times. The duration of the intervals can vary from as short as 15-20 seconds up to five minutes for some endurance athletes. I'd note that women do tend to show less fatigue and faster recovery during HIIT than men, meaning that they may be able to do more total intervals and use a shorter rest-period during their workouts.

The adaptations to interval training span a fairly large range depending on the exact type of workout that is done, primarily depending on the duration of the intervals themselves. This can include improvements in something called VO2 max, the ability to tolerate high levels of acid within the muscle (this causes a burning sensation) and many others. For reasons I will discuss later in this book, HIIT may be especially beneficial for women to improve their fat loss.

Traditionally interval training was used predominantly by performance athletes but in recent years. there has been much interest in interval training for improving general health and fat loss as well (4). This is primarily due to the time efficiency of interval training which, under some conditions, may be shorter than a traditional aerobic workout while generating similar benefit. As I'll discuss more in Chapter 28, this has to be weighed against the intensity and discomfort of HIIT along with its potential to add too much stress to a woman's workout routine. Like high-intensity aerobic training, excessive amounts of HIIT (and studies typically use 2-3 sessions per week at an absolute maximum) can over-stress the body. While HIIT has it's place, it must be used in moderation.

Sprint Training

In a way, sprint training is sort of a sub-category of HIIT. Many actually use the terms interchangeably although this isn't really correct. A true sprint refers to activities lasting ~10 seconds or less and is usually done at 100% effort. Due to the short duration and intensity involved, much longer rest intervals are also taken with sprint training compared to HIIT. For example, a track sprinter might run 30-60 meters all out and then take 3-6 minutes rest and sprint training workouts tend to be very long with most of the time spent standing around. This makes sprint training very non-time efficient compared to HIIT or traditional aerobic work.

The primary goal of true sprint training is to improve maximum or top-end speed and it is used by all types of athletes for this goal. Athletes who are involved in sprinting events such as the 100m in track and field or the match sprint in track cycling do a tremendous amount of this type of work but in almost all sports, having a higher top-speed tends to be beneficial as it generally allows faster speeds at any longer distance. It's simply the amount of total sprint training that is done in any given sport that varies.

Due to the high-skill nature (and relative time inefficiency) of sprint training, along with the injury risk for certain types of activities (especially running), I don't think true sprint training should be used by anyone but highly trained athletes. The risk is too high and the benefits too small for most. If anything other than aerobic training is done, it should be HIIT and I will provide recommendations later in this book.

Jump/Reactive Training

Since it tends to be strongly associated with sprint sports, I want to mention jump or reactive training (sometimes called plyometric training). I imagine most readers know what jumping entails and reactive training is simply a specific type of jumping where someone will jump, land, and then jump again as quickly as possible (jumping rope is one example). Jump training improves the body's ability to generate muscular power and for sports that require the athlete to react quickly, this improves that ability. There are endless numbers of drills that are available ranging from simple, low-intensity exercises such as jumping rope to intermediate exercises (such as bounding) to very high-intensity activities (such as depth jumps). Typically the total amount of jumps that is done and the amount of rest taken goes up with increasing intensity. Skipping rope can be done for extended periods while no more than 5 maximal depth jumps might be done with several minutes rest between each.

For most of the time they have been around, jump training has been used exclusively by performance athletes. Lately there is some interest in plyometric type training in the general public. There are plyometric classes in some gyms where a variety of plyometric activities are done, usually with insufficient rest to do them properly, and these are potentially dangerous. Jumping while fatigued puts trainees at risk of jumping or landing poorly which can put women specifically at risk for injury. For reasons that are somewhat unclear, many physique competitors have started to utilize jump training either in their training or during their dieting period. Outside of the potential to improve BMD, I see little point to this. Not only is it ineffective but it is potentially very dangerous.

The issue here is incredibly female specific and one that I will go into great detail on in Volume 2 but women are roughly 3-9 times more likely than men to tear their Anterior Cruciate Ligament (ACL), which acts to stabilize the knee. Not only are women far more likely to sustain this type of injury, it tends to occur in a distinctly different way than in male athletes. In contrast to men, who typically sustain ACL injuries during collision or combat sports, women tend to have it occur when they jump, land or cut from side to side. There are a number of reasons for this some of which are related to biomechanical differences. A woman's wider hips, differences in the speed and pattern with which her muscles fire and the impact of estrogen and progesterone on tendon and ligament strength along with others all play a role (coordination can also change during the menstrual cycle with injury potentially changing in different weeks). But this interacts enormously with the social fact that women have traditionally been less likely to do sports at a young age. They tend to have lower levels of fitness overall and a general lack of training background.

Women's knees will often break in during jumping or landing (you see the same type of thing during certain weight training movements such as squats and leg presses, discussed next) and this throws enormous stresses onto the joint and ligaments. If this type of knee movement occurs beyond a certain point during jumping, landing or cutting to the side, it can cause an ACL tear to occur. In recent years, specific programs aimed at improving jumping mechanics and muscle firing have been developed; that along with proper basic fitness training is showing benefit for reducing knee injuries (5). Group plyometric classes or programs being given to dieters are unlikely to provide this type of basic training, putting women at risk for injury. I will note, and discuss further below, that jumping has a large impact on improving BMD. It simply must be done correctly and safely.

Resistance/Weight Training

The next type of exercise I want to discuss is resistance or weight training (aka lifting weights) and I will use those terms interchangeably. While weight training can technically be considered a type of interval training, in that it alternates short periods of high-intensity exercise with some rest, it's best to consider it separately as it not done using the traditional types of aerobic exercise modes. For years, resistance training was more or less ignored in terms of its potential to improve health and fitness but it's now become recognized that proper weight training should be part and parcel of literally all exercise programs due to the benefits it offers.

At its simplest, weight training is any activity that requires the muscles of the body to work against a high resistance and this is typically done for fairly short periods of time (anywhere from 1 second to perhaps 60 seconds at the maximum). In a typical set, the resistance (which can come free weights to machines to rubber tubing, etc) is lifted and then lowered some number of times (I will use a range of 1-20 repetitions for the most part) before resting for some duration and then performing the next series of repetitions or exercise.

Weight training has a primary goal of improving muscular strength and size. Increased muscular strength tends to make activities of daily living easier and even small increases in muscle size tend to improve appearance and body shape. Resistance training not only helps to limit lean body mass (LBM) during a diet but may actually increase it under certain conditions. For reasons I will discuss in Chapter 14, weight training can also improve women's fat loss. In recent years, there has also been the realization that age related muscle loss (termed sarcopenia) can be disastrous. Proper weight training coupled with proper diet can prevent this so resistance training is, in some ways, that much more important for the peri- or postmenopausal women.

Despite the enormous benefits of weight training for women, there is often a resistance to it. Either women refuse to lift weights at all or, when they do, they only use very light weights which never really challenge them. The major fear comes from the idea that women will become muscularly bulky by doing so, a misconception created by pictures of steroid using bodybuilders in some forms of media. But the reality is that women's normally low levels of testosterone prevent this from occurring. In most studies of beginner women, a total muscle gain of 3-4 pounds over 6 or more months is common. Putting it another way, men (with their higher testosterone levels) are trying their hardest in the weight room to get as big as possible and most are failing. It simply doesn't happen to women without the use of drugs.

Some women do report feeling bulky in the first few weeks of a proper resistance training but this is due to increased water and carbohydrate being stored within the muscle and this effect goes away after several weeks. A potential exception to this are women with elevated testosterone levels as seen with PCOS or subclinical hyperandrogenism. At least relatively speaking these women have a greater potential to gain muscle size and strength (which is why they are commonly found in certain sports that require those) but even there, muscle growth is always a slow process.

In addition to the other listed effects, one of the major benefits of proper resistance training is its positive effects on BMD. By proper here I mean using challenging/heavy enough weights on exercises that stress the bones of the body sufficiently. Either by itself or in combination with jumping, weight training can help premenopausal women to achieve peak bone density earlier in life. Weight training has even been found to limit bone loss or even increase bone density in postmenopausal women (5). Proper nutrition and nutrient intake, discussed in Chapter 20, is critical to maximizing this effect.

Weight training can be divided somewhat into different types of training. This will be discussed in great detail in Volume 2 but I will look at the topic somewhat in Chapter 28. I will only finish by addressing the concept of toning up; this usually refers to using high repetitions and short rest intervals, or even specific exercises that are meant to tone (rather than grow) a muscle. This is often suggested to women to explicitly avoid becoming bulky which, as I mentioned above, isn't a realistic fear in the first place. Being "toned", at least in the popular use of the word, simply refers to having a reduced level of body fat along with some degree of muscle size. Reducing body fat is primarily a result of diet (and aerobic/HIIT exercise) and increasing muscle size is accomplished far more effectively with proper resistance training than high repetitions. Combined with changes in diet, those will generate a "toned" physique far more quickly than the approaches so typically recommended to women

Technical Training

Technical training describes any type of training explicitly aimed at improving technique, usually in some specific sporting movement. It is generally only used by athletes although beginning exercisers should focus on improving technique when they begin exercise, especially in the weight room. For physique athletes, posing practice might be considered a type of technical training. Like stretching, technical training is frequently done as part of the workout (generally as part of the warm-up, discussed next) although specific separate technical sessions may be done by many athletes.

The primary changes that occur in response to technical training are in the brain and nervous system, although muscles are certainly worked (any physique athlete knows that posing practice can be very hard work). Technical training is generally (or at least can be) done fairly frequently since it is primarily about teaching the brain and nervous system to do the movement properly. Here, more frequent practice should be done for shorter periods of time than the reverse.

As well, technical training should usually be done when the athlete isn't tired although high-level athletes may do this in order to ensure technique stays stable when they fatigue in competition. Technical training sessions are typically fairly limited in duration; the time spent on any one drill is also usually limited as endless repetition tends to cause athlete's to lose focus. Performing shorter technical sessions more frequently is generally superior for this reason. Alternating between different drills back and forth tends to have better results as the athlete has to think and focus more when they switch from one drill to another and back again.

Warming Up

Let me next discuss warming up; any activities done before a workout and has as it's primary goal preparing the body for the workout session. Most typically a warm-up routine would include some type of low-intensity activity to generally raise body temperature (and this is more important when exercise is being done in the cold) which might be followed by some amount of stretching (if needed), technical training (if needed) and then progressively more intense exercise as the workout itself begins.

The specific types of warm-up activities done depend very heavily on the type of workout being done with the importance of the warmup increasing as the intensity of the workout goes up. A low intensity aerobic workout may need no specific warm-up while a maximum sprint workout might require 45-60 minutes before the actual workout begins. Warm-ups for weight training workouts can vary enormously depending on the type of workout being done. Very heavy training tend to require the most warm-up which is usually done by performing multiple sets of the same exercise with progressively heavier weights. Specific technical drills may be done in certain types of activities as well. For more traditional muscle growth or general fitness training, less warm-up is generally needed.

Although I'm not aware of any research on the topic, anecdotally women seem to require more warm-up than men for high-intensity activities, especially those that are highly technical. This could be due to differences in their nervous system and some have suggested that differences in the muscles and ligament themselves may be responsible. Regardless, women involved in high-intensity activities such as strength/power or sprint training may need to experiment with their warm-ups, performing more total work at progressively increasing intensities until they determine how much they individually need to perform at their best.

Cooling Down

Conceptually related to warming up is cooling down and the goal here is to facilitate the body's return to normal after an intense workout. This occurs through a number of mechanisms including allowing heart rate to return to normal levels (primarily for aerobic training), to help clear waste products from muscle (for high-intensity aerobic, HIIT or weight training workouts) and, importantly to lower body temperature back to normal. Women differ here from men, taking longer for their body temperatures to decrease to normal following a workout. For women exercising in the heat, and especially during the luteal phase and/or for women on certain types of birth control (when body temperature is elevated to begin with), avoiding excessive heat buildup during training along with bringing it back down more quickly is important for recovery. I will discuss this in more detail in Chapter 22.

Typically a cool-down will consist of 5-20' of very low intensity aerobic activity (130 heart rate or lower) as this type of active recovery brings heart rate down gradually while helping to remove waste by-products from muscles. This may be followed by light stretching if needed as this can help the body generally relax so that it can start the recovery processes. The amount of cool-down necessary depends on the intensity of the workout. Low-intensity workouts may require little to no cool down as the workout itself is at a recovery heart rate while a HIIT workout might require 10-20' of low intensity activity.

General Training and Diet Goals

While I suspect a large majority of women reading this book will have changes in body composition (specifically fat loss) as their primary goal, I want to look at some of the individual goal or sport categories that women might be interested or involved in. For each goal/sport I'll first describe what it represents before looking at the typical combination of types of exercise that might or might not be done. For the individual sports categories, I will primarily be grouping them based on their requirements for strength, power, muscle size, endurance, etc. along with the types of training that are most commonly done. Since I can't include every possible sport in this chapter, readers will have to compare the primary training they perform for their sport with what I have described. One type of sport I won't describe is pure skills sports such as archery or pistol shooting where the training is almost exclusively of a technical nature.

Bone Health

Due to the importance of bone health (bone mineral density or BMD) to women I want to discuss it both first and separately from the other goals. As I will discuss later in this book, women have until roughly their mid-20's or so to develop peak BMD. Most of the gain occurs during puberty but this isn't the target readership for this book and there's little that can be done in hindsight. At most parents of young girls who are reading this book can ensure that everything is being done after puberty to maximize BMD in terms of activity and nutrition. Past the mid-20's, there is typically a slow loss of bone density that accelerates at menopause, especially if hormone replacement therapy is not undertaken (the effect is due to the lack of estrogen which is also a contributor to the loss of BMD in amenorrhea). The increased rate of loss in women along with starting at a lower peak BMD is part of why osteoporosis is much greater risk for women than men (differences in average life span is also important here as men typically die before their bone density drops far enough for it to be an issue).

I say typically above as emerging evidence finds that proper exercise and nutritional intake (discussed in Chapter 20) is able to increase BMD even past the mid 20's. Perhaps more importantly, some research suggests that even postmenopausal women can either slow/eliminate the age-related loss of BMD or gain small amounts of BMD outright. The effect is smaller in this population: while the post-pubertal female may gain 2-5% BMD per year, the gain is only 1-3% per year past the mid-20's and into menopause. This is still significant in that even avoiding the typical loss of BMD helps to avoid problems later in life: a postmenopausal woman who gains 1.5% BMD instead of losing 1.5% BMD is still 3% ahead.

The key factors in developing or maintaining BMD are activity and proper nutritional support including adequate calories, calcium, Vitamin D and others. Since I will discuss nutrition in detail in Chapter 20, I will focus on the exercise component here. In short, the primary requirements for exercise is that it generates high peak forces and is brief and intermittent in nature. Higher levels of activity are generally associated with higher BMD but the type of exercise done makes an enormous difference in the overall effect of BMD, both in terms of the change and where that increase is seen (researchers typically focus on the lower leg, hip, spine and wrist).

Studies have found that athletes in sports with a large amount of jumping such as gymnastics, volleyball and basketball, tend to have the highest BMD (at least in the lower body). Athletes who lift weights have the next highest BMD with explosive lifters such as Olympic lifters having higher BMD than powerlifters who lift more slowly. Sports with less of a high-impact or explosive component tend to have lower levels of BMD. Surprisingly, endurance athletes, especially those who's sport generates no impact forces (i.e. cycling, swimming, cross country skiing and others) often have lower BMD than sedentary individuals with running being slightly higher. These observations, combined with a number of direct studies has led to the conclusion that the best types of exercise for improving BMD are weight training and jumping activities which are high-intensity, generate high peak forces and are done intermittently (5,6). In contrast, running or walking, which generates low peak forces and is done continuously is not as effective in improving BMD except perhaps in postmenopausal women who have very low BMD to begin with. Sprint running does improve BMD but, as above, requires good technique to be done safely.

Weight training, which can be used to load all bones of the body is superior in some ways to jumping which only stresses the lower body (jumping may also have no effect on BMD in postmenopausal women). So far as weight training, a key aspect is that the weights be heavy enough and put stresses on the bone directly or in unusual ways. Studies finding a benefit suggest that loads higher than 80% of maximum (roughly 8 repetitions to fatigue) are required in younger women while slightly lighter weights (12-15 repetitions to fatigue) are sufficient after menopause. Amazingly, one study in postmenopausal women used one set of upper body and one set of lower body exercises for 10-12 and 12-15 repetitions to fatigue twice weekly and that alone (perhaps 5 minutes of training) improved BMD. Since it is high peak forces that improve BMD, gradually moving to faster lifting speeds may be beneficial but it must occur gradually and be done safely. A recent study used extremely heavy loads (sets of 5) in post-menopausal women and found amazing improvement in BMD but this must be worked up to gradually.

While a recent study found that jumping was beneficial for older women, most has shown that it is mainly effects before menopause. Perhaps most surprisingly is how little it takes. As few as 10-20 maximal vertical jumps (a jump where the knees are bent, the person jumps as high as possible and lands) with 15-30 seconds between repetitions done 3-6 times per week has a significant impact on BMD. This means that as little as 5-10 minutes of activity three times per week can improve BMD, at least in the legs.

Given the differences in the effect of exercise and BMD in different age groups, choices of exercise should be population specific. For pre-menopausal (but not very young) women a combination of heavy, full-body weight training along with small amounts of jumping seems to be ideal. Postmenopausally, running (if it can be done safely) and heavy weight training would be an optimal combination. If a postmenopausal woman already has low bone density, the amount and intensity of training must be brought up gradually to avoid overstressing the already weakened bones. It's unclear how the other hormonal modifiers impact on this. I mentioned that birth control may negatively impact on BMD and the research on PCOS seems to have an overall beneficial effect and I would expect exercise to add to this.

General Fitness and Health

While the reality is that many, if not most, women are interested in weight or fat loss at most points in their life, there may be some female readers who are simply interested in improving their overall health and fitness. This includes improving their overall quality of life, improving bone density (or at least limiting it's loss), avoiding age-related muscle or function loss and others. Achieving these goals can be done with roughly three hours per week of exercise which should include a minimum of two days per week of resistance training along with at least three days per week of aerobic training. HIIT is optional but may be useful for variety. Premenopausal women would want to add a small amount of jumping for bone health and older women should add flexibility training. Even when changes in body composition are not the primary goal, they often happen in the early stages of beginning an exercise program.

Improving Body Composition/Appearance

While athletes of varying types frequently want to improve their body composition (this will be defined in detail in the next chapter), here I am talking about the woman who is not an athlete and who has no goal of competing in any sporting activity but who wants to improve her appearance to one degree or another. In the most general sense, her training will look very similar to what I described for the woman seeking general health and fitness although she will probably be performing proportionally more exercise overall. Three to four days of proper resistance training with as many (and potentially more) days of some type of aerobic work would be common; HIIT could be done for one or two sessions per week. Stretching has little impact on appearance but can be done as desired. While it doesn't really impact on appearance, jumping should be done by premenopausal women to improve BMD.

More specifically, changing body composition entails two primary goals which are gaining lean body mass (LBM, defined in more detail in the next chapter) and losing body fat. Gaining LBM occurs in response to proper resistance training (discussed in Chapter 28 of this volume and in detail in Volume 2) along with sufficient dietary protein. While a slight caloric surplus maximizes gains in muscle mass, beginning trainees often find that they gain small amounts of LBM while eating at maintenance or losing fat. Since women in this category don't generally desire enormous gains in LBM, the need for an explicit muscle gain phase would be unlikely to be included in this goal.

While gaining LBM (or at least not losing it) helps to improve overall shape and appearance, losing body fat always has a much more profound effect on lowering BF% (I will show why this is the case in Chapter 7) and realistically will be a more primary goal for most women looking to improve body composition. The obese/PCOS women may wish to lose small amount of fat to improve their overall health and/or fertility as well. As I will discuss in Chapter 8, fat loss is primarily driven by the creation of a long-term imbalance between calorie intake and energy expenditure. Calories can be reduced, activity can be increased or the two can be used together. Which approach is taken tends to depend on several factors such as how much exercise is being done along with the dieter's current body weight/body fat levels and I will discuss these specific situations later in the book. Now let me look at specific sports.

Physique Sports

This category includes women's bodybuilding, physique, figure and bikini. All are judged primarily on appearance with factors such as overall muscularity, symmetry and body fat levels playing a role in competition results. Posing is a critical aspect of competition as well. Each subcategory of the physique sports has its own requirements for either muscularity or leanness. Typically the amount of muscularity required goes down from bodybuilding to physique to figure with bikini requiring the least. Similarly, the requirement for leanness decreases with bodybuilding/physique requiring the lowest levels, fitness being somewhat variable but generally being slightly higher and bikini usually requiring the least. I will give more specific numbers in the next chapter.

The physique sports are unique in that the primary type of training that is done is not performed in the actual competition (posing is the only component has any relevance to the competition). For all physique sports, weight training tends to be the primary activity and is done both to increase muscularity (either in general or specific muscle groups) or to maintain muscle while dieting. As I mentioned above, jumping has become popular for unclear reasons but some would be valuable from a BMD standpoint. Aerobic and HIIT is done in varying amounts at different parts of the year. Typically, less aerobic/HIIT work is done when increasing muscularity is the goal while proportionally more will be done when dieting. Posing practice is typically ignored until the contest diet has begun and, even there, it may not be done in large amounts until fairly close to the contest.

Strength/Power Sports

This category includes sports where the competition is geared around maximal or near-maximal, often single, efforts lasting a very short time (often no more than a few seconds). This includes powerlifting, Olympic lifting, and some of the throws (shotput, discus) in track and field. Due to the similarities in terms of training to the other sports, I'd include female strongman competition here as well although it's events are typically longer (60-75 seconds) and it might realistically be included in the next sport I will discuss. All pure strength/power sports are predicted on some degree of muscle size, strength and power production along with technique. True endurance (outside of the ability to complete long workouts) is not required.

As such, the training for these sports revolves almost exclusively around resistance training, explosive training and technical work. The types of resistance training that is done can vary but typically includes a large amount of heavy/low-repetition training (heavy weights for sets of 1-5) with some amount of higher repetition work to increase muscle mass as needed. Explosive training may include jumping exercises along with others such as medicine ball work or explosive lifting. Technical work tends to vary the most and will depend heavily on the sport in question. In powerlifting and Olympic lifting, the weight room is the sport although specific technical work may be done as needed. Female strongman competitors perform some combination of traditional weight room work along with practicing with the implements while throwers typically lift and throw and lift and throw and then lift and throw some more.

As it can hinder the development of strength and power, true aerobic work outside of the lowest intensity activity (i.e. brisk walking) is almost never done. At most what is often called work capacity or general physical preparation (GPP) is done and might involve pulling a sled or performing barbell complexes (a series of exercises done continuously). HIIT would be universally inappropriate (except perhaps for female strongman) and true sprinting would make more sense for athletes in these sports. At the same time, the technique requirements are high and the impact can be a danger for heavier athletes.

Several sports in this category have weight classes which means that athletes cannot continue to gain weight unless they intend to compete in a higher class. With one exception, weight class athletes tend to maintain a reasonably but not excessively low BF% as this lets them carry more muscle at any given body weight. Depending on their weight class and how far away they are for it, short dieting phases are sometimes required. Since they can manipulate water weight within a fairly small range (about 3% of total body weight), the total amount of fat that needs to be lost is decreased. The lack of true aerobic work in strength/power sports along with the fact that weight training burns proportionally fewer calories than other types of training can make fat loss relatively more difficult since it's hard to increase calorie expenditure without harming performance. This means that reducing calorie intake/adjusting the diet itself tends to be the best approach for fat loss. The exception to the above is weight class sports have a super heavy weight class where any weight above a certain point is allowed an some sports have no weight class. Athletes in this group often carry a significant amount of body fat as it often improves their leverages and allows them to eat enough to support their training. Fat loss is rarely a goal until these athletes retire from competition.

High-Intensity Performance Sports

Although all sports tend to require a high-intensity in both training and competition, I am using the term to refer to sports that still have a large requirement for strength, power and explosiveness but which is lower than the pure strength/power sports. Speed is often a requirement and for certain events, there may be some endurance component although it is not very large. Some of the sports that might be included here are the 100m/200m sprint in track and field, some track cycling events (i.e. match sprint), sprint swimming events (50-100m) along with others of that rough duration.

Other sports where the competition event falls between roughly 20 seconds and 1 minute would be included here. Cheerleading figure skating, and gymnastics also fall into this category. While the duration of the competitions tends to be longer (i.e. the free skate program is 4.5 minutes and gymnastics routines vary in length) the requirements for the sports are more similar to the other sports in this category than not. Generally they revolve around strength, power and explosiveness and alternate between near maximal explosive efforts (i.e. a jump in figure skating) and relatively easier recovery. As described above, athletes in these sports often show the highest bone density due to the explosive nature of their sport.

In addition to a usually staggering amount of technical work, sports in this category tend to focus more on strength, power and explosiveness than much else. Many of these sports have a high requirement for maximum speed and this makes up a large amount of training as well. While relatively more endurance is require for these sports, the amount of true endurance training tends to be at least somewhat limited or done in very specific ways. Track sprinters almost never perform true aerobic training and use specialized workouts for both general and speed endurance. Track cyclists often ride their bikes at low intensities for an hour a few days per week but this is for recovery (or possibly to reduce body fat slightly), is non-impact so it doesn't harm recovery or hinder improvements in their performance. As well, cyclists simply enjoy riding their bikes. For most of the described sports, true HIIT is rarely done although pure sprint training is part and parcel of the training due to the requirements for a high top speed. Cheerleaders and figure skaters may do minimal true aerobic work as much of their conditioning comes from practicing routines/skills; HIIT may also be done.

Depending on the sport, increasing amounts of muscle mass can be relatively more or less beneficial; the same goes for reducing BF% Track cyclists and swimmers tend to carry the most muscle since their body weights are being supported and, within limits, BF% is often somewhat higher. In contrast, excessive muscle mass can potentially slow down a track sprinter although their body fat levels tend to be very low. Sports such as figure skating or gymnastics have an aesthetic component that can't be ignored and excessive muscle mass and body fat can be detrimental to performance. At the same time both sports have a large strength and explosiveness component which needs to be trained. Typically a fairly large total amount of training is done in these sports and that alone is often sufficient to keep women who do them fairly lean. If fat loss is desired, it may be possible to add low-intensity work (i.e. extending warm-up and cool-downs) to burn extra calories while adjusting diet slightly. I'd mention and will discuss again that athletes in many of these sports already habitually undereat and if diet is adjusted at all, it may actually be to increase food intake.

Mixed Sports

I will use the term mixed sports to refer to activities that require a relatively even balance of strength/power along with endurance. Explosiveness and speed are often important as well. The majority of team sports such as basketball, ice hockey, netball, field hockey, volleyball and softball and others fall into this category but individual sports such as the middle distances (400-800 m) in track and field or many swimming events along with mixed martial arts or boxing would be included here as well. Athletes needn't be as strong as athletes in the strength/power or high-intensity performance sports but need more endurance than either (but less than endurance athletes discussed next).

Given the nature of these sports, the training tends to be far more balanced in terms of the different types of training which are done. A balance of weight training (the amount of which varies from sport to sport), explosive training, sprint training and general aerobic/cardiovascular training may all included and they all tend to be performed at some point in the week. Alternation of higher intensity days with lower intensity days is a common pattern and there is often also the need for technical along with tactical training, especially in the team sports. Generally, different aspects of training are emphasized at different parts of the year moving from more general conditioning to more specific competition work as the season approaches. In the team sports especially, competitions may occur weekly with the competition season lasting for several month at a time.

Developing optimal muscularity along with maintaining a reasonable BF% is also typically an aspect of these sports. As with some strength/power sports, MMA and boxing have weight classes which may require explicit dieting and/or water manipulation to make the weight limit. To at least some degree, the sheer amount of training being done tends to keep these athletes lean but losing fat may become somewhat of a goal at certain times of the year. Due to the large amount of training being done it can be difficult to add more although slight increases in aerobic activity can burn significant calories. Since there is a limit to how much training can realistically be done, changes to the diet may be the only option for fat loss.

Endurance Sports

Finally are the endurance sports which refers to any activity where the competition lasts 4 minutes or more (most competitions are much longer than this). Examples include running, cycling, mountain biking, rowing, the longer swimming races, triathlon, cross country skiing, race walking and others. Events can last from just over 4 minutes (in the 1500m in track and field) to 6-7 minutes (rowing) up to several hours (the marathon/ultra-endurance running, cycling and triathlon). There are even ultra-endurance events where the athlete may be in more or less continuous movement for many hours at a time and women actually outperform men in ultra-endurance running events longer than 52km (32 miles).

As the name suggests, the primary determinant of performance is aerobic endurance although there are others such as lactate threshold (this has other names but can be thought of as the maximum speed which can be maintained for an hour), efficiency and technique. Top speed is also important either to improve speed at lower intensities or to give the athlete the ability to catch a competitor or sprint at the end of the race. Even in the shorter events such as the 800m (which may last no more than 2 minutes), the predominant type of training (up to 80%) done in endurance sports is relatively low- to moderate-intensity aerobic work complemented by relatively small amounts (perhaps 20%) of HIIT of varying durations. Small amounts of true sprint work may also be done. Aerobic work may be done daily (some sports train more than one time per day) with HIIT typically done no more than twice per week (especially for runners). Some endurance sports such as swimming and rowing are highly technical and specific technique workout are often done.

With the possible exception of rowing, which requires a good deal of strength at the start of the race, weight training does not typically make up a large amount of training for endurance sports. Excessive muscle mass can be detrimental in most cases although swimmers and rowers tend to be more muscular than other athletes as their sports require proportionally more power and they don't have to go up hills. For this reason, it would be almost unheard of for an endurance athlete outside of a rower or swimmer to explicitly try to gain muscle mass. It's actually not unheard of for endurance athletes to want to lose muscle mass, especially in muscles that don't contribute to performance (i.e. the upper body muscles in running or cycling). While some research has found that weight training and jumping may improve performance (especially in running), both types of training tend to be relatively de-emphasized for most endurance athletes (again, rowing, swimming and cross-country skiing being notable exceptions). At most it is generally used in the of-season, especially for athletes who live in wintery areas and can't train easily. Once the competition season approaches, it is eliminated from training as often as not.

While this is logical in a purely competition sense, it is actually a large problem in terms of developing or maintaining optimal BMD. Only running puts any type of impact stress on the bones (and there only in the lower body) but it is not a high peak force and the effect is not large. Swimming and cycling not only have no impact forces but the body is supported and they may show poorer BMD than sedentary individuals. One study even found that cyclists lost bone density during their 4-month competition season despite the inclusion of weight training and jumping. All of these factors, when combined with issues such as menstrual cycle dysfunction or outright eating disorders, has the potential to not only harm these athlete's BMD in the short term but set them up for problems much later in life. Not only are endurance athletes not building BMD during the critical years, they may be losing it.

For this reason, the inclusion of weight training with some jumping in at least the off-season of training (coupled with proper nutrition as described in Chapter 20) should be considered mandatory for all female endurance athletes. This may not be optimal in the sense that it is only done for part of the year but the realities of high-level competition are that compromises have to be made. If possible, it would be ideal to maintain at least some amount of that type of training during the competition season but that may not be realistic due to the competition demands and amount of training that must be done to meet them.

With few exceptions, endurance athletes tend to maintain a low body weight and body fat levels. Body fat is, in a very real sense, dead weight that costs energy to move (especially up hills) without contributing to performance. Runners are typically the leanest of all as they have to project their bodies across gravity with cyclists carrying slightly more fat due to being supported on the bike. Swimmers often carry slightly more body fat than cyclists. Not only does this not harm performance it may help because it makes the athlete float more easily which means that less of their energy goes to staying on top of the water. Cold water swimmers (another sport where women outperform men) tend to carry more fat as well, not only to help them float but because it acts as insulation.

Rowing is unique among endurance sports in that it has two weight classes and female rowers may have to actively diet to reach the weight cutoff. Since dehydration tends to harm performance, it cannot always be used and this means that fat loss may be the only approach to make the weight cut off with some women being unable to realistically reach the lower weight class. From an energetic standpoint, with the possible exception of ultra endurance events, body fat is never limiting for any endurance event and in the sense that it is effectively deadweight, reducing it within limits does tend to improve performance. At the same time, reaching extreme levels of leanness and what is required to do so can cause a number of problems. These will be discussed in Chapter 12.

When fat loss is desired, endurance athletes have the benefit of already burning a large number of calories in training. But that also means that adding more activity may not be possible without being too much and it can be a fine balance. A small increase in low-intensity work (i.e. lengthening warm-up and cool-downs for harder workouts) is often possible but adjusting the diet may be the only realistic approach in many cases.

Chapter 5: What is Body Composition?

Having examined the normal menstrual cycle and the most common hormonal modifiers, I want to discuss the topic of body composition for the next several chapters. There are two primary reasons I want to do this. The first is that the differences in body composition between women and men (detailed below) tend to underlie many of the differences that are seen in terms of apparent gender differences in fat gain, fat loss and exercise performance. Hormonal differences (and the changes that occur) clearly play a role but the difference in body composition tends to explain a great deal of the differences that are seen.

The second has to do with a topic that will take up a large portion of this book which relates to dieting and what I will for now call weight loss. I mentioned that women are generally more likely to be dieting than men and this is true whether the general population or an athletic population is being examined. There are still many long-held misconceptions and simply poor ideas about dieting and many of them relate to a misunderstanding of the differences between body weight, body fat and body composition.

Because while many who pursue dieting tend to still think in terms of weight loss itself, looking at body composition is not only far more accurate but far more important. This isn't to say that the scale doesn't have it's uses or that weight is irrelevant in all situations (i.e. weight class athletes who must reach a specific weight). But there are a number of potential problems with it by itself. To nobody's surprise, there are a set of issues that women face in this regard that men really don't. Understanding body composition, what it means, along with the differences between body weight and body fat, are a key aspect of improving women's results in everything from dieting in general to improving their athletic performance.

Women's Body Composition

So what is a woman's body actually made of? The answer is a whole bunch of different things including bones, skeletal muscle, organs (heart, liver, kidney, brain, etc.), water, stored carbohydrate, blood, minerals and of course there is body fat. For simplicities sake, these different components of the human body are typically divided into two categories. The first is fat and includes, well, all of the different types of fat that I will discuss in some detail below. Everything that is not fat will be called lean body mass (LBM) and you'll sometimes see this called Fat Free Mass (FFM). For all practical purposes they are interchangeable and I will use LBM throughout this book.

What is LBM and What is it For?

While many, especially in the athletic community, tend to equate LBM with muscle, this isn't really accurate. Rather, LBM refers to everything that isn't fat and this includes a number of distinct tissues which are structurally very different. The brain has a very specific structure as do the various organs (including a woman's reproductive organs). Bone is it's own tissue as is skeletal muscle. Water, minerals and carbohydrates are all distinct as well. Every type of LBM in the body tends to have a fairly specialized purpose. The heart pumps blood, kidneys filter waste, the liver is involved in tons of different biological processes, bones provide the body with a physical framework, skeletal muscle generates force for movement, reproductive organs exist for reproduction, etc. All are important although, as you'll see later in the book, some are relatively more important than others in terms of short-term survival. They are all important but as I'll talk about below, only a few are really that relevant in terms of what can or cannot be impacted on by diet (or training) and what is really worth paying attention to in the short term.

While the amount of bone, or rather how dense bones are, is critical to women's health, the primary type of LBM that is important in terms of altering body composition is skeletal muscle. Other types of LBM can change, water and glycogen for example, but changes in the amount of muscle are key here. Skeletal muscle is made up of a number of different types of tissue. The actual muscle fibers are made of protein but this is only about 25% of the total in muscle. The rest is a combination of water, minerals, stored carbohydrate (called glycogen), intra-muscular triglyceride (IMTG, fat stored within the muscle itself) and the various cellular machinery involved in muscular metabolism.

What is Body Fat and What is it For?

In contrast to LBM which is made up of a number of very distinct tissues, body fat tends to be fairly similar in its chemical structure with one exception. The technical term for body fat is adipose tissue and most types of body fat fall under description of white adipose tissue (WAT) although it's really more of a milky beige color. Whether they know it or not, when people want to lose "weight" or improve their appearance, it's WAT that they want to lose. All WAT is made up primarily of stored triglyceride (TG), and this makes up 85-90% of the total fat cell (the rest is water and cellular machinery). A TG is the combination of three fatty acids attached to a glycerol molecule. When people talk about saturated or unsaturated fats they are actually referring to the chemical structure of the fatty acid chains. The fat found in food is nothing more than TG and I'll talk about how women's bodies handle dietary fat in Chapter 10.

The exception to the above is what used to be called brown adipose tissue (BAT) but is now thought to be brite or beige adipose tissue in humans (the distinction isn't that important here and I'll call this BAT as well). Sort of a reddish color, BAT stores very little triglyceride and exists to burn other fuels for energy and to produce heat (1). It's currently not clear how much of a real world impact on calorie expenditure BAT has at this point. As well, since BAT tends to be primarily activated under conditions of chronic cold exposure, which most in the modern world try to avoid, the relevance of BAT is questionable.

So what is body fat for beyond making people unhappy about their appearance? The earliest ideas held that body fat was nothing more a relatively inert place to store energy and clearly that is certainly one of it's primary purposes. During certain types of exercise or when there is insufficient food (as in dieting or starvation), stored fat is mobilized to provide energy to the body. While carbohydrate can also provide energy, fat stores are especially suited to this role as they provide 9 calories per gram while carbohydrates only provide four. As importantly, the storage of carbohydrate requires a large amount of water with 3-4 grams of water being stored for every gram of carbohydrate, while fat does not. A fairly lean individual might store 100,000 calories of fat, enough to sustain them for weeks or months without any food. To store that much energy as carbohydrate would be impossible and the actual stores of carbs (as glycogen in the muscle an liver) is fairly limited.

For women especially, it's clear that lower body provides a fuel source during pregnancy and for breastfeeding. As I mentioned in Chapter 2, women's hip and thigh fat is actually used preferentially for this purpose being stored in preparation for pregnancy and being used for energy in the later stages of pregnancy and during breastfeeding. Relatedly to this, at least part of a woman's body fat distribution is probably related to sexual selection and attraction, providing the curves and other female characteristics that are found to be sexually appealing. But there is far more to body fat than that.

Body fat turns out to be crucial in both immune system function and inflammation with both too little and too much body fat causing problems. Too little fat means that the immune system may not function as well as it could while too much means that the immune system is overactive. Excessive body fat also causes an inflammatory state. Body fat may also play a role as a physical cushion in the body or act for insulation against cold (and women do handle heat and cold differently than men). Body fat is also a place where the body stores glucose; in a variety of disease states, it becomes impossible for the body to store incoming carbohydrate in muscle and fat cells can take up the slack at least for a little while.

As I mentioned in Chapter 2, fat cells are also a place where local metabolism of hormones can occur. A great deal of women's estrogen is actually made from the conversion of testosterone within the fat cell (in postmenopausal women, almost all of her estrogen is made this way). Fat cells also can impact on cortisol (a stress hormone) metabolism, converting active cortisol to inactive cortisone and vice versa and there are other numerous effect occurring with more being discovered almost continuously. Perhaps one of the most newly recognized aspect (newly here means since the mid 1990's) is that fat cells, produce a host of chemicals and hormones that drastically impact on physiology. Leptin, which I mentioned in Chapter 2 and which I will talk about in great detail later, was the first to be discovered and the list continues to grow almost weekly.

My point here is primarily to point out that, as much as people dislike body fat (for appearance reasons) and while excessive amounts certain cause health problems, fat cells are critical for overall health and function. Too little can be just as bad as too much and in odd disease states, where people make no fat cells, a number of health problems crops up. It's simply an issue where thinking of fat cells as "good" or "bad" is mistaken (3).

Types of White Adipose Tissue
While the above applies to all types of WAT generally, it turns out that fat stored in different parts of the body can act very differently. Different distributions of fat (i.e. upper versus lower body) can impact on overall health and there are large differences in the rate of blood flow through the fat cells, how easily or not the fat cells store fat along with how easily or not they release that fat back into the bloodstream. There are also clear gender differences that I will discuss in a later chapter. For now let me look at the different types of WAT in the body.

The first type of fat is essential fat, fat in the body that is essential for both life and normal function. This includes fat around the brain, around the internal organs (different from visceral fat, discussed next), in the nervous system (sheaths around nerves are made of fat) and in the brain. In general, essential fat is taken as 3-4% for men and 10-12% for women with the difference being attributable to what is called sex-specific fat (breast tissue is included here). You can't lose essential fat and if you did, you'd be dead.

Visceral fat, which many readers have probably heard of, refers to a type of fat found primarily in the gut that surrounds the organs (it is different than essential fat, though). Visceral fat is highly metabolically active meaning that, while it stores fat fairly easily, it also releases fat easily. This is probably to provide a rapid source of energy to the body but excess amounts of visceral fat is associated with insulin resistance and increased heart disease risk (4). Visceral fat is deep within the body and not really visible outside of making the stomach stick out (and often feel quite hard to the touch). When it is lost, while the stomach may be flatter (or easier to suck in) there is no major change in appearance. Testosterone tends to promote visceral fat accumulation and between having low testosterone and elevated estrogen, women do not generally store much. However women with PCOS/hyperandrogenism or who become very overweight tend to store visceral fat. After After menopause, visceral fat levels increase if HRT is not begun which contributes to the increased risk of heart disease seen in women under those conditions.

Subcutaneous fat is fat found underneath the skin which makes it visible in a way that essential and visceral fat is not. Whether they know it or not, when people talk about losing fat (or even weight to some degree), they are really talking about losing this type of fat. While subcutaneous fat used to be considered a single type of tissue, it's now known that fat in different parts of the body are physiologically distinct (I will discuss this in more detail in Chapter 6). Upper body fat is more similar than not and represents everything above the waist including fat on the face, shoulders, chest (except breast fat), upper and lower back and abdominal area (which can be further subdivided into deep and superficial and upper and lower). Lower body fat refers to everything below the waist including the glutes/hips, thighs and calves.

Since they have less visceral fat, women tend to carry more subcutaneous fat with more of the total being stored in the lower body (PCOS/hyperandrogenism, obesity and the postmenopausal woman on HRT tend to carry more upper body fat). Relative to visceral fat, subcutaneous fat is more difficult to lose although this depends on the area being examined and whether women or men are being examined. Subcutaneous fat is less metabolically active than visceral fat which means that it tends to have less of an impact on disease risk. Carrying more fat in the lower body, which is particularly metabolically inactive, lowers heart disease risk which is why women are typically protected until after menopause.

What is Body Composition?

With the above background, I can finally address what body composition actually represents. Fundamentally it refers to the ratio of all of the different tissues in the body that I mentioned above. So assume we could determine how much of a woman's body was made up of every kind of tissue that is present. We might find that she had 40% muscle, 25% body fat, some percentage of brains, liver, kidneys, reproductive organs. Bones would make up some other percentage, water, minerals, stored carbohydrate another percentage. When all of this was added together, it would equal 100%. Let's also assume that we could determine the weight of each tissue. If we took the weight of each tissue and added them together, it would add up to her total bodyweight. So of her 135 lbs, 40% or 54 pounds would be muscle, 25% or 34 lbs would be fat, and the same would hold for every other tissue in her body.

And that breakdown, the percentage of her body that was represented by every type of tissue present would be her body composition. As I mentioned above, few go to this level of detail and it's more common to delineate the body into fat and everything else (LBM). This is important for a number of reasons not the least of which is that weight may remain the same even if body composition is changing. Of more relevance to the next section, it's important because weight gain or loss can occur over different time frames and in response to the gain or loss of a variety of different tissues.

Losing and Gaining Weight: What is Being Lost or Gained?

Although it has been changing in the last decade or so, the reality is that most people (women or men) tend to focus only on changes in body weight. If weight goes up, that's usually bad (unless it is an athlete trying to gain muscle) and if weight goes down that's usually good. For the sake of example, let's say someone starts a diet and a few days later their scale weight has dropped by a few pounds. Most would consider that a success but I would ask the following question: What was lost? Was it water, stored carbohydrate, muscle, fat, bone, organs? Perhaps the person just had a big bowel movement.

The scale can't answer this question in any meaningful fashion and this presents a rather large problem. And this becomes an enormous practical problem as many people, especially if they are dieting, not only focus solely on the scale to track their progress but often obsess over the changes (or lack thereof). They may weigh multiple times per day (or before and after going to the bathroom) and often over react completely to small day-to-day changes in bodyweight. A frequent pattern is that if weight goes down, that means it's time for celebration. Bring on the cake. But if weight goes up, it's time to reduce food intake even more and add an extra hour of exercise to the gym. As you'll see below, these types of short-term changes are relatively meaningless overall although daily weighing can still be useful so long as it is approached correctly. Women, primarily the normally cycling female but also others, have an added problem here that I will discuss below.

When looking at weight loss or weight gain, there are usually some safe assumptions that can be made about what is being gained or lost. Surprisingly, there can actually be some small changes in organ size but these are impossible to measure, happen rapidly an probably don't represent much total weight in the first place. Bone density can change in both directions but these changes tend to be fairly slow and don't represent a large amount of weight. During weight loss, bone loss is at most 1.6% of the total loss and gains in bone density might be in the realm of 2-3% over 6-12 months with proper training and nutrition. Since the changes are so small over any reasonable dieting time frame and can't be measured easily (only one method of body composition measurement, discussed in the next chapter can track bone density), this usually isn't worth worrying about either.

Practically this means that the only bodily tissues worth worrying about are water, the carbohydrate stored within muscle (which is actually related to water storage), digesting food, fat mass, and the part of total LBM that is represented by muscle. Food residue, the undigested food moving from the gut through the colon before excretion can actually make up 3-7 lbs (~1.5-3 kg) depending on the diet (high-fiber diets tend to produce more food residue) and this can be a significant portion of a woman's total bodyweight in some cases. But over most realistic time frames (i.e. the months that most diets will last), those are really the only tissues that need to be worried about. And the basic bathroom scale can't differentiate between them (a special kind of scale discussed in the next chapter attempts to do this). Two pounds of water loss and two pounds of fat loss will show up identically here in terms o the weight change. This works in reverse for weight gain where an increase in scale weight can't give any indication of what is being gained.

That said, there are some general comments that can be made regarding the relative contribution that changes in food, water, carbohydrate, muscle and body fat may be making changes in body weight and over what time frame.

Water/Glycogen/Food Residue

Almost without exception, very short-term changes in scale weight tend to represent changes in water, glycogen or food residue (a good bowel movement can cause a 1-2 pound weight loss in some cases). Even small changes in the diet can cause scale weight to change pretty significantly in a fairly quick period of time. Someone on a low-sodium diet who eats high-sodium meal may bloat up for a day or two, gaining several pounds of water weight. Chronic stress can also cause water retention due to the increase in cortisol which, as I mentioned in Chapter 2, binds to the receptor involved in water retention.

Dietary carbohydrate intake can enormously impact on water weight. Through a variety of mechanisms, when carbohydrates are lowered, the body tends to lose a lot of water; losses of 1-15 pounds in a few days have been seen in studies of low-carbohydrate diets. Many diet books use this to their advantage. By lowering or eliminating carbohydrates from the diet, body weight drops enormously in a few days and this can be very rewarding to the dieter (5). It can also backfire when dieters get frustrated that the rapid losses don't continue indefinitely. They may lose 5 pounds in the first week due to water loss and then lose "only" 1-2 pounds per week after that.

This works in the opposite direction as well: someone who has been on a low- or even lowered-carbohydrate diet who eats a lot of carbs for one reason or another can see their weight spike fairly significantly (large individuals may gain 7-10 pounds in one or two days). Every gram of carbohydrate stores 3-4 grams of water with it which explains the big increase in body weight. As I mentioned in Chapter 4, this partially explains why women often "feel bulky" when they start weight training. Their muscles start storing more carbohydrate and this causes them to store more water. But it goes away within about a week.

While all of the above is true for both women and men but normally cycling women have the added issue of the menstrual cycle (recall that some forms of birth control can cause water retention and PCOS women may experience issues at nearly random times). Most women are familiar with how wildly their body weight may change throughout the month. I discussed the hormonal reasons why in Chapter 2 but the late follicular and late luteal phase tend to be the worst and body weight changes of 5-10 lbs (~2.5-5 kg) are not unheard of. This tends to generally drive women crazy (even women well versed with body composition can be affected psychologically by this) but it gives women an additional factor in tracking changes that men don't have. This is discussed in Chapter 6.

And it's absolutely critical for readers to realize that all of these changes, small or large, don't represent anything meaningful in terms of reaching their goals. Rather, given the actual rate of change in levels of body fat and muscle mass, these rapid changes can only represent the gain or loss of water, carbohydrate, food in the gut, etc. As I will discuss in a later chapter, storing a pound of actual body fat takes about 3,500 calories over maintenance which makes a true loss or gain of 4 pounds of fat a physiological impossibility as it represents 14,000 calories of energy. To eat that many excess calories or burn that many calories through exercise in one day would be impossible.

The above should not be taken to mean that body weight is meaningless or that the scale is useless. Rather, it must be understood that short-term changes in bodyweight don't represent anything meaningful in terms of what people are trying to lose (or gain). As well, the scale can still have its place to track progress, it must simply be used appropriately. As well, in at least one case, body weight does still matter. This is for those weight-class athletes who have to be at a specific body weight for their competition. In this case, manipulating water, glycogen and food residue it useful but with the understanding that it is only a short-term change to achieve a specific goal. I don't know that this represents a majority of this book's readership and the reality is that, under most circumstances, the focus of dieting (or weight gain for athletes) should be on the changes in either body fat or LBM (specifically muscle).

Fat and Muscle

As short-term changes in body weight always represent water, glycogen, etc. they don't particularly count in terms of actually changing body composition. Certainly it may change a little bit with water or glycogen loss (both of which count as LBM), but overall changing the ratios of body fat and skeletal muscle is how body composition changes. When trying to lose (or gain) weight, individuals should really be focused on the changes in either fat or skeletal muscle that are occurring. Fat loss will be best achieved by losing fat while either maintaining, or even slightly increasing, the amounts of muscle while muscle gain should ideally come with as little body fat gain as possible (it's usually impossible to avoid it completely).

I'd note that the scale still can't differentiate changes in fat and muscle either, they do occur over a much larger time scale than changes in water, glycogen or food residue. So while a 2-3 lbs (~1-1.5 kg) change in body weight over a day will assuredly represent nothing more than water weight or food in the gut, that same change over multiple weeks is far more likely to represent a "real" change in body composition. Even that conclusion can be problematic depending on when body weight is actually measured. If someone only measures once per week (i.e. on Monday) the change from the first to the second measurement might represent a real change or might not. I'll talk about tracking in the next chapter.

For now I just want to emphasize my primary point which is that short-term changes in body weight don't represent anything real while longer term changes generally do. The short-term changes can only be water weight, etc. while the long term changes are far more likely to represent real changes in the amount of fat or muscle someone is carrying. That said, when females want to improve their appearance, health, etc. the goal should not only be to lose (or gain) weight. Rather it should be to improve their body composition, to lose fat, gain muscle or some combination of the two.

Body Fat Percentage

While the overall concept of body composition has to do with the fact that the human body is made up of different amounts of different tissues, since we are dividing the body into only LBM and fat mass, it's more useful to think in terms of body fat percentage (BF%). This represents the percentage of someone's total weight that is made up by fat (by definition everything else is LBM). If someone has a BF% of 30%, the other 70% is LBM. If their BF% is 20%, they have 80% LBM. I'll present some representative numbers later but this percentage can range from a lower limit of 10-12% in the leanest women up to 50-60% in cases of extreme obesity. And while body composition in the most general sense is more associated with appearance and health than weight per se, BF% is arguably even more related to both. A woman at 25% body fat will not only have a different appearance but is likely to be healthier than one at 45% body fat I'd mention again that the distribution of body fat is also relevant here and a more typical female fat patterning (gynoid or pear shaped with body fat in the lower body) is metabolically healthier than the typical male fat patterning (android or apple shaped). In this vein I'd note that, even more than body weight per se, body composition is far more related to overall health. If someone loses fat and gains some amount of muscle, their health will improve even if their body weight per se is unchanged (6).

Within the context of this book, perhaps the larger attention to be more worried about BF% and body composition is that it will be a much larger determinant of appearance (and performance) than just body weight (again, weight class athletes may also have to worry about a specific weight). Two women at the same weight with a different BF%/body composition may look totally different. So consider two women who both weigh 130 pounds. The first is an athlete at a relatively lean 18% body fat while the second is inactive with 28% body fat. Their weight is the same but their body composition is different and the athlete will be visibly more muscular and leaner than the inactive woman.

And while body weight can change due to shifts in water weight or food residue without any real changes in BF%/body composition occurring, it's entirely possible for body weight to stay the same while body composition is improving. So consider a beginning exerciser who gains 2 lbs of muscle while losing 2 lbs of fat. Her weight will be unchanged although her body composition will have improved. Or consider a more extreme example where a woman starts at 130 lbs and 25% body fat and 6 months later she is 130 lbs at 20% body fat. She may look completely different while weighing the same. Related to this, the predicted weight loss (or gain) may be lower than expected due to changes in body composition. If a woman gains 2 pounds of muscle while losing 4 pounds of fat, she will have only lost 2 pounds on the scale although her fat loss is double that (this will come up again when I talk about gender differences in weight loss in response to exercise in Chapter 11). Her weight will only go down by two pounds but the impact on her body composition, health, appearance and how her clothes fit may change significantly.

Finally, this can work in the opposite direction. If body fat is gained while muscle is being lost, BF% may increase and body composition worsen despite no change in weight. I mentioned an example of this in Chapter 3 when I discussed how some forms of hormonal birth control can cause a slight loss of muscle and gain in fat despite no real weight change. The same occurs at menopause without hormone replacement therapy, even if a woman's body weight doesn't change much, she will start to lose LBM while gaining fat (along with a shift in fat distribution). Weight is unchanged but body composition is worsening.

For athletes or those actively trying to gain weight, the above concept works exactly in reverse. Here short-term changes in weight up or down are still equally meaningless and tend to represent shifts in water weight, etc. Only longer term changes in body weight indicate that either muscle/LBM or fat is being gained. In general, when people try to gain weight it's in an attempt to gain LBM while limiting the amount of fat that is gained and tracking changes in body composition is more meaningful than changes in weight per se. There are exceptions, those recovering from true eating disorders or after an extreme diet, where weight gain must come with an increasing amount of body fat (along with regaining lost LBM).

Because regardless of what is or isn't happening to body weight itself, if BF% is changing (up or down), the actual body composition is also changing. This could be a change in the total amount of fat, the total amount of muscle mass or both. And outside of those weight class athletes who have to reach a specific goal weight, it's those long-term changes in body composition that really matters. Having a measurement or estimate of BF% is important for many reasons. With that and body weight it is possible to calculate the total amount of fat and LBM in pounds or kilograms. A variety of calculations can also be done with these numbers and I will present them throughout this book. As well, some aspects of diet such as protein intake are better set relative to LBM so being able to calculate or at least estimate this is important. Finally, these measurement and calculations allow someone to much more accurately track what is changing in their body than they would be able using body weight alone. Let me note that for the rest of this book, I will refer almost exclusively to BF% as it is the value with the most real use.

Chapter 6: Measuring and Tracking Body Composition

Continuing from the last chapter, I want to now look at some of the practical aspects involved in both measuring and tracking changes in body composition or body fat percentage (BF%). I will be discussing a number of methods but it's important to realize that none provide more than an estimate. Every method has pros and cons and while I will use that estimate to determine many aspects of diet setup later in the book, from a tracking standpoint, changes are more important than absolute numbers. Since they can also be relevant, I will also be looking at some non-body composition methods of tracking progress in this chapter and will make recommendations for combinations of those methods that can be used. I'll also examine the issue of what "good" BF% might be for different situations, introduce the diet Category system I will use in this book and look at some female specific issues relevant to the topic.

True Body Composition Measurements

The first set of methods I want to discuss are true body composition measurements in that they measure (or estimate) some aspect of actual body composition. They vary in their accuracy, difficulty of use and availability and I will describe them more or less in order from least to most complex.

Body-Mass Index (BMI)

The BMI is a fairly old measurement which relates an individual's body weight to their height. More technically BMI is defined as weight in kilograms divided by height in meters squared but this can be converted to inches and feet for Americans. For decades BMI has been used to indicate general health or some kind of ideal weight and insurance companies use some version of it to determine how much to charge you per month. A high BMI tends to correlate with health risk and a BMI greater than 25 kg/m^2 is defined as overweight and a BMI greater than 30 kg/m^2 is considered obese. Very low values are equally problematic with a value below 18.5 kg/m^2 is considered unhealthy or malnourished (possibly indicating an eating disorder or wasting disease). Between 18.5 and 25 is considered optimal. It's critical to note that these are only averages and it's been established that individuals with a high BMI can be healthy while those in the optimal range may be unhealthy.

Part of the reason for this is that BMI is not strictly speaking a measurement of BF% and doesn't indicate body composition or how much fat or LBM someone is carrying. Two females who are 5'7" tall and who weigh 150 pounds have the same BMI. If one is an athlete with 20% body fat and the other is inactive at 35% body fat, not only is their body composition different but so are their relatively health risks. It's also not uncommon for active individuals, generally males, to be told that they are overweight due to a high BMI score although they are relatively lean and simply carry more muscle mass. This leads to active individuals to often suggest that BMI should be thrown out for being useless but this is an over reaction. BMI was never meant to be used in an athletic population.

In the general public, it is simply not that common to find people with high BMI who also have a low BF% although people with a low BMI often have a fairly high BF% (they are often called skinny fat). It's also possible to have a high BMI and be metabolically healthy or a low BMI and be unhealthy (1). But no body composition method is perfect and BMI is not useless, it's limitations simply have to be acknowledged. For that same group, BMI will give at least a rough indicator of general health risk along with giving a fairly easy way to track changes from diet and exercise (technically since height is not changing, tracking body weight would provide the same information).

And while BMI has primarily been used to track overall health trends, it turns out that it can give a rough estimate of BF% (2). A calculator to determine BMI can be found here:
http://www.cdc.gov/healthyweight/assessing/bmi/adult_bmi/english_bmi_calculator/bmi_calculator.html

That BMI value can be used to estimate BF% here:
http://healthiack.com/body-fat-percentage-calculator

Due to its easy of use, I have used this method in my books for over a decade. And while inappropriate for athletic individuals, I think it is probably the easiest approach for people first starting out. It's quick and easy, provides a good starting point and can be used to track changes over time. Once someone has been working out consistently for 6+ months, I would not consider BMI to be accurate and they should use another of the described methods.

Tape Measure/Circumference Measurements

Although decidedly low-tech, it is actually possible to get a decent estimate of BF% with nothing more than a tape measure. The military has often developed a lot of these equations since they need to be able to measure a lot of people quickly and easily. There are online calculators that estimate BF% in this fashion that generate results that are at least similar to more complicated methods which can be found here:

http://www.freeweightloss.com/caclulators/

Even if they are not used to track body composition per se, tape measure measurements still provide another way to track general progress while dieting (or attempting to gain muscle). During a diet, a decrease in circumference measures (i.e. diameter of the hips or arms) generally indicates body fat loss and it's not uncommon to see this occur even in the absence of much weight loss. Muscle is denser and takes up less space than body fat so someone gaining some muscle while losing fat should still see a reduction in their tape measure measurements. Taking a variety of measurements including arms, bust, waist, abdomen, hip and thighs can provide a general indication of whether fat is being lost and specifically from where. Even a single trouble spot (i.e. arms or thighs) could be tracked in this fashion.

Whether used for BF% estimation or just as a general tracking method, the tape measure is not without problems. First and foremost it's critical to always measure at the same spot, around the largest part of the bust or halfway down the thigh or what have you or the values can't be compared to each other. This is not always easy and even slight differences in where the measurement is taken can make them inaccurate. It's also important to at least try to pull the tape measure to the same tension every time, neither too tight nor too loose. This can also be very difficult to do and there are tape measures with a spring on the end such as the Gulick II which will improve the accuracy of measurements.

Waist/Hip Ratio (WHR)

The waist/hip ratio is exactly what it sounds like, that is the ratio of the waist (measured with a tape measure at the narrowest part) and the hips (measured with a tape measure at the widest part). Technically the WHR ratio is not a measure of body composition but a measure of body fat distribution and health risk. On average, women tend to have a lower WHR than men but WHR can go up with menopause, PCOS/subclinical hyperandrogenism and in obesity. A WHR calculator can be found here:

http://www.healthcalculators.org/calculators/waist_hip.asp

As with circumference measures, it's important to not overtighten the tape measure.

Skinfold Calipers

Possibly the most commonly used method of BF% measurement are skinfold calipers, a small plastic device that is used to squeeze fat at different parts of the body. The measurements go into an equation that then estimates BF%. A variety of sites ranging from 3 to 7 (or more) can be used and numerous different equations exist. Typical sites for women's measurement are the back of the arm, chest, iliac crest (above the hip) and thigh. Calipers give a BF% estimate that is usually close to much more high-tech methods at least in the hands of a trained user. Trained is a key word here as using calipers correctly takes a good deal of practice and many do not have it (this can be a big problem at commercial gyms with a high employee turnover). My general experience is that most trainers are hesitant to grab as much fat as they should. Many women have a thigh skinfold that is nearly impossible to measure accurately in many cases. This can lead to drastically underestimated BF% values.

While generally accurate when used properly, calipers do have an inherent error of about 2-3% in either direction (note that all methods have some degree of inherent error). This means that they may not be able to pick up smaller changes in BF% to begin with. Fat cells do store water and changes in water retention (that will usually show up as changes in scale weight) can impact on skinfold measurement. The equations can be problematic as well. A host of assumptions are being made about bone density (which differs between women and men, can vary with training, etc.) which can cause them to give some strange values, even if the skinfold measurements are accurate. The equations will occasionally put women well below the 10% lower limit for essential fat, men have been estimated at 1-2% and, due to differences in bone density, black male athletes are occasionally given a negative number. Although it doesn't give an estimate of BF%, some recommend just tracking the skinfold changes. If the thigh skinfold goes down from 25mm to 22mm, fat has been lost.

There are many different calipers on the market ranging from very cheap one site click types (which I do not recommend as they are very inaccurate) to $400 clinical calipers used in research. The best one I've found in terms of the price to accuracy ratio is the Slimguide caliper. At $29.99 it's as accurate as the more expensive models and only a little more than the cheaper models which can be incredibly inaccurate. They are indestructible and any reader who wants to be able to track at least some of their own skinfolds could pick up a set and practice on themselves.

Underwater Weighing/Bod Pod

Underwater weighing is an older method of estimating BF% and often considered the "Gold Standard" for measuring body composition in that it was thought to give the most accurate value (other methods were usually compared to it in research). Underwater weighing requires getting dunked into water in a bathing suit and is essentially based on the rather simple concept that fat floats. First the person is weighed on land and then again underwater and this allows BF% to be estimated. While reasonably accurate, underwater weighing facilities are not commonly found outside of research laboratories and can be expensive. Similar to underwater weighing, a fairly new technology is the Bod Pod; it measures how much air a person displace and represents a similar concept to the above. It is done on land and in clothes but the machine is very expensive and not commonly found. There is also some recent question as to the Bod Pod's overall accuracy and I mention it only for completeness.

Due to the cost and difficulty of access, it's unlikely that either underwater weighing or the BodPod will be particularly useful in most situations readers of this book might encounter. Tracking fat loss or muscle gain requires that measurements be made at some reasonable frequency and using either method frequently is somewhat unrealistic. One approach that could be used would be to get an estimation via underwater weighing and compare it to a simpler method such as calipers or the taper measure. If two measurements 4-8 weeks apart can be obtained, it will indicate how close the simpler method is to the supposedly more accurate method both in terms of absolute values and changes. Then only the simpler method would be used going forwards.

Bioelectrical Impedance (BIA)

I mentioned in the last chapter that some scales at least attempt to estimate BF%, rather than only measuring body weight, and BIA scales represent the primary approach to this. BIA works on the basic concept that fat and LBM have different amounts of water. It works by running an electric current through the body and this can be foot to foot (scales), hand to hand (little handheld devices) or hand to foot (specialized equipment) and using the speed of measurement to estimate body water and BF%. While quick and easy, BIA is extremely sensitive to water balance in the body. Drinking a large glass of water or having a large urination can change the values and some devices have an athlete and non-athlete mode that will give different BF% values for the same person measured at the same time. If hydration status is controlled extremely well, BIA might have some role but this tend to be uncommon outside of research. Change's in body weight and water throughout the menstrual cycle would make this method almost impossible due to shifting amounts of water weight although women with one of the hormonal modifiers would have less issue in this regard. Overall I do not recommend BIA.

Infrared Reactance/Bodymetrix/Skulpt

Infrared reactance (IR) is an old method where a device was put against the biceps (front of the arm) and measured how quickly a beam bounced back as this was meant to indicate how much muscle and fat was present. Not only is measuring at that single site not very useful as it has no relationship to the rest of the body, the method was originally developed to get a rough estimate on cattle for farmers. It's not very accurate and I do not recommend it. There are two related devices which are the Bodymetrix and Skulpt which claim to measure skinfolds without having to use calipers or pinch the person. Both work by bouncing a beam through the fat and back to determine its thickness and this is used to estimate BF%. Both are kind of cool and high-tech and use multiple measurement sites. The devices are somewhat expensive and I doubt that any but the highest end commercial gyms would have one. I also haven't seen any validation of their accuracy. They are worth watching but at the current time I can't recommend them.

Dual-Energy X-Ray Absorbitometry (DEXA)

DEXA, relatively speaking, is both one of the newer and higher tech methods of measuring body composition, using some fairly high technology to make a head to toe toe full body scan. In doing so, and in contrast to the other methods I've discussed, DEXA can determine a person's body composition beyond just fat and LBM. Most importantly to readers of this book, and this was the purpose for its original development, DEXA can measure bone mineral density (BMD). Currently it is the only method that is able to do this. While DEXA machines have been expensive and relatively difficult to find in the past, their availability is increasing while the the cost of a measurement is decreasing.

While the ability to measure DEXA is reason enough to consider it, it will also estimate BF%, killing two birds with one stone. While it gives an overall measure of BF%, DEXA is unique in that it will provide a BF% for the upper and lower body separately. So it might tell a woman that her upper body is 20% body fat and her lower body is 27% body fat. While this can be useful to track the changes in regional body fat levels (i.e. upper body might drop by 3% but lower by only 1%), for the purposes of this book, only the whole body BF% will be important.

I do need to make an important point about DEXA relative to other methods as it pertains to how information later in this chapter and book will be presented. In many cases, I will recommend specific aspects of diet set up or other issues be based on starting BF%. And the values I have traditionally used came from older methods such as calipers or rough visual assessment. This is important as DEXA seems to give systematically different numbers than those older methods, in the realm of 3-6% higher (3). Demonstrating this, a number of top physique competitors have been measured via DEXA in contest shape and invariably the values are at least 3% more than what calipers would put them at (i.e. a woman might be calipered at 10% but DEXA would say she is 13% or higher). I don't honestly know what is responsible for this difference and I don't think it matters in a practical sense. It simply needs to be recognized. When I provide some rough BF% for different goals below and present my Category system I will provide both the older method values along with adjusted DEXA values.

While the price is decreasing, DEXA does cost more than other methods and would be generally inappropriate for regular tracking of a diet or muscle gain program. Measurement simply have to be made too frequently to be cost effective or practical under most conditions. Which doesn't mean that DEXA shouldn't be considered, due to its ability to track changes in BMD. As BMD changes far more slowly than body fat, an annual DEXA measure would probably be more than sufficient. When it is done, it could be correlated with a simpler method such as calipers or the tape measure with the simpler method being used for most short-term tracking.

Other Tracking Methods

While having some initial estimate of BF% is important for many topics in this book, and is important to track on some level, there are other methods of tracking progress on a diet (or when trying to gain muscle). None estimate body composition per se but in conjunction with one of the methods above, they have their use. Tape measure measurements are one of these but were discussed earlier.

The Scale

Hopefully after reading the last chapter, you understand that short-term fluctuations in scale weight don't represent anything real (in terms of the gain or loss of actual body fat or LBM). I should mention one major exception. For women who are carrying a significant amount of body fat (what I will call a Category 3 dieter, defined below), assuming even the most basic exercise and nutrition program is in place, almost all weight lost will be body fat outside of the initial drop in water weight. In this case, the scale may be all that is necessary to track progress. This is especially true as many of the true BF% methods tend to become inaccurate at the extremes of high or low body fat. For women not in this situation, the scale can still provide useful information but only if the person using it can accept that day-to-day changes are meaningless and they should not make poor lifestyle choices based on those changes.

In recent years, there has been a good bit of backlash against the scale, especially for women. Some of this is based on what I've discussed already in terms of it not representing changes in body composition or what have you, that the day-to-day changes make the practice useless. While I have made similar arguments above, the key to weighing is to do it daily and use those measurements to create a 7-day rolling average (this just means that every new day's number will replace the value from 7 days ago). This approach smoothes out the daily fluctuations (one higher day is offset by a lower day) and creates a trend line that is either flat, downwards or upwards representing no change or a real loss or gain of some type of body tissue (the scale still can't say if it's fat or muscle). It also eliminates the inaccuracy of measuring once weekly where a single day's fluctuation can give a very inaccurate picture of what is actually occurring in the body.

Recent research has found that daily weighing actually helps people to adopt new health habits, probably by focusing their attention to those goals (4). If a woman weighs daily, it acts as an immediate reminder that she is attempting to change her eating or activity habits and that along helps with adherence. Daily weighing and feedback was also shown to help college aged women avoid the normal freshman year weight gain that tends to occur by giving them better feedback (5). Regular monitoring of body weight has also been shown to help with long-term weight maintenance, a topic I will discuss more in Chapter 31 (6). While short-term fluctuations should still be ignored, a true increase in weight of perhaps 3-5 pounds should indicate that the dieter is backsliding and that more focus needs to be placed on eating and activity patterns (7). Regarding psychological stress, while some women might be impacted, overall the practice of daily weighing has not been shown to cause psychological problems (8).

While body weight can be tracked with a spreadsheet, there are apps such as <u>Happy Scale</u> and others that can do it. Even some recent bathroom scales will keep a built-in rolling average of weight. Whether dieting or attempting to gain weight, it is ideal to weigh at the same time of day under the same conditions. This usually means in the morning, preferably after using the bathroom. Weight can be taken naked or clothed although naked will give more consistent values (clothes can weigh 1-2 lbs or 0.5-1 kg or so). Clearly if any given woman finds that daily weighing is causing her psychological stress, it should be abandoned. But overall, so long as the scale is used properly, it is a useful tool with daily weighing being the superior approach overall. I would mention that even this approach to using the scale can be a problem for the normally cycling woman as the weekly changes in body weight will make the averages inaccurate. I will discuss this issue below along with how to take it into account/work around it.

The Mirror/Pictures

Along with the tape measure and the scale, another non-body composition method that can be useful to track changes is to simply use the mirror or pictures. The reality is that most people (women or men) who want to lose weight/fat or change body composition do it primarily to look better (specifically to look better naked). This is actually critical for physique athletes who are judged on their appearance but even performance athletes who want to alter body composition for their sport are often concerned with their appearance as well. This is especially true for women due to the societal pressures that are present here. The mirror or pictures can be useful in this regard but there are some issues that I want to address.

One problem is that the mirror or pictures can lie. Or, perhaps more accurately, the person's brain can lie to them about what they are seeing. This is most pronounced in many eating disorders where an extremely skinny individual will still "see" a fat person in the mirror (males tend to see a skinny body even while heavily muscled). Even outside of that extreme, most people will tend to focus on what they perceive as their specific trouble spots or simply see a different body that is actually there. As I'll discuss somewhat later in the book, it's extremely common for dieters who have reached an extremely low level of body fat to see themselves as fat even when they are at a BF% that is fairly low.

There is an additional issue which is that there are often differences in mirrors or lighting that can impact drastically on a person's visual appearance. In general, very bright lights tend to worsen appearance as it washes everything out and slightly darker lights (within limits) improve it. Every gym seems to have one particularly magic mirror that makes people look significantly leaner or more muscular than they actually are. Using the same mirror under the same lighting will avoid this problem.

Similar to the mirror, pictures can provide not only a way of tracking but a record of the changes that have occurred. In some ways, they may be better than the mirror in that they are taken less frequently. Over short periods of time, unless someone is extremely lean (here I am talking about certain types of athletes), visual changes just don't occur that quickly. Looking in the mirror daily, someone is highly unlikely to see any visual changes occurring and this can be demoralizing. Even if those changes are occurring, they tend to be too small on a day-to-day basis to be noticeable. In contrast, taking pictures every 4-8 weeks will tend to show more visual changes, especially if they are compared side by side.

As with all aspects of tracking changes, it's critical to take pictures under the same conditions. This means that the same clothing (or something very similar should be worn), the same lighting, distance from the camera, etc. should be used. If this is not done, the pictures will not be comparable to one another. It's a dirty little secret in the fitness and diet industry that many of the before and after pictures being used to sell a product may be taken on the same day. Changing the lighting from harsh to lowered, tanning, having the person wear a more flattering outfit, change their posture, go from frowning to smiling makes a staggering difference in no time at all. If you look closely the person may be standing slightly differently, twisted at the waist to narrow it, etc.

Clothing Fit

Similar to the use of the tape measure and circumference measurements, another approach to tracking progress is to go by the way clothes fit. In some ways this is actually superior to the tape measure in that the issue of measuring the exact same place is eliminated. If a specific piece of clothing is fitting more loosely, body composition is improving and if that same piece of clothing is fitting more tightly, it may be worsening. I say may as those athletes focusing on gaining muscle may still find some clothes fitting more tightly due to the increases in muscle mass. Even after the dieting is done, when long-term maintenance is the goal, clothing be used to catch problems before they get out of hand (this is just another method of monitoring like using the scale). If a specific piece of clothing starts to get tight again, weight regain may be occurring and the individual will know to become more focused on their eating and exercise habits.

Choosing From the Different Methods

Having looked at a variety of ways of either estimating BF% or tracking progress while attempting to alter body composition (whether losing fat or gaining muscle) I want to make some more specific recommendations about how to integrate them. Once again, every method has its pros and cons, benefits and drawbacks. None are perfect and most are best used to track progress over time rather than being considered as a one-time measurement. Regardless of the specific measurement, if it is changing in the goal direction (i.e. down for fat loss, up for muscle gain), that is what matters most. As well, except for some of the methods I explicitly stated were inaccurate (i.e. BIA, Infrared), the differences in the values given by most methods should all be fairly close to another. If one method gives a BF% of 22% and another a BF% of 25%, that's simply not meaningful. It certainly won't significantly impact on most of what I will present in this book.

Perhaps the best way to offset any given method's cons is to use some combination of methods rather than relying exclusively on one (perhaps the lone exception to this is the woman carrying significant fat for whom weight loss will almost always indicate fat loss). That way, any changes that are not picked up by one method will become apparent by another. So consider a woman who we know lost 2% body fat at (roughly 2.5 lbs/1.2 kg for a 130 lb/59 kg woman). The error inherent in calipers might not be able to measure that but a 7-day rolling average of her scale weight certainly would. If she were very lean, she might also notice visual changes in the mirror. I think you get the idea.

In terms of specifics, despite their limitations, scale weight (combined with some measure of BF%) will be required in order to do the calculations that I will present in this book. Again, a 7-day average or at least measuring at specific times of the month along with ignoring small daily variations are the key to making this method useful. Used properly, calipers are surprisingly accurate but tend to have problems at the high and low extremes of body fat. Paying attention only to changes in the values can be useful here although this doesn't provide a BF% estimate. As well, without a helper, only a handful of sites can be measured unless someone is a contortionist. BMI is quick and easy and can either be used as a general indicator of health or to estimate BF%. It is not appropriate for athletic or well-trained individuals. Tracking the WHR ratio may be useful for women who are carrying large amounts of fat around the midsection since it indicates the loss of visceral fat which indicates an improvement in health. The tape measure can be surprisingly accurate to estimate BF% as well as tracking changes in inches overall.

To one or more of those methods that tracks or semi-tracks some aspect of body composition, the mirror or pictures (or a test piece of clothing) can be added. Basically the combination of a BF% estimate, possibly another method that tracks regional changes in body composition (WHR or tape measure) and at least one non-BF% method of tracking progress will probably give the best combination in terms of providing enough different data points to truly track changes. Some may not even need all of those and I can't cover every possible circumstance to make recommendations. I'd only reiterate, at the risk of beating a dead horse, is that short-term changes in any of these measurement methods tend to mean very little in the big scheme. Focusing on larger changes is the key to making any of them work.

Let me finish by making an often under appreciated point which is that changes in body composition or even weight are generally not only slow but rarely happen in a constant or linear fashion. Weight or BF % may drop, then remain unchanged for a week or two before dropping significantly (seemingly overnight), etc. The same tends to occur for those trying to gain weight with weight going up, stalling, going up some more. There are a number of reasons for these plateaus and stalls that I'll discuss in Chapter 25 but women must understand that a lack of change for a week or two means nothing.

Body Composition Numbers

Having looked at the concept of body composition/BF% in the last chapter and methods of estimating/tracking it above, I want to address the question of what a good or appropriate BF% might be. The answer to that question depends entirely on the situation. The optimal BF% for basic health will differ than that for optimal athletic or appearance goals. While healthy levels BF% have been thrown around, it's now becoming clear that it is possible to be healthy while carrying significant body fat or to be unhealthy while being lean. Much of this comes down to activity levels and active individuals with more fat are often more metabolically healthy than those who are lean but inactive. Which isn't to say that there isn't a general relationship between increasing BF% levels and health, simply that it is not universal.

While excess body fat tend to be highly associated with health risks, it's equally possible to carry too little body fat for optimal health. At the lower extremes of BF% (10-12% for women) as seen among some athletes or in anorexia, a woman's physiology is severely negatively impacted in terms of her hormone levels, menstrual cycle function, etc. This will be discussed in great detail in Chapter 12. This just means that there is some happy medium to be had between too little and too much in terms of health status. I would mention that, even in those cases where a woman might not be able to achieve a supposed "healthy" BF%, even a 5-10% fat loss from her current level drastically improves health and fertility.

Moving to sports performance, what represents an optimal BF% can vary enormously depending on the sport and I discussed at least some of this in Chapter 4. Some sports, especially those that require the body to move across or against gravity tend to be both lighter with a lower BF% than those that don't. Runners tend to be lighter/leaner than cyclists who are lighter and leaner than swimming while rowers are larger and may carry more fat overall. In some sports, shotput for example, higher levels of body weight and BF% may improve performance through a variety of mechanisms.

Athletes in weight class sports tend to be relatively lean as this allows them to carry more muscle at any given bodyweight; many have a Superheavy weight class where weight is unlimited and the athletes often carry significantly more fat. In some of these sports, it's common to train at a higher body weight and BF% before reducing body fat and manipulating water weight at the last minute to make their class. A large number of women's sports such as gymnastics, ballet and figure skating tend to have an aesthetic component emphasizing extreme thinness and BF% tends to be low in those sports. The physique sports of bodybuilding, physique, figure and bikini have requirements that range from the lowest limits of women's BF% to slightly below the average/healthy range.

I would note that even in sports where a lower BF% is common or where losing body fat may improve performance, this does not imply that lower is always better. As I'll discuss in detail in Chapter 12 and touch on throughout this book, a woman can develop hormonal, metabolic, physiological and other problems from the dietary and exercise requirements to get super lean and this can have the contradictory effect of harming performance. Outside of those sports, such as the physique sports, where a specific BF% is required, performance athletes should strive to reach an optimal BF% rather than a minimal one.

In terms of non-athletic appearance goals, the types of bodies that are often held up as societal ideals are perhaps 18-20% for women or a bit higher, generally with less muscularity. To put this into perspective, women tend to get visible abdominal muscles (the 6-pack) around 15-17% or so and this is leaner than many want to be outside of specific athletic subcultures. While many skinny and/or light women might appear lean, they often have a high BF% which is called being-skinny fat.

I've presented some relatively average values for BF% for different situations below and you will see two values. The first represents numbers derived from older BF% methods while the second is their DEXA adjusted equivalents.

Situation	Older	DEXA
Lower Limit	10-12%	16-18%
Extreme Obesity	50%+	56-58%
Average	21-28%	27-34%
Recommended for "health"	18-25%	24-31%
In Shape by Mainstream Media Standards	~18-20%	~23-26%
Physique Athletes*	10-18%	16-26%
Performance athletes	Varies	Varies

*Physique represents bodybuilding, physique, figure and bikini and the degree of required leanness varies between them.

Readers who want a rough visual idea of what the above numbers represent can see examples of what women at different BF% look like here (note that the listed percentages are based on the older methods rather than DEXA):

https://www.bodyrecomposition.com/fat-loss/female-body-composition-examples.html/

In addition to giving some context for the numbers in the above chart, the pictures at that link can provide somewhat of a reality check for the estimated or assumed BF% a person may have. It's not uncommon for online fitness forums to give people body fat estimates based on visual assessment and many are being given bad information in that they are being told that they are 14-16% body fat when they are really 25%. For physique athletes especially, this causes enormous problems as women underestimate their dieting time and get nowhere close to reaching their goals.

Diet Categories

While estimating BF% is important for many reasons, at least one of those is for readers to determine what dieting category they are in. This is a delineation I have used for many years now and is based around the fact that a woman's physiology is changing to one degree or another based on her current BF%. I won't detail those here but those physiological changes impact on many practical aspects such as how much protein she might need while dieting, her relative risk of menstrual cycle dysfunction, how rapidly she will be able to lose weight or fat, her relative risk of muscle loss and others. When I look at the research relating to women's body fat issues, it will be important to recognize what category the subjects being studied are in. I've presented my categorization system using both older BF% methods and adjusted DEXA values below.

Category	Older Methods	DEXA
1	24% and lower	27-30% and lower
2	25-34%	28-40%
3	35%+	38-41%+

While I have presented the table with rather discrete cut off points, please realize that this is a continuum. My cutoff points are based on underlying physiology but it's not as if physiology changes completely from one category to the next. A woman at 35% body fat (41% via DEXA) is far closer to a Category 2 female physiologically than a woman at 45%. Similarly, a Category 2 dieter at 25% is essentially the same as a Category 1 dieter. But some sort of delineation is required to make the system work and I'll only suggest that women at the very low end of one Category should consider themselves in the next lower category in terms of the rest of this book. So a woman at 35% body fat (41% by Dexa) should consider herself in Category 2 in terms of her diet set up, etc.

Some Category Comments

Before looking at some last practical issues, I want to make some brief comments about the Categories above and who might typically be found within them. In general, the Category 1 female tend to be involved in some degree of training. They could be in one of the physique sports, a performance sport or be what I will call a serious trainee (possibly workout out intensely 5-6 times per week but not competing). In many cases, either for performance, competition or appearance, these women will want to lose some amount of body fat As frequently they may want to gain muscle. The physique athlete may wish to bring up weak bodyparts and many performance sports benefit from increased muscle mass. I'd note that there can be a Category 1 female who is not active or training. They frequently are genetically lean although they still want to lose weight. Weight gain is a rare but very occasional goal.

Category 2 tends to span the broadest range of possible situations since it matches up with relatively average BF% for women to begin with. Athletes may be in this group as many sports do not require extreme leanness, many recreationally exercising women may also be in this group. It's possible for a physique athlete who let their body fat get away from them in the off-season to be here although that can cause a lot of problems when it's time to diet down for a contest. The serious trainee might fall here if here diet isn't set up correctly such that, despite all of the training, she is not losing body fat or maintaining a lower body fat effectively . It's just as likely for women to be in Category 2 who are sedentary or only minimally active. Fat loss is likely to be the primary goal in this group.

In general, Category 3 women are the least likely to be involved in any sort of training program or sports although there are certainly exceptions. As I've mentioned, in some sports such as the throws in track and field or the super-heavyweight classes of some strength/power sports, athletes benefit from being heavier and athletes may carry a significant amount of body fat despite being involved in intensive training. While it's atypical for them to want to lose fat until they are done competing, they frequently desire to increase their muscle mass to improve performance. Overall, it is far more likely for the Category 3 women to be relatively sedentary. In this case, fat/weight loss and/or improving health and fertility is likely to be the exclusive goal.

A Female Specific Issue for Tracking Body Composition

With the understanding of what body composition/BF% is and how to measure and track it, I want to address a female specific issue that goes unconsidered by most that the normally cycling woman must contend with (women with a hormonal modifier have less of an issue with this). That issue is the often considerable changes that occur throughout the menstrual cycle in water retention. This not only impacts on scale weight but can also impact on other methods of tracking (9). Both calipers and the tape measure measurements can readily be altered during different weeks of the month and, depending on its degree, water retention can make women feel or look puffy in the mirror or in pictures or make clothing fit differently. As I described in Chapter 2, the late follicular and late luteal phase (Weeks 2 and 4 respectively) tend to be the worst in this regards with the early follicular (Week 1) generally showing the lowest body weight and early luteal (Week 3) being somewhere in-between.

This causes several problems. The first is that it can exacerbate the normal issues many have with the scale. The woman who is already fixated on the small day-to-day changes can be driven mad by the weekly changes as she will be adhering to her diet and exercise program and almost over night, her weight spikes by several pounds or kilograms. Hopefully readers will avoid at least this issue now that I have pointed out what those types of fluctuations mean but I've even known female trainees who, despite knowing full well the difference between body composition and body weight, still getting affected by these types of weight shifts. Even taking a rolling average as I recommended above doesn't eliminate this because the average value and trend line will be shifting up and down each week. Within any given week, the rolling average will be useful but from week to week it will not be. An added issue is that it makes tracking changes more difficult for the normally cycling woman compared to women with most of the hormonal modifiers or men since comparing different weeks of the cycle to one another won't give any accurate indication of what is happening in response to her diet or exercise program.

To better illustrate this, I've shown a hypothetical month of average weekly body weights and how they might change in different weeks of the cycle along with month to month. These numbers are for illustration only and any individual woman may see smaller or larger changes from week to week.

Phase	Month 1	Month 2	Month 3
Early Follicular	143 lbs	141 lbs (-2)	140 lbs (-1)
Late Follicular	147 lbs	145 lbs (-2)	144 lbs (-1)
Early Luteal	145 lbs	143 lbs (-2)	142 lbs (-1)
Late Luteal/PMS	150 lbs	148 lbs (-2)	147 lbs (-1)

You can see that average body weight is changing from week to week during the month with the lowest value occurring in the early follicular phase and the highest in the late luteal phase. I might go so far as to suggest women avoid any measurement during the last week of the cycle due to the large increase that can occur which can be extremely psychologically stressful. In practice that would mean only tracking for three weeks out of the month. Perhaps the bigger point of the table is that comparing any individual week of the cycle to any other individual week is rather pointless due to the water weight shifts that are occurring. Weight goes up from the early to late follicular phase, goes down to a different number in the early luteal before increasing again in the late luteal phase. The week-to-week shifts in hormones and body weight make any comparisons useless. The same holds for other body composition methods.

At the same time, you can see that it is possible to compare one week of the month to the same week of the following month. Bodyweight or BF% could be compared between the early follicular phase of Week 1 and the early follicular phase of Week 2 and this will give some indication of what is actually happening over time. The same would hold for the late follicular to late follicular, early luteal to early luteal and late luteal to late luteal. So from Month 1 to Month 2, body weight goes down 2 lbs in each week of the phase. The numbers are all still different from each other but the absolute change is the same. I've shown a similar result from Month 2 to Month 3. The changes might not be this consistent in the sense that every week might not show the same 1 or 2 pound loss and I'd expect the late luteal phase to be the most variable. But overall, comparing only like weeks of the cycle to each other will give a much better indication of what is happening than trying to compare weeks within the same month.

This does raise the question of what a woman's "real" weight or BF% both for her own peace of mind as well as within the context of the calculations that will appear late in this book. That is, which week's numbers should a woman use when setting up her diet or protein intake or what have you? In one sense it doesn't matter so long as the same week of the month is used to make any changes. In another sense, since any increase in water weight from week to week isn't "real" in the sense of representing a true change in body composition, measuring in a week where water retention is known to occur makes no sense. As water retention is likely to be at its lowest during the early follicular phase, I'd generally recommend using the average body weight, BF% estimate, from that week. Usually weight will be at its lowest roughly 3-4 days following menstruation and this would give the best indicator of a woman's true weight. There is another reason that using the early follicular phase to set up a diet is important related to when it's best for the normally cycling woman to actually start her diet that I will discuss in a later chapter.

How Often Should Measurements be Taken?

The final question I want to address regarding tracking body composition is how frequently measurements should be taken, either for general tracking purposes or to know when some aspect of the diet may need to be adjusted. In general, outside of the daily weighing/rolling average I described, most people probably take measurements too frequently. Even with the scale, this is true and people will weigh when they wake up, before and after they go to the bathroom, with and without clothes, in the evening with the goal of getting the lightest weight possible (this is of course the correct value). At any gym you can see dieters weighing before and after the workout to see how much they've lost. Even with other methods, people go a little bit nuts. They'll break out the calipers or tape measure daily or multiple times daily and just drive themselves crazy by doing so. Measurement error and the small day-to-day changes I described make this pointless and even actual body composition changes are far too slow for this to be useful.

The only possible exception to the above is the very lean Category 1 female who is nearing the end of her diet where appearance and even skinfolds may be changing very rapidly. This will never happen in the Category 2/3 female and the reason has to do with the total amount of fat being lost relative to how much is left to lose. A 130 lb female at 14% body fat with 10% essential fat only has 4% fat or 5 pounds of fat that she can lose. A half-pound fat loss represents 10% of that value and the measurable or visible changes my be profound. In contrast, a 200 lb female at 40% body fat with 10% essential fat has 60 lbs of fat that she could potentially lose. A 2 pound fat loss is only 3% and simply won't be visible or measurable. But outside of that singular population (lean Category 1 females), obsessive and constant measurement only adds to the inherent stress of dieting (stress is discussed in Chapter 13).

At the other extreme, it is possible to measure too infrequently. Whether trying to lose fat or gain muscle, if the diet and training program are set up effectively, changes should be occurring within some reasonable time frame (even if the normally cycling woman has to wait a month to accurately judge it). Waiting endless months before realizing that no progress is being made is wasted time. At some point, some aspect of the diet or exercise program has to be changed if nothing is happening.

Somewhere between those two extremes is a happy medium and I've provided some general guidelines based on the dieter's Category (since that will impact how rapidly significant changes occur). These values should be applied to every form of tracking except for daily weighing which is, by definition, done daily. Since the normally cycling woman may have to wait a month to gauge if changes are occurring, she should use 4 week multiples. Women with any other hormonal modifier can measure anywhere within the recommended range.

Category	Frequency of Measurement
1	Every ~2-4 weeks
2	Every 4-8 weeks
3	Every 8-12 weeks

As the Category 1 dieter is generally an athlete or is on a specific time schedule to reach their goals, they will need to measure the most frequently to ensure that they are not falling behind in their progress. The changes here tend to be small (i.e. fat loss may be no more than 0.5 lbs/0.22 kg per week) but still must be tracked.   Technically speaking, if a woman is normally cycling she will still be having shifts in water weight that mean she can only realistically compare changes every 4 weeks.   If a woman loses her menstrual cycle (assuming it was present to begin with), which is likely to happen if she diets to the lower limits of Category 1, this will cease to matter. With the development of amenorrhea, the normal cyclical changes in hormones will disappear and measurement can be made as often as necessary.

As a woman enters Category 2 or 3, the duration between measurements increases for reasons already mentioned. While changes may occur proportionally faster here (a woman who is heavier or carrying more fat can often lose more quickly), it's still important to avoid too frequent assessment of body composition as there may not be a sufficient enough change to maintain motivation.   But that duration can't be too long or a complete lack of results might be missed. Once again, daily weighing really eliminates this problem as an average trend downwards in weight over time will indicate if the diet or exercise program is effective. It's simply that measurable changes in BF% or visible changes are unlikely to occur that rapidly.

A Basic BF% Calculation

Wrapping up the discussion of BF%, I want to present an equation that will serve as the base calculation for many different aspects of this book (other calculations will be shown in later chapters). That calculation is how to determine, based on body weight and some estimate of BF%, how many actual pounds (or kg) of fat or LBM a person is carrying. Since I will be referring to her throughout this book, I will use a sampler dieter who weights 150 pounds at 22% body fat (Category 1).

Step 1: Convert BF% into a decimal
To do this take the BF% value and divide by 100.
22% / 100 = 0.22
Step 2: Determine Total Pounds of Fat
Next multiply bodyweight by the value in 1 to get pounds of fat.
150 pounds * 0.22 = 33 pounds of fat
Step 3: Determine LBM
Subtract the total pounds of fat from weight to get pounds LBM.
150 pounds total weight - 33 pounds of fat = 117 pounds of LBM.

So she weighs 150 pounds with 33 pounds of fat and 117 pounds of LBM.

This same calculation can be used in reverse to determine BF% based on their LBM and fat mass. I've shown this in the box below for a woman with 30 lbs of fat and 120 lbs of LBM

Step 1: Determine Total Weight
Add the total pounds fat to total pounds lBM
120 lbs LBM + 30 lbs fat = 150 lbs total bodyweight.
Step 2: Determine BF%
Divide total bodyweight by pounds fat and multiply by 100 to get
30 lbs fat / 150 lbs total weight = 0.20 * 100 = 20% body fat

---

It's fairly uncommon to have information on the total pounds of fat or LBM to do the above calculation. Rather, the first equation is generally used to determine the starting point on fat mass and LBM while the second is used to see how changes in either will alter BF% or body composition.

Chapter 7: Altering Body Composition

With an understanding of what body composition represents along with various methods of measuring/tracking it and some representative numbers for body fat percentage (BF%), I want to look at some specifics related to altering body composition. Certainly this won't be the goal of every reader (and I will address general health and fitness later in the book) but, realistically, most women do want to change their body composition either for performance or appearance. I'd note again that there are times when manipulating water and body weight may be relevant for specific athletes or situations but here I will focus on making "real" changes to body composition or BF% in terms of altering the amount of LBM (here referring to muscle mass) and body fat someone is carrying.

In this chapter, I will be looking at a variety of different topics. I will start by looking at how alterations in LBM or fat mass can potentially alter BF% before looking at specific situations where someone might want to alter how much of either that they have. I'll also look at the physiological underpinnings of each process.

The Best Way to Alter Body Composition

Technically, any given reader of this book could have one of two primary goals. The first would be to gain muscle. While the process may be difficult in terms of what is required in terms of training or nutrition, changes here are relatively simple in the sense that gaining muscle will cause muscle to be gained. Losses of body fat may alter how someone looks for any given muscle mass but cannot increase the total amount of muscle mass that someone is carrying. Generally speaking, here the goal is to gain muscle without gaining excessive amounts of fat. In contrast, since it represents the ratio of fat to total bodyweight, gaining or losing LBM or fat can impact on overall BF% although in slightly different ways.

If someone gains LBM without gaining fat, BF% will go down as they are now heavier with the same total amount of fat (only the BF% has changed). Even if some fat is gained, so long as more LBM is gained than fat, BF% still goes down. If fat is lost, BF% goes down almost without exception and in this case a woman will have less total pounds/kg of fat. If fat is lost with no muscle loss, BF% will go down. Even if some muscle is lost (and women are less likely to have this occur), so long as more fat than muscle is lost, BF% will go down. Finally, if someone gains LBM while losing fat, BF% will go down.

This works identically in reverse in terms of BF% going up and body composition worsening. If LBM is lost with no change in total fat, BF% will go up due to fat making up a larger proportion of total weight. If fat is gained either without a change in LBM or in excess of LBM gains, BF% will also go up. In the case where LBM is lost while fat is gained (as occurs in some diseases, with certain drugs and with some types of birth control), BF% will go up and this may be true even if weight doesn't change.

Since it is rare outside of a few specific situations for someone to want to increase their BF%, and since dieting is a far more prevalent goal, I will be focusing primarily on lowering BF% here. And the reason that I am discussing this is due to an oft heard suggestion that, rather than dieting and focusing on fat loss per se, the goal should be to focus on increasing LBM. This idea generally revolves around two primary claims. The first is the fact that muscle burns calories even at rest and that increasing the amount of LBM will raise metabolic rate. Old studies suggested that a single pound of muscle could burn 40-50 calories per day but this is drastically incorrect with the real value being closer to 6 cal/lb or 2.7 cal/kg (1). For perspective, a pound of fat burns roughly 2 cal/lb or 0.9 cal/kg meaning that three pounds of fat will burn the same number of calories as one pound of muscle. The consequence of this is that only the most extreme gains in muscle mass have even the potential to raise energy expenditure meaningfully.

Consider that, over the first 6-7 months of training might gain 3-4 pounds of muscle which amounts to 18-24 calories extra per day burned. Two different studies have found that women show perhaps a 30 calorie per day increase in resting metabolic rate when they gain 4.5 pounds (2 kg) of muscle over 12-24 weeks (1a,1b). A gain of 10 lbs of LBM has the potential to burn 60 calories per day and a massive 20 pound gain in muscle might burn an additional 120 calories per day. Every bit adds up but, in the short-term especially, gains in LBM have no meaningful impact on energy expenditure. It does take energy to synthesize muscle but even there the relatively slow rate of muscle gain in women makes this fairly insignificant. It takes roughly 2,700 calories to synthesize one pound of muscle so a woman gaining one pound of muscle per month might burn ~100 calories extra per day. Any actual increase in energy expenditure from the process of gaining muscle will primarily come from the training involved but long-term increase in metabolic rate from muscle gain are more or less irrelevant under all but the most extreme circumstances.

The second idea behind gaining LBM to lower BF% revolves around the mathematical fact that BF% will go down if pure LBM is gained and body weight goes up. As described above, here the total amount of fat a woman is carrying will not change but, since her total weight has increased, the relative percentage of fat will go down. While this is certainly true, as I'll show in the chart below, the effect of gaining LBM pales in comparison to the process of losing fat in terms of its impact on BF%.

I will be starting with a sample dieter who weighs 150 lbs with a BF% of 22%. The first calculation in the last chapter can be used to determine that she has 117 lbs of LBM and 33 lbs of fat. All I will be doing below is to manipulate the amounts of LBM, fat or both and recalculating BF% (using the second equation from the previous chapter) for each change. All I've done here is recalculate BF% by dividing the total weight by the total amount of fat. I will be making one simplifying assumption which that 100% fat is being lost or 100% LBM is being gained. While this isn't always the case, it makes the math simpler and the differences in the results don't change that meaningfully without that assumption.

First I'll look at moderate changes of either a 5 lb gain in LBM or a 5 lb loss of fat with no other change. I'll also look at what happens if someone gains 5 lbs of LBM while losing 5 lbs of fat (this isn't common and I'm showing it mainly to make a point). I'll also look at the extremes of gaining 20 lbs of LBM (roughly a woman's maximum potential) or losing the same 20 pounds of fat. Finally, just for illustration, I'll show a 10 lb loss of fat.

	Fat (lbs)	LBM (lbs)	Weight (lbs)	BF%	Change
Starting Point	33	117	150	22.0	N/A
+5 pounds muscle	33	122	155	21.3	-0.7
-5 pounds fat	28	117	145	19.3	-2.7
-5 lbs. fat/+5 lbs. muscle	28	122	150	18.7	-3.3
+ 20 lbs muscle	33	137	170	19.4	-2.6
- 20 lbs fat	13	117	130	10.0	-12.0
- 10 lbs fat	23	117	140	16.4	-5.6

The primary message of the above chart is that, in every case, compared to gaining LBM, losing the same amount of fat has a far more pronounced effect on lowering BF%. In the first case, gaining 5 lbs of LBM only lowers BF% by 0.7% while losing the same 5 lbs of fat lowers it by 2.7%, nearly four times as much. Gaining 5 lbs of LBM while losing 5 lbs of fat generates a larger result (3.3% vs. 2.7%, basically the individual results added together) but the major effect is still from losing fat. At the extremes, gaining 20 pounds of LBM only reduces body fat by 2.6%, almost the same as losing only 5 pounds of fat. But losing 20 pounds of fat reduces BF% by 12% from 22% to 10% (the lower limits of what a woman might achieve). Even a 10 pound fat loss causes over twice the reduction in BF% (- 5.6% vs. -2.6%) than gaining 20 pounds of muscle. Half as much fat loss as LBM gain has twice the impact on BF%.

Hopefully the above shows that the impact on BF% by gaining muscle isn't even close to that of actually losing fat. The fact that even smaller amounts of fat loss have a greater effect than enormous gains in LBM shows that; when the numbers are equal, fat loss may have four times the overall effect. Even if this weren't the case, there is an additional issue that must be considered which is the time frames involved.

Because in almost all situations, the fact is that gaining muscle is a grindingly slow process, even moreso for women than men. In contrast, fat loss can occur relatively quickly. So while gaining even 5 pounds of muscle might take 6 months of effort (and might come with a small amounts of fat gain), that same 5 pound fat loss might take only 5-10 weeks. As the numbers get larger, so do the differences. A 10 pound gain in muscle might take a woman a year or more. The same 10 pounds of fat loss might take 10-20 weeks. Gaining the extreme of 20 lbs of muscle is a career goal for most women and might take 3+ years if it is achieved at all. That same 20 lb fat loss might take 6 months for a lean female and less than that for someone in my Category 2 or 3. Even if it took a full year to lose that 20 lbs of fat, it's still one third of the time it would take to gain the same amount of muscle with far greater impact on BF%.

I'll finish this section by noting that everything discussed above works the same in the opposite direction. That is, losing LBM tends to have a relatively small overall impact on increasing BF% while fat gain always has the much more profound effect. Without putting it in chart form, if the sample dieter loses 5 lbs of LBM with no change in her total fat her BF% only increases from 22% to 22.7%. If instead she gained 5 pounds of fat with no change in LBM, her BF% would increase from 22% to 24.5%. Regardless, increasing LBM or preventing it's decrease is still important for other reasons, discussed next.

Gaining and Losing LBM

Irrespective of the fact that gains and losses in LBM have minimal effects on either metabolic rate or BF%, there are still many reasons for women to be concerned about how much LBM they are carrying either in terms of increasing it or preventing its decrease. For general fitness and health, carrying some amount of muscle mass along with some degree of increased muscular strength tends to improve health, strength and overall physical function (i.e. the ability to carry heavier objects). Even small increases in muscle size, especially in women's proportionally weaker upper bodies, can have a huge impact on function and the importance of increasing LBM and strength has finally been recognized by most authorities.

While this is important for all women, it becomes especially critical with aging as there is often a loss of LBM that harms both health and function. I would mention that much of this age related loss is related primarily to changing activity levels. Studies of female master's athlete show a significant retention of LBM compared to their sedentary peers. Women have the additional factor of menopause where LBM loss accelerates significantly, especially if they decide not to go on HRT. This often sets up a vicious cycle where a loss of muscle leads to a loss of function/decrease in activity which causes more muscle to be lost.

For the physique athlete, muscular size is part and parcel of their competitive requirements although the amount of muscle required depends on sport (decreasing from bodybuilding to physique to figure to bikini). Symmetry and balance among muscle groups is key and frequently these athletes only need to gain muscle in specific areas. For performance sports, gaining muscle can improve strength and power production, improving performance in many sports. In others, too much muscle mass can be detrimental. A weight class athlete may not be able to realistically make their weight class if they carry muscle mass beyond a certain point although they may simply move into the next higher weight class. Many endurance sports have performance harmed if excessive muscle is carried, especially in muscle groups not relevant to the sport (i.e. the upper body for runners). I would mention that, due to their generally reduced ability to gain muscle mass, female athletes don't have nearly the concern here as male athletes (who often get a bit overzealous in the weight room in the off-season) but there may be situations (discussed below) where muscle loss is actively sought.

LBM loss is, in general, not good although there are occasional situations where it may be actively desired. Outside of the normal aging process and menopause, probably the most common situation a woman will encounter where LBM loss is a risk is during a diet. Again I'm focusing only on actual muscle mass loss as the early water and glycogen loss is technically LBM. The relative risk of LBM loss depends on a few factors. A primary one is body fat percentage with leaner dieters being at greater overall risk. Category 3 dieters may lose zero actual LBM while Category 2 dieters are at a slightly higher risk and Category 1 female dieting to the extremes the most risk. Other factors play a role here, with the exercise program and diet playing a major role in whether or not LBM is lost. I'd point out again that women are much less likely to lose LBM than men and studies I will describe near the end of the book found that female physique competitors who were performing resistance training and eating sufficient protein lost essentially zero LBM while reaching the lower limits of BF%.

There are a number of reasons to limit LBM losses while dieting. One is that even if BF% is decreasing, the loss of LBM can lead to less than hoped for visual improvements. Dieters end up being slightly smaller versions of their previous self. Maintaining LBM or even increasing it slightly has a profound impact here providing the much sought after "toned" appearance that represents sufficient muscle size coupled with a reduction in BF%. Weight training, in addition to both increasing muscle mass or preventing its loss, can indirectly improve fat loss as well. This is discussed in Chapter 14. A second reason is that avoiding LBM loss while dieting helps to limit the normal drop in metabolic rate (discussed later in the book) that can occur (2).

Additionally, it's recently been found that LBM sends a signal to the brain that can increase hunger; losing LBM while dieting results in more hunger than would otherwise occur. The main risk here is for the Category 1 dieter. So long as they are active and eating sufficient protein, there is little to no problem but I described a subgroup of lean Category 1 females who are inactive who are often attempting to lose weight. As they tend to diet without exercise (especially resistance training) or sufficient protein, they often lose LBM. This leaves them with more rebound hunger than they would otherwise experience which puts them at the risk for rebounding and ending up at a higher BF% than they started at (3).

There are rare occasions where LBM loss may be accepted or even desired. I mentioned one above which is the endurance athlete who may be carrying excess muscle, especially in non-relevant muscle groups, that is harming their performance. Losing that muscle reduces body weight and this often improves their performance. Outside of that there are two primary situations where actively losing LBM or at least avoiding further increases may be appropriate. The first is in PCOS or Category 3 women (and remember that the two are often linked) who has gained a large amount of undesired LBM as they gained weight. Losing that extra LBM during a diet may be an appropriate goal either from an aesthetic point of view or to allow bodyweight to be reduced to the most significant degree.   Similarly those women with PCOS/subclinical hyperandrogenism who are not interested in sports performance (and who tend to put on LBM at a slightly faster rate than other women) may want to explicitly avoid the types of training that tend to increase LBM to the greatest degree. There are still benefits to weight training such as improved health but the program will have to be modified in this situation.

But outside of those very few exceptions, the majority of women should put at least some effort into either increasing their LBM or at least preventing its loss and this is true whether fat loss or simply general health is the goal. I'd note that the type of training that best accomplishes this turns out to be the type of training that either increases or prevents/slows the loss of bone mineral density.

The Physiology of Gaining and Losing Muscle

Without getting into unnecessary complexity, I want to look briefly at the process of either increasing or maintaining muscle (the overall processes tend to be more or less identical). Muscle fibers can technically increase in number (called hyperplasia) or size (called hypertrophy). The latter represents the majority of the increase or decrease in muscle and I will focus only on it. In the simplest sense, subjecting skeletal muscle to certain types of stress causes it to adapt. In the case of muscle gain that generally means weight training (discussed in Chapter 4) where it is forced to work against a heavy weight for relatively short periods of time. This stimulates growth and now amino acids (from dietary protein) must be provided in sufficient quantities as the building blocks of new muscle tissue. Sufficient calories are also required and the best muscle gains will always occur when proper resistance training is combined with sufficient dietary protein and a slight calorie surplus (4). Since their rate of growth is relatively slow, women never need a large calorie surplus and I will give specific recommendations in a later chapter.

The amount of muscle someone can gain is based on a number of factors. There are genetic factors but arguably the most important is the level of reproductive hormones. Testosterone is the key player here although recall that estrogen plays an important role in muscular remodeling as well. Progesterone has a negative effect on muscle growth through various mechanisms.   Due to their lower testosterone levels, women start out with less muscle mass, gain it more slowly, and have less potential in terms of the total amount of muscle that they might gain.   In response to training, at least in beginners, women do gain a similar percentage of muscle as men, the amount is simply smaller in an absolute sense due to starting out with less. Women with elevated testosterone levels due to PCOS/subclinical hyperandrogenism do tend to have more muscle, gain it relatively more quickly and have a higher potential gain that they might achieve. Quite in fact, differences in testosterone levels between women directly predict the amount of muscle and strength that they gain from training (4a).

The process of losing muscle, called atrophy is effectively the opposite of gaining it. Here the muscle fibers are broken down to provide amino acids and energy to the body.   While this can happen in a number of disease states, the most common situation for readers of this book will be dieting. Hormones such as cortisol increase to mobilize fuel and one of its impacts is to break down muscle tissue to provide energy to the body.   Excessive aerobic exercise can cause this as well. This breakdown of muscle is especially prevalent if the diet has insufficient protein and no resistance training is present to "tell" the body to maintain the muscle that it has.   For the record, while it was long felt that extreme caloric deficits caused more muscle loss, this is generally untrue if the diet is set up appropriately. Most very low calorie diets did not use exercise and contained far too little protein and that, rather than the calorie intake per se, was the problem. There are other situations that muscle loss can occur under as well. The loss of estrogen signaling after menopause is one (although resistance training and sufficient protein can at least off set this) and I've mentioned several times that certain forms of birth control can cause this.

Why Gain or Lose Fat?

In addition to the fact that changes in the amount of body fat have a more pronounced effect on changes in body composition and BF% than changes in LBM, the reality is that a large percentage of women are either currently dieting or have dieted at some point in their life. And while their goal may have only been to lose weight, hopefully it's now clear that the goal should actually be losing fat. As I also expect the majority of the readers of this book to be interested in fat loss, for whatever purpose, I will spend proportionally more time on it.

First let me look at the issue of gaining body fat. Certainly body fat gain is, for most people, not an explicit goal but rather a consequence of their lifestyle and environment. The modern environment has been termed obesogenic, meaning that we are surrounded by readily available, high-calorie palatable foods that are easy to over eat with a lifestyle that requires very little activity for most people. That said, there are a small handful of situations where someone might have fat gain as a goal. Fat regain would be a more accurate description as, outside of some specific disease states beyond the scope of this book, it will generally only be a goal after someone has lost a significant amount of fat to begin with. This would include the Category 1 female who had dieted to or near the lower limits of female BF% (~10-12% by older methods). Whether it was done for physique competition or performance, she will need to regain body fat to some level to normalize her hormonal status, physiology, menstrual cycle function, etc. There might also be the occasional performance athlete who had reduced their weight or fat to the point that it harmed performance or health for whom regaining some amount weight and fat might actually improve both. Finally are women with eating disorders that cause them to achieve extremely unhealthy body weight and body fat levels and for whom regaining both weight and fat is part of their recovery. This must be medically supervised and I include it only for completeness.

In terms of sports performance, there are a handful of situations where carrying more body fat can be useful. One is in the types of strength/power sports such as throwing or Olympic lifting (in the unlimited class) where overall body size plays a role in performance simply due to the increased body mass. Since there is a limit to how much LBM can be gained, typically gaining fat is the only real way to increase overall size and weight at some point. Gaining fat not only increases their leverages but allows these athletes to eat enough to support heavy training. Even athletes who have to make a weight class often train at a higher body weight and body fat level and then reduce fat and manipulate water before a competition. They may diet down slightly for a competition before deliberately raising weight and body fat to optimize their training before the next competition.

Moving to the topic of fat loss, there are numerous reasons why a woman might want to lose body fat. Generally, carrying excess body fat tends to be unhealthy although, as I mentioned in Chapter 6s, this relationship is not as cut and dry as many think. Body fat distribution plays a role and I mentioned that carrying more fat in the lower body is healthier than carrying more in the upper body. It is also possible to carry more fat and be metabolically healthy or carry less and be metabolically unhealthy. Activity levels are a major factor here (i.e. being fatter but active may be healthier than being leaner but inactive) but, in general, carrying excess body fat is associated with a variety of health risks. Both insulin resistance and fertility problems are common with obesity (and PCOS which is often associated with it) and even losing small amounts of fat ends to drastically improve these health parameters.

Arguably the most common reason that women will want to lose fat is for appearance reasons. Many people will pay lip service to wanting to improve their health (and this is often true when the issue of fertility is a concern) but, right or wrong, the reality is that most want to look better. In some cases, and this is especially true for women who are fixated on body weight rather than body composition, the goal is to reach some (usually) arbitrary goal weight or lose some (usually) arbitrary amount of weight. If it does nothing else, hopefully this book will demonstrate that body composition is the far more important end goal than body weight per se and that attempting to lose some number of pounds or reach some specific goal weight is not the best way to approach things.

For athletes, body fat reduction may be a goal for performance reasons, appearance reasons, or both. As I mentioned in Chapter 6, reducing body fat can improve performance at least up to a point. Beyond that point, between the hormonal and physiological changes that occur, along with the amount of food restriction and exercise required, performance is often harmed (along with other changes I will discuss in Chapter 12 when I talk about menstrual cycle dysfunction). As I've mentioned, the physique sports have appearance as a primary goal and, whether healthy or not, reducing BF% is part and parcel of competition. There are also some performance sports with an aesthetic component, where the athletes are expected to look a certain way and may be penalized if they do not meet the appropriate requirements. Even for those performance sports without an explicit appearance component, female athletes are often still under pressure from an appearance point of view due to wearing skin-tight outfits in competition or simply those common social pressures that exist for women (but rarely men).

Gaining and Losing Fat: Introduction

In Chapter 5 I mentioned that fat cells are primarily made up of stored triglyceride (TG, three fatty acid chains connected to a glycerol molecule) with a bit of water and the cellular machinery involved in fat cell metabolism and hormone production. Since the glycerol part of the TG isn't that relevant to the discussion, going forwards I will only be focusing on the metabolism of the individual fatty acids (FAs). I am also only going to describe the system generally here as gender differences are discussed in detail in Chapter 10. At any given time, fat cells are both storing fatty acids within the fat cell (called lipogenesis) or releasing them (called lipolysis). It's a fairly continuous process and while this might seem wasteful, it gives the body the ability to rapidly adjust to changes in energy needs. That is, if fatty acids are needed for energy, they are already available for use rather than having to be mobilized first.

In terms of fat gain, it is the balance of these two processes that determines what happens to a fat cell. If more fat is being stored than released (and burned for energy), fat will be gained. If more fat is being released/burned for energy than is being stored, fat will be lost. There are actually two ways that fat can be gained, through an increase in fat cell size or an increase in fat cell number (this runs contrary to old ideas that said fat cell number was set at birth and never changed). When fat is gained, fat cells can increase either in size or number. In contrast, when fat is lost, fat cells will only decrease in size. This is important as, when Category 2 women and men were both overfed, upper body fat cells increased in size while lower body fat cells increased in number (5). Short of surgery, the new fat cells can't ever be lost again.

Both fat gain and fat loss are more generally controlled by what is called energy balance, the difference between calorie intake (from food) and calorie expenditure (from a number of different factors). It is more complicated than this with the balance of nutrients (protein, carbohydrates, fat and alcohol) all having slightly different effects. Since protein is rarely if ever stored as fat and alcohol has only indirect effects on fat gain, I will be focusing almost exclusively on carbohydrates and fat metabolism below.

With that basic background, I want to look in some detail at the physiology of both gaining and losing fat in the same way as I looked at the physiology of gaining and losing muscle. Given that it is relatively more complicated, and given the general focus on fat loss for women (along with some gender specific issues), I will spend much more time on fat loss than fat gain.

Gaining Fat

As I mentioned above, in the most general sense, fat gain occurs when calorie intake exceeds calorie expenditure. As more calories are available than are required, any that can't be used for immediate energy are stored for later use. This can actually include increased carbohydrate storage within muscle or liver as glycogen or fat within the muscle as Intra-Muscular Triglycerides (IMTG) but at least some will go into fat cells. And in this regard, there are a number of gross misconceptions and ideas about what causes fat gain. Since fat cells are made up of the exact same chemical structure found in the fat in food, many assume that eating fat will lead to fat gain. In recent years, the idea that carbohydrates are the cause of fat gain has become popular (usually based on the increase in the hormone insulin).

And it turns out that there is truth to both of ideas in that both carbohydrate and fat can contribute to fat gain; they just happen to do it through different mechanisms (6). Dietary fat contributes to fat storage directly and any that isn't burned for energy or stored as IMTG will be stored in fat cells (under extreme circumstances fat can be stored in places such as the pancreas or liver). In contrast, dietary carbohydrates cause fat gain indirectly by affecting how much fat the body is burning overall. When more carbs are eaten, the body burns more carbs for energy which means it burns less fat. Whatever dietary fat is being eaten is likely to get stored. Similarly, if less carbohydrates are eaten, the body burns more fat for fuel which means less fat may be available for storage.

An often heard claim is that excess dietary carbohydrate is converted to fat and stored (a process called De Novo Lipogenesis or DNL) but this is a process that happens very rarely in humans. Generally it takes massive intakes of carbohydrates (700-900 grams per day) for multiple days to stimulate DNL. Under most circumstances, DNL contributes minimally to fat gain (7). I want to make it clear that this in no way means that a low-carbohydrate diet automatically prevents fat gain. Since they are typically associated with higher total fat intakes, the overall effect may be no different than a higher carbohydrate/lower-fat diet. I would mention only briefly that protein is essentially never stored as fat and alcohol acts very much like carbohydrate in terms of its effect on fat storage. When alcohol is consumed, it must be burned off for energy so anything else that is consumed is more likely to be stored. If alcohol is consumed with fatty foods, this can readily contribute to fat gain. All of that said, an actual net gain in fat can only occur if calorie/nutrient intake exceeds requirements.

While the full details of how fat is stored is incredibly complex, I only want to focus on two key enzymes (both mentioned in Chapter 2) that are involved in storing dietary fat. After it has been eaten, dietary fat goes through complex metabolism in the stomach whereby it is repackaged into something called a chylomicron. These go into the lymphatic system and eventually move past the fat cells. Here an enzyme called Lipoprotein Lipase (LPL, also found in muscle) breaks fatty acids off of the chylomicron for storage within the fat cell. While LPL was thought for decades to be the only key player in this process, it is now known that Acylation Stimulating Protein (ASP), which I mentioned in Chapter 2 is a far more potent stimulator of fat storage, especially in women. For years, it was thought that storage of ingested dietary fat was the only way that fat cells could store fat but there is actually another which is being called the direct pathway (8). Here, fatty acids that have been released from fat cells and which are floating through the bloodstream can be stored directly in fat cells and this occurs without the activity of LPL. More importantly, fatty acids released from fat cells in one place in the body can be stored in fat cells in a different part. I'll talk about the implications of this for women in Chapter 10.

There are a tremendous number of factor which determines how likely or not someone is to store (or lose) fat although many of them are outside of our control. Both the type and amount of exercise play a role here and there are clear genetic differences with some people being more prone to store fat than others. Hormones are key players with insulin playing a primary role in both stimulating fat storage and inhibiting fat mobilization although I'd mention that eating pure dietary fat will stimulate fat storage (via ASP) without the need for insulin to increase. Other hormones tend to play a more modulating role here. Clearly both estrogen and progesterone have an impact on both how easily and where fat is stored. Cortisol, which I have not discussed but will detail in Chapter 13, has an odd impact on fat metabolism in that small pulses of cortisol increase fat mobilization but chronically elevated levels can increase fat storage (especially if insulin levels are high).

The hormonal modifiers can also play a role. I mentioned that birth control can play a role although it seems to be small overall along with the effect depending heavily on the specific type of BC in question. PCOS/hyperandrogenism can contribute to fat gain along with impacting on where that fat is stored. The general aging process along with a shift in women's hormones as she ages also plays a role with menopause causing both weight and fat gain along with a shift in fat patterning unless HRT is begun. While all of these play clear mediating roles in whether or not fat gain occurs, the primary factor is still the balance between calorie intake and expenditure which are about the only two factors that most people have any sort of control over.

Losing Fat: Introduction

As I realistically expect most readers of this book to be primarily interested in fat loss, I will be spending proportionally more time on the topic. Once again, here I will discuss primarily general concepts as female specific issues/gender differences are discussed in detail in Chapter 10. Just as fat gain occurs when more fat is being stored than mobilized in a fat cell, fat loss occurs when more fat is mobilized and then burned for energy that is being stored. And, just as with fat gain, the primary cause of this will be when there is a long-term deficit between calorie expenditure and calorie intake.

In that situation, the body must find an alternative source of energy (or adapt metabolically, discussed in detail in Chapter 9) to make up for the deficit. That means using fuels already stored within the body and that includes stored body fat. If that deficit is maintained for a sufficient time period, the net effect will be that fat is mobilized from fat cells and "lost". I would note again that while fat gain can occur through increases in fat cell size or number, fat loss always occurs through a decrease in fat cell size. Outside of surgery (i.e. liposuction, cryolipolysis), the removal of fat cells (a process called apoptosis by which they actually die) generally only occurs under very extreme conditions.

While the above paragraph more or less sums up fat loss, I want to delve a bit further into the physiology involved as this will be important when looking at some of the gender differences that occur in fat distribution and fat loss itself. To do so I will ignore many of the more minor or less important aspects of the fat loss process and focus only on three: mobilization, transport and oxidation (the actual burning of fat). Let me now look at each in sequence.

Mobilization/Lipolysis

While all of the steps in fat loss are important, arguably the single most critical is that of the actual mobilization and release of fatty acids (called lipolysis) from within the fat cell. I say most critical as, short of surgery, if the fat is never mobilized from the fat cell, it can never be lost. Lipolysis describes the process by which the stored TG is broken down into three FAs and a molecule of glycerol by a variety of enzymes. Those fatty acids and glycerol are released from the fat cell into the circulation around the fat cells and how easily or not this occurs depends on a number of different factors.

One is the actual size of the fat cell. Larger fat cells release FAs more easily than smaller fat cells and this is part of why fat loss becomes more difficult as people get leaner. This actually means that, contrary to belief, people carrying more body fat have an easier time using fat for fuel during a diet (this is part of why they lose less muscle as well). Their fat cells are typically more full and there may be more of them in total and this adds up to an easier time mobilizing fat for energy. One odd factor is the actual type of fat stored in a given fat cells. Here I am talking about saturated and unsaturated fats (this is just a description of their chemical structure and I will discuss them more in Chapter 18). Saturated fats are more difficult to mobilize than unsaturated and it turns out that lower body fat is more likely to store saturated fats. This often make it hard to the touch compared to fat in other parts of the body which is softer or squishy.

The primary enzyme in fat cells that is responsible for lipolysis is Hormone Sensitive Lipase (HSL), which breaks fatty acids off of its glycerol backbone for release into the bloodstream. There are other enzymes of importance but HSL ultimately controls whether or not fatty acids are mobilized. When HSL activity is high, fatty acid mobilization is high and when HSL activity is low, fatty acid mobilization is low. While there is more complexity to the system, HSL activity is ultimately controlled by hormone levels which can either increase or decrease the amount of HSL present or increase or decrease its activity.

There are three primary hormones and multiple secondary hormones that play the major role in either stimulating or inhibiting fat mobilization (9). The secondary hormones here are growth hormone (GH), cortisol and the reproductive hormones, testosterone, estrogen and progesterone. GH directly stimulates lipolysis but the effect is delayed, taking about 2 hours after a surge in levels to stimulate fat mobilization. Women do have higher GH levels than men both at rest and in response to exercise. I mentioned cortisol above and will repeat that it's effects depend on whether or not it is released in short pulses (which mobilizes fat) or is chronically elevated (which may cause fat storage). I detailed the reproductive hormones in Chapter 2 and will only say here that their effect tends to be somewhat indirect, modifying the level of enzymes or receptors that impact on fat metabolism.

The three primary hormones, in that they have direct effects, involved in regulating lipolysis are insulin, the catecholamines and a relatively new hormone called Atrial Natriuretic Peptide (ANP). The first two have been known for decades to have an impact but ANP was not only discovered relatively recently (in 2000) but stimulates lipolysis through a completely different biochemical pathway than other hormones utilize (10). ANP will come up later in the book not only because there are gender differences in how levels respond to exercise but because it has potential to help women with lower body fat loss.

Insulin is arguably the single most important hormone in terms of fat mobilization in that even small increases it can inhibit lipolysis by up to 90%. Even the amount of insulin present in the bloodstream after an overnight fast inhibits lipolysis by 50% from its maximal levels. This prevents an excessive release of fatty acids, as might be seen in Type I diabetes, that can be damaging to the body. In addition to its effects on inhibiting lipolysis, increase in insulin also stimulates fat storage so its effect is two-fold in terms of the fat cell (note that insulin is a general storage hormone also increasing carbohydrate and protein storage elsewhere in the body). Insulin has this effect by binding to the insulin receptor which both activates LPL and inhibits HSL.

Prior to the discovery of ANP, the catecholamines, adrenaline and noradrenaline (or epinephrine and norepinephrine) the fight or flight hormones, were the only hormones thought to directly affect lipolysis. As I mentioned in Chapter 2, adrenaline is released from the adrenal gland and works throughout the body while noradrenaline is released from nerve terminals and only works locally where it is released. Levels of both increase in response to various types of stress although exercise is the one that we tend to have the most control over. The type, amount and intensity of exercise determines how much of each hormone is released with adrenaline primarily being released at lower intensities and noradrenaline not being released in significant amounts until much higher exercise intensities are reached. The catecholamines have their own specific receptors called adrenoceptors (or adrenoreceptors) which are found almost everywhere in the body including the heart, skeletal muscle, liver, fat cells, etc. Here it gets slightly complicated as there are two primary types of adrenoceptor which are called alpha- and beta-adrenoceptors which have roughly opposite effects in the body. There are also multiple subtypes of each such as alpha-1, alpha-2, beta-1, beta-2 and beta-3 which are found in different levels in different parts of the body.

The simplest way to think of beta-receptors is as accelerators of some physiological process. When catecholamines bind, this causes an increase in heart rate, blood pressure, or fat mobilization. In terms of fat cell metabolism, only the beta-2 receptor is relevant and when it is activated, HSL activity will increase, mobilizing fat. In contrast, think of the alpha-adrenoceptor as a brake. When activated, it slows some process, lowering heart rate, blood pressure, calorie burning or decreasing lipolysis. Only the alpha-2 receptor is relevant to fat cells and when it is activated, it will decrease the activity of HSL, decreasing lipolysis. While this may seem needlessly complex, I am discussing it as fat cells in different parts of the body can have different ratios of beta-2 to alpha-2 receptor and this has an enormous impact on the relative ease or difficulty of mobilizing fat. Fat cells with more alpha-2 receptors than beta-2 are more difficult to mobilize than fat cells with the reverse distribution. This actually means that the catecholamines can technically stimulate or inhibit lipolysis depending on the receptor ratio and I will discuss this more below.

In terms of their overall effect on lipolysis, insulin and the catecholamines basically oppose one another. Insulin inhibits HSL activity, inhibiting lipolysis, while the catecholamines (broadly) stimulate HSL activity and stimulate lipolysis. Generally speaking, when insulin is high, as after a meal, the catecholamine levels will be low with nutrient storage being stimulated. In contrast, when the catecholamines are high, as between meals or during exercise, insulin is low with fat mobilization being stimulated. In the rare situations where both insulin and the catecholamines are elevated, insulin's effects will dominate and fat cell lipolysis will be decreased.

Finally there is ANP which, bizarrely, is released from the heart and which is primarily involved in regulating blood pressure and water balance but also stimulates lipolysis. As stated it works through a different overall pathway than insulin and the catecholamines although the end result is still to increase HSL activity. A number of factors regulate ANP with exercise being the one that we can most control. Of some interest ANP can maintain lipolysis even in the face of high insulin and there is some indication that its effects may depend on the specific region of body fat (i.e. upper vs. lower body).

Transport

While the mobilization of fatty acids is the critical step for ultimately losing fat, it isn't sufficient to guarantee fat loss. Quite in fact, a large number of fatty acids that are released turn right back around to be stored within the fat cell a gain, a process called re-esterification. Fat cells can't burn fat for energy which means that any mobilized fatty acids must be carried somewhere in the body that can. The critical step here is the rate of blood flow past the fat cell. If it is high, mobilized fatty acids will be carried away from the fat cell. If it low, they will not and are more likely to be stored again. As it turns out, the same basic factors that control lipolysis tend to control blood flow with insulin, the catecholamines and ANP playing the major role. Insulin has the odd effect of increasing blood flow to fat cells but its overall effects are still to inhibit lipolysis. The catecholamines work identically with beta-receptor activation increasing blood flow and alpha-receptor activation inhibiting it and the ratio of receptors determining the overall effect. ANP improves blood flow to fat cells. Finally, fat mobilization and blood flow tend to be related: fat cells that are resistant to mobilization have poor blood flow and vice versa (11).

Once a fatty acid has been mobilized and transported away from a fat cell, it has a number of potential fates. One is that it can be stored in a different fat cell by the direct pathway I mentioned above. Fat may also be stored within skeletal muscle as IMTG for later use or, in the case of severe obesity, stored in the pancreas or liver. While that storage still technically reduces the size of the fat cell that the fatty acid came from, the fat is not truly lost from the body until the final step in the process has taken place.

Burning/Oxidation

The final step in fat loss is the actual "burning" or oxidation of the fatty acid. This can occur in many tissues of the body including the heart and liver although I will primarily focus on skeletal muscle. Ignoring complex details, the fatty acid is transported into the muscle cell, entering the mitochondria (the powerhouse of the cell) where it reacts with oxygen (hence oxidation) and is broken down to provide energy, water and carbon dioxide (which are then excreted from the body). At this point, the mobilized fatty acid is now truly gone from the body.. And while this process is always continuously occurring, in the situation where more fatty acids are being burned than stored, fat will be lost.

A number of factors impact on the body's ability to use fat for energy. Skeletal muscle contains two fiber types which are Type I which tend to use more fat for fuel and Type II which uses more carbohydrate The relative ratios within a muscle thus impact on the use of fat for fuel. The level of enzymes and density of mitochondria within skeletal muscle also impact on fat burning and both are increased with regular exercise, increasing fat burning potential. As I discussed in Chapter 2, estrogen directly stimulates fat oxidation in skeletal muscle. A major factor impacting on fat burning capacity is the storage of other fuels in the muscle. When muscle is full of carbohydrate, it will burn more carbohydrate for energy. If it is full of IMTG, it will use those for fuel. Lowering levels of carbohydrate or IMTG within the muscle will enhance the use of body fat derived fat for energy. I will discuss this more in Chapter 14.

71

Different Types of Fat

When I described the different types of body fat in Chapter 4, I divided it into multiple types with visceral and subcutaneous fat being the only types of importance here. Visceral fat is a deep type of fat surrounding the organs while subcutaneous fat is underneath the skin and can be subdivided broadly into upper and lower body fat. This division is important as it's now recognized that where fat is found in the body impacts on it's physiology. It's insulin sensitivity, alpha-2:beta-2 adrenoceptor ratio, blood flow, type of fat stored, etc. can all vary which impacts on how easily or not fat is stored or lost from that area.

Even those generalizations are gender specific with women and men often showing not only different but effectively reversed physiologies in different areas of the body (12). Genetic programming very early in life along with levels of reproductive hormones tend to be the indirect causes of these differences which ultimately determine to how the fat cells or blood flow responds to insulin, the catecholamines and possibly ANP. This, along with differences in how women and men metabolize different nutrients (discussed in Chapter 10) ends up explaining a major part of the differences in body composition.

Of all the type of fat, visceral fat is the most metabolically active overall. It does store fat easily after a meal but is generally resistant to the anti-fat mobilizing effects of insulin with more beta- than alpha-receptors and good blood flow. This adds up to a type of fat that is easily to mobilize overall. When visceral fat is present (and in many women it will not be outside of the previously mentioned hormonal modifiers), it is lost readily in response to diet or exercise. Since it is deep within the body, this loss doesn't drastically improve appearance although people will report "feeling" leaner.

In a general sense, subcutaneous fat is generally more sensitive to both the fat storage and anti-fat mobilizing effects of insulin and less sensitive to the fat mobilizing effect of the catecholamines; it also has lower blood flow than visceral fat. This adds up to a type of fat that is relatively easy to store fat in but proportionally harder to mobilize fat from. But key to this section, the degree of ease of storage/difficulty of mobilization varies significantly with the type of fat being examined. Overall, upper body fat stores fat fairly effectively but releases it at a slower rate than visceral fat. It's blood flow is less than visceral fat as well and this adds up to an area of fat that is only moderately difficult to lose overall. Upper body fat, especially abdominal fat, can be even further subdivided into deep versus superficial fat and even an upper and lower superficial area. Deep abdominal fat is similar to visceral fat in that it is easy to lose with upper superficial slightly more difficult and lower superficial the most difficult.

But all of these pale in comparison to fat in the lower body which shows the most resistance to mobilization and loss (how fat is stored after a meal is complex and will be discussed in Chapter 10). This is due to it being very sensitive to the anti-fat mobilizing effects of insulin, having up to a 9:1 ratio of alpha- to beta-receptors and has poor blood flow (often being cold to the touch). Finally I should mention breast fat. There is shockingly little data on fat cell metabolism here with most revolving around breast cancer. Overall, breast fat shows a metabolism similar to upper body fat both in terms of fat storage and fat mobilization (13). Typically a woman's breasts get larger if she gains fat and often shrink when she loses fat. There is at least some indication fat cell number may be reduce in breast fat while dieting. Anecdotally, female who diet to extremely low levels often lose breast tissue that may never return.

Although ANP is turning out to play an important role in fat mobilization, there isn't as much research on how it impacts on different areas of body fat. Given its mechanism of action, it should avoid the entire region specific fat cell metabolism. This makes the manipulation of ANP (primarily through exercise) a potential way to sidestep the problems normally associated with losing lower body fat.

I've summarized the above information in the chart below:

Type of Fat	Storage	Mobilization	Blood Flow	Ease of Loss
Visceral	High	High	High	Easy
Upper body	Medium	Medium	Medium	Medium
Breast	???	Medium	???	Medium
Lower body	Complex	Low	Low	Difficult

Regardless of the details I presented, the fundamental aspect of fat loss or gain still primarily comes down to the energy balance equation. I say primarily as there are situations such as certain types of birth control or menopause where fat is gained while muscle is being lost regardless of energy balance. Diet and exercise also plays a role here, mainly in terms of impacting on what is lost or gained. But the overriding factor is still energy balance, discussed in the next chapter.

Chapter 8: Energy Balance

Continuing with the discussion of changing body composition, I want to expand on what I wrote about energy balance being the fundamental controller of changes in body composition. Once again, there are exceptions that I mentioned such as birth control, the changes at menopause, where the ratios of lean body mass (LBM) and body fat may be altered negatively for purely hormonal reasons without any change in energy balance. It's simply that anybody who is actively trying to alter their body composition must do so by altering their energy balance (along with other factors). There are two major reasons I want to delve into the details here. The first is that there are many misconceptions about how the energy balance equation does or should work, typically based on a very simplistic and superficial understanding of what it represents and I want to clear them up. Of perhaps more importance is that this chapter provides necessary background for the next chapter on metabolic adaptation which will lead into a thorough discussion of the issues surrounding women's fat gain and fat loss.

Energy Balance

As it's most basic level, energy balance (EB, also called the energy balance equation) represents the relationship between energy intake (EI, from food) and energy expenditure (EE, the number of calories expended during the day). In the US, it is often described as calories in versus calories out (other countries use kiloJoules). This relationship of EI and EE determine the changes that occur in the body's overall energy stores. Please note here that I have not said change in body weight but energy stores and this is a critical distinction that is often ignored and contributes to the misconceptions that surround EB. Its importance is due to the fact that gaining or losing a pound of fat represents a different change in the body's energy stores than gaining or losing a pound of muscle. This is discussed in more detail below.

The main concept to grasp at right now is that long-term imbalances between EI and EE lead to changes in the body's energy stores. If EI exceeds EE, the body's energy stores and bodyweight will increase. If EE exceeds EI, the body's energy stores and body weight will decrease If EI equals EE over the long term, weight will be stable with no meaningful change in the body's energy stores. A key concept here is that of long-term imbalances. Most people have small imbalances between intake and expenditure on a day-to-day basis but they tend to cancel each other out over time which is why most people remain at a fairly stable weight and body composition over fairly long time periods. It's a long-term imbalance that causes meaningful changes in the body's energy stores and body weight or body composition.

I want to make it absolutely clear that energy balance alone is not the only factor of importance in terms of what changes do or do not occur in body composition (the idea that this is the case is a common criticism of EB). The composition of the diet in terms of protein (especially), carbohydrates and fat are important as is the amount and type of exercise that is or isn't present. But these factors, discussed later in the book, only operate within the energy balance equation itself. For now let me look at the individual components that comprise both EI and EE.

Energy Intake (EI)

The energy intake side of the equation is fairly simple to explain as it represents the calories provided by the food being eaten each day. Proteins, carbohydrates, fat and alcohol all provide energy to the body in varying amounts with the standard values being given as 4 cal/gram for protein and carbohydrates and 9 cal/gram for dietary fat. Alcohol provides 7 cal/gram and fiber, often said to contain no calories, actually provides 1.5-2 cal/g to the body. These values can and do vary slightly for different foods (i.e. protein may vary from slightly below to slightly above 4 calories per gram) but the difference tends to be fairly minimal. Outside extreme variations in diet, differences in one direction are likely to be cancelled out by differences in the opposite direction.

Without detailing the process, the above values (often called the Atwater factors) are determined by burning foods in the laboratory and it's often claimed that this is not representative of how they are used within the body and that differences in nutrient metabolism in the real world makes those values meaningless. It's true that foods are not absorbed with 100% efficiency from the human stomach (and factors such as cooking and processing can impact this) with some percentage escaping digestion to be excrete. Proteins can vary from 80-95% absorption efficiency with animals proteins being utilized much more effectively than vegetable source proteins. Carbohydrates fall within the same ranges with high-fiber foods often being absorbed more poorly. Fats are absorbed at about 97% efficiency regardless of type. But this has already been factored in and only those calories absorbed/digested are counted to begin with.

Energy Expenditure

While energy intake simply represents the calories and nutrients absorbed from foods, energy expenditure (which I will refer to as Total Daily Energy Expenditure or TDDE) is made up of four distinct components that I will describe separately. Those four are resting metabolic rate (RMR), the thermic effect of food (TEF), the thermic effect of activity (TEA) and a relatively new factor called Non-Exercise Activity Thermogenesis (NEAT). When all four are added up, this represents TDEE.

Very strictly speaking, researchers define BMR (basal metabolic rate), representing the number of calories burned at complete rest (typically during sleep) and RMR (resting metabolic rate) which are the number of calories burned once someone is awake. RMR is about 10% above true BMR but it easier to measure, more commonly used and I will use it going forwards in this book. RMR typically makes up 60-75% of TDEE although the percentage may be much lower if activity is very high. RMR is primarily determined by the amount of LBM and here I mean all type of LBM, not just muscle. Brain, kidneys, liver and other organs actually contribute over half of a day's RMR despite being only 7% of the body's total weight. Skeletal muscle, burning only 6 cal/lb, only contributes about 20% of RMR despite being almost half of the total LBM. While LBM explains a majority of RMR there are other factors. Age, gender, genetics and the levels of hormones such as leptin, thyroid and the catecholamines are all important. Two people of the same weight and body composition may have a slightly different RMR although the difference is usually fairly small. Additionally, and contrary to what is often believed, RMR increases with bodyweight with heavier (i.e. overweight) individuals having a higher RMR than lighter/leaner individuals (1).

TEF refers to the number of calories burned during the digestion and utilization of food by the body and this varies for each nutrient. Protein may have a TEF between 15-25%, carbohydrates 6% and fat only 3%. For a mixed diet, TEF is generally estimated at 10% of total calorie intake so a diet of 1800 calories would have a 180 calorie TEF. This average 10% can change, high protein intakes may increase it to 15% (so 240 calories on an 1800 calorie diet). Overall, TEF is a relatively small overall part of TDEE and is actually often ignored completely. TEA refers to the energy burned during formal exercise and this can vary enormously between two people. A sedentary individual may burn zero calories via TEA while a trained athlete may burn hundreds or thousands of calories during exercise. When activity is a large proportion of TDEE, the relative contribution of RMR will be lower than 60-70%.

Finally is NEAT, a relatively newer component of TDEE which represents calories burned in all activities that are not formal exercise (2). Originally, it was thought that NEAT mostly represented fairly unconscious types of movements such as fidgeting or moving from sitting to standing. Many readers will remember that one kid in school who was always bouncing their leg up and down and this represents NEAT. In more recent years, NEAT has started to encompass voluntary activities so long as they aren't formal exercise. Gardening, walking up stairs, walking from the car to the store, moving from sitting to standing and basically anything beyond sitting down is now considered NEAT. Even gum chewing counts as NEAT and burns a few calories.

The importance of NEAT in TDEE cannot be overstated in terms of its potential impact on TDEE, fat gain or fat loss. When people are locked into a room where they can't move around much, NEAT may burn 100-600 calories; low levels of NEAT are also predictive of both weight and fat gain over time. More importantly, variations in NEAT end up explaining the majority of the differences in TDEE between two people, at least when neither is performing large amounts of exercise. From the highest to lowest levels, NEAT can vary by 2000 calories per day for two people of the same weight and body composition and any large scale differences in TDEE are due to variations in NEAT (3). RMR and TEF simply don't vary that much and while TEA can contribute significantly to calorie expenditure if large amounts of exercise are done, only trained athletes can usually accomplish this. For non-athletes, and outside of some specific disease states, there is no such thing as a slow metabolism (i.e. RMR), only low levels of NEAT.

In addition to explaining most of the difference in TDEE between individuals, NEAT is probably the place where changes have the greatest potential to alter TDEE. In the modern world, most people have a low requirement for the activities which generate NEAT on a daily basis. Sedentary lifestyles coupled with the ability to drive and a variety of household time and energy savers add up to a low level of NEAT on a day-to-day basis. Finding ways to increase NEAT is not only critical to increasing TDEE but has the potential to have an even larger impact than formal exercise.

Consider a situation where someone would normally be burning about 1 calorie per minute, just sitting down. If they moved to standing up, perhaps with a standing desk, that might increase to 2 calories/minute. While that seems small, that would burn an additional 60 calories per hour; over an 8 hour work shift that would be an additional 480 calories per day. This is the rough equivalent of 45-60 minutes of exercise. Using a treadmill desk and increasing calorie burn to 3 cal/min would double that value to 960 calories per day over an 8 hour work shift; this is the rough equivalent of 90-120 minutes of moderate exercise per day. As importantly, increasing NEAT in this fashion takes an almost insignificant effort relatively speaking. I would note that a large part of NEAT appears to be genetically determined with some people automatically doing more of it than others. Practically this means that increasing NEAT will take conscious effort for most people (3). Even here, small effects can add up significantly over time.

Changes in Energy Stores

The final component of the energy balance equation is the change in the actual energy stores of the body which, as mentioned, is not identical to changes in body weight. This can get a bit complex but understanding the difference is a key to understanding some of the major misconceptions that surround weight and fat loss. Recall from chapter 5 that the there are a variety of tissues in the body; each of those is made up of varying amounts of protein, water, fat, minerals, etc. and each contains a different amount of energy stored within them. The energy stored within a pound of brain is different than that stored in a pound of muscle or fat. Since changing body composition in a real way means altering the proportions of fat and muscle, I will focus on those. It's also important to consider the energy value of water and stored carbohydrate as these can change fairly rapidly. I've shown the energy content per pound (0.45 kg) in the chart below.

Tissue	Calories/Pound
Water	0
Glycogen	~1800
Skeletal Muscle	~600-700
Fat	3,500

The above numbers represent the number of calories "stored" within them and changes in the amounts of each are what the phrase "changes in energy stores" is referring to. So the loss of gain of any amount of water causes zero change in the body's energy stores which is why changes here have no meaning in the context of energy balance. The loss or gain of one pound of glycogen represents the loss or gain of 1800 calories of energy stored within the body. As I discussed earlier, since glycogen can be cycled on and of the body fairly rapidly, this doesn't have much real meaning either. Gains or losses of a pound of skeletal muscle represents a change of 600-700 calories in the body's energy stores although it's important to realize that the building of a pound of muscle requires far more calories than the 600-700 it contains. Finally, the gain or loss of a pound of fat represents a change of 3,500 calories in the body's energy stores. I suspect most American readers are familiar with that value and this leads me to perhaps the largest misconception about the energy balance equation, one that has led to an astonishing number of incorrect criticisms.

The 3,500 Calorie "Rule"

Perhaps the most enduring rule of weight loss is that losing one pound requires a total calorie deficit (i.e. imbalance between energy intake and expenditure) of 3,500 calories. This value, originally derived only for body fat derives from the following. One pound of fat is 0.454 kilograms or 454 grams of tissue of which 85-90% is actual stored triglyceride (TG). Multiplying 454 grams by 0.85 or 0.90 yields roughly 395 grams of actual stored TG. Since each gram contains 9 calories, that means that the pound of fat contains 395 grams * 9 cal/g = 3554 calories per pound of fat, the magical value.

From this follows a simple mathematical approach to weight loss. To lose one pound per week, all that is requires is a 500 calories/day imbalance between energy intake and expenditure. This could entail reducing food by 500 calories per day, increasing activity by 500 calories per day or some combination. A 500 calorie/day deficit times 7 days is a 3,500 calorie total deficit and one pound should be lost. To lose two pounds would require a total deficit of 7,000 calories or 1000 calories/day and you get the idea.

The problem is that it doesn't work with the mathematically predicted and real-world weight and fat losses rarely being the same. This leads many to conclude that the energy balance equation is flawed or does not apply to humans or what have you. This too is incorrect and there are a number of reasons that the predicted and actual weight/fat loss are rarely the same. One is simply a lack of adherence to the diet or exercise program. But even assuming that adherence is perfect, it's very rare for the predicted real-world changes to occur where a 3,500 calorie deficit yields the loss of exactly one pound of weight (5). There are a number of reasons for this and I want to look at each.

What is Being Lost or Gained Revisited

As I stated above, the energy balance equation states that long-term imbalances cause the body's energy stores to either increase or decrease. And while this usually means that weight will also change, the concepts are not identical due to the differences in energy content of different tissues in the body and the loss or gain of one pound of muscle (~600-700 calories) represents a difference change in bodily energy stores than the loss or gain of one pound of fat (~3,500 calories). This distinction is important as the original 3,500 calories equals one pound was only ever meant to apply to body fat. Somewhere along the way this was forgotten and people reached the conclusion that a one pound change in bodyweight represented 3,500 calories regardless of what was being gained or lost.

This misunderstanding is what has led to a major criticism of the energy balance concept. Since changes in body weight seem to occur in amounts that have no relationship to the 3,500 calorie/pound value, the rule appears to be violated. This leads people who simply don't understand the equation or the rule to conclude that it is incorrect. This is part of why I spent so much time discussing body composition and how changes in it are more important than weight per se. Because just as changes in water, glycogen, food residue, fat and muscle can impact on how much weight is gained or lost and over what time frame, those same changes determine the actual change in energy stores that are occurring or what surplus or deficit is needed to generate them. As I did in Chapter 5, let me look at each again.

Water, Glycogen and Food Residue

As I mentioned above, water contains no calories and gains or losses here really have nothing to do with the energy balance equation. This is why changes in water weight, frustrating as they may be, don't represent anything real. A four pound gain in water weight over night doesn't represent the caloric surplus of 14,000 calories (4 pounds times 3,500 calories per pound) anymore than a four pound fat loss over night represents a 14,000 calorie deficit. This misunderstanding is one of the reasons that people thought that low-carbohydrate diets had a metabolic advantage. Studies in the late 60's and early 70's would put subjects on low- or high-carbohydrate diets at the same calorie level and often see a several pound weight loss in the first few days in the low-carbohydrate group. But since this rapid loss was simply water, it represented a zero calorie change in the body's energy stores.

As described, the body's carbohydrate stored can change fairly rapidly in both directions and this also leads to some apparent contradictions of the 3,500 calorie rule. Certainly storing carbohydrates in the body (as glycogen in the liver or muscles) does increase the body's energy stores but it also increases water weight (every gram of carbohydrate stores 3-4 grams of water). Someone storing 400 grams of carbohydrate (1600 calories of energy) might gain as much as 4.5 pounds of actual weight due to water but those 4.5 pounds only contains 1600 calories of energy. The same holds when glycogen and water are lost: 4.5 lbs of weight may be lost if those 400 grams of carbohydrate are depleted from the body. Since the 3,500 value only applies fat, there is still no violation of the energy balance equation.

I mentioned in Chapter 5 that food residue in the gastrointestinal tract can also contribute to body weight changes but here there is no energy to consider. Since energy balance only applies to food that was actually digested and absorbed, any undigested food, or the energy that it represented, simply doesn't count in this regard as it never actually contributed to the body's energy stores.

Fat and LBM Changes

It should be clear from the chart above that one pound of fat and one pound of muscle contain a different amount of stored energy. In the case of muscle, one pound contains 600-700 calories while only one pound of body fat actually represents the 3,500 calorie rule value. Put differently, if someone created a 3,500 calorie deficit and lost 100% fat they would lose exactly one pound of body weight. If they lost 100% skeletal muscle, they would actually lose 5-6 lbs of total weight (3500 calories/600-700 cal/lb = 5-6 lbs). Both represent 3,500 calories of energy lost but the total weight loss is clearly very different. Here it gets slightly more complicated.

Because while it is possible for weight loss to come 100% from fat or weight gain to be 100% from LBM, it's more common to lose some proportion of each. Since fat and LBM contain different amounts of energy, the proportion gained or lost will determine the actual energy value that change represents. So let's assume that someone creates a 3,500 calorie deficit and the composition of their weight loss is made up of 90% fat and 10% muscle. The 10% of energy from muscle will represent 350 calories or roughly 0.5 lbs of muscle while the 90% from fat will represent 3150 calories or about 0.9 lbs of fat. The total weight loss in this case will be 1.4 pounds (0.9 lbs fat + 0.5 lbs muscle), higher than the 3,500 calorie rule would predict.

This has two major implications. The first is that scale weight will go down faster if skeletal muscle LBM is lost due to the differences in how much energy it contains. I actually strongly suspect that the reason that many rapid weight loss centers recommend against exercise as it limits the loss of LBM while dieting. By deliberately allowing LBM loss to occur, the number on the scale will drop more quickly than if muscle were not lost even if body composition is not improving as much as it should be. If that approach is combined with a low-carbohydrate diet, the weight losses that are achieved can be extremely large due to the amount of water loss that will occur. The number on the scale will drop rapidly although the changes that are actually occurring are either irrelevant (water) or negative (LBM loss).   Similarly, and I will discuss this in detail in Chapter 10, is the fact that actual weight loss will always be slower when a larger proportion of fat is being used. That is, at 100% muscle loss, a 3,500 calorie deficit will generate a 5-6 pound weight loss. At a ratio of 90% fat:10% muscle, the same deficit will cause a 1.4 lb fat loss. In the case of 100% fat loss, that same 3,500 calories will only cause one pound of weight loss.

The second implication is that losing one pound of fat will require a slightly larger deficit than the 3,500 calorie value assigned to it. If only 90% of the total deficit is coming from fat energy, that means that an additional 10% (the same 350 calorie value that comes from LBM above) will be required to lose one pound. So the total deficit to lose one pound of fat in this case will be 3,850 calories (3,500 + an additional 350). This still doesn't violate the 3,500 calorie per pound rule. It's simply that a larger total deficit is required to actually achieve the 3,500 calorie per pound of fat deficit that is necessary.

Summing Up
Due to the differences described above in terms of the energy content of different tissues in the body, the 3,500 calorie rule will hold to varying degrees at different times in a fat loss diet. In the early stages of a diet, when primarily water and glycogen are being lost, the rule won't hold and weight loss may be much larger than predicted.   Just as several pounds of water can be gained overnight, it can be just as easily lost. Since that water contains no energy, it is irrelevant to the 3,500 calorie rule.   This will remain true even if some LBM/muscle is being lost later in the diet. The same 3,500 calorie deficit will cause more than one pound of body weight to be lost although fat loss will be slightly slower than predicted.

If and when fat loss represents 100% of the weight being lost, the 3,500 calorie/pound value will finally become accurate with a 3,500 calorie deficit generating both 1 real pound of weight loss and fat loss (6). For the Category 3 and 2 woman it is relatively trivial to lose 100% fat although Category 1 women can also do this with a proper diet and training set up. The early rapid weight losses will still seem to violate the rule (and monthly water weight changes for the normally cycling woman will appear to violate them weekly) but, over time, the 3,500 calorie per pound of fat lost rule will basically hold.

Summarizing the Above
Putting the above in a slightly different way, any changes in weight can be thought of as having two phases, a rapid phase and a slow phase. The rapid phase, occurring over days, represents the loss of water, glycogen and food residue while the slow phase represents actual changes in body composition. If more fat and less LBM is lost, weight loss will be slower than if more LBM is lost. I've shown this below.

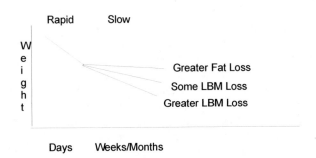

Weight Gain
Just as the predicted and real-world weight losses often don't match, the predicted and actual weight gains often do not either. As some readers of this book, likely athletes, often desire to gain weight, I want to address this briefly. For the most part, the same comments I made above holds in reverse here. The 3,500 calorie per pound rule is still only valid for body fat although it is slightly more complicated here. Because while mobilizing and burning energy off the body only provides the calories stored within

whatever tissue is being lost, gaining weight often takes more calories than just the energy stored within the tissue being gained. Storing fat doesn't actually take much more than the 3,5000 calories it stores but it's still not 100% efficient. So the necessary calorie surplus to gain fat will be at least slightly higher than 3,500 calories. This assumes that 100% fat is being gained and this is often not the case. If LBM is being gained, the total weight gain for any given calorie surplus will be lower than predicted.

This is due to the fact that while a pound of muscle may only contain 600-700 calories when broken down for energy, it takes roughly 2400-2700 calories to synthesize that pound of muscle. So while a 3,500 calorie deficit where 100% muscle were lost would result in a 5-6 pounds weight loss, a 3,500 calorie surplus where 100% muscle were being gained would not result in a 5-6 pound muscle gain. Rather, due to the high calorie cost of making muscle, it might yield a 1.3-1.4 lb muscle gain (3,500 calories/2400-2700 calories = 1.3-1.4 lbs). Since it's relatively rare to gain 100% muscle with no fat gain, the actual total surplus to gain one pound of muscle will be higher than the 2400-2700 calorie value.   If fat makes up 30% of the total weight gain, the actual surplus to gain one pound of muscle will be 30% higher than predicted which is actually very close to 3,500 calories per pound (2700 * 1.3 = 3510 calories). I will use this value later in the book when I talk about setting up diet for muscle gain.

The Equation Changes

In addition to all of the issues discussed above, there is an arguably even more important factor, one that is critical for the understanding of the dynamics of weight/fat loss or gain. This is that both sides of the energy balance equation can and do change in response to changes in food intake, activity levels and the actual changes in weight or body composition. I can't tell if this fact is unknown or simply ignored by those who deny the energy balance equation but it is critical to both understand and accept. As I will discus thoroughly in the next chapter, in response to weight/fat loss, the body will adapt and both increase hunger/appetite (in an attempt to get people to eat more) while it decreases TDEE. This also occurs in response to weight gain although it seems that the body is better at defending weight/fat loss than weight and fat gain under most conditions.

Ignoring this fact has led to some wildly inaccurate ideas about the energy balance equation and how weight and at loss should occur. Because people seem to assume that TDEE will remain static throughout a diet and that the created deficit will be unchanging with weight and fat loss continuing indefinitely. Obviously this does not happen and, as the body adapts, what once was a 500 cal/day deficit becomes 400 then 300 then 200 until the body comes more or less into balance. Below I've shown what people predict or hope the loss should be versus what actually occurs.

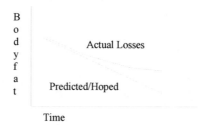

Many of the very simplistic ideas regarding weight gain and weight loss can be easily explained by this reality. For example, it is claimed that removing even 100 calories per day (one apple) will cause a large fat loss (around 10 lbs) over a year's span. But over time this 100 calorie deficit will be reduced and by the time the body has lowered TDEE by 100 calories, no more fat loss will occur with much less than 10 lbs having been lost. The same holds in reverse and the idea that a mere 100 calorie/day surplus will generate a large fat loss is untrue as the body will increase TDEE over time until the surplus is eliminated.

Simply, any discussion or prediction of weight and fat loss that does not factor in the changes in TDEE is guaranteed to be wrong and will lead to many disappointments (7). For any fixed diet and exercise program, not only will the total losses be lower than predicted, but they will occur more slowly than expected. Understanding this is important for many reasons, not the least of which is motivation and adherence. When dieters expect fat loss to occur at some rate and the real world changes are less than this, this tends to hurt motivation. The effort involved is simply too far out of step with the results being generated. It's equally important for athletes who must reach a certain goal BF% (8). This is true for both the active dieting phase (i.e. to estimate actual dieting time) along with dealing with the "aftermath" of the diet. Now let me continue from the above to discuss the metabolic adaptations to dieting in detail.

Chapter 9: Metabolic Adaptation

As the last chapter of background information before I start looking in detail at gender differences and women's physiology in terms of fat gain and fat loss, I want to look in some detail at the topic of metabolic adaptation. While there are other reasons the the predicted and real-world changes in weight or body fat tend to differ, this is a primary one as the energy balance equation will change in response to alterations in food intake, activity levels or actual bodyweight and body composition changes. This can happen in both directions with energy expenditure decreasing with food restriction and fat loss and increasing with increased food intake and bodyweight gain (the increases in response to weight gain often being less than those in response to weight loss). The practical effect of this is that fat and weight loss will almost always be slower than predicted although the predicted weight gain tends to also be less than expected.

Readers may be familiar with the concept of setpoint, representing the idea that the body will attempt to regulate (or "defend" as it is sometimes described) a specific body weight or body fat percentage (BF%), accomplishing this through changes in either energy intake or expenditure. While there is ample data that this exists in humans, there is a related concept called a settling point where the body settles at a given weight and BF% based on activity and diet. While the relative importance of each has been debated for years, the best models incorporate both. A person's overall lifestyle are part of the settling point but it's clear that the body adapts metabolically to both weight loss and gain (the setpoint).

This will be one of the longer and potentially most complicated chapters in this book and the large amount of information I want to examine will make it a bit disorganized. One reason is that there are technically three different situations that I need to examine. The first is weight or fat loss which tends to be the simplest. The second is weight or fat gain which has to be examined in terms of someone gaining weight/fat from their current body weight or gaining weight and fat back after having lost it. This is made more complex as initial BF% has a fairly large impact on what adaptations are or aren't seen and to what degree. The Category 3 woman may see a distinctly different response than the Category 1 woman. And this is true both in response to fat loss and fat gain. There can also be an enormous amount of individual variation in all of the above with some showing a much larger or smaller response in either direction. While other factors are involved, some people objectively do gain fat more easily or lose it with more difficulty and vice versa. Finally, all of the adaptations (in both directions) tend to be incredibly inter-related since the same basic systems in terms of hormones and physiology are controlling both energy intake and expenditure.

My goal with this chapter will not only be to at least outline/semi-detail the adaptations that can occur in different situations but also to address the potential magnitude of those changes, along with individual variation (and do so for the various situations I described above). I'll also look at the mechanisms controlling the system. Much of this chapter's information will be coming from the enormous number of review papers that have been written although individual studies will be used to fill in the gaps (1-7). To avoid needless repetition and since I will be referring back to them frequently throughout this chapter, I want to first detail two of the studies from which much of the information in this chapter derives.

The Minnesota and Leibel Studies

The first is considered a seminal study on both starvation and refeeding and is called the Minnesota Semi-Starvation Study (or just the Minnesota study). Done in the 50's, it took 32 normal weight men and placed them on 50% of their maintenance calories with a fairly low protein intake and no exercise beyond forced daily walking. This was meant to mimic what might occur in a concentration camp environment and it gathered data on a staggering number of topics including body weight, body fat percentage, hunger and energy expenditure, all of which were measured in great detail (8).

At the end of the study, the men had lost 25% of their starting weight and reached 4% body fat, the lower limit for men. At this point the men were allowed to eat again under either controlled or uncontrolled conditions so that increases in body weight, BF%, hunger, etc. could be measured as weight was regained. While probably the most comprehensive study ever done on the topic, the fact that only men were studied makes direct extrapolation to women impossible. Due to when it was done, the technology was crude by today's standards and concepts such as NEAT did not even exist and were not directly addressed. Despite this the data is still valuable and other research exists to address those limitations.

The second study, headed by a researcher named Leibel, is more recent and looked at the topic of both weight loss and weight gain. In it both lean and obese men and women were carefully fed or dieted to either gain 10% of their starting weight or dieted to 10 or 20% below their starting weight with full measurement of all components of energy expenditure being measured to see how they changed (9). In addition to including both women and men (and both lean and obese), it had access to potentially more accurate technology along with measuring components such as NEAT. Between those two studies, along with others, an overall picture of the types of adaptations that can occur can be drawn and that's what I'll do. Since it is relatively less complex, let me start with energy intake (EI), the calories consumed from food, in terms of how it can, or at least tries, to adapt in response to changes in body weight/body fat.

Energy Intake (EI) Regulation

Let me start by addressing the energy intake (calories in) part of the energy balance equation. Once again this represents the calories from the food we eat and I'd reiterate that only the food that is actually digested and absorbed matters here. Let me make it clear at the outset that human food intake is impacted by a staggering number of factors many of which are purely environmental (at most they interact with the underlying biology). Since people's environments don't tend to change enormously without conscious effort, I will only only focus on the biological factors that impact on EI and what changes occur there.

Broadly speaking, there are two major systems that are relevant to food intake and researchers refer to these as the homeostatic and hedonic systems respectively (9). The homeostatic system is meant to regulate food intake based on the actual nutrient requirements of the body (i.e. if blood glucose falls, people get hungry for carbohydrates to raise it). This system is also affected by the body's overall energy stores. Body fat is a key player in this although LBM/muscle is turning out to have a role as well. These two factors work to control hunger which is purely a short-term response (someone will get hungry, get eat, get full and stop eating) and appetite (the overall desire for food). If the distinction is unclear consider older individuals who will get hungry (eating a meal and stopping) but eat little total food overall.

The hedonic system is related to the fact that eating is pleasurable and biologically rewarding. Highly palatable, typically high-sugar/high-fat foods, tends to cause the largest response here but eating of any sort tends to have an effect here. This system is involved in any number of rewarding activities (such as sex) and it's interesting to note that the pathways seem to be related to those that control drug addiction (10). This is mediated by dopamine (DA) in the brain along with the opiod hormones both of which impact on how rewarding or enjoyed food (or other activities) are. For genetic reasons, many appear to start with a more responsive or sensitive hedonic system (i.e. they enjoy eating certain foods more than others). This is often found in obese individuals and is part of why they are more likely to gain weight in the modern environment (11). The naturally lean individual simply may not enjoy these foods as much.

While the two systems above are somewhat distinct, they are also inter-related in terms of the factors that are regulating them. Here the system gets very complex with an absolutely staggering number of different things sending a signal to the brain. The levels of glucose, amino acids and fatty acids in the bloodstream play a role here and even the physical stretching of the stomach after a meal sends a signal to the brain to signal fullness. There are also an enormous number of hormonal signals, many sent from the stomach itself that play a role here. Cholecystokinin (CCK), peptide YY, glucagon-like peptide 1 (GLP-1) and others are released in response to food intake with the proportion and amounts of each hormone being related to the size of the meal and the amounts and type of nutrients consumed (12). Protein, fat and fiber have the biggest impact on CCK, for example with protein being the most filling nutrient of all.

Of all of these, perhaps the most important hormone released from the stomach is ghrelin. When ghrelin goes up, it stimulates hunger (it is the only hormone to do so) and ghrelin levels actually increase before habitual meal times. Ghrelin has other roles related to the control energy expenditure as that I will discuss below. The hormone leptin, released primarily from fat cells plays an enormous role here although it tends to be somewhat more indirect, changing how the brain responds to the other hormones. But all of these hormones send an integrated signal to the brain (specifically the hypothalamus) that ends up influencing hunger and appetite. Many, if not most of these hormones, also impact on the hedonic system usually by altering the levels of dopamine (DA) in the brain to one degree or another.

Adaptation to Diet and Fat Loss

When someone reduces food intake or in response to dieting, there is a fairly stereotyped response in the above systems. Due to less total food being eaten, less of the fullness hormones such as CCK, PYY, etc. are released. Ghrelin levels are also increased overall and don't decrease as much after a meal. Leptin, released primarily from fat cells, decreases which means that the brain responds even less to those hormone signals. The increase in leptin and decrease in ghrelin, along with the other hormonal changes, has a potent overall effect which is to increase appetite and hunger along with decreasing how full people get after a meal (at the extremes, dieters may be hungry shortly after finishing the previous meal). Those same hormonal changes also impact on the hedonic system with DA levels dropping (leptin plays a major role here) along with other changes. This makes tasty foods taste even better (think of how much better a cookie or piece of cake tastes when you're hungry) and dieters even notice and pay attention to palatable foods that much more easily. These changes can make dietary adherence more difficult.

In addition to any short term changes in hunger, there are also longer term changes as fat is lost. In overweight individuals, for example, hunger increases by 5% and fullness decreases by 3% for every 2.2 lbs (1kg) of fat lost (13). The more fat is lost, the greater the effect. Although not well studied at the extremes of low BF%, hunger and appetite may be relentlessly high. In the Minnesota study the men became absolutely obsessed with food, talking about little else, near the end of the diet. This can be seen online in the behavior of lean athletes who are dieting who talk about looking at or posting pictures of tasty foods (which they call food porn) on social media.

In that same Minnesota study, when the men were given free access to food, they ate with abandon, rapidly regaining weight and body fat. In fact, their hunger remained elevated long after their body fat was restored and didn't return to normal until their LBM was also regained (13). They ended up with a higher BF% than they started for this reason. It's now known that LBM sends an independent signal that drives hunger which makes preventing it's loss during a diet along with restoring it as rapidly as possible after a diet critical to avoiding fat regain (the combination of resistant training and sufficient protein, both of which were absent in that study, is the key to both goals).

While the above primarily refers to food restriction per se, since it is possible to increase calorie expenditure to generate fat loss and I want to look at the impact of exercise in this regard. In the most general sense, at least in the short-term (1-2 days), exercise seems to have at most a small effect on increasing hunger. Even when people do eat more, it's usually less than the humber of calories that they burned during exercise. So someone might burn 400 calories with exercise and eat 150 more calories in a day than they otherwise would. The exercise still has an effect of creating a deficit, it's just smaller than would be expected (14). I'd mention that this short-term effect may not be representative of a long-term effect. Hunger often takes 3-4 days to even begin to increase on a diet and, over time, a deficit is a deficit and fat loss is fat loss. Eventually hunger will increase in response to exercise. I'd also note that the increase in hunger after exercise is hugely variable with some people showing a larger increase in the palatability of foods which may cause them to eat more than others following exercise (15).

In leaner individuals the situation is somewhat more complex. While you would expect exercise to stimulate hunger more due to the lower BF%, in some cases, exercise may blunt hunger, causing athletes to unconsciously undereat. This may be related to the performance of higher intensity exercise and seems to interact with their diet (16). Finally I'd mention that there can be a psychological impact of exercise on eating whereby people may justify eating more (i.e. "I did an hour of aerobics, I deserve a cheeseburger.") There is a related phenomenon called disinhibition that I will discuss in a later chapter.

Ultimately, it should be clear that food restriction, to some degree exercise, and fat loss tends to stimulate hunger and appetite along with making people desire/enjoy more palatable foods. However, these tendencies should only be seen as biological urges as they can clearly be overcome to one degree or another. People clearly do control their food intake both during and after a diet (I'll talk about other strategies to help deal with this) so there is no guarantee that food intake will increase. For this reason, it's relatively more important to look at the adaptations to energy expenditure.

Energy Expenditure Regulation

Moving to the topic of energy expenditure, recall from the last chapter that there are four distinct components of what is called Total Daily Energy Expenditure (TDEE): Resting Metabolic Rate (RMR) which are the number of calories burned at rest, Thermic Effect of Food (TEF) which are the calories burned in digesting and utilizing food, the Thermic Effect of Activity (TEA) which are the calories burned during formal exercise, and Non-Exercise Energy Expenditure (NEAT) which are the calories burned during activities which aren't exercise. As expected, all four of these both can and do change in response to dieting/fat loss. Logically, this would be expected if for no other reason that the fat loss alone. A smaller body will burn less calories at rest (RMR) and during activity (TEA, NEAT) and a reduced food intake will mean that TEF is reduced. And this certainly occurs. However, when the changes in each component are examined, there are often reductions in TDEE or each component that are greater than would be predicted on the change in weight alone. This additional decrease is called the adaptive component or adaptive thermogenesis (AT).

So if someone lost weight and their TDEE was predicted to drop by 100 calories but is measured to have dropped by 150 calories, that extra 50 calories is the adaptive component, another mechanism that works to slow fat loss and restore body fat levels after the diet is over. As with other components of this system, the adaptive component can be hugely variable between any two people causing one to lose fat or weight more quickly than another even on an identical diet and exercise program. This adaptive component can occur very rapidly during a diet, long before any measurable fat loss has occurred. In one study, TDEE dropped by 100 calories (ranging from 0-250 calories) within the first week. For someone on a 500 cal/day deficit, this could reduce it to 250-400 cal/day reducing fat loss immediately. After that initial rapid drop, there is a slower more gradual decrease as fat is lost. At the low extremes of BF%, the adaptive component increases enormously a although the major drop in TDEE is still from the total weight/fat loss. Finally, the adaptive component is much greater during active dieting but decreases when the diet is over.

The Adaptive Decrease in TDEE

Although I will look at the individual components below, I want to start by looking at the size of the adaptive decrease in TDEE first. As with the changes in hunger, much of this is determined by initial and ending BF% along with the total amount of weight and fat that is lost. In the case of the Category 3 dieter losing a moderate amount of weight, the total adaptive reduction in TDEE might be no more than 15% below the predicted level which might amount to 150-250 calories per day. This can range from zero to 500 calories per person with people showing the larger adaptive drop both losing fat more slowly and being more likely to regain it after the diet is over. At the extremes of fat loss, much larger drops have been measured. In the Minnesota study, the men showed a total drop in TDEE of 50-55% or 1800 calories per day (and large variance between the men) as they lost 25% of their total weight (and an enormous amount of LBM). This means that 25-30% of the total drop, or 450-600 calories, was due to the adaptive component while the other 1200-1350 calorie drop was due to the weight loss.

More recently, and supporting the above numbers, a male bodybuilder was followed as he lost 28 lbs (14% of his initial body weight), losing 22 pounds of fat and 6 lbs of LBM (17). His TDEE dropped by 1300 calories or 37% from baseline. As 14% of that drop was due to the loss of weight, the other 23% is due to AT, broadly supporting the Minnesota study numbers. Anecdotally, both female and male physique competitors, who meticulously track their calorie and activity levels before and during a diet have reported a roughly similar drop in TDEE. These two values, 10-15% (150-250 calories) for moderate fat loss in Category 2/3 individuals and up to 25-30% (450-600 calories) for extreme fat loss in the Category 1 dieter will represent the low and high extremes for the adaptive component.

The causes of the adaptive component of metabolic rate decrease are primarily hormonal. Among other changes when calories are reduced or fat loss occurs, hormones involved in energy expenditure such as the catecholamines (adrenaline/noradrenaline) and active thyroid hormones (T3) go down (the latter is due to impaired conversion of T4 to T3 in the liver). The catecholamines and thyroid hormones interact, each making the other work better and the drop in the two is a major part of the adaptive drop in metabolic rate. There are other hormones that change with dieting. Leptin, discussed below, is a major one but there are also changes in growth hormone (GH) and cortisol. The total change tends to be related to the loss of fat: greater fat loss to a lower BF% means a greater drop in hormones and larger adaptive component. In addition, estrogen, progesterone and testosterone all change with fat loss and the impact of this depends very heavily on diet Category. For the Category 3 female, the changes may actually improve her health and fertility. In Category 2, the changes are fairly inconsequential. But in Category 1, menstrual cycle dysfunction is common in women (males may reach castrate testosterone levels) as they reach the lower limits of BF%. Now let me look at each component of TDEE individually.

Resting Metabolic Rate (RMR)

The total decrease in RMR in response to a diet is due to two factors: the actual loss of body weight and the adaptive component described above. Here the adaptive component is due to the body become more efficient and burning less calories per pound of tissue. So not only is there less of that tissue overall but what is left is more efficient. As I mentioned in Chapter 8, RMR is predominantly related to the amount of LBM someone has. Here I am referring to all types of LBM, not just skeletal muscle. Recalling that organ, brain, etc. burns far more calories than skeletal muscle, the loss of organ mass would be expected to reduce RMR significantly. And this actually happens with a recent study (mimicking the Minnesota study for 3 weeks) found a loss of organ mass in the first week of dieting that explained most of the drop in RMR (18). There was still an adaptive component, mind you, it was simply smaller than had been seen previously.   Given the importance of LBM in determining RMR, it's usually been felt (and at least some studies find) that preventing LBM while dieting is the best way to limit the a reduction in metabolic rate (adaptive or otherwise). While there is at least some truth to this, the fact is that RMR tends to drop in response to large-scale fat and weight loss even if LBM is maintained (19). And this is due to the fact that body fat is sending the primary signal to the brain in terms of how it should adapt to dieting.

Looking at the magnitude of the drop, a primary factor is still BF%. In the Category 3 individual losing a moderate amount of weight, the total adaptive drop may be no more than 150-250 calories. Of this decrease, perhaps 10-15% is due to the changes in RMR and this amounts to roughly 15-40 calories per day, an insignificantly small number. Even the dieter who experiences a 500 calorie total decrease will still only see the RMR drop making up 50-70 calories per day. At the extremes the picture changes with the Minnesota study being on of the very few data points available. Above I mentioned that the total adaptive drop was 1800 calories per day. Of that drop, RMR dropped a total of 40% (720 calories) of which 450 calories was due to the loss in weight an an additional 270 calories (roughly 4-5 times the drop in the Category 3 individual) was due to the adaptive decrease in RMR. This means that the majority of the total drop in TDEE, 60% or 1100 calories came from the other components of total energy expenditure.

If the total adaptive adaptive drop in RMR only represents 10-15% of the total in the Category 3 individual and perhaps 25% for those who lose extreme amounts of fat, the majority of the drop must be explained by changes in the other components.   I make this point as it's common to hear people talk online about how dieting has ruined their metabolism or put them into fat storing mode, at least broadly referring to the supposed changes in RMR.   For the overweight individual, this is clearly untrue and, even at the extremes, it contributes less than half of the total drop (adaptive or otherwise) in energy expenditure.

TEF, TEA and NEAT
As the total drop in RMR can only explain a relatively small proportion of the total drop, that leaves TEF, TEA and NEAT as the possible contributors (these are sometimes grouped as Non-Resting Energy Expenditure or NREE). TEF is the simplest and ends up only being impacted by the overall decrease in food intake with no adaptive component. Since TEF is only 10-15% of total calorie intake to begin with, the change here is always fairly small. A 500 calorie food reduction only reduces TDEE by 50-75 calories while a 1000 calorie reduction in total food intake has the potential to reduce TEF by 100-150 calories. While this is certainly part of the overall adaptation to dieting and fat loss, it is clearly not a major part of the decrease in total energy expenditure.

Moving to TEA, I'd first note that many studies examining weight loss and metabolic rate adaptation do not use exercise making changes here irrelevant. Only those dieters who are already on exercise programs or who are athletes will face adaptations here and there are three that might occur. The first is simply that people will be less motivated to exercise in general or be unable or unwilling to maintain the same exercise intensity. Assuming this is not the case and the exercise program is maintained, there are still two adaptations by which TEA will be reduced. The first is due simply to the reduction in body weight; a smaller body takes less energy to move. If muscle mass is lost, this effect could be even more pronounced as the dieter will find it more difficult to maintain their previous intensity in terms of running or cycling speed, weights lifted, etc. Fewer calories will be burned even if the same total amount of exercise is done.

There is also an adaptive component where muscular efficiency may increase, causing 25% fewer total calories to be burned (i.e. someone burning 100 calories will now only burn 75), especially during low intensity activity (21). In premise, wearing a weight vest to restore the weight loss has some potential to reverse this but it can only partially do so (21a). In order to burn the same amount of calories, either more total exercise or exercising at a higher intensity will be required. While these adaptations occur, both for the non-exerciser (for whom the above is irrelevant) or the trainee, the changes still cannot explain the majority of the adaptive drop in TDEE.

If RMR, TEF and TEA cannot explain the majority of drop in daily energy expenditure, only changes in NEAT are left. And, just as it represents the larger contributor to the variance in TDEE between people, changes here turn out to explain the majority of the drop that is seen with dieting. Ignoring the unconscious aspect of NEAT (fidgeting, changing posture), which may decrease, and focusing on the most conscious NEAT types of activities, reduction in calorie expenditure can occur here for a few reasons. The first two are identical to what happens with exercise: a smaller body burns fewer calories and there is the increased muscular efficiency that occurs.   Since that efficiency primarily impacts on low-intensity activities, and many NEAT activities are low-intensity by definition, the change here could potentially have an even larger impact than it does on TEA.

Larger than either of those is the fact that that NEAT levels typically go down with calorie restriction. People not only perform less of the activities which burn calories via NEAT but unconsciously perform less of higher-intensity activities. Clearly demonstrating this is a study where calorie restriction from 10-30% below maintenance resulted in daily reductions in NEAT from 100-500 calories per day (22). There was a 100-200 calorie per day variance between subjects with the people showing the larger drop being the ones who lose fat more slowly/regain it more rapidly. While not studied to my knowledge, given the fact that NEAT is often very low in overweight individuals, NEAT could potentially increase somewhat with weight loss as it becomes easier to move. As well, it's possible that those individuals with a lower initial level of NEAT see a smaller reduction simply because there is less to reduce. Regardless, the overall picture is that NEAT goes down when dieting. To put this into further perspective, I'd mention the Biosphere 2 study which accidentally turned into a 2-year long diet (23). While reaching a very low BF%, the subjects (both women and men) experienced an insignificant 2.7% decrease in RMR while their daily NEAT was reduced by half (23).

Looking back at the Minnesota study, as I noted above, the drop in RMR can only explain 40% of the total drop (and most of that was from weight loss) leaving 60% or 1100 calories to be explained by TEF, TEA or NEAT. TEF can only explain perhaps 150 of those calories leaving TEA and NEAT. While we might debate if it counts as formal exercise, the men were forced to walk for 2 hours/day but performed no other exercise. Even the decreased calorie burn here still can't explain the largest part of the decrease. While not directly measured (since the concept and technology didn't exist), this means that NEAT the remainder of the day must have been reduced enormously due to fatigue and exhaustion. At the extremes of low BF%, exhaustion sets in causing people to unconsciously move around as little as possible if they are not forced (or are forcing themselves) to exercise. Maintaining normal exercise intensity is difficult enough under these conditions and keeping NEAT from falling excessively can be nearly impossible.

All of this points to the simple fact that while changes in RMR, TEF and (if exercise is present), TEA are part of the overall adaptation they cannot explain the majority of the change. Just as differences in NEAT explain most of the variation in daily energy expenditure between any two people, changes in NEAT explain most of the drop in energy expenditure that occurs while dieting. And while a large part of this reduction in NEAT is assuredly in the unconscious part of it, this at least gives dieters the possibility of seeing less of a drop in energy expenditure by working to maintain NEAT.

In this vein, people who sit more while dieting (meaning a lower NEAT) have been found to lose less weight on a diet than those who sit less (24).   By deliberately choosing to engage in activities that increase NEAT such as parking further away from the store, using a standing or treadmill desk, etc. NEAT levels will either be better maintained or even potentially increased.   New technology holds promise here with apps and activity trackers which give daily feedback on NEAT (indicating when it needs to be increased). Even a pedometer can be used and targeting a specific number of steps per day will increase NEAT.

There is also formal exercise to consider.   On the one hand, increases here could possibly offset the decreases in NEAT and work to maintain daily energy expenditure. On the other, exercise itself has the potential to decrease NEAT in some situations and it's been argued that human energy expenditure may be genetically set with increases in one component being offset by reductions in another (25).   In one study, subjects performed 400 calories per day of exercise but only increased daily energy expenditure by 250 calories due to a reduction in NEAT at other times of the day (26). The impact of exercise on NEAT seems to be most pronounced in beginners and older individuals although trained athletes often reduce NEAT after particularly exhausting workouts.

This effect tends to go away as fitness improves and the exercise isn't as fatiguing but this actually makes a case for lower intensity activity being a better choice in many circumstances. So consider the situation where a dieter performs a hard 400 calorie workout which causes them to reduce NEAT later in the day by 150 calories for a net 250 calorie increase. Compare that to a dieter who performs a more moderate 250 calorie workout who sees no reduction in NEAT. Both have burned the same 250 extra calories per day but the second achieved it with a much more enjoyable and sustainable approach. In this regard, the activities that increase NEAT are generally low intensity yet have the potential to greatly impact on TDEE. As I showed in the last chapter, increasing calorie expenditure from even 1 to 3 cal/min during an 8 hour work shift can burn nearly 1000 extra calories per day without causing undue fatigue. It would require 90 minutes of exhausting exercise to do the same and some of the calorie burn might very well be offset by reductions in NEAT later in the day.

Other Metabolic Adaptations to Dieting

In addition to the changes described above, there are a host of other adaptations that occur in response to dieting/fat loss. One that is often unconsidered is sleep which can become disrupted with dieters either having trouble falling asleep or staying asleep (I'd remind readers that women's sleep can become disrupted during the late luteal phase of the menstrual cycle to begin with). A large amount of research has recently linked shortened sleep, below 6 hours/night, with increased hunger and appetite along with reduced energy expenditure due to fatigue (27). This is regulated through a chemical in the brain called orexin which regulates sleep and energy balance along with being involved in how much NEAT someone performs (28).

Moving away from the energy balance equation per se, other changes occur that serve to both limit further fat loss and encourage fat gain if food intake increases. In Chapter 7 I mentioned that it become more difficult to mobilize fat from the fat cells as they shrink and they become less sensitive to fat mobilizing hormones. Along with this is an increase in fat cell insulin sensitivity meaning that insulin has a greater impact on inhibiting fat mobilization. Enzymes involved in fat storage also increase. As it becomes more difficult to mobilize and use fat for fuel, the proportion of LBM being lost increases (29). This can become significant as dieters reach the lower levels of BF% and I described previously how loss of LBM on a diet can increase hunger both during and afterwards (recall that women lose less LBM than men which is one of their fewer advantages in this regard).

While all of the adaptations I have described are popularly referred as the body going into fat storage or fat hoarding mode (or in some cases metabolic damage), they really represent a completely normal and logical adaptation to dieting and fat loss. During the diet they work to slow fat loss and may even cause it to stop if energy expenditure decreases until it matches energy intake. However, claims that people start regaining fat while still in a calorie deficit are nonsensical. Rather, the body is simply primed to store fat at an accelerated and more efficient rate if and when calorie intake increases.

How Long Do the Adaptations Last?

A question that is often asked regarding the above adaptations is how long they last after someone has lost some amount of fat and kept it off. And the answer, depressingly, is effectively forever. Research has examined this over time periods ranging from 7 months to 7 years of post-diet weight maintenance and at least some amount of adaptation to TDEE is still present (30). So long as bodyweight and body fat are maintained below the pre-diet level, energy expenditure will never return to where it was prior to the diet. As with the initial adaptations themselves, much of this is due to maintaining a reduced bodyweight and food intake with RMR, TEF, TEA and NEAT all being reduced for that reason alone. But at least some proportion of the adaptive component also remains. It is reduced compared to during the phase of active dieting but it is still present. The question then becomes how much of an impact it has.

And the answer is, at least for Category 3 individuals, not very much. In one study, the total drop in TDEE was 500 calories per day there was only a 3-5% adaptive decrease in RMR present (31). This amounts to perhaps 40-70 calories per day and again changes in RMR really aren't responsible for the large scale changes that are occurring. Adaptive changes in the other components have not been studied to a great degree but it is likely that they are maintained to one degree or another. Certainly the motivation and ability to exercise can increase when food intake is raised and it's possible that NEAT will recover or increase once the person is no longer active dieting. But the fact remains that TDEE will always be reduced with some degree of the adaptive component still being present. At least some increase in hunger and appetite is also usually seen although, once again, it will be less than during the period of active dieting since more food is being eaten and at least some hormonal recovery will have occurred. Most dieters report some fairly permanent degree of residual hunger and loss of fullness even if they are no longer dieting.

Since they aren't often included in diet studies, very little work has been done on lean individuals in terms of how much change in TDEE or the adaptive component is occurring. When they are done they either examine eating disorders such as anorexia where extremely low body weights or are comparing female athletes with menstrual cycle dysfunction to those without (I will discuss this in detail in Chapter 12). Regardless, someone who is attempting to maintain a very low bodyweight/BF% is likely to experience all of the adaptations to an even greater degree in terms of a large scale reduction in TDEE, a relatively large adaptive component (that never disappears) along with increased hunger and appetite.

Ignoring the fact that it is not generally healthy for people, women moreso than men, to maintain extremely low BF% for extended periods, it's worth addressing whether the above can be addressed or dealt with. Here exercise, especially for the general dieter has the potential to play a huge role. There are several reasons for this. One is that increased exercise can help to offset the metabolic adaptations which are still present. It will also allow for more calories to be eaten, offsetting some of the issues with hunger and appetite, while still maintaining energy balance. Regular exercise is also often associated with better adherence to the diet which provides another benefit when maintenance is the goal. In this vein, while exercise do not generally improve weight or fat loss per se, it has been shown to improve long-term weight maintenance, assuredly for the reasons listed above (32).   It's worth mentioning that, in direct contrast to the above, many who maintain a lowered bodyweight/BF% for extended periods often report that it becomes easier with time. Since it's clear that some amount of metabolic adaptation will always be present (and that the "Setpoint" never goes down), the reason is assuredly behavioral with people's new activity and eating patterns becoming more and more ingrained and automatic.

Adaptations to Overfeeding and Weight/Fat Gain

Having looked at the adaptations that occur to dieting, I want to look at what can or does happen in reverse, when people overeat and gain weight and fat. There are two situations here, one when someone gains weight from their current weight and the other when someone regains weight after a diet.

Overeating from a Baseline Weight and Body Fat

Looking first at what happens when people gain weight or fat from their current weight, I'll first say that if bodyweight/body fat are regulated in any meaningful way, it would be expected that the adaptations that occur with dieting would occur in reverse with weight gain.   Appetite, hunger and the rewarding nature of food should decrease while TDEE should increase.

 In response to a 10% weight gain, RMR has been shown to go up about 20-25% (~150-250 calories with large variation) with 10% being due to the weight gain itself and the rest the adaptive component. Surprisingly this was seen in both women and men and lean and overweight subjects. Other studies, usually providing 1000 calories over maintenance, have found broadly similar results with at most an increase in RMR of perhaps 100 calories (34). TEF also increases in all situations due simply to eating more calories. This increase clearly can't offset the total calorie surplus and an 8-9 fat gain is common. At best it helps a little and makes it slightly easier to return to the pre-overfeeding body weight. Assuming formal exercise is being done, TEA would be expected to increase.   A larger body burns more calories and, if muscle is gained, higher power outputs, running speeds, weights being lifted, etc. should allow more calories to be burned. Muscular efficiency also decreases with weight gain so that more calorie are burned. If weight gain is excessive, this can make exercise more difficult so there is a limit to this effect.

As with dieting, that leaves NEAT as the place where potentially the largest impact might be seen. The same effect on bodyweight and muscular efficiency will be present here leaving the question of whether or not NEAT will increase with overfeeding. And the answer is that it does for some individuals. In the study that first identified NEAT, women and men were placed in a metabolic chamber before being overfed by 1000 calories per day (36). Based on the calorie surplus, fat gain should have been enormous but ranged from 3 to 15 pounds between subjects. And while there were small increases in RMR and TEF (exercise was not allowed), the major difference was in NEAT. Subjects who increased NEAT the most gained the least fat and vice versa. In fact, some subjects increased NEAT by an incredible 700 calories per day (leaving 300 to be stored) while one female subject actually decreased her NEAT. The impact was not only potentially enormous but enormously variable.

The cause of the adaptive response to overfeeding is, once again, hormonal with hormones moving in opposite directions as seen with dieting. Levels of active thyroid increase as do the catecholamines with reproductive hormone levels improving and cortisol and GH levels going down. At some point, this does go awry, with obesity, both women's and men's hormone levels become dysregulated. But with moderate weight gain, the impact on hormones is generally positive in terms of increasing TDEE via an adaptive component with NEAT still playing the potentially major role.

Overeating and Regaining Fat After a Diet

Let me now address what happens when people begin overeating and regaining weight and fat after having previously dieted down and this occurs for two primary reasons. The most common is that people succumb to the increased hunger, appetite and attention/enjoyment of palatable foods and start overeating again. The second is the athlete who has dieted to a low BF% for temporary (usually competition) reasons who needs to deliberately regain fat afterwards. In both cases, the starting situation is relatively identical in that hunger and appetite will be increased while daily energy expenditure will be decreased. As discussed in the sections above, what primarily differs is in the degree of changes seen with greater adaptations in both being seen as BF% goes lower. And in both situations, at least in the broadest sense, hormones, hunger, appetite and the various components of energy expenditure will recover and finally reach baseline when the dieter reaches their pre-diet BF% and body composition levels. Whether this happens quickly or slowly depends only on how quickly or slowly that pre-diet body composition is reattained.

I'd mention that, despite various claims of "reversing metabolic damage" there is no practical way to restore TDEE (except perhaps by drastically increasing activity levels) without regaining the lost body fat to pre-diet levels. Since fat sends the primary signal here, it has to be regained to restore physiological normalcy. Recall from above that LBM is involved here and the system will not reach true normalization until both fat and LBM have been restored. Demonstrating this, in the case study of the male bodybuilder, since less LBM was lost and he was training and eating sufficient protein as he regained weight and fat, no excess body fat was gained. His metabolism (and presumably his hunger levels) returned to 100% of it's starting value at the same BF% (~15%) he had started at. I will discuss several case studies of female physique athletes in Chapter 34 where the same phenomenon was seen.

Just as with the recovery in energy expenditure back to baseline, the changes in hormones with overeating from a reduced bodyweight/body fat will be recovery back towards normal. Levels of active thyroid hormone will increase back towards baseline as will the catecholamines and reproductive hormones. Cortisol will decrease as well. Just as energy expenditure won't recover until the previous level of body fat is reattained, neither will hormone levels (as well they will go above normal if body weight/body fat overshoots it's starting place).

Individuality and Interrelationships

In several of the sections above, I mentioned that there is a fairly large variation between any two individuals in the adaptive response of metabolic rate to either dieting/fat loss or overeating/fat gain. As it turns out, these responses are inter-related, partially explaining why some people seem to remain naturally lean in the modern world while others do not. For example, the people who increase energy expenditure in response to cold exposure also raise it the most in response to overfeeding (37). There is also huge variance here with the increases ranging from 38 to 380 calories per day. Similarly, there is a direct relationship between the increase in energy expenditure with overfeeding and the drop with dieting (38). People with a spendthrift metabolism raise TDEE the most with overfeeding and have it decrease the least during dieting; they gain weight with difficulty but lose it easily. In contrast, those with a thrifty metabolism show the least increase in TDEE with overfeeding and the largest drop while dieting; they gain weight easily and lose it with more difficulty.

Does Yo-Yo Dieting Permanently Impair Metabolism?

A commonly heard claim is that the process of losing weight/fat and then regaining it, often called Yo-Yo dieting (or weight cycling) can cause a permanent impairment of metabolic rate or make fat loss more difficult in the long run. I want to address both how this might occur and whether or not it has been found to happen. One way this might occur would be due to body composition worsening after a cycle of weight loss and regain. If someone lost a significant amount of LBM due to poor dieting practices and failed to regain it after the diet, they would end up at a higher BF% (even at the same weight) which could potentially impact their energy expenditure. However, considering the small difference in calorie burn between muscle and fat (replacing 5 lbs of LBM with fat only changes RMR by 30 calories), the only real way this might occur would be if organ mass was lost and not regained (39).

Another that might cause this, especially for women, is if the distribution of body fat changed. If fat were lost from a relatively easy to lose area but regained in a more difficult to lose area, this might have a long-term negative effect. This might actually occur to a small degree and I will discuss this in the next chapter. There could also be some sort of permanent change in the brain, how it responds to the various hormones that are released that regulate metabolic rate but this is poorly studied at this point. It's far more likely that those people with thrifty metabolisms are starting off with a biology that makes fat loss more difficult although it might get worse with repeated cycles of dieting. Alternately, one of the hormones that regulates metabolic rate might never recovery fully.

That said, direct studies show that repeated cycles of weight loss and regain seem to have no long lasting impact on most components of energy expenditure (40). The changes when weight and fat are lost are reversed with the weight and fat are regained. While not the target audience of this book, this may not be the case in younger individuals. Wrestlers who weight cycled ended up with a 15% lower RMR (250 calories per day) than those who didn't and this is significant (41). Given the common tendency for women to start dieting at fairly early ages, it's possible that repeated cycles of fat loss and regain could have negative long-term effects. Even here, women recovering from anorexia (perhaps the most extreme example) completely normalize their metabolic rate when their body weights are normalized (42). A very small amount of data has documented a permanent 5% reduction in NEAT with weight cycling. Two of those are case studies in arctic explorers and the same occurred in the Biosphere experiment I mentioned above. Nobody knows why but this shows that NEAT is still the major place where changes occur.

Anecdotally some dieters do report greater difficulty in subsequent diets but this is likely due to issues with adherence. This isn't to say that there couldn't be a long-term metabolic effect but it simply hasn't been seen in the research to date. At the same time, physique athletes often report finding that getting very lean becomes easier with repeated diet cycles, likely due to the combination of good dieting practices and determining how best they should implement their own diet.

Hormonal Responses

I want to wrap up this chapter by examining some of the hormonal response to both fat loss and fat gain in slightly more detail than above, primarily focusing on the hormones that were not discussed in previous sections. I mentioned the concept of a setpoint early in the chapter, a body weight or body fat that is regulated or defended by the body. For this type of system to work, the body would need to know how much someone was eating or how much fat/weight they were carrying so it would know how to adapt. The relevant structure here is called the hypothalamus and you can think of it as integrating signals that are coming into the brain from all over the body. Depending on what it senses, it tells a gland called the pituitary gland, a glad that controls other glands, what to do. So the hypothalamus might signal the pituitary to tell the thyroid gland to produce more or less thyroid. The pituitary also regulated reproductive function via LH and FSH. But it's the hypothalamus controlling the entire system.

A huge number of signals "tell" the hypothalamus what is going on in the body. I already mentioned some of them above, CCK, PYY, GLP along with changes in blood glucose, amino acid and fatty acid levels all signal the brain about nutrient intake. Insulin sends its own signal to decrease hunger although this only occurs in men. Ghrelin is a key player already mentioned with increases causing hunger and decreases indicating fullness. Ghrelin tends to be both a short-term signal, responding to meals although it also shows long term changes with fat loss (increasing) or fat loss (decreasing).

But the real player in the entire system is leptin, which I talked about briefly earlier in the book and will discuss again. Released primarily from fat cells, leptin's discovery in 1994 changed the face of obesity research as it showed that fat cells were an active player in controlling metabolism. In terms of this chapter, leptin provided a signal to the brain about not only how much someone was eating but how much fat they were carrying. Leptin levels are directly related to subcutaneous fat levels (insulin is related to visceral fat levels) and women product 3-4 times the leptin as men. Leptin changes in response to both short-term food intake (dropping by as much as 50% in only 7 days of dieting) and fat loss (dropping much more slowly). Leptin can increase just as rapidly, increasing with as little as 5 hours of overfeeding. Overall, leptin is a major part of the signal to the hypothalamus that someone is either losing or gaining fat.

And leptin ends up coordinating the entire system that is involved with appetite, hunger, etc. It impacts on how well hormones such as CCK and PYY work, directly controls the signals sent by the hypothalamus to the pituitary and directly inhibits cortisol release. Leptin plays a role in controlling brain levels of DA and serotonin along with directly impacting on fat mobilization and fat burning in muscle. When leptin levels are normal, the system works more or less correctly. I say more or less as the obese may be resistant to leptin's effects. Initial studies attempted to generate weight loss with leptin injections but they mostly failed. This is because leptin primarily coordinates the adaptations to dieting; when it decreases all of the adaptations described above occur with the degree of adaptations being related to the drop seen (43). Quite in fact, after someone has dieted, leptin injections will mostly reverse the adaptations seen (44). Basically, falling leptin induces metabolic adaptation but increasing levels above normal do not.

This raises the question of why the Leibel study showed the same metabolic rate increase to weight gain in the lean and the obese. It's been suggested that some other signal than leptin is working when weight is gained but nobody knows for sure (45). Even that doesn't explain why the system appears asymmetrical with weight gain being easier than weight loss at least for some people (46). Most likely the effect here is due to the environment where the hedonic system can easily overwhelm any metabolic effects. Even animals who normally regulate body fat well become obese if fed the modern diet and humans are no different. Regardless, let me now finally turn my attention to gender issues in these systems to address why women seemingly gain fat more easily and lost it with greater difficulty.

Chapter 10: Women, Fat Gain and Fat Loss: Part 1

Having examined a great deal of background information in the previous chapters, I want to now examine in some detail gender differences and women's specific issues in terms of fat gain and fat loss. For every topic I will discuss there is generally at least one difference between women and men and while research continues to unravel the specifics and details, the major distinctions have been established. Since there is a great deal of information to cover, I have decided to split it into two chapters. This chapter will focus primarily on the underlying physiological differences while the next chapter will examine the direct research on weight and fat loss along with some other related topics.

For consistency, I will be organizing this chapter to follow the overall flow of the previous 5. I'll look at differences in body composition first before looking briefly at gender differences in the risk of obesity, disease, fat loss and starvation. The different components of energy balance will be discussed next including differences in hunger, appetite and food preferences along with gender differences in energy expenditure. Next I'll examine how the different nutrients are used both after and between meals as well as during and after different types of exercise. Finally I'll look at the topic of what is being lost (i.e. LBM vs. fat) during a diet and address the issue of weight loss and regain and how it can impact on body fat distribution. As needed, I will look at the impact of hormonal modifiers on all of these issues.

Due to the large amount of information I want to examine, this chapter will jump around a bit between topics and a large amount of the information will come from a number of recent review papers. While all look at effectively the same topic in broadly the same way, each takes a slightly different approach to the issue which is why I'm including them all (1-9). Individual references will be included as needed.

Gender Differences in Body Composition

While I discussed body composition, the relative proportions of fat, LBM, etc. in general terms in Chapter 5, I want to first look at specific gender differences in this regard. Women and men differ in nearly every aspect here and I'd note that the grand majority of changes do not show up until puberty. At this point, the increase in reproductive hormones interact with genetics and early physiological programming to generate the differences that are seen.

On average, women are both shorter and lighter than men. But at the same Body Mass Index (BMI, discussed in Chapter 6), women carry approximately 10-12% more total body fat than men, some of which is sex-specific fat such as breast tissue (9a). Women also have more total subcutaneous fat and less visceral fat than men. In addition to carrying more total body fat, there are significant differences in body fat distribution between women and men with women carrying more fat in their lower bodies. Despite this, women often have more total fat (in pounds of kilograms) in their upper bodies than men. Women also have more total fat cells than men in both the lower and upper body. Finally, women also store more Intra-Muscular Triglyceride (IMTG, fat within the muscle) than men.

Given that women have 10-12% more body fat than men, by extension they carry 10-12% less lean body mass (LBM and here I am talking about all LBM, not just muscle). Of that total LBM, women carry about 5% less total muscle mass (47% vs 51%) than men due to having slightly more organ mass (9b). Proportionally more of a woman's muscle is carried in her lower body compared to her upper body as well. For comparison, I've shown a woman and man at the same BMI in terms of their average body composition along with a woman "scaled up" to the same weight as a man.

	Woman	Man	Scaled-Up Woman
Weight	150	165	165
BF%	22%	12%	22%
Total LBM/Muscle*	117 lbs/55 lbs	145 lbs/74 lbs	129 lbs/60.5 lbs
Total fat	33 lbs	20 lbs	36 lbs

*Assumes 47% of total LBM is muscle for women and 51% of total LBM is muscle for men

Let me reiterate a point I made in the first chapter which is that the above represents only averages and only when comparing women and men under the same circumstances. Any individual woman may be taller or heavier than any individual man; on average they are not. A highly trained female athlete might have more LBM and less BF% than a smaller untrained male but this is not a fair comparison. When comparing an average female to male or athletic female to male, the above generalities will hold.

Clear that the average gender differences in body composition are fairly significant. Of more importance, these differences alone end up explaining away a great number of the supposed gender-based differences in physiology. Early studies made a common mistake of comparing women to men and just measuring some outcome in absolute terms. So consider a piece of research that determined that women burned 7 cal/min and men burned 10 cal/min doing the same task. This looks like a clear gender difference and the simplest conclusion would be that some physiological or hormonal difference was the cause. Except that you'd fundamentally expect women to burn less calories performing a given task simply due to being smaller on average.

And when you correct for those differences in weight or body composition (and there is a great deal of technical argument about what the best way to do this), most of the differences disappear completely. It's not always all of them but most of them. Put differently, say you took the above values of 7 and 10 cal/min and then divided it by the women and men's body weights. So you might take the 7 and 10 cal/min values and divide by total LBM, finding that both women and men burned 0.25 cal/min/lb of LBM or something (the numbers are just for illustration) causing the gender difference to disappear. This is due to the fact that, with minor exceptions, a woman's body tissues are the same as a man's. Under a microscope, her muscle tissue looks more or less identical to a man's. She simply has less of it. Her liver would look more or less identical to a man's. Hers is just smaller. And this holds for most tissues in the body. Perhaps the biggest difference here is in the fat cells due to difference in women and men's fat distribution and the differences in how fat cells in different parts of the body either store or lose fat. Her larger amount of lower body fat will be more difficult to lose than his greater amount of upper body fat.

Phrased differently, if a woman and a man had an identical body composition in terms of weight, total LBM and muscle mass and BF%, their physiologies would be almost indistinguishable in many ways. It's simply that this is almost never the case unless someone is comparing a highly trained muscular/lean female athlete and an untrained male. In practice, there will always be some apparent gender differences between women and men, even if a large portion of it is related only to body composition differences. Which isn't to say that there aren't still other differences in physiology outside of just body composition. There are with most of these being driven by the differences in reproductive hormone levels between women and men along with any changes that are occurring throughout the month.

I'd add that even if these differences in body composition explain many of the perceived or measured differences, they still have enormous practical implications for diet and fat loss. I mentioned one of these in Chapter 1, how carbohydrate loading becomes nearly impossible for female endurance athletes because the amount of carbohydrate needed may exceed their daily calorie intake levels. The same holds true in other domains. Due to having lowered calorie requirements, women often can not alter their diet to the same degree as a larger man would be able. I'll discuss in the next chapter that, to burn the same number of calories with exercise, women have to exercise more or at a higher intensity due to being lighter.

Effect of Hormonal Modifiers on Body Composition

While a woman's average body composition develops at puberty, it can be impacted to one degree or another by the hormonal modifiers. In general, PCOS women are at a higher risk of being overweight to begin with. As well, those PCOS women with elevated testosterone levels (and to a lesser degree women with subclinical hyperandrogenism) tend to have a more male-type fat patterning with more fat around the midsection and an increase in visceral fat. They frequently carry more skeletal muscle/LBM than other women although their BF% will still tend to be higher as well. As mentioned in Chapter 3, by and large hormonal birth control (BC) doesn't seem to have a major impact on body composition although some types may cause a small increase in fat with a small loss of LBM. Depo-provera is an exception and is associated with the greatest weight and fat gain.

As obesity is defined by BF% to begin with, obviously overall BF% is higher approaching 50% or more of total weight at the extremes. With increasing weight there is some increase in LBM although this eventually hits a maximum with all further weight gain being from body fat. With aging, there is often a worsening of body composition some of which is due to age and most of which is due to reduced activity levels. As women approach or enter menopause, there is often a significant worsening and change in body composition if hormone replacement therapy (HRT) is not undertaken. Both total weight and body fat increases with fat patterning moves to a more male pattern (increasing relative disease risk) and LBM is lost. HRT appears to reverse the majority of this (9b).

Women, Obesity, Disease, Fat Loss and Starvation

While a great deal of the perceived gender differences in physiology more or less disappear when the differences in body composition are taken into account, it's also clear that there are differences that cannot be explained solely by this. I'll address the specific physiology below but first want to look at a number of observations that have been made that show quite clearly that women and men differ in both their propensity for fat gain and fat loss.

On top of carrying a larger percentage of body fat (and often more total fat) than men, women are far more likely to become obese than men with the biggest difference seen after women go through menopause. As well, women are three times as likely to be found in what is called the super obese category, marked by the highest extremes of BF%, in some cases as high as 50-60%. Clearly, within the context of the modern environment, women's bodies do respond differently in terms of their propensity to gain fat. Despite this, women are relatively more protected against developing certain diseases such as diabetes/insulin resistance (PCOS women excepted) and heart disease which are often associated with excessive body fat levels, especially when they are younger. This is due to having more subcutaneous fat in general and more fat stored in their lower bodies in specific (this pattern being more metabolically healthy overall). In contrast, men tend to carry more visceral fat which is where the health risks lie. When women start to gain visceral fat (as occurs with elevated testosterone levels, at menopause or in obesity), their risk of those same diseases increases.

Looking at weight and fat loss, it's generally felt or argued that women have more trouble losing weight and fat than men. Either they lose less total weight/fat or lose it more slowly. I'll discuss this in more detail in the next chapter and will only say here that, in at least some situations, women's bodies clearly do regulate energy balance/homeostasis differently than men. An interesting observation in this regard is that women are more likely to survive starvation or famine than men. This was never studied directly, of course, and the data comes from situations in the early 20th century such as war and famine but the pattern was clear with women showing a higher survival rate. And this is due to physiological reasons that make women's bodies better able to handle a lack of food, better conserving energy for survival in the long-term. I'll look at the mechanisms and reasons (in an evolutionary sense) in the next chapter. For now let me look at potential gender differences that could contribute to the overall differences that are seen.

Differences in Appetite and Hunger (10)

As I have with previous chapters, let me start by looking at gender differences in terms of total food intake, food preferences, appetite and hunger. In terms of overall calorie intake, women generally eat less than men a large part of this is due to simply being smaller. At the same time, there are clear hormonal influences at work. As testosterone stimulates hunger and appetite, women's much lower levels are another part of why they eat less than men overall. Women's bodies also show a difference in how they respond to the hormonal signals involved in fullness. For example, women show higher overall levels of ghrelin (which recall stimulates hunger) and experience a smaller drop when they eat. As described in the last chapter, both leptin and insulin play a role in regulating hunger. Here there is another gender differences with women's brains responding more potently to leptin and men's brains responding more potently to insulin. As leptin is related more to subcutaneous fat (found in greater amounts in women) and insulin is related more to visceral fat (found in greater amounts in men), this makes some degree of sense. But while insulin changes rapidly in response to a meal, leptin does not and this might be another part of why women's hunger does not decrease as much after a meal. Finally, women do not see the same reduction in hunger when they eat more meals while men do (this is discussed more in Chapter 23).

Women's taste buds differ from men's and they experience foods as sweeter and creamier than men do. Women also often prefer the taste of carbohydrates and fats while men prefer protein and fats (11). Somewhat related to this, while obese women show a relationship between their total carbohydrate and fat intake and their body fat levels (lower carb/higher fat intakes meaning a higher body fat level), men show no such relationship (12). Women frequently lament that the same high-fat, high-calorie foods that cause them to readily gain body fat don't cause the same in men and I'll explain why this is below.

It's important to remember that most, if not all, of the above changes to one degree or another during the menstrual cycle with hunger and appetite being the most controlled in the follicular phase (especially in the days before ovulation) while increasing in the luteal phase (along with this comes an increased cravings for carbohydrates and fats). Meals also digest more quickly during the luteal phase, meaning that women will not stay full as long and may be more likely to overeat (12a). As already discussed, this is due to the changes in estrogen and progesterone which are occurring.

A final issue to consider is more psychological than physiological and has to do with what researchers called restrained eating, which is similar but not identical to dieting, and disinhibition (which I mentioned briefly previously). Restrained eaters are those who are concerned with their bodyweight and overall food intake while disinhibition refers to a situation where environmental triggers such as stress, being around others who are eating or being around highly palatable foods causes them to break their diet and overeat (13). Restraint can actually be rigid or flexible which actually have very different effects in this regard but I will discuss this in a later chapter. I bring up the topic here as women are not only more likely to be concerned about their weight and/or be actively dieting but tend to have higher dietary restraint than men (14). If they are rigidly restrained, they may be at risk for disinhibition and overeating.

Effect of Hormonal Modifiers on Food Intake
Looking briefly at the potential effects of the hormonal modifiers, I mentioned in Chapter 3 that, overall birth control doesn't seem to increase hunger or appetite. This depends on the generation of progestin with first and second generation progestins potentially increasing hunger and appetite while the third and fourth generation lack this effect. Due to the hunger stimulating effect of androgens, women with subclinical hyperandrogenism or PCOS may experience greater hunger and appetite overall. PCOS women have also been found to eat more highly refined carbohydrates and saturated fats and that their bodies do not regulate hunger as well as they should (15). Finally, women with PCOS are also more prone to binge or other types of disordered eating (15b, 15c). As I mentioned the obese often show a hunger, appetite and reward system that isn't working well in the first place although this may be as much a cause of them becoming obese as a consequence. Regardless there is often a dysregulation of the systems involved in hunger and appetite that contributes to the problem. Given the role of estrogen in decreasing hunger, any situation where estrogen levels are decreased would be expected to increase hunger. This includes the loss of menstrual cycle (amenorrhea) and it's known that hunger and food intake increase at menopause (moreso if HRT is not begun). Along with other changes in physiology, this all contributes to age-related gains in weight and fat.

Differences in Energy Expenditure
Moving to the energy expenditure side of the equation, I want to look at each of the four components which make up Total Daily Energy Expenditure and will do so separately. It's been known for some time that, on average, women have a lower Resting Metabolic Rate (RMR) than men. And for many years this was felt to represent an inherent gender difference related to some aspect of physiology. But as I described above, almost all of the difference ends up being related to the differences in body composition. As RMR is related predominantly to LBM, women's lower levels will mean a lower RMR. When RMR is normalized for LBM, the difference disappears (16). As noted above, women's tissues burn the same number of calories per pound as a man's, they simply have less of them. That said, research has found that women may have slightly lower or higher energy expenditures relative to their LBM than men. In the follicular phase, it may be slightly lower while in the luteal phase it may be slightly higher. In both cases, the difference is only a few percentage points either way which is insignificant.

Overall women do show a lower Thermic Effect of Food (TEF) but this is primarily due to eating less total food. Limited research shows that, as a percentage of total calories, women have a slightly lower TEF than men although the differences is quite small (16a). TEF does change throughout the menstrual cycle, being slightly lower during the luteal phase but the effect is only about 3 calories per meal (16b). One unstudied, but potential gender difference, could be related to the choices of foods. As dietary protein has the highest thermic effect, women't tendency to undereat protein relative to carbohydrates and fats might lead to a somewhat lowered TEF as well. Any effect here will only be for the most extreme dietary comparisons and the overall small effect of TEF overall make gender differences fairly insignificant.

Moving to activity, women have been found to be less physically active than men at all ages although it's difficult to tell if this is an actual biological difference or driven more by environmental and social factors (17). What is clear is that women often exercise for different reasons than men with women being driven by more external factors such as body weight and physical appearance. Women also tend to emphasize aerobic training while men emphasize resistance training. In terms of the energy expenditure of formal exercise (TEA), women generally burn fewer calories during exercise than men for two primary reasons. The first is due to simply weighing less as it takes more calories to move a heavier body. The second is related to body composition with women's lower levels of muscle resulting in lower running speeds, power outputs, weights lifted, etc.

Finally there is Non-Exercise Activity Thermogenesis (NEAT) which has not been well studied in terms of gender differences. As with formal exercise, women will burn less calories during NEAT due to simply being smaller. Since most types NEAT are low intensity, it's debatable if differences in LBM will contribute further. The unanswered question is whether women show lower levels of NEAT than men or not. What little data exists suggests that it depends more on societal factors in terms of what tasks women do or do not perform. On the Ivory Coast, where women perform 95% of domestic and 30% agricultural duties, their NEAT is higher than men's. In Australia, Canada and the UK, women's levels of NEAT may be 1/3rds that of men's. In the United States, women and men's NEAT appear to be roughly equal (18). This doesn't indicate if there are any true gender differences outside of environment for NEAT. At most there is the indirect observation that the four worst responders in the overfeeding/NEAT study I described in the last chapter were women. But more research is necessary.

Effect of Hormonal Modifiers on Energy Expenditure

There tends to be limited data on the hormonal modifiers and their effects on the different components of energy expenditure. At least some forms of birth control can actually increase a woman's RMR by about 5%, similar to what is seen in the luteal phase, due to the progestin component. Amenorrhea, discussed in detail in Chapter 12, is associated with a significant decrease in RMR, similar to what is seen at the lower limits of BF% in men. Women with PCOS appear to have a normal RMR compared to non PCOS women with a similar body composition although they do show a slightly reduced TEF (perhaps 30 calories per meal) in response to a meal (18a). Overall, their total energy expenditure relative to standard prediction equations is normal (18b). Women do show a greater age related decrease in energy expenditure than men, roughly 143 calories/decade versus 34 calories, probably related to changes in body composition (19). At menopause energy expenditure goes down due to both the loss of LBM and an apparent decrease in energy expenditure in the organs; this is reversed with hormone replacement therapy (20).

Two Implications of the Above

Before delving deeper into the physiological gender differences, I want to address two practical implications of the above sections relative to fat loss (and I will mention these again). The first is that, for the most part, due to their lower energy expenditure and food intake, women are frequently unable to achieve the same degree of calorie restriction as men. For a woman with a maintenance calorie level of 1700 calories to reduce her food intake by 500 calories per day (a 30% decrease) is drastically different than for a male with a 3000 calorie to do the same (only a 16% decrease). Not only will this impact her more hormonally but, practically, it may make adhering to the diet impossible due to the low total food intake. This can be less of an issue for heavier Category 3 women as their higher starting food intake allows a greater reduction with fewer problems. The second is related to exercise with the same issue arising. Due to being smaller and having less muscle, a woman will burn less calories during any given workout. She will have to exercise more or at a higher intensity to burn the same number of calories.

Differences in Nutrient Metabolism

In addition to the global differences in hunger/appetite and energy expenditure, women's metabolism of the different macronutrients (protein, carbohydrates, fats and alcohol) differs from men's to one degree or another and this is true both after a meal is eaten, between meals and both during and after exercise. In many cases, the differences are related to body composition but in others it's clear that they represent a true physiological difference. Given the differences in body composition and fat patterning, it would be surprising if this were not the case. At the same time, many early (or logical) assumptions about nutrient metabolism are turning out to be incorrect with some surprising things occurring.

As I will be focusing predominantly on carbohydrate and fat metabolism in the next sections, I want to address dietary protein and alcohol here first. Both at rest and during aerobic exercise, women use less protein for fuel and this is clearly due to the effects of estrogen (21). Quite in fact, if men are injected with estrogen, their metabolism changes to mimic that of a woman's. Practically this means that a woman's protein requirements relative to her LBM will be lower than a man's. This does change slightly from the follicular to the luteal phase when increased progesterone increases protein breakdown but this effect is extremely small and can be safely ignored (21a). There is limited research on the impact of hormonal modifiers here although any loss of estrogen signaling (i.e. amenorrhea, menopause without HRT) has the potential to negatively impact on protein metabolism. Aging also plays a role here and protein requirements are now known to be increased significantly in older individuals.

Women's bodies also metabolize alcohol differently than men, reaching a higher blood alcohol level if they ingest an identical amount of alcohol. Some of this is related to differences in body composition (having less total body water to dilute the alcohol) but women also have lower levels of the liver enzymes that metabolize alcohol (22). While I won't discuss alcohol much in the context of overall diet in this book, there is an interesting gender difference worth mentioning. In general, alcohol intake doesn't seem to generate the weight or fat gain that would be expected based on the calorie values and some calories seem to be "missing". There is also a gender difference here where women show a lower Body Mass Index (BMI) with increasing alcohol intake while men show an increasing BMI (23). Put differently, alcohol intake leads to lower body weights in women but higher body weights in men. This appears to be mostly a social phenomenon since women frequently drink instead of eating while men commonly drink in addition to eating high-calorie, high-fat foods. Type of alcohol also plays a role with wine being associated with a lower BMI and hard liquor associated with a higher BMI. This may be interacting with gender differences in alcohol preference that may be present. I mention this only for completeness and am in no way recommending women attempt to drink themselves thin (BMI is also not a perfect indicator of BF%).

Nutrient Metabolism After a Meal

First let me look at differences in how nutrients, focusing on carbohydrate and fat, are metabolized following a meal. Here I'll be assuming a mixed meal containing some combination of protein, carbohydrates and fats. These enter the stomach where they are digested and absorbed, eventually reaching the bloodstream. This puts the body into a storage mode where the nutrients are either burned for energy or stored for later use. Carbohydrate is stored in muscle or liver as glycogen while dietary fat can be stored within muscle as Intra-Muscular Triglyceride (IMTG) or within fat cells.

After a meal, women burn roughly 14% less fat than men for energy, their bodies using more carbohydrate. I'd note that as she will generally be eating less total fat per meal than a male, the total amount of fat stored may be less in absolute terms even if the percentage is higher. A large part of this is due to the average differences in body composition. As women have roughly 12% more total body fat than men, they store just over 12% more of the total fat eaten (with no apparent difference between the follicular and luteal phase). An additional factor is that women's subcutaneous fat is more sensitive to the anti-fat mobilizing effects of insulin; the hormonal response to eating shuts off fat mobilization. In contrast, men's visceral fat is more resistant to insulin and continues releasing fatty acids into the bloodstream after a meal, causing more to be used for energy. Any fat not burned for energy is stored primarily in her subcutaneous fat but this raises a seemingly silly question of which area (i.e. upper vs. lower body fat) that fat is stored.

Given the difference in body fat distribution, readers might assume (and researchers did the same) that women's bodies would preferentially store fat in the lower body while men did so in the upper body but that turns out to be wrong. Rather, after an average sized meal, both women store roughly twice as much fat from the meal in the abdominal/upper body area as in the lower body. Women also store double the dietary fat in both areas as men (who store relatively more dietary fat in visceral fat). This does depend somewhat on a woman's body fat patterning. Women with a more upper body fat patterning (as occurs in obesity or with elevated testosterone levels) tend to store relatively more fat in the upper body while women with a lower body fat pattern store relatively more in their legs. There is one exception to the above. When women eat a very high-calorie and high-fat meal (in this case 100 grams of fat), those excess calories will be stored directly in lower body fat cells (24). An old saying, at least in the US is "A moment on the lips, a lifetime on the hips." and the combination of this type of direct lower body fat storage along with a general resistance to loss shows that it is basically true.

Irrespective of that one exception, most of the post-meal fat storage is in the upper body fat areas in both women and men. Given the differences in body fat patterning, this came as a bit of a shock to the researchers. Stranger still, research found that the post-meal storage pattern did not predict where fat was gained in the long term (25). Despite storing fat in their abdominal area immediately after a meal, women still gained fat in the lower body over time, raising the question of how this process occurred. The answer, as detailed below, has to do with what happens in-between meals.

Nutrient Metabolism Between Meals

Several hours after eating a meal, the nutrients that were eaten will all have been burned for energy or stored and the body will begin to rely more on stored calories such as muscle and liver glycogen, IMTG or fat. The same occurs after an overnight fast to a more pronounced degree. This effect is hormonally driven. As storage hormones such as insulin drop and nutrient mobilizing hormones increase, fatty acids will be released from fat cells to be used for energy. The liver will also break down stored glycogen to glucose (or produce it from other substances in the body) which is released into the bloodstream to maintain blood sugar. Of the fat being released into the bloodstream, 80% comes from upper body fat cells and the remaining 20% from lower body fat cells and this occurs in both women in men. This provides the reason that both women and men store fat in the upper body after meal: these fatty acids can be used for energy more quickly between meals. If women (or men) stored fat in the lower body right after a meal, there might not be enough fatty acids available to provide energy to the body between meals. But this still doesn't explain a woman's lower body fat patterning. If fat is stored in the upper body after eating why or how does it eventually "end up" in the lower body?

Surprisingly, women show up to 40% higher rates of fat mobilization than men although this is primarily coming from the upper body. They also show 15% higher levels of fatty acids in the bloodstream. Given the general pattern of having higher body fat overall and a greater difficulty losing fat, this makes very little sense as women would be expected to mobilize less fat than men, rather than more. This becomes even more confusing when two more contradictions are considered. The first is that high blood fatty acids tend to cause insulin resistance which can lead to diabetes or the Metabolic Syndrome. Yet, as I mentioned above, pre-menopausal women are generally protected from this disease. Women have higher levels of fatty acids in the bloodstream without the negative effects that would normally occur.

The second is that, in general, the more that a given nutrient or fuel is available, the more it tends to be used for fuel. When carbohydrates are available, the body burns more carbohydrates and when fat is available, it burns more fat. Yet women, who have 15% higher levels of fatty acids end up burning 10% less total fat than men and less total fat grams per hour or day than men. Once again this is primarily related to differences in body composition. Since women have a lower total energy expenditure, they burn less of all nutrients (in absolute terms) than men. Since they have 10-12% less LBM, they burn less total fat for fuel as a percentage. This means that, regardless of anything else they will burn less total fat grams per day than a male, despite having more total fat on their bodies (26).

So now we have a situation where women have higher rates of fat mobilization which leads to higher levels of blood fatty acids which isn't matched by either the negative health effects or increase in the use of fat for fuel that would be expected. If fatty acids are being released but not burned for energy, this means that they must have another fate which they do. This is called non-oxidative disposal which just means that the fatty acids are disposed of somewhere in the body without being burned (oxidized). And this happens to a greater degree in women (27). Recall from earlier in the book that after mobilization, a fatty acid can simply turn back around to be stored back in the fat cell, a process called re-esterification. This process is 64% higher in women than men which means that most of the fatty acids being released into the bloodstream are just being stored back within a fat cell. While being sort of wasteful (it's called a futile cycle), this gives women the benefit of being able to shift to using fat for fuel more readily (as during exercise, discussed below).

But there is no law that says that fatty acids release from one fat cell have to be re-esterified into that same fat cell. If blood flow is sufficient, those mobilized fatty acids can be transported elsewhere in the body. While they may be used for energy, they can just as easily be stored in a different tissue. This could include the situation where they are stored within muscle as IMTG. As I've mentioned, in cases of extreme obesity, fat is stored in inappropriate tissues such as the liver or pancreas. Of relevance to the topic of fat patterning, readers may remember the direct fatty acid storage pathway I mentioned in a previous chapter, a pathway by which fatty acids released from one fat cell can be stored/re-esterified in a different fat cell. Which is exactly what is going on here. Fatty acids which have been released from the upper body fat cells, but which are not burned for energy, can eventually be stored in lower body fat cells. This occurs more in lean women than in lean men and to the greatest degree in obese women, probably due to the increased amounts of total fat and fat cell number in the lower body.

And this final piece of the puzzle explains all of the above observations. After a meal, women not only store more total dietary fat but that fat is predominantly stored in upper body fat cells. After a meal, women show higher rates of fatty acid release (especially from the upper body) but burn less of it for fuel due to a lower energy expenditure and having less LBM. Those unburned fatty acids are either stored back in the fat cells they came from or are redistributed to other areas of the body, including lower body fat cells. And it is this long-term redistribution of fat from the upper body to the lower body that explains both the development and maintenance of women's lower body fat patterns. I'd note that this primarily occurs in the case where body fat is being gained as, during weight maintenance, any fat stored should be burned off for energy before being redistributed to other areas.

Nutrient Metabolism During Exercise

Continuing from the above, I want to look at gender differences both during and after exercise as this also helps to explain some of the differences seen in fat loss and fat patterning. While I discussed many types of exercise in Chapter 4, I will only be focusing on three types in the following sections. The first is aerobic exercise, any continuous whole-body movement done for 20 minutes or more. The second is High-Intensity Interval Training (HIIT) which alternates short bouts (15-90) seconds of very high-intensity activity with similar durations of low-intensity activity. Finally is weight or resistance training where muscles are forced to work against a high resistance with the goal of increasing muscular strength or size. Most of the research I will be discussing in the following sections has focused on aerobic exercise although I will address the limited work on other types of exercise (especially as HIIT and weight training have some potentially enormous benefits or women's fat loss).

Fuel Use During and After Exercise

Perhaps surprisingly, women actually use a larger percentage of fat for fuel during low- and moderate intensity aerobic exercise than men. This effect is even more pronounced during the luteal phase when insulin resistance due to elevated progesterone limits carbohydrate use further. Women also start using fat for fuel more rapidly than men during aerobic exercise, a consequence/benefit of the futile cycle I mentioned above. At higher exercise intensities, women and men use roughly the same amount of fat and carbohydrate although there are still some small differences present. I say surprisingly as this would seem at first glance to contradict women's generally lower rates of fat loss. But there are several factors at work here to explain this.

The first is that, except for highly trained athletes, exercise typically makes up a very small part of the overall day's energy expenditure. Unless extremely large amounts of activity, hours per day, are being done, the total number of calories and fat burned during exercise is quite small. This is doubly true for women as they burn less calories than men during exercise due to being smaller. As a singular example, in one study, women and men performed 90 minutes of exercise at a fairly hard intensity (75% of maximum heart rate). The women burned 660 calories while the men burned 985 calories (33% more). Of those 660 calories, women burned 36 grams of fat (less than one tenth of a pound) while the men burned 45 grams of fat (28). Since one pound of body fat contains 454 grams of fat, it would take women nearly 13 workouts to lose one pound while men would require only 10. This assumes that 100% of the fat being burned was coming from body fat in the first place which turns out not to be the case.

I mentioned earlier in the book that women's muscles store more fat within their muscle (called IMTG) and it turns out that women's bodies use more IMTG for fuel than men during aerobic exercise (29). This reduces the total amount of body fat burned during exercise and, when all is said and done, of the total fat women use for fuel, only 12% of it comes from fatty acids mobilized from fat cells. Of the 36 grams of fat used for fuel during exercise, only 4 of that would be coming directly from fat cells and most of that will be coming from upper body fat cells to begin with. I'd note that the depleted IMTG will eventually be replaced and this can technically come from either body fat or dietary fat. In a dietary deficit, where more fat is being burned than eaten, the body should take fat from fat cells and transfer it it into the muscle as IMTG. Even this will be coming primarily from upper body fat meaning that a woman's lower body fat will remain even as her upper body is losing fat. I want to finish by mentioning an absolute insane oddity about women's fat metabolism during exercise. Which is that, via the direct pathway I mentioned, women can actually store fat in their lower bodies while they are walking (30). That is, even while using fatty acids for energy, women's bodies are still finding a way to store fat in their hips and thighs. However, the effect is insignificant with perhaps 1/10th of a gram of fat being stored in an hour of exercise.

Regardless of the specific numbers, the fact is that the impact of any reasonable amount of exercise on the use of fat is quite small. And this compounded by the fact that, following exercise, women shift back to using more carbohydrates for the rest of the day. In contrast, while men use less total fat for fuel during exercise, this causes them to use more fat for fuel the rest of the day. So while women may burn slightly more fat (as a percentage) during an hour of exercise, they will use more carbohydrate for energy the remaining 23 hours of the day. In contrast, while a man may burn a smaller percentage of fat during that same hour of exercise, he will use more fat for energy the other 23 hours per day. And it should be clear that the non-exercise part of the day is far more important than the small amount of fat burned during exercise itself. Adding to this is the fact that women rely more heavily on blood glucose during exercise while depleting their muscle glycogen to a lesser degree than men which has further consequences for nutrient metabolism during the day.

This difference in fuel use during exercise actually explains a great deal of the post-exercise differences as well. As a general rule, the more glycogen stored within a muscle, the more carbohydrate and less fat it will use for fuel and vice versa (if glycogen is depleted, the muscle will use more fat for fuel). Because they deplete less of their glycogen during low- and moderate-intensity aerobic exercise, women use less fat the rest of the day while men show the opposite pattern, using more glycogen to fuel exercise and using more fat for the rest of the day. Supporting this is the observation that if men eat before aerobic exercise, they use more glycogen for fuel and this increases their use of fat for energy to an even greater degree of the rest of the day (31). While not studied in women, I would not expect this to be effective due to women's greater reliance on blood glucose to begin with (i.e. eating will not increase muscle glycogen depletion in women as it does in men). I would mention in finishing that while the above would certainly seem to represent an inherent gender differences in terms of physiology (and is to at least some degree), a primary factor is simply the differences in body composition. Being smaller, women burn less calories during exercise, less total fat during exercise and less total fat the rest of the day.

I should mention that it's somewhat debatable if what is burned during exercise is particularly relevant to what is being lost from the body in the long-term. Certainly it plays a role but the calorie deficit is a much larger component of generating fat loss. So long as there is a long-term deficit, some amount of fat will have to be mobilized and used for fuel. The above is primarily addressing the issue of why women lose seemingly less fat than men. I'd mention again that part of the above is clearly just related to the lower calorie expenditure seen overall. In the one study I mentioned, despite using a higher percentage of calories as fat, the women burned not only less total calories but less total grams of fat. To even equal the same absolute amount of fat burned (in grams) requires a longer exercise sessions or a higher intensity. I will discuss in Chapter 14 the potential benefits of higher intensity exercise on women's fat loss.

There is another factor to consider in the above which is the potential extra calorie burn that occurs after exercise. Popularly called the afterburn effect, the technical term is Excess Post-exercise Oxygen Consumption (EPOC). Simply, this represents the number of calories burned after exercise, with most of them coming from fat. EPOC is related to both the duration and intensity of the exercise. Longer durations raise EPOC linearly but higher intensities can raise it exponentially. I would mention that the actual calorie burn during high-intensity exercise is often far lower than during low-intensity since it cannot be maintained as long. So even if the EPOC is potentially higher, the total calorie burn may be lower.

Following aerobic exercise, women show a lower EPOC than men for the same amount and intensity of exercise, burning less total calories and fat after exercise than men (32,33). EPOC and fat oxidation are both higher during the luteal than follicular phase although the difference in EPOC is only 40 vs. 60 calories over 6 hours (33a). This may not be the case following sprint exercise (30s all-out) where women and men show an identical EPOC although the total effect is still quite small, roughly 50 calories burned over 2 hours (34). As I'll discuss in a later chapter, resistance training may also induce a greater EPOC. Although the menstrual cycle data suggests a biological difference, a large part of the difference is once again related to women being smaller with less LBM (35). This prevents them from generating the same power outputs and running speeds as men with less metabolic stress in general but still means that they will show a lower absolute EPOC in addition to a lower calorie burn during exercise. Women also generally exhibit more precise homoeostatic control, returning to their baseline physiology more quickly than men.

Effects of Hormonal Modifiers

Looking at hormonal modifiers, in women with PCOS, fat mobilization is decreased significantly at rest which may be part of their predisposition to weight gain. Weight loss in general along with aerobic exercise can overcome this, possibly through increased sensitivity to the hormone ANP I discussed previously (36,37). BC is complex in that it seems to increase the rate of fatty acid mobilization but also increases the rate of re-esterification during aerobic exercise although this doesn't seem to impact on the use of fat for fuel (38). In the obese, there are often high levels of fatty acids in the bloodstream but this is coupled with a tendency to burn carbohydrates for fuel at rest. Exercise reverses this (39). At menopause, there is a decrease in both fat mobilization (reversible with caffeine) and fat burning during exercise with postmenopausal women showing fuel use like that of older men. Oral forms of HRT appear to decrease the use of fat for fuel (by impacting liver metabolism) while transdermal forms increase it (40).

The Composition of Weight Being Lost

In Chapter 7, I talked about altering body composition and how the proportion of fat, muscle, water, etc. being gained or lost impacts on not only the changes in body weight but the caloric equivalent of those changes. Focusing only on the proportion of fat and LBM being gained or lost, I'd mention again that women tend to lose a lower proportion of LBM (often 1/3rd or less as much) and more fat than men for any given amount of weight loss (41). Since a pound of fat contains more energy and requires a larger deficit than the loss of a pound of LBM, that loss will always be slower. This is compounded by the fact that, due to being smaller with a lower food intake women cannot generally create the same daily deficit as men. Imagine a woman on a 300 calorie/day deficit who loses 100% fat and a man on a 600 calorie/day deficit losing 80% fat and 20% muscle. Over 7 days, she will create a 2100 calorie deficit, losing 0.6 lbs of fat while he creates a 3,500 calorie deficit and loses 1.8 lbs of which 0.8 lbs is fat and 1 lb is muscle. He will need perhaps 2 more days to lose a full pound of fat while she will need 5. By losing a greater proportion of her weight as fat, she ends up losing both weight and fat more slowly (42). This works in the opposite direction with women gaining more fat and less LBM than men such that their weight goes up more slowly.

Regional Fat Loss and (Re)Gain

To wrap up the discussion of the physiology underlying women's fat gain and loss, I want to expand on a topic I mentioned in the last chapter when I talked about Yo-Yo dieting. This had to do with the potential for a redistribution of body fat when and if fat was regained after a diet was over and the potential of this to make future dieting efforts more difficult. So consider the possibility where a woman loses fat from the easier to mobilize upper body fat but regains it in the more difficult to lose lower body fat. Even if she ends up at her pre-diet BF%, she might have more trouble losing that fat during later diets.

I described a study earlier in the book where Category 2 women and men were overfed, gaining 6.5 lbs of fat over 8 weeks. Of that, 4 lbs of fat was gained in the upper body with the fat cells increasing in size, with the other 2.5 lbs being gained in the lower body and fat cell number increasing (over time, the gained upper body fat would be redistributed to the lower body). During a second 8 week time span, they were put on a diet and lost 6 lbs of fat with 5 lbs coming from the upper body and 1 coming from the lower body (43). Presumably if they had kept dieting they would have lost the remainder of lower body fat but this points out that, in both women and men, upper body fat is both easier to gain and lose overall. In a related vein, Category 2 women performed 6 months of combined aerobic exercise and weight training; they lose 3% body fat with no fat loss from the legs (44).

This is problematic as several studies suggest that when and if fat is regained, fat distribution can and does change. In one, women who regained weight after a diet were found to increase their thigh body fat levels by 102% (2% over where it started) despite only regaining 83% of the lost weight (45). Had they regained all of the lost weight, presumably this would have gone even higher. Another found that despite a 93% total fat regain after dieting, women increased their hip fat by 6% over where it had started (46). While not measured, it's conceivable that lower body fat cell number also increased in both cases.

Summing Up

Putting the above data together leads to the following overall picture. When women gain fat, it tends to be in both the upper and lower body with the gained upper body fat being redistributed to the lower body over longer time frames. When they lose fat, proportionally more of that fat will come from the upper body as it is easier to mobilize (as discussed in Chapter 7). When fat is regained, there may be a proportionally greater increase in her lower body fat with levels increasing above their pre-diet levels. Over several cycles of Yo-Yo dieting that alone has the potential to lead to proportionally greater lower body fat levels.

If a woman diets poorly (insufficient protein, no resistance training, rigid, she may lose LBM along with the fat (coming from the upper body with the LBM representing muscle). Her diet become unsustainable and she begins overeating in the face of lowered energy expenditure. As she regains body fat, she will gain proportionally more in the lower body (potentially increasing fat cell number) and this will be more true if she is eating a large amount of high-calorie, high fat foods which are preferentially stored there. Since she will not be regaining the lost LBM, her hunger will remain higher than it would otherwise and she may end up with not only a higher BF% but proportionally more hip and thigh fat. This situation potentially worsens with each cycle of fat loss and regain.

This all points not only to the importance of using proper dieting practices but is critically important for those women attempting to diet to a very low BF% and who typically do lose their lower body fat in doing so. When they regain fat (as they eventually must) they must ensure that there is no body fat overshoot or proportional increase in the amount of lower body fat present. Because while the above is mostly in Cat 2/3 women, there are at least anecdotal reports of increased lower body fat in Cat 1 women after a diet, especially if the post-diet phase includes bingeing on high-calorie, high-fat foods.

Chapter 11: Women, Fat Gain and Fat Loss: Part 2

Continuing from the discussion of physiological differences between women and men in the last chapter, I now want to look at the direct research that has been done in terms of fat gain and fat loss. It's generally accepted that women lose less fat (or lose it more slowly) than men in response to diet or exercise and there is certainly some truth to the idea. At the same time, there are a number of pitfalls to this type of research that need to be addressed and that I want to discuss. Following those comments, I want to first look at research that has compared women and men in terms of their response to specific weight/fat loss interventions. As most research is done on overweight individuals, I will address potential differences between lean and obese women. I'll finish by looking at gender differences in energy homeostasis (how the body regulates energy balance) along with a brief look at the evolutionary reasons those differences exist.

Direct Research on Weight/Fat Loss: Introduction

When I discussed some of the difficulties in doing comparative gender research in Chapter 1, I touched briefly on the issue of how women and men should be matched in the first place. That is, within the context of this chapter, how should diet studies be set up or how should the results be compared. Should the women and men weigh the same (in which case a woman's BF% will be much higher), should they have the same BF% (in which case the men's weight will be much higher), or should they be at the same BMI (in which case weight and BF% will differ)? If you do match them in some way, the question remains as to whether or not that will reflect the real world (where weight, BMI and BF% may all differ).

Once that has been addressed the next question is how should the results be compared. There are two primary ways of doing this: you could compare the total amount of weight or fat lost in absolute terms (i.e. women and men lost 4lbs and 5 lbs respectively) or you could compare the percentage of weight or fat lost relative to their starting point (i.e. both women and men lost 5% of their starting weight). The second approach is probably the more valid one as a relatively lighter woman would be expected to lose less total weight than a man regardless of any other differences. So consider a woman who weighs 250 lbs and loses 12.5 lbs and a man who weighs 300 lbs and loses 15 lbs, both losing 5%. Her absolute loss was smaller but, once initial body composition was taken into account, her relative loss was identical.

Even if most studies use it, weight loss per se isn't the ideal goal or even the best result to look at in the first place. Changes in body composition are far more relevant and, as I've discussed, the relative changes there impact on both total weight loss and the rate at which it occurs. As discussed, women lose less LBM and more fat than men under most conditions which means less total weight loss (but often more total fat loss) along with that weight loss being slower. In many exercise studies, women often gain some LBM (due to starting out with less than men) even if they lose similar amounts of fat. They may lose less total weight but their fat loss is identical and their body composition has improved.

Finally is the issue of individual variability. Most studies only report the average result but, just as it did with the issue of birth control and weight gain, this can mask the results that any given individual might experience. There is actually some evidence that women are more variable than men in their response to diet or exercise interventions and this acts to cancel out some of the changes that would otherwise be seen. Finally there is the fact that most research on weight and fat loss is done in Category 3 individuals for what should be logical reasons. While they certainly experience metabolic adaptation, it becomes more pronounced into Category 2 and Category 1 and the results between women and men may differ.

With those potential pitfalls addressed, I want to look at the direct research that has compared women and men in terms of their response to various weight loss interventions. I'll separate these into two sections, the first will include diet only and diet plus exercise, while the second will focus on exercise only studies. I'd note only for completeness that there is some indication that women may do better than men when they include weight loss medications in the program but this is beyond the scope of this book.

Diet Alone or Diet Plus Exercise (1)

I want to start by addressing studies looking at diet alone or diet plus exercise. These tend to vary enormously in how they are set up and might compare low- to high-protein, low- to high-carbohydrate, low- to high-fat or look at the Mediterranean diet or any other number of possible combinations (I will provide my recommendations in Chapter 19). If exercise is included, it may be low-intensity aerobic exercise, high-intensity aerobic exercise, resistance training or a combination of one or more (there might also be diet plus aerobic exercise compared to diet plus resistance training). This can make comparing the results of different studies very difficult.

Variations in the calorie intake or the side of the deficit relative to maintenance may also differ. This is important as it ties into the baseline differences in energy expenditure that are present. If both women and men are placed on some fixed calorie level such as 1200 or 1500 calories per day, the woman will have a smaller daily deficit since her total energy expenditure is lower to start with. If calories are reduced by some percentage below maintenance, the same will occur. If a woman and man with maintenance levels of 1800 and 2700 calories respectively reduce that by 25%, her deficit will be 450 cal/day while his will be 675 cal/day. Of course she will lose less weight (and lose it slower) than him. The only time that you'd expect a woman to lose the same amount as a man would be if both created an identical daily deficit. If both women and men reduced their calorie intake by 500 calories/day or increased their exercise by 500 calories/day this would be expected to generate the same results. This raises the practical issue where it may be impossible, or at least very difficult, for women to be put on the same intervention as men.

With all of that said, in the aggregate, the research shows that women do in fact lose less total weight than men in response to various types of interventions. The difference actually isn't enormous with women losing roughly 12.5 lbs (5.5 kg) and men 18 lbs (8.5 kg), a mere 4.5 pound (2kg) difference. But this would be expected for all of the reasons discussed above. Looking at the results in terms of the percentage loss, the difference is much smaller with women losing 7% of their starting weight and men 8%, a mere 1% difference. I would mention in this regard that some studies find that women show a slower initial loss of weight than men which could be related to men having more of the easy to lose visceral fat. Since they are smaller, women might also be losing less body water and glycogen. Finally, since women are losing less LBM than men, their total and rate of weight loss will be slower (it's hard to see men's greater loss of LBM as a benefit). Perhaps surprisingly, women appear to show slightly better long-term weight maintenance than men and this may actually be due to a slower initial rate of weight loss (2). Most studies find that maximum weight loss occurs at about the 6 month mark (supporting all of the research from the last chapter on how the body starts fighting back) but women may continue to lose past that point. Their slower initial losses may be offset by more continued losses over the long-term.

While exercise alone has not been shown to be terribly effective for weight loss (this is discussed below), its inclusion in a weight loss program has been shown to provide benefits. Of perhaps the greatest importance is that diet alone can cause a loss of bone mineral density while the inclusion of exercise prevents this (3). Other potential benefits of exercise are improved adherence to the diet along with preventing the loss of LBM that might occur (gains in LBM sometimes occur as well). Weight training far more so than aerobic exercise can prevent the decrease in LBM with fat loss but ultimately diet is the major driver on fat loss. A recent study in Category 3 pre-menopausal women showed this by comparing a diet only to weight training only to diet with weight training in terms of fat loss (3a). Weight training increased LBM with no impact on fat loss while diet decreased fat loss without altering LBM. The diet plus weight training group lost fat while increasing LBM and avoided a drop in metabolic rate.

In diet plus exercise studies, there are some gender differences but they tend to be somewhat smaller than see in diet only studies. On average women lose 11 pounds (5 kg) to a man's 14.5 lbs (6.5 kg), a 3.5 lb (1.5 kg) difference. This is actually a smaller total weight loss than in the diet alone studies but this is where only looking at changes in body weight becomes misleading. If LBM loss is reduced or LBM is gained due to exercise, total weight loss will be reduced even if fat loss is not. When the above results are expressed as a percentage, women seem to show slightly worse results with women losing 3.6% of their starting weight and men 5.2% (a 1.6% difference vs. 1% for diet alone). This is assuredly a consequence of the impact of exercise on LBM. Since women start out with less LBM than men, they gain it more easily with exercise. They may lose less weight but lose as much fat while improving body composition.

Exercise and Weight and Fat Loss

While it is slightly out of order to address exercise in the absence of any dietary control or modification, I have done so for two reasons. The first is that exercise alone is often recommended as being nearly magical for both weight and fat loss, even in the absence of dietary control. The reality here is far different with exercise being generally ineffective in terms of its effect on weight or fat loss for both women and men. There are a number of reasons for this but a main one is that the amount of exercise that all but highly trained athletes can realistically do is usually fairly small. This is double true for women due to their being lighter and smaller. The calorie burn from exercise is simply too small to matter. More important to the topic of this chapter is that the impact of exercise on weight/fat loss is the place where the largest apparent gender differences in terms of total losses or the adaptations and compensations that occur to limit losses show up.

Looking at the topic observationally, early research showed no relationship between a woman's activity levels and her BF% while men who were more active had a lower BF%. Similarly, when women increase NEAT, they show no loss of fat, presumably due to increasing their appetite while men's BF% does decrease (4). Perhaps shockingly, in response to 5 months of half-marathon training, women showed no overall increase in their Total Daily Energy Expenditure probably due to decreasing NEAT while men's TDEE did increase (5). In contrast to the above, and supporting the importance of weight training, a recent study found a moderate relationship between the weight training frequency and intensity and women's BF% (5a). Specifically, for every day of added exercise, BF% was reduced by about 1.5% and LBM increased by 1.5 lbs. The overall difference was fairly small, however with non-exercisers having a BF% of 32.3% vs. 30% in the weight training group.

Moving to more direct research, a number of early studies that I will not detail generally observed that women did not lose significant amounts of weight with exercise alone (almost always aerobic exercise) while men did. This led to the general conclusion that exercise without diet ineffective for women (6). Indirectly supporting this was research showing that women's fat cells did not increase their response to fat mobilizing hormones in response to 20 weeks of training while men did (7). This is probably an artifact of women already mobilizing more fat than men which means that they have less improvement to make. Similar results have been seen for the impact of exercise on insulin sensitivity where women show no improvement from exercise while men do. But this is simply due to women being more insulin sensitive to begin with and having less room for improvement.

Women also show a large amount of variability in weight loss or gain both in general and compared to men in terms of their response to exercise (8,8a). Some women have been found to be weight-loss "responders", losing as much weight as predicted (and showing less of a reduction in NEAT) while others are "non-responders", losing less weight than predicted due to greater reductions in NEAT (9). There is likely to be variability in the changes in hunger, appetite or the enjoyment of palatable food between any two women. It's also likely that women who show the greatest reduction in NEAT show the greatest increase in hunger, appetite, etc. As I noted earlier in the chapter, this variation can make reporting of average results a problem. In one study on exercise and weight loss, women showed about an equal distribution of weight loss and weight gain while all the men lost at least some weight during the study. This made the average weight loss appear much smaller for the women.

As I mentioned above, exercise has generally been found to be ineffective for weight and fat loss due, among other reasons, to the relatively low numbers of calories that can be burned. Even studies using larger amounts of exercise,generating significant amounts of weight loss in men, usually fail to have the same effect in women. At best women avoid weight gain or gain a small amount of weight (10). Coupled with a woman's smaller body size and muscle mass along with a greater tendency to decrease NEAT or increase food intake, exercise alone is simply that much less effective for woman than men (11). While the above conclusion, that exercise alone is ineffective for causing weight loss in women, seems well supported, there are some problems with it, some of which I already mentioned. One is the reporting of average results, mentioned above. Another is that most exercise studies generate very little weight loss in in women or men. Finally is the fact that changes in body weight can mask changes in body composition.

One commonly cited study on this topic demonstrates this well. In it, women and men were trained over 40 weeks to complete a half-marathon and the study concluded that men but not women lost weight but this is misleading (12). On average, women lost just under 2 lbs while men lost just over 2 lbs. The women's loss wasn't statistically significant while the men's was but neither group lost very much in the first place. The body composition changes also paint a very different picture. Here the women lost 5.5 lbs (2.5kg) of fat while gaining 2.6 lbs (1.2 kg) of LBM while the men lost 8 lbs (3.5 kg) of fat and gained 3.5 lbs (1.5 kg) of LBM. The fat loss represented 3% of the women's starting body fat and 4% of the men's. Certainly the women lost less total fat (as would be expected) and a smaller percentage (similar to the diet and diet plus exercise studies) but the increase in LBM in both groups made the actual change look far smaller than it was. Focusing on the small change in weight loss per se leads not only to a poor conclusion but misses the point about the much more important changes in body composition. Although NEAT was not measured, the women's food intake did tend to increase about halfway through the training program while the men's didn't, once again suggesting a difference in how women and men regulate energy balance.

Even more importantly than the above is the fact that not all studies find that women lose less weight (or fat) than men. A recent analysis of short-, medium- and long-term studies finds in some studies women lose less weight/fat than men but in others they do not (13). It also pointed out a number of potential factors that might cause the results to be so mixed. A major one has to do with the generally small amount of total weight loss that is seen in the first place, often no more than a few pounds. In many cases, the measured changes are well within the normal day-to-day variation in body weight and that alone could obscure the true results. Many earlier studies also failed to control for the women's menstrual cycle and that alone could easily explain the differences. As mentioned, in several studies women gained LBM while men did not meaning that their total weight (but not necessarily fat) loss will be lower.

But there are two much larger issues at work here. The first has to do with adherence and whether or not the exercise program is being followed in the first place. In studies where the exercise program is supervised by the researchers, weight loss is always greater than when it isn't. Quite simply, many people, regardless of gender, show poor adherence to the exercise program. The second, and far more important issue has to do with an issue I've mentioned several times which is that women will always burn fewer calories than men for any fixed amount of exercise. Studies that give exercise based on frequency, time and intensity (i.e. 5 days/week for 45 minutes at 70% of maximum heart rate) will always generate a lower calorie expenditure in women than in men and that alone would predict lower amounts of weight and fat loss. In fact, this may be the primary factor in the differences that have been seen to date (14).

This raises the question of whether or not women and men will lose the same amount of weight and fat if they burn the same number of calories during exercise. In one study of Category 3 women and men, this appears to be the case (15). In it, the subjects performed supervised exercise five days per week working up from 150 calories burned per workout to either 400 or 600 calories burned per workout over the first five months of training. They maintained that level for an additional five months. In the 400 calorie/day exercise group, there was no difference between women and men in either weight or fat loss: the women lost 8.4 lbs (3.8 kg) and the men 9 lbs (4kg) of weight and almost 100% of it was body fat. In the 600 calorie per day exercise group, the results were slightly different. Here the women only lost 8.9 lbs (4 kg) or 0.5 lbs (0.2 kg) more than in the 400 cal condition while the men lost 13.5 lbs (6kg) or 4.5 lbs (2.2 kg) more. For statistical reasons the results were considered identical but suggests a trend where performing more exercise was less effective for women. It's impossible to tell if this is just a statistical blip or if the women's bodies started to compensate at the higher energy expenditures.

Regardless, this study points out that if women and men burn the same number of calories in exercise, their fat loss is effectively identical. It also suggests that the results of previous studies had less to do with actual gender differences and more to do with women simply being smaller and burning fewer calories overall. I'd note that this study did use a fairly large amount of fairly intense exercise although it was built up to gradually over many months (this is important for reasons I'll discuss in later chapters). But there is another point to consider which is that, in burning the same number of calories during exercise, the women had to exercise longer than the men (50 vs. 32 minutes in the 400 calorie/day group and over an hour vs. 42 minutes in the 600 calorie group). Other research supports this observation. In one, women and men who burned the same number of calories with supervised exercise lost identical amounts of fat, but the women had to exercise for 54 minutes to the men's 43 minutes (16). Indirectly supporting this, when women burn the same 400 calories as men during low- or high-intensity exercise, they burn more fat both during and after exercise (relative to their LBM) than men (17). This effect is especially pronounced after high-intensity exercise but means that the apparent gender differences in fuel use after exercise may simply be due to burning fewer calories. As with the other studies, the women had to exercise significantly longer to achieve this (120 vs. 89 minutes for low intensity exercise and 86 vs. 50 minutes for high-intensity).

These studies make two primary points. The first is that, at least in overweight women, a major cause of the apparent gender difference in weight loss is that women simply burn fewer calories for any given amount of exercise. When they burn the same number of calories as men, their fat losses become essentially identical with the drawback being that they have to exercise for anywhere from 20-35% longer than men. Presumably this could be partially offset by women exercising at a higher intensity (and I will discuss other potential benefits of including high-intensity training for women in Chapter 14) but that brings up other potential issues having to do with excessive amounts of intensive exercise overstressing women's bodies. This will be discussed in detail in the next two chapters. The same general conclusion will hold for diet in that women will more or less lose the same amount of fat as men if the same deficit is achieved. But, practically it is more difficult for them to do so.

Lean Versus Obese Women

The above issues, whereby it is more difficult for women to achieve the same calorie deficit with diet or calorie burn with exercise becomes even more pronounced as women are lighter and leaner. Not only is it more difficult for the woman to even achieve the same degree of calorie reduction or exercise energy expenditure as men as they become lighter, but many of the adaptations and compensations start to become more pronounced in leaner women.   While studies done in obese individuals may not find significant differences in terms of weight and fat loss (assuming a few conditions are met), this stops being the case as women enter Category 1 or try to reach lower limits of female BF%. It not only becomes effectively impossible for a woman to achieve the same daily calorie reduction or exercise energy expenditure as men but, even when they can, their results still come more slowly.

This difference between categories makes perfect sense within both the context of the general adaptations to dieting along with the specific issues that pertain to women (discussed at the end of this chapter). Fundamentally a Category 3 woman is not at risk of starving to death as she has plenty of fat to lose in the first place. Even here, there may be differences based on body fat patterning. Women with a male-like upper body fat pattern lose fat from exercise alone while women with a lower-body fat pattern do not (18). Perhaps bizarrely, while upper body obese women and men lost fat in response to exercise, lower body fat women actually gained fat (19). This suggests that the effect is as much due to total body fat/Category as it is to fat distribution and patterning (recall from the previous chapter that 6 months of exercise training caused fat loss in the arms but not legs). The Category 3 woman with the upper body fat pattern has easily lost visceral fat (like men) along with relatively easier to lose upper body fat; the woman with a lower body fat pattern does not.

This is important to this discussion due to the fact that women with a typical body fat patterning tend to lean out effectively from the top-down. Their upper bodies, face, breasts, shoulders and even abdominal area (in the mid to high teens of body fat) will become lean while their lower body fat may not have changed significantly. The greater the relative proportion of the difficult to mobilize lower body fat, the less of an effect any intervention will tend to have. Studies find that while exercise generates at least some fat loss in both obese women and men, it has no effect in lean women (20). In one study, three months of exercise caused fat loss in obese women and men but didn't generate fat loss in women who had been matched for body fat to the men (21). An interesting observation in this study was that men with smaller but more fat cells lost no fat while men with larger but fewer fat cells did (recall that fat cell size is a determine of how easily fat can be mobilized and lost). As women's lower body fat is typically made up of smaller but more fat cells, this probably explains the lack of exercise alone.

Other factors could be involved here. One is the potential for food intake to increase after exercise, which has been shown to occur to a greater degree in lean than obese women. When exercise alone is used, lean women will exactly increase their food intake to cancel out the calories burned from exercise while obese women will not (22-23a). Lean women also report an increase in the sensory attractiveness of food (i.e. food becomes more appealing) after exercise that men do not (24). This seems to contradict what I wrote in an earlier chapter about exercise not increasing appetite or hunger. While true in the short-term, it's clear that women do in fact increase their calorie intake in response to exercise over the long-term (25). This occurred in the half-marathon training study I mentioned above but ultimately means that, in lean women, exercise alone is unlikely to be effective for generating fat loss if the diet is not controlled. The lean woman's body will simply adapt and cancel any effect of the exercise. I would note again that, in highly trained female athletes, the above may reverse itself and hunger may be blunted in response to exercise (26,27). This can cause a different problem where female athletes are chronically undereating.

Regardless of that, the fact is that all of the adaptations that are occurring in the leaner female dieter will act to slow fat loss, frequently to rates lower than that of men. While little research has been done on this (researchers don't often do diet studies in lean individuals), anecdotally, Category 1 women always lose fat more slowly as they approach the lower limits of BF% than men, even if they are on broadly similar exercise programs and calorie deficits. This could be due to greater reductions in NEAT or some other component of energy expenditure but occurs nonetheless. For reasons I will discuss next, the adaptations are always more pronounced in leaner women (and often moreso than in leaner men).

Gender Differences in Energy Homeostasis (28-30)

As readers may remember from science class, the concept of homeostasis is that the body will, to one degree or another, attempt to maintain some relatively fixed or stable level. Body temperature is one where the body will shiver if someone becomes to cold or sweat if they become too hot. The bodyweight or body fat set point is another with the adaptations in the different components of energy balance at least attempting to maintain homeostasis. And while much of the difference in weight or fat loss can be explained by differences in initial body composition, it's still clear that women's bodies, to one degree or another, regulate energy balance and homeostasis differently than men. Their adaptations are, in many cases larger along with being more variable. They return to baseline faster after high-intensity exercise and there are other examples of this. One has to do with how well or poorly women handle heat or cold stress compared to men. Under some conditions, women handle heat better during exercise (although they cool down more slowly afterwards) and start shivering later (saving energy expenditure) in response to cold. These do point to physiological differences between the and all ultimately point to women's bodies being more efficient at storing calories when they are available while limiting their use for fuel when they are not. While many of those differences appear to be less important in overweight women, larger effects start to become far more prevalent as women become leaner. Given what the system is "trying" (in a biological sense) to accomplish, this all makes sense. Before addressing that, I first want to look at what end up being the physiological controllers of the differences in energy homeostasis.

As I've focused on some of these already, I'll be focusing here on insulin, leptin and estrogen. Both leptin and insulin play numerous roles in the body but, specific to energy homeostasis, they are both related to levels of body fat and food intake. Leptin is related mostly to subcutaneous fat and changes very slowly over time (i.e. hours or days) while insulin is related to levels of visceral fat and changes relatively quickly (i.e. minutes). Given women's greater amount of subcutaneous fat you would expect it to be a more important signal compared to men for whom insulin might more important given their larger amount of visceral fat. In animal models this is true and one study has shown that men reduce their appetite and lose weight in response to inhalable insulin while women do not (31).

Since leptin appears to be the more important signal for women, I want to look more at some of the gender differences here. First and foremost women have four times the leptin levels of men. Some of this is related to having more total fat but women's fat cells produce more leptin per pound of fat or kg as well. This is a direct effect of estrogen with testosterone reducing leptin production. At the same time, due to having more leptin to begin with, women are relatively more leptin resistant than men overall (32). Recall that leptin sensitivity also changes during the menstrual cycle, being relatively higher in the follicular phase and relatively lower in the luteal phase. And while not studied in humans, the hypothalamus (the structure that senses the changes in leptin and other hormones) of female animals is more sensitive to the changes in leptin compared to when it has been masculinized during fetal development. All of this means that the same drops in leptin levels between women and men are likely to send a stronger signal and generate greater adaptations in women.

Adding to this difference is the act that women's levels drop both faster and to a greater degree than men's in response to both diet and exercise. For example, in obese women, leptin levels drop nearly as much in response to three days of fasting as in men who lose 21% of their starting weight (33). In older individuals, a similar degree of weight loss in both women and men reduce leptin by 45% in women but only 21% in men (34). Finally, in response to exercise alone, a week of regular exercise will reduce a women's leptin levels by 61% compared to a 38% drop in men (35). While not my focus, the hormone ghrelin increases to a greater degree in women in response to exercise and this occurs even if calories are raised to prevent a deficit from being created (36). This combination of changes would tend to stimulate hunger and food intake, even in the absence of a calorie deficit.

Moving on to estrogen, I mentioned many of the effects that it has back in Chapter 2 and it's clear that it plays a major role in positively regulating women's energy balance (37). Recapping only briefly, estrogen is involved in all aspects of fat storage and oxidation while also blunting appetite. The loss of estrogen signaling at menopause has a number of significantly negative effects including increases in bodyweight, body fat and a shift in fat patterning all of which are reversed by HRT. While estrogen clearly has effects on fat and muscle cells themselves, much of this effect is due to estrogen's effects in the brain. As I discussed in Chapter 2, estrogen only sensitizes the brain to the effects of leptin but sends it's own leptin-like signal. This explains why the estrogen peak before ovulation (and more generally estrogen being the primary hormone during the follicular phase) has such a profound effect on reducing hunger and appetite. Relative to energy homeostasis, estrogen levels drop (along with progesterone) when calories are reduced and fat loss occurs in premenopausal women (38).

All of these changes, along with others I'll discuss in the next chapter on menstrual cycle dysfunction, explain why the system works differently in women (especially lean women) compared to men. Essentially, in response to any sort of energetic stress, calorie reduction, exercise, or the combination there will be a drop in leptin levels. This drop will be occurring on a background of already higher leptin resistance causing the drops in leptin to have a more potent effect. This combines with the decrease in estrogen levels which will have an impact due to both estrogen's direct effects along with its effects on leptin signaling. These changes will all signal the hypothalamus to begin the adaptations to dieting and fat loss that I described in such detail in Chapter 8. The adaptive component to RMR, TEA and NEAT will all occur along with an overall increase in hunger. The latter is primarily due to the changes in levels of serotonin and dopamine with dieting, similar to what occurs already during the luteal phase. And since the overall hormonal signals are more potent, you'd expect the adaptations to be both larger and faster.

Why is it Like This?

To wrap up this chapter and topic, I want to briefly look at some of the explanations that have been offered to explain why all of the gender differences in fat storage, loss, and and energy homoestasis exist. By explanation, I don't mean the physiological or biological reasons that I've already explained but rather the speculative evolutionary reasons that caused these differences to develop in the first place. Usually this means what benefits these changes might have had during evolution for survival in one way or another. The basic idea here comes down to the difference in reproductive roles between women and men and the idea that women were far more important for the survival of the human race, necessitating the differences that are seen (39).

Women's bodies produce a singular highly energetically costly egg on a monthly basis while men's bodies produce large numbers of relatively low energy value sperm all the time. If and when pregnancy occurs, women bear an enormous energetic cost to support the development of the fetus in utero to begin with coupled with the energetic cost of breastfeeding after birth. While the cost is not enormous (perhaps 300-400 calories/day), it does add to her calorie requirements. Finally, women were tasked with raising the child after birth to the point that it was most likely to survive (about age 5). This necessitated being able to survive along with provide sufficient resources for the child.

All of this added up to a woman's body needing to be relatively better at storing calories when they were available along with storing them in the relatively more difficult to mobilize hip and thigh fat (which recall are used preferentially at the end of pregnancy and to support breastfeeding). If food was not available in sufficient amounts, she had to be able to resist nutritional stress to a greater degree. I mentioned that women are more likely to survive a famine in the last chapter and it's interesting to note that women can generally maintain normal breast milk production in the face of insufficient food. In addition to storing calories more effectively, they are better at resisting nutrition stress and caloric insufficiency. Since dieting is just controlled starvation on a longer time scale, these same effects occur.

Men in contrast faced none of these demands. Having provided their relatively low cost sperm to the reproductive process, they are not required further. Certainly it can be helpful if they are around in terms of providing resources or protection. But in the case where food is not available, I might argue that it is better for men to die earlier as this will leave more resources available for the pregnant mother and unborn child. But ultimately these differences in reproductive requirements between women and men drove the development of the differences by increasing reproductive success. Women who were more able to store calories or survive food shortages passed on their genes to the surviving children while those women who weren't did not.

In keeping with the above ideas, it's worth considering the entire structure of the menstrual cycle as a whole as it is effectively geared towards a woman's both becoming pregnant and sustaining that pregnancy (the long-term adaptations to metabolic rate are more for long-term survival). The early follicular phase is, in one sense, the tail end of the previous cycle as the system starts to develop the follicle and prepare for the remainder of the cycle. But going into the late follicular phase, prior to ovulation, several changes occur as the follicle is about to be released and implanted. First is the small spike in testosterone levels which likely exists to increase sex drive. The large spike in estrogen is when a woman's appetite and hunger are at its lowest and it's been suggested that, by decreasing her desire for food and drink, a woman's desires for pleasures of the flesh will increase (40). A recent study supports this hypothesis, showing an inverse relationship between hunger and sexual interest: when hunger is highest, sex drive is lowest and the lowest hunger/highest sexual interest occurred when she was most fertile (41a).

Adding to this, a number menstrual cycle of women's behaviors change around or at ovulation, more or less subconsciously that are geared towards reproduction. She becomes more physically attracted to masculine looking men (presumably with better genetics), becomes more receptive to sexual advances and her hips even swing in a way that is meant to be more sexually attractive (41-43). This is clearly being driven by the hormonal changes during the menstrual cycle as the use of birth control has been shown to modify or alter these. Specifically, women's preferences in terms of physical attraction change when they are on birth control as her body effectively "thinks" she is pregnant (44).

Entering the luteal phase after implantation of the egg, more changes occur to ensure that, if pregnancy occurs, there will be sufficient calories available. Hunger and appetite both increase with total calorie intake and cravings for carbohydrate and fat occurring. The increase in consumption of those foods, along with progesterone's direct effect on fat storage in the legs, all acts to ensure calorie and fat storage in the hips and thighs. If pregnancy occurs during a given cycle, her physiology will change completely as her storage of calories in her lower body will increase further, helping to ensure sufficient calories are available to support the later stages of pregnancy and breastfeeding. If pregnancy does not occur, her system will wind everything down to expel the un-implanted egg and endometrial lining during menstruation as the cycle starts all over again. A tangential question in this regard is why women's bodies to through the seemingly wasteful process of expelling the endometrium monthly rather than just allowing it to remain. This seems to be yet another adaptation to reduce energy expenditure. At least part, if not most, of the increase in energy expenditure during the luteal phase is due to the calorie needs of the endometrial lining and shedding it monthly will save her body 100-300 calories per day during the duration of the follicular phase compared to maintaining it for the entire time (45).

I want to mention, simply for completeness, that many of the gender differences are not only driven by the reproductive issues mentioned above but by sexual selection. That is, many aspects of the body were selected due to being sexually or physically attractive. In most cases, these external manifestations were also indicative of her underlying physiology in one way or another (46). This includes such factors as her waist to hip ratio (indicative of her estrogen to testosterone ratio and overall reproductive potential), hair and skin (indicative of overall health), and permanently enlarged breasts (indicating her hormone levels, genetics as well as acting for sexual attraction), along with others. Some of these such as her hair/skin or breast size and shape even change throughout the menstrual cycle in concert with the changes in estrogen and progesterone.

While the reasons appear to be manyfold, it's fairly clear that a woman's physiology is truly geared around her overall reproductive role (I'd note that so are men's, they are just set up differently). This is seen in her general tendency to store fat more effectively while losing it with greater difficulty and in a different general pattern than men. Her body shows overall energy conservation in both directions as she is more likely to become super obese as well as to survive famines. Even the monthly shedding of the endometrial lining is an adaptation to conserve energy, saving several thousand calories per month. If the menstrual cycle is lost completely, the normal increase in metabolic rate during the luteal phase will be lost and this can conserve 30,000 calories per year. Quite in fact, the dysfunction that can occur in menstrual cycle function may be one of the clearest indicators of differences in energy homeostasis regulate between women and men. This is discussed in detail in the next chapter.

Chapter 12: Menstrual Cycle Dysfunction

Continuing from the last chapter, I want to look at the issue of menstrual cycle dysfunction. Not only does this represent one of the myriad ways that a woman's body can adapt to conserve energy, but it also represents a potentially very damaging physiological change that often occurs in response to diet, fat loss, exercise and stress. I want to re-emphasize that there is no such thing as a truly "normal" menstrual cycle to begin with. There is a general structure and pattern that occurs but this can vary enormously between any two women or even in the same women from month to month or throughout her age. I mention this as some of the dysfunctions (i.e. anovulatory cycles) that I'm going to describe may happen from time to time under otherwise normal conditions. This chapter is only addressing chronically occurring dysfunction.

There can be quite a number of medical reasons that menstrual cycle dysfunction can occur but those are far beyond the scope of this book. The only one that potentially falls under a medical heading is frequent oligomenorrhea that is often seen with PCOS or elevated testosterone levels. Rather I will be focusing on four types of menstrual cycle dysfunction that are seen to occur in a dieting, exercising or athletic population. In that context, these dysfunctions would represent a change from the otherwise normal cycle. While each of these can absolutely occur in any woman, they are found at a many times greater frequency in the athletic/dieting population which points to a clear link between the two.

In addition to looking at the different types of menstrual cycle disorders that can occur, what they represent and their physiological consequences, I will look in some detail at their causes. As there are many older ideas still floating around, many of which are incorrect, I'll look both at those older ideas along with what is felt now to be the primary cause of menstrual cycle dysfunction. One of those causes, stress, is so important that I will discuss it in detail in the next chapter. The majority of what I will be discussing in this chapter applies only to Category 1 women who are normally cycling to begin with.

Certainly there can be menstrual cycle dysfunction for women in Category 3 but these are related to hormonal changes that occur with obesity (or underlying PCOS) or other medical disorders. For the most part, the presence of hormonal modifiers removes the possibility of menstrual cycle dysfunction although there are exceptions. The oligomenorrheic woman with PCOS/hyperandrogenism can develop amenorrhea and even women on birth control (BC) report increased breakthrough bleeding or other changes. There are also other hormonal changes of importance that occur in all Category 1 women that I will describe.

Types of Menstrual Cycle Dysfunction

While early work on menstrual cycle dysfunction identified only oligomenorrhea and amenorrhea, which were often grouped together as oligo/amenorrhea (this was prior to the realization that many athletic women were oligomenorrhea as a consequence of elevated testosterone), more recent work identifies four distinct dysfunctions that may occur. These are luteal phase defect/deficiency, anovulation, oligomenorrhea and amenorrhea which will all be described shortly. Luteal phase defect and anovulation are referred to as subclinical menstrual cycle disorders due to the fact that they aren't directly apparent as the menstrual cycle appears normal in duration and menstruation still occurs. Except for the inability to become pregnant (if that is the goal), there is no real reason for a woman to suspect she has either and the determination can only be made through medical workups. In contrast, oligomenorrhea and amenorrhea are termed clinical disorders as they do have external manifestations. In oligomenorrhea, the cycle is longer than 35 days and in amenorrhea it is completely absent.

Luteal phase defect or deficiency refers to a situation where either the luteal phase itself is shortened to less than 10 days (the follicular phase lengthens here) or remains the same length with insufficient progesterone being produced. Estrogen levels may be low and this used to be called follicular phase deficiency (modern descriptions seem to group luteal and follicular phase defect together). In the case where estrogen is low, the egg may or may not be viable in the first place but some amount of endometrial tissue still develops (causing menstruation). Even if the egg is viable, there is insufficient progesterone to support implantation of the egg and infertility results. As noted, the cycle looks normal but is not

Anovulatory cycles, which are far more common than realized under normal conditions, refers to the situation where an egg itself is not released from the follicle for implantation. Estrogen remains lower than expected during the follicular phase and the normal increase in FSH (causing the follicle to burst) and LH (stimulating hormonal production) do not occur. There is still some development of the uterine lining which must eventually be shed, causing menstruation. Again, the cycle looks normal but is not.

Oligomenorrhea is defined as infrequent menstruation with a cycle only occurring every 35 to 90 days. Here, estrogen and progesterone levels show an erratic pattern. On some days an oligomenorrheic woman's hormonal profile may be identical to a normally cycling woman's but these days will not fall on the expected days of the month. On other days, the hormonal profile will show a completely different pattern from any day in a normal menstrual cycle. As in the subclinical disorders, infertility is common in oligomenorrhea but it is also outwardly clear that the cycle is abnormal due to it's length. While both represent oligomenorrhea, I want to mention that two types of oligomenorrhea can be distinguished here based on what is causing them The first is in women with overt PCOS or subclinical hyperandrogenism who's elevated testosterone levels are the cause of the lengthened cycle. In this case, the oligomenorrhea is likely to have been present from a very early age.   The second type of oligomenorrhea is seen in the woman who were previously normally cycling and who developed oligomenorrhea in response to the causes I will discuss below. It is this second type that I will primarily focus on in this chapter

Finally there is amenorrhea which is most generally defined as a lack of menstrual cycle but which is typically divided into two types. Primary amenorrhea has occurred if a woman does not begin menstruating (termed menarche) before age 15. As it's not likely to be that relevant to most readers of this book, I will only mention it briefly again below.   Secondary amenorrhea occurs when a woman who has begun menstruating does not menstruate for more than 90 days and/or there are fewer then three cycles per year. Among other changes that are present below, amenorrhea is marked by both low estrogen and progesterone, neither of which show the normal cyclical changes. In this case, no egg is released, no uterine lining develops and menstruation does not occur.

As I mentioned above, secondary amenorrhea can occur for a number of medical reasons but these are beyond the scope of this book. Rather I will be focusing solely on a specific type of amenorrhea that is marked by changes in both Follicle Stimulating Hormone (FSH) and Leutinizing Hormone (LH), which I mentioned briefly in chapter 2. Not only are both hormones low but they lose their normal daily and monthly release patterns.   FSH and LH are released from the pituitary gland under control from the hypothalamus, the brain structure I talked about in some detail in Chapter 9. Since the dysfunction can ultimately be traced to the hypothalamus, the specific type of amenorrhea I will be discussing is often termed Functional Hypothalamic Amenorrhea (FHA) or sometimes just Hypothalamic Amenorrhea (HA).

For some time it was unclear if the four menstrual cycle dysfunctions described above occurred more or less at random or represented a progressive continuum of dysfunction. The current belief is that women do in fact move progressively normally cycling to luteal phase defect to anovulation, potentially through oligomenorrhea (this seems to occur less commonly) to amenorrhea as the final end point. In that sense, the earlier dysfunctions can be thought to represent "warning cycles" before the menstrual cycle is lost completely. The problem here being that the subclinical disorders have no external manifestations. Until a woman develops oligomenorrhea or amenorrhea, there is no indication of a problem. The four menstrual cycle dysfunctions I described are all broadly related in many ways, not the least of which is that they all represent a low estrogen condition (1). The various hormonal and metabolic changes I will describe below are all present in varying degrees with each type of dysfunction and all become progressively worse as the cycle becomes more disrupted. Luteal phase defect has the least effect, anovulation the next, oligomenorrhea the next and amenorrhea the most profound effect.

Rates of Menstrual Dysfunction

While various types of menstrual dysfunction can occur in all women to one degree or another, the above dysfunctions are seen at a significantly higher rate in exercise women/athletes although the type of menstrual disorder and the rate at which they occur depends on a host of factors, especially the sport being examined. I'd mention that determining exact rates of menstrual cycle dysfunction is problematic for a number of reasons. Early studies, based on self-reporting by female athletes, only indicated the presence of oligomenorrhea and amenorrhea as there would be no way for a woman to notice of report the presence of a subclinical disorder. Only more recent direct research, using bloodwork and other methodology, has been able to identify the presence of the subclinical disorders which are also seen with increased frequency.

In a general sense, higher rates of menstrual cycle disorders have traditionally been found in sports with large aesthetic components or where a low bodyweight and thinness is an important criteria. This includes sports such as gymnastics, ballet, figure skating and many endurance sports such as running or cycling where lower body weights improve performance. Sports requiring larger amounts of training show increased rates of menstrual disorder and younger athletes are at a higher risk for them for reasons discussed below. More specifically primary amenorrhea is found with less than a 1% incidence in the general population but may occur in up to 7.4% of collegiate athletes and at rates of 22% in cheerleading, diving and gymnastics. Rates of secondary amenorrhea in the general population is roughly 2-5% but may occur in up to 60% of distance runners with the rates going up as training volume goes up (and bodyweight decreases). Oligomenorrhea is also found in up to 40% of distance runners and 60% of rhythmic gymnasts (again this may be a consequence of elevated testosterone levels in some cases). While subclinical menstrual disorders only occur in 5-10% of sedentary woman, studies find that even recreationally exercising women may show them at a rate of 50-80% (2). Perhaps more shocking than the rate itself is that the difference between exercising and non-exercising women is only two hours per week. This indicates just how sensitive women's bodies are to stress and leads into a discussion of the cause of FHA.

Causes of Menstrual Cycle Dysfunction: Introduction

The high frequency of menstrual cycle disorders seen in athletes led to speculation for years as to what the cause or causes might be for them. Most of these were observational in nature but at least seemed logical based on what was seen in female athletes. Researchers proposed that a low amount of body fat/ high amounts of muscle, attention to food intake (or outright eating disorders), a large amount of intensive training and others were causes. Perhaps the most amusing theory was that the bouncing of a woman's breast during certain activities had an effect similar to nursing, releasing the hormone prolactin which inhibits normal menstrual function (nursing, done properly, is an extremely effective form of birth control).

A problem with early studies of menstrual cycle dysfunction is that there were invariably based on surveys of high-level athletes rather than direct intervention studies. That is, they had women report their training, diet and rate of menstrual disorders rather than subjecting women to a given diet or amount of training and seeing what happened. This type of self-reporting has a number of problems. One I mentioned is that only oligo/amenorrhea could be identified. Another is the possibility that the increased rate of menstrual cycle disorders is less related to the training or diet itself and more to women with certain physiologies or body types tending to choose or succeed at certain sports.

I've described one of these already, the fact that oligomenorrhea is often found in certain sports being due to women with PCOS/elevated testosterone being more likely to be found in and succeed in those sports. Similarly, women who start menstruating later in life (i.e. primary amenorrhea) often end up with a more linear physique with longer limbs which is beneficial in sports such as dancing, running or gymnastics. As a final example, women who are prone to low body weights or with an eating disorder that causes a low weight might be drawn into sports requiring thinness. In all of these cases, it would be the underlying disorder that led the women into sport rather than involvement in the sport causing the disorder. You would also expect the dysfunction or disorder to be present from a very early age.

This is in distinct contrast to a woman who starts to move through the progression of subclinical to clinical menstrual disorders from a normally cycling state which would clearly indicate a change due to some aspect of sports involvement. And this has been shown to occur in a variety of intervention studies, where women are exposed to certain combinations of diet, exercise, etc. with menstrual cycle function measured, usually through bloodwork, ultrasound and other highly accurate methods. So while self-selection for certain sports may contribute to the relatively high occurrence of menstrual cycle dysfunction in active women, there is clearly some aspect of involvement in sport or training that is causing the increased levels of dysfunction.

Body Fat Percentage (BF%)

Perhaps one of the earliest, and certainly the most commonly held reason for the development of amenorrhea (whether primary or secondary) was related to body fat percentage (BF%). As most women with amenorrhea showed low levels of BF%, this seemed logical. Based mostly on observational data, it was felt that a woman needed 17% body fat (which is still very lean for a woman) before she would start menstruating and reach menarche (3). The underlying idea was that until a woman had sufficient body fat to potentially sustain pregnancy, her body would not become reproductively active in the first place. Given the role of fat stored calories to support pregnancy, this makes a great deal of logical sense. Related tangentially to this is that the age of menarche has been progressively dropping in most western societies. At least one theory to explain this is that, due to increasing rates of childhood obesity, girls are crossing the critical BF% threshold sooner. It's also been proposed that compounds in the environment which act like estrogen may be having an impact. I will bring this up again when I talk about soy and phytoestrogens in Chapter 24. That said, it was shown early on that girls started puberty at varying BF% levels and that the idea of some critical absolute threshold level was incorrect. At the same time, females in sports where primary amenorrhea was seen frequently do start menstruating after retirement when they gain body fat so there may still be some linkage between the two (I'll come back to this below).

The system was assumed to work the same way in reverse: a woman needed a certain amount of body fat to sustain pregnancy and if her BF% fell below that, indicating that there was insufficient food or she were starving, she would cease menstruating. The critical threshold here was suggested to be 26-28%. Given the frequency with which amenorrhea was seen in sports which placed a primacy on thinness for either performance or aesthetic reasons, this made sense (and many still think it to be the case). But this also turned out to be incorrect as studies easily identified female athletes at identical body fat levels where one group still had a menstrual cycle (although often indicators of subclinical dysfunction) while others had developed amenorrhea. At best, amenorrheic women have a slightly lower average BF% (about 2%) but the variance in BF% between women who are and are not cycling is much larger. Other studies found that some women lost their menstrual cycle at relatively high BF% levels compared to other women who were still cycling at very low body fat levels. As a final point on this topic, women who undergo bariatric surgery have been found to develop amenorrhea in some cases, even when BF% is still very high.

Certainly there is individual variation in which women do or do not maintain normal menstrual cycle function (or avoid amenorrhea) even given identical conditions but it was clear that the idea of some singular critical threshold for BF% in either direction was incorrect. I will show later that BF% can play an indirect role in menstrual cycle dysfunction and, the exception noted above, leaner women are at far more risk than woman carrying more fat. But BF% levels alone simply cannot explain the high incidence of menstrual cycle dysfunction seen in active women or athletes.

Menstrual Cycle Adaptation and Stress

Although I've been discussing changes in the menstrual cycle as a dysfunction or disruption (which it is), it might be better to think of it in terms of being an adaptation, in the sense of occurring for good reasons, rather than a dysfunction. I mentioned one of those reasons in the last chapter which is to conserve energy. The decrease in progesterone/shortening of the luteal cycle and/or decreased in endometrial proliferation may save 1000 or more calories per individual cycle. These savings will increase as the cycle becomes progressively more impaired with greater energy savings occurring as hormones drop, the egg is not released and the endometrial lining doesn't develop at all. By causing infertility, the incredible calorie expenditure of pregnancy is avoided. Logically this would tend to occur under conditions (such as a low BF%) when those calories aren't available although, as above, that is clearly not the only explanation.

In a more general sense, these adaptations might be expected to occur when a woman's body is under high levels of chronic stress. Under such conditions, the chance of a successful pregnancy is likely to be impaired and it makes sense that a woman's body would reduce the chances of this occurring since it would represent an enormous caloric risk for a potentially negative outcome. This isn't to say that stress is bad per se, only that chronically stressful situations are. But what is stress? For now I will define it as the response to anything that tries to push the body out of homeostasis (the relatively fixed level at which the body tries to maintain itself). This causes the body to mount some type of defense in an attempt to restore balance, called the stress response. There are almost endless types of stressors possible and, as I'll detail in the next chapter, not only do they all tend to generate the same general response, they have a cumulative effect on the body, adding together to determine the total stress (called allostatic load) on the system (4). Relevant to the topic of this chapter is the fact that exercise stress, diet/energetic stress and psychological stress not only have independent effects on menstrual cycle function, the combination of one or more of those stresses has an even greater impact (5) Since all of these are frequently found to one degree or another in dieting and/or active women, they all need to be examined.

Exercise and Diet Related Stress

As amenorrhea (and later subclinical menstrual dysfunction) was seen in hard training female athletes, it was logical to assume that the inherent stress of exercise, especially intense exercise, was playing a role in menstrual cycle dysfunction (6). Observationally, for example, as body weight decreased and training volume went up, the frequency of amenorrhea increased in runners. At the same time, direct studies on the topic found varied and mixed results (note again that subclinical disorders had not been identified and were not looked for). One early study in younger women found that a percentage showed menstrual cycle disruption while two others, in older women, found no disturbances over a year of endurance training (7-9). In all three studies, exercise was gradually increased over the study period and this is critically important as the body can gradually adapt to stress. For example, in one case study of a female marathoner, the training load that caused menstrual cycle dysfunction in the first year didn't in the second year as she had adapted to the training (i.e. it was less stressful to her body).

110

In perhaps one of the most frequently cited studies, young girls were immediately exposed to an enormous training load including 4.5 hours of exercise per day consisting of 10 miles of running per day with 3.5 hours of other activities which was increased over time and most of the girls showing some degree of menstrual cycle dysfunction (10). A similarly done study found that even 2 weeks of intensive exercise can cause some degree of menstrual cycle impairment (11). In both cases, the girls had no time to adapt to the training. When training loads increase more gradually and intensity is not excessive, dysfunction is less likely to occur (12). Another aspect of that study was that one group of girls lost weight while another mostly maintained their weight. In the group that lost weight (who were effectively dieting), there was a 95% rate of menstrual cycle disturbance while the group that didn't "only" showed a 75% rate of disturbance. These studies make two points. The first is that performing a large amount of intense exercise without a build-up may cause problems in it's own right. The second is that adding additional stresses such as dieting and weight loss worsens the problem.

And this is relevant as dieting alone can cause menstrual cycle disruption to occur, especially in "normal" weight women (women carrying more fat rarely suffering dysfunction). The more weight which is lost and the younger the women, the more likely menstrual cycle disturbance is to occur (13). There is also an odd a delay in the change in menstrual cycle function and weight loss, maintenance or regain. One study found that the majority of menstrual cycle disruption occurred after weight loss had stopped and did not resume for some time period even when weight was regained (14). The reasons are unknown and I'll mention it again when I talk about the factors involved in recovering from menstrual cycle dysfunction.

Energy Availability (EA)

A difficulty in drawing conclusions from the above studies is that there were often multiple factors at play including the amount of exercise, intensity of the exercise, diet and weight/fat loss per se. This makes it impossible to draw a conclusion about any single factor as the cause. However, there is a more general concept called Energy Availability (EA) which can effectively tie them all together.

To understand what EA represents conceptually, consider that even at rest the human body is using energy to sustain an incredible number of processes. It takes energy to keep the heart beating, the brain functioning, to circulate blood, to keep the organs functioning properly, to build bone, to grow hair or nails or to keep the reproductive system working. But these processes are not equally important as some are required for immediate or long-term survival while others are not. If the heart stops beating or the kidneys or brain stop functioning, a person will die. In contrast, if the body stops producing bone, hair or nails, shuts off reproduction or decreases immune system function, there is no immediate negative effect. Losing these functions may not be ideal but they will not cause death. Note that, outside of the body's baseline functioning, exercise is the primary activity that will also require energy.

EA simply represents the amount of energy to fuel the body at any given time and is practically defined as energy intake from food minus exercise energy expenditure. Since lean body mass (LBM) is the primary calorie using tissue in the body, EA is divided by LBM and can be expressed as:

$$EA = (\text{Calorie Intake} - \text{Exercise Energy Expenditure})/LBM$$

Conceptually, if EA falls below a certain level, the body will adapt, shutting down non-essential processes to ensure that there is sufficient energy to maintain the essential ones (14a).

While this can get a bit confusing, it's critical to understand that EA and energy balance are not the same. Energy balance represents the difference between calorie intake and total daily energy expenditure (TDEE) while EA is the difference between food intake and exercise energy expenditure. This means that energy balance may change as a woman's body shows the metabolic adaptations discussed in Chapter 9 while her EA may be unchanged over time. Even if the difference in her calorie intake and TDEE is decreasing, if her calorie intake and exercise energy expenditure are the same, her EA will remain the same. This can lead to a situation where a woman is no longer losing fat or weight while her EA is unchanged (and potentially too low to sustain all bodily functions).

Calculating exercise energy expenditure is a bit more complicated than just determining how many calories were burned during exercise. This is due to the fact that the number of calories that would have been burned at rest (which represent the body's normal requirements) and used regardless of exercise must be subtracted out. So consider a woman who burns 400 calories in an hour of exercise but who would have burned 60 calories during that same hour at rest. Her exercise energy expenditure is only 340 calories over normal and it is this value that should be used to calculate EA. A sample EA calculation appears below.

A female weighing 150 lbs at 20% body fat has 120 lbs of LBM and 30 lbs of fat.
She is eating 2000 calories per day and performing 340 calories per day of exercise.

EA = 2000 calories - 340 calories = 1660 calories per day/LBM
EA = 1660 calories/120 lbs LBM = 13.8cal/lb LBM (30.3 cal/kg LBM)

If she were to increase her activity to 450 calories per day her EA will change as shown
EA = 2000 calories - 450 calories = 1550 calories/120 lbs LBM = 12.9 cal/lb LBM (28.4 cal/kg)
If she eats 1550 calories with no exercise, her EA will not change as shown
EA = 1550 calories - 0 calories = 1550 calories/120 lbs LBM = 12.9 cal/lb LBM (28.4 cal/kg)

In cases where an extreme amount of exercise is being done while few calories are being consumed, it is actually possible to have a negative EA. This isn't unheard of in sports such as ballet and gymnastics where women train up to 8 hours/day on very low calorie intakes.

EA and Menstrual Cycle Dysfunction

As I mentioned above, while the early studies on dieting and/or exercise were suggestive of the factors underlying menstrual cycle dysfunction, the lack of control or number of variables made drawing specific conclusions problematic. Was it the diet, the amount of exercise, the intensity or some combination. This would be addressed in what are typically referred to as "elegant" studies, referring to their design, by a research group headed by Ann Loucks. Each study, lasting 5 days to ensure complete control, manipulated either food intake, activity or both to provide a specific EA to the women. And over a series of studies, Loucks clearly demonstrated that a low EA is one of the primarily causes of menstrual cycle disturbance and/or FHA (15). More specifically she showed that when EA falls, a number of negative physiological changes occur. A primary one is a reduction in LH levels along with a reduction of their normal release pattern (termed reduced LH pulsatility).   Along with this are other hormonal changes indicative of energy conservation such as reduced insulin, leptin and active thyroid (T3) levels along with increased cortisol and growth hormone (GH) levels.

Reduced LH pulsatility had been seen previously in response to dieting which is, by definition a lowered EA state (16). The other hormonal changes in response to low EA are also identical to the changes that occur in response to dieting and fat loss per se. Loucks also found that strenuous exercise caused no changes in LH pulsatility so long as calories were maintained at maintenance levels (17). Over the short-term at least, the primary stress of exercise in terms of negatively impacting menstrual cycle function is due to creating a low EA state rather than to any inherent effect of the exercise itself. An earlier study had made a similar observation: women who performed 3 days of exercise (90 minutes per workout) after eating at maintenance showed no change in hormones while the same amount of exercise after 6 days of dieting impaired LH pulsatility (18). This data does seem to contradict the study I mentioned above where young women exposed to large amounts of intense exercise still showed menstrual cycle dysfunction despite maintaining their weight and the reason for this is unknown.

What may be most surprising about all of this is just how quickly all of these changes occurred. With as few as 5 days of low EA, there are measurable decreases in LH pulsatility, insulin, leptin, and active thyroid hormones along with increases in cortisol levels. That isn't to say that the menstrual cycle will become disrupted in this time frame but that hormonal adaptations begin to occur that quickly. In the long-term, this will eventually lead a woman through the menstrual cycle changes potentially to full-blown amenorrhea with the full cluster of hormonal effects that goes along with that.

Somewhat unexpectedly, Loucks' group found that a low EA generated by exercise had slightly less of an effect on reducing LH pulsatility than calorie restriction. They proposed that carbohydrate availability more than EA per se, might be the issue as the brain is responding to glucose availability in terms of many of the adaptations seen (in the short-term leptin is also more sensitive to carbohydrate intake). In the exercise group, due to a shift towards burning fat for fuel, more dietary carbohydrate was available to the brain due to food intake being higher and this wasn't the case when calories were restricted. While this might argue for the use of exercise rather than diet for fat loss, I'd note that the difference in the change in LH pulsatility were small. Practically, the Category 1 female for whom this is mostly relevant, will invariably have to use some combination of dietary restriction and exercise to reach her goals.

The Critical EA Threshold

In the original studies on EA, two extremes of EA were compared to see if there was an effect. Not only were the values used generally unrealistic, they give no indication of how a woman's body responds to different levels of EA or if there is some threshold where problems begin. This was done in the next set of studies with women subjected to a variety of different EA levels from low to high. And these studies identified that there were two critical EA thresholds. The first was the threshold at which LH pulsatility (and by extension menstrual cycle function) and the other hormones such as thyroid, cortisol, estrogen, etc. started to be negatively impacted. This occurred at an EA of 13.6 cal/lb LBM or 30 cal/kg LBM (19). At a slightly lower threshold, of EA, 11.3 cal/lb LBM or 24 cal/kg LBM, the changes in hormones become progressively worse and bone density began to be negatively impacted (20).

Effectively, 13.6 cal/lb LBM (30 cal/kg LBM) seems to represent the lowest EA that is compatible with maintaining normal reproductive function and this corresponds roughly with RMR. I'd note that a sufficient EA (in terms of supporting both health and training) is thought to be 20.5 cal/lb LBM (45 cal/kg LBM). This is really only for high-performance athletes engaged in a large amount of training and somewhere between the two values would be ideal for most although it represents somewhat of a gray area. In the long-term, an insufficient EA can compromise training intensity and adaptation even if the critical threshold is not crossed. Again these values represent EA, not energy intake per se. Whatever exercise energy expenditure is being performed must be added to the calculated goal EA to determine total calorie intake. I've shown the different EA values representing the two low thresholds along with the high level of adequate intake for different amounts of LBM in the chart below.

LBM	Bone Density Threshold 11.3 cal/lb LBM	Menstrual Cycle Threshold 13.6 cal/lb LBM	Adequate Intake 20 cal/lb LBM
100	1130	1360	2000
110	1243	1496	2200
120	1356	1632	2400
130	1469	1768	2600
140	1582	1904	2800
150	1695	2040	3000

So consider a female with 120 lbs of LBM who is attempting to stay right at the 13.6 cal/lb LBM (30 cal/kg LBM) critical threshold during a diet. Her baseline EA is 1632 calories assuming no exercise. If she performs 300 net calories per day of exercise, she will have to eat 1932 calories to avoid falling below the threshold. If she increases her exercise energy expenditure to 400 calories, she will have to raise her food intake to 2032 calories to maintain the same net EA of 1632 calories per day.

There are a few issues with the studies I've described that are worth mentioning. One is that they were all done on untrained women and it's possible that trained women would respond differently. Another is that they are all purely short-term, only showing hormonal changes that would be expected to lead to menstrual cycle dysfunction rather than menstrual dysfunction itself which would take far longer to occur. Indirectly supporting the critical EA threshold are studies which find that female athletes, almost without exception, who are amenorrheic have an EA below the 13.6 cal/lb LBM (30 cal/kg LBM) threshold (21). At the same time, female athletes who still have some menstrual cycle function can be found with an EA below the critical threshold although they typically have some form of subclinical dysfunction. Put differently, all women who are amenorrheic have an EA below the critical threshold but all women below the critical threshold will not develop amenorrhea. Adding further to this idea is that raising calories above the critical threshold causes a reversal of the metabolic changes along with restoration of menstrual cycle function. In contradiction to the above are two longer studies showing that menstrual cycle dysfunction can occur with an EA above the critical threshold although none presented with amenorrhea (21a,22). In the second, women below the critical threshold were still 50% more likely to have a dysfunction. Most likely this represents the longer-term adaptations that will occur to a lowered EA regardless of the exact level. I would expect women who cross the critical threshold earlier in a diet to have more problems sooner.

While a discussion of gender differences may seem odd here (since men have no menstrual cycle to lose), there has been recent interest in the issue of low EA among male athletes along with its potential consequences. Observationally at least, broadly similar effects on hormonal status and reproductive function has been seen in men's sports that emphasize leanness (22a). While very little direct research has been done but it appears that men's critical EA thresholds are lower than that of women. One study found that an EA of 6.8 cal/lb LBM (15 cal/kg LBM) lowered insulin and leptin with no effect on thyroid, IGF-1 or testosterone (22b). Another found that while an EA of 6.8 cal/lg LBM (15 cal/kg LBM) negatively impacted bone health in women, it did not in men (22c). Based on limited data, it has been suggested that men's critical EA threshold may be as low as 9.1-11.4 kcal/lb LBM (20-22 cal/kg LBM) before hormonal or reproductive status is negatively impacted (22d). Regardless of the specific numbers, this all points to the fact that women's physiologies are more sensitive to low EA than men's, inducing adaptations much earlier. This is on top of potentially more severe consequences, discussed later in the chapter.

Before moving on, I want to address an idea that came out of the research above in terms of actual dieting practices. Some dieting extremists took the existence of the above critical EA threshold as an admonition to never increase activity or lower calories to the point that the threshold was crossed. While this is a wonderfully idealistic viewpoint, it is not practical in many situations. The Category 1 woman attempting to diet to the extremes of low BF% will realistically have to cross the critical threshold at some point, potentially risking menstrual cycle and other hormonal dysfunction. Otherwise she will simply not reach her fat loss goals. I will offer a variety of dietary strategies to at least limit the problems that tend to occur in a later chapter but crossing the critical threshold is an unfortunate requirement in many cases.

The Role of Leptin in FHA

Before looking at some other potential factors involved in causing menstrual cycle disturbance (or at least contributing to low EA), I want to look at some of the underlying mechanisms behind why low EA plays such a primary role. Not only will this provide some suggestion of how to potentially improve the situation (in dietary or exercise terms), it will also explain my comment above about BF% still playing somewhat of an indirect role in FHA even if there is no critical BF% threshold where problems occur.

In the early days of research into amenorrhea, when the original ideas about body fat thresholds were being conceptualized, nobody really knew how or why body fat might be a player in all of this (the same was true regarding the setpoint). It was just an observation which seemed to have some degree of logic to it. One theory I mentioned above had to do with the ratio of fat to LBM. Since a large amount of a woman's estrogen is produced in fat cells via conversion of other hormones, it was thought that too little body fat would lower estrogen to such a point that menstrual cycle function was impaired. While I'm sure other ideas were proposed, it should come as no surprise (given it's role in coordinating other dieting adaptations), that leptin plays a major if not primary role in all of this (23).

Returning again to menarche, until leptin crosses a certain level, puberty will not occur and menstruation will not begin. Similarly, the reduction in leptin due to low EA are a primary signal to the body to adapt not only generally but to reduce menstrual cycle function. Very directly, leptin levels in female athletes correlate with both reproductive and hormonal function (24). Low leptin levels also correlate strongly with the loss of the menstrual cycle and there may be some critical level of leptin that is required to maintain normal function (25). And just as leptin injections can reverse some of the other dieting adaptations, in at least some women, they can reverse amenorrhea (26). Effectively, by raising leptin levels artificially, the brain is tricked into thinking everything is normal. While this is one of the very few approved uses of leptin, it comes with its own set of problems, namely that low EA is causing a cluster of other hormonal and physiological problems that simply replacing leptin will not fix. In fact, leptin could cause appetite and calorie intake to go down, further exacerbating the problem.

As leptin is highly correlated to BF% levels in the first place, this would seem to provide some link between BF% and the menstrual cycle as was originally proposed. However, recall that leptin is also linked directly to calorie (and especially carbohydrate intake), decreasing rapidly when either are reduced (also recall that leptin may work differently in women than men). In Loucks' original EA studies, no significant amount of fat could have been lost in only 5 days but there would have been a rapid reduction in leptin, sending the signal to reduce LH pulsatility and induce the other adaptations.

At most, women starting with a lower BF% will have a lower level of leptin to begin with which will drop rapidly in response to a low EA/lowered calorie intake. If there is a critical leptin level below which problems start, a leaner women will cross it much sooner than a woman carrying more fat. When the individual responses to low EA are examined, leaner women always have a larger decrease in LH pulsatility (27). As I mentioned before, women in Category 2 and 3 almost never experience menstrual cycle dysfunction due to low EA. The lone exception being women who undergo bariatric surgery who have EA drop to effectively zero almost immediately.

Psychological Factors in FHA

Having examined some of the physiological stresses that can contribute or outright cause FHA, I want to look at other causes/contributors starting with psychological stress (discussed in great detail in the next chapter). Psychological stress is just as real to the body as physiological stress, often generating the same hormonal responses. Cortisol is a key player here; not only is it released in response to psychological stress (also going up with low EA) but chronically elevated levels can independently inhibit menstrual cycle function. Observationally, women with FHA often report increased interpersonal stress with friends and family (28). More directly, researchers have identified a subgroup of women with FHA who are not dieting or exercising excessively but who still show signs of menstrual irregularities or FHA (29).

When psychologically tested, these women show a common cluster of behaviors including pre-occupation with their weight and a high degree of perfectionism (traits that are often found in female athletes or dieters to begin with). Along with this is high dietary restraint, discussed previously, describing a pre-occupation with food intake and body weight. Not only is dietary restraint more likely to be found in women than in men, women with menstrual cycle dysfunction show higher degrees of dietary restraint than women without (30). Other research has found that these women show an overall high stress responsiveness, marked by dysfunctional attitudes, difficulty coping with daily hassles, subclinical depression or anxiety and others (30a). While these women often report some slight differences in their food intake (described below), it does appear to be a case where nothing more than mental stress, and the chronically elevated cortisol responses that occur, is causing FHA (31).

Further supporting that this is a psychologically driven issue is the fact that Cognitive Behavioral Therapy (CBT), which aims at teaching coping skills and alternate modes of thinking, has been shown to reverse FHA in these women (32). In one study, 87.5% of women who underwent CBT regained menstrual cycle function while only 25% of women who did not go through CBT did (32a). Analysis of that same group showed that CBT alone was able to reduce cortisol levels and increase leptin levels, removing the negative impact of chronically elevated cortisol on the system (32b). Even if the above only describes a subset of women with FHA, it's clear that stress is a major player. As well, recall that all stress adds up in the body and a woman who may be dieting, exercising and have a certain psychological profile has more total stress than a woman without one or more of those. I'll discuss this more below.

Other Dietary Factors Contributing to Menstrual Cycle Dysfunction

I mentioned above that, in a group of women who were not dieting/exercising but who showed FHA, there were some subtle differences in their food intake and these do partially contribute to the problems that may be occurring. The women with FHA were eating slightly less than those without but they were also found to be eating significantly less dietary fat (16% or 29 grams compared to 32% or 58 grams) and more fiber. This is relevant as, independent of calories, changes in fat and fiber intake have been found to alter a woman's hormonal profile.

Specifically a low-fat/high-fiber diet lowers levels of both estrogen and progesterone compared to a high-fat/low-fiber diet (33). To little saturated fat has a similar effect on hormone levels. The effect isn't enormous with estrogen being reduced by 7% or more depending on how low fat intake is taken but it does exist. This is certainly beneficial from a health standpoint, in terms of reducing the risk of breast cancer (34), but it could contribute to the risk of menstrual cycle dysfunction as estrogen will be dropping from a lower starting point under such conditions.

The studies on this topic are problematic in that they generally compare changes in both dietary fat and fiber, making it impossible to know if it's the fat, fiber or combination having the effect. As well, they typically compare fairly extreme intake levels of 20% to 40% dietary fat, making it impossible to know what might be happening between those two values or if there is some cutoff point below which estrogen decreases. I would mention that the same 20% fat intake has been shown to reduce symptoms of PMS and this is likely due to the lowering of both estrogen and progesterone in the first place (35). The same low-fat diet, over a 2-year span, has also been shown to reduce breast density (36).

In that they are typically low in fat and high in fiber, vegetarian and vegan diets have the potential to cause menstrual cycle dysfunction (37,38). In one of the studies I cited above, while dieting itself increased the risk of menstrual cycle disorders, women on vegetarian diets were more likely to experience them. Perhaps surprisingly, the generally considered to be healthy Mediterranean diet (based around moderate protein, high-vegetable and relatively low-fat intakes) can have the same negative impacts on menstrual cycle function (39). While a low-fat/high-fiber intake may be a partial cause, there are other reasons that vegetarian/vegan diets could be contributing to menstrual cycle dysfunction. One is that the nature of the diets often lower calorie intake, which could take women below the critical EA threshold (especially if they are active). Limited intake of specific foods such as red meat might also cause nutrient deficiencies (i.e. iron and zinc). In one early study, 25% of amenorrheic women were vegetarian and 100% of them ate no red meat (40). They also consumed far less calories so a lowered/low EA was also present.

The above is not mean to necessarily argue against a low-fat/high fiber intake. Clearly it is beneficial for improving some health markers, reducing symptoms of PMS and reducing breast cancer risk. At the same time, it may not be optimal for athletes or lean/exercising women in terms of maintaining normal menstrual cycle function. Optimal fertility might also be harmed with certain dietary patterns and women seeking to become pregnant should look at their overall diet in this regard. This is also a potential area where a typical male approach to dieting (especially for the Category 1 individual) with a very low-fat and high-fiber intake might not be ideal for women. Men's hormones can certainly be impacted but they have no menstrual cycle to lose and clearly don't suffer the same overall consequences.

Having looked at the potential impact of low-fat/high-fiber diets, I want to look at the other extreme and talk about high-fat/ketogenic diets. These are diets typically containing moderate or high protein intakes, low levels of carbohydrate (50-100 grams or less) with relatively higher fat intakes. Anecdotally at least, there are reports of leaner women who had lost their menstrual cycle regaining normal function when they follow such diets. I tend to think that this is related to these types of diets being higher in fat and often lower in fiber by definition but what little research exists is mixed. In obese women with PCOS, ketogenic diets have been shown to cause weight and fat loss and improve menstrual cycle function but almost any weight loss in this population has similar effects (41,42).

In leaner, women I'm only aware of a single study. In it, women were placed on a ketogenic diet for the treatment of adult epilepsy (this is one of the uses of the diet) and, despite being at maintenance calories, 100% of them showed some degree of menstrual cycle dysfunction (43). This is not an ideal model for dieting women, mind you. The ketogenic epilepsy diet is set up differently than the fat loss version and the presence of epilepsy (or use of medications) could have interacted somehow. However, ketogenic diets effectively mimic starvation while eating food but the same overall hormonal responses to starvation are typically seen. Adding to this, the female brain requires roughly 80 grams of carbohydrate per day (in contrast to a male's 100-120 grams) and ketogenic diets automatically provide less than that. If the brain's carbohydrate availability, rather than EA per se, is a controller of LH pulsatility, the lack of dietary carbohydrates (along with the brain's shift to using ketones for fuel) might contribute to menstrual cycle dysfunction. Ketogenic diets can be modified to address this issues.

Overall, the above research points to a situation where extremes of diet are potentially problematic for lean female athletes at risk for suffering menstrual cycle disruption. It would appear that both sufficient dietary fat and carbohydrate are required for a woman's optimal hormonal and physiological function to at least one degree or another (sufficient carbohydrate is also necessary to support high-intensity training). And this bring up an issue I have mentioned throughout the book: during a diet, due to women's smaller sizes, there is often not enough room to include both in sufficient amounts while keeping calorie intake low enough to generate fat loss. There are solutions to this addressed later in the book but this represents another situation that men often don't have to face. Due to being larger and having higher energy expenditures, their diet often allows more than enough room for all the nutrients.

Causes of a low EA

While there are other potential contributors to menstrual cycle dysfunction, it's clear that, by and large low EA is the primary cause. And while the amount of exercise being done certainly contributes this, I want to look briefly at some of the reasons that a woman's food intake might be insufficient to prevent her EA from falling below the critical threshold (44). The first are conscious reductions in food intake, usually aimed at decreasing BF%. As I've mentioned previously, performance athletes often benefit from a reduced BF% although this can harm performance if taken to the extreme. In the physique sports, a low BF % is part of the competition itself and reductions to very low levels represents a necessary evil. So while it might be debatable if a female endurance athlete needs to reach 10-12% for optimal performance, a female bodybuilder or physique competitor will have to do this to be competitive. Beyond even competition reasons are the simple fact that women are currently and have always been under more social pressure to be thin which, as often as not, pressures them to diet. This is true in the athletic realm as well as in the general public with relatively "normal weight" women often wanting to lose weight or fat.

Tied in with the issue of the diet itself is the impact of exercise, especially high-intensity exercise on appetite that I discussed in a previous chapter. I mentioned that this impact can be variable often increasing hunger but that, in trained athletes, intense exercise may actually blunt hunger. This effect is increased on a high-carbohydrate, high-fiber, low-fat diet and this combination can cause highly active females to unconsciously undereat relative to their daily requirements (another reason to maintain adequate fat intake). Women with menstrual cycle dysfunction have also been shown to choose foods low in calories for their volume (low energy density), this keeps them full with insufficient calories to support their training (44a).

Finally is the often high-prevalence of overt eating disorders (EDs) in both women in general and female athletes in specific that cause women to deliberately reduce their food intake, often to extremely low levels. The term anorexia athletica is often used and, even when full-blown EDs aren't present, subclinical forms may be. This is especially true in those sports requiring low body weight/body fat levels and which are focused on thinness (45). I'd remind readers that the presence of ED's may be part of the reason that these women are successful in sport to begin with, rather than being a consequence of involvement. I'd even argue that, especially in the physique sports, the presence of a subclinical ED can be seen as a competitive "advantage" in that it helps the person sustain the extreme diet that is required to be successful. These comments are in no way meant to diminish the huge damage that EDs, whether overt or subclinical, do or that they should be ignored without treatment.

Who Keeps Their Cycle?

While amenorrhea is obviously fairly common among lean female athletes, it is also clearly not universal with female athletes reaching very low levels of BF% and body weight without losing their cycle (though most probably have subclinical menstrual cycle dysfunction). Some of this could be due to better overall dieting or eating practices such that the critical EA threshold is not crossed (or is crossed later before being raised once the fat loss goal has been reached) but females are also found below the critical threshold who are not amenorrheic. The question is why and the answer is only somewhat known.

Researchers often refer to the concept of robustness in terms of menstrual cycle function when discussing this topic. The basic idea is that, in the same way all biological systems can vary between people (i.e. some people break bones easily and others do not), some women's reproductive systems and/or hypothalamus are more robust than others. The same degree of low EA, weight/fat loss or exercise simply does not affect them as much as it does other women. Going back to the issue of women and famine is the fact that, even during the most extreme situations (i.e. starvation/concentration camp victims), some women are still able to conceive and bear children. Presumably their systems are more robust. Practically this becomes an issue when any individual woman (who may have a more robust system) is able to diet or reach a certain BF% without problems and assumes this applies to all women (who are not as robust).

Sadly, in almost all of the discussions of the topic I've found, nobody has offered any actual reason for these differences. As is usually the case there may be genetic contributors to the relative risk of FHA occurring (45a). At least some studies have found that women with pre-existing luteal dysfunction are at risk of losing their cycle completely. Given the progressive continuum of menstrual cycle disturbances that can occur, this most likely represents them already starting out with some degree of psychological stress or low EA. Women who start dieting with a pre-existing dysfunction will simply get worse.

Outside of genetics, only one factor has been directly identified that can limit menstrual cycle disruption and that is a concept referred to as reproductive or gynecological age. In contrast to biological age, which is how long a woman has been alive, reproductive age represents the number of years since she began menstruating. If a woman starts menstruating at age 15 and is now 25 years old, her reproductive age is 10 years. If she is 30, her reproductive age will be 15 years. Women reproductive systems are often very unstable when they first reach menarche but becomes more stable with age. Full reproductive maturity appears to coincide with the time that her pelvis stops developing and this occurs at roughly a 14-16 year reproductive age. And it has been shown, again by Ann Loucks, that the impact of a low EA on LH pulsatility disappears in women after they reach a reproductive age of 14 (46).

The same changes still occur in thyroid, insulin, IGF-1, leptin and cortisol so this is just an issue of her reproductive system having become more robust. This protection is only partial, however, and women of a higher reproductive age can become amenorrheic, especially if they are leaner to begin with (47). The women in Louck's study were at 26% body fat, just above my Category 1 cutoff and this may have contributed to the lack of change in LH pulsatility. The reproductively mature Category 1 woman attempting to diet down to the extremes of leanness is still at risk for menstrual cycle dysfunction. And while not a topic of this book, the reality is that many female athletes are well below a 14 year reproductive age, putting them at the greatest consequence for stress/low EA on their reproductive systems.

Putting It All Together

I've discussed a lot of information in the previous sections and I want to try to put them all together into a cohesive model of menstrual cycle disturbance. After years of study, it's clear now that the primary factor that causes menstrual cycle dysfunction is a chronically low energy availability (EA) with a proposed critical EA threshold existing below which problems begin (some studies find dysfunction near but above this threshold). Genetics and reproductive age play roles outside of EA per se. And this explains all of the previous observations of menstrual cycle dysfunction. Dieting itself is, by definition, a low EA state even if exercise is not being performed and it has been shown that greater dietary deficits predict a higher frequency of menstrual cycle dysfunction although they do not predict the severity (48). Exercise may have its own independent effect if an excessive amount is done without a build-up and dieting/weight loss further increase the effect. Those two factors alone explain the earlier studies with reproductive age explaining why younger women are more likely than older to have problems.

In all cases, more problems occur in relatively "normal-weight"/lean women where heavier women or those carrying more body fat are far less likely to have problems. Which brings things full circle to the role of BF% in this. At least until such a time as the body adapts by lowering energy expenditure, a low EA, by definition will be creating a caloric deficit, causing both weight and fat loss. It's most likely that the low EA/calorie deficit is causing the low BF% seen rather than low BF% causing the dysfunction. This would explain the fact that menstrual cycle dysfunction doesn't occur at any specific or critical body fat percentage (BF%). In addition to genetics or reproductive age, a woman at a higher BF% could be experiencing a chronically low EA while a leaner woman might not be. Even here, while related to BF%, leptin is far more sensitive to changing calorie (and carbohydrate) intake meaning that it will be impacted most by a chronically low EA. And, regardless of the other contributory factors, it is that chronically low EA that eventually causes a woman from normally cycling to luteal phase defect to anovulation to oligomenorrhea and, potentially at least, to full-blown amenorrhea.

Psychological factors such as personality profile or other stress may also play a role. It can be difficult to separate out energetic from psychological stress and I will discuss this more in the next chapter. Both factors can contribute independently, interact or act as a driver for the other (i.e. many people will exercise to relieve psychological stress but exercise can cause energetic stress). In a practical sense all of these factors are often clustered together. Women with a certain psychological profile who are exercising excessively while chronically undereating/eating in specific patterns are creating a perfect storm to generate menstrual cycle dysfunction. If certain genetic factors or a low reproductive age are present, the problem worsens. Having looked at the causes of menstrual cycle dysfunction, let me look at the consequences.

The Effects of Amenorrhea

As I mentioned earlier in the chapter, it's now known that the various menstrual cycle dysfunctions represent a progressive movement from a normal menstrual cycle to the complete loss of cycle and the changes that occur in a woman's metabolism is progressive as well. Since it represents effectively the "endpoint" of menstrual cycle dysfunction, and has the most extreme impact on all aspects of a woman's physiology, I will discuss FHA first with the understanding that the lesser degree of menstrual cycle dysfunction represent lesser degrees of the same effect. As a low EA is often a consequence of dieting and fat loss, there is at least some overlap between FHA and the normal adaptations to dieting.

As I mentioned in Chapter 3, a primary change in amenorrhea is an overall decrease in a woman's reproductive hormones. The normal cyclical changes in LH and FSH are also lost which means that no egg develops or is released, no corpus luteum develops and there is no menstruation. Estrogen may be reduced to 33% of normal with progesterone at 10% of normal and no cyclical changes occurring. Given the profound effect of these hormones on a woman's body, this drop has an enormous number of effects.

Some of these effects could be looked upon as somewhat of a positive. The loss of progesterone signaling means that its effect on stimulating fat storage via ASP are lost. As well, the lack of cyclical changes in a woman's hormones means that the typical shifts in water weight and retention disappear. This can make tracking a fat loss diet easier and may reduce the mental stress in female dieters that comes from their bodyweight jumping up and down. Women who suffer from PMS often see a reduction in those symptoms along with the loss of menstruation. Even that has a small benefit in that it reduces a woman's monthly iron loss, reducing her risk of developing anemia. While the above do represent potential positives of amenorrhea (and some women speak of "banishing the estrogen", actively embracing the loss of the cycle), I cannot overstate that the negative effects are both more numerous along with being far more potentially damaging to a woman's physiology and long-term health.

Looking first at the drop in estrogen, a number of metabolic effects will be seen. The lack of estrogen signaling means that hunger will no longer be well controlled as both its direct effects and leptin sensitizing effects will be lost. Along with this will be the loss of estrogen's anti-inflammatory effects, anti-oxidant effects and beneficial effects on muscular remodeling Metabolically, the positive effects of estrogen on fat mobilization and oxidation will be lost with the consequence that the use of protein for fuel during aerobic exercise may be increased and a topical estrogen patch can reverse this (49). The cortisol response to exercise is also increased by 50% (49a) Contrary to what might be expected, insulin sensitivity increases, shifting fuel use towards carbohydrates and away from fat. Again, the loss of progesterone signaling means that the normal increase in metabolic rate that would occur during the luteal phase is lost significantly reducing monthly calorie expenditure. This is in addition to the normal dieting adaptations.

Other hormonal changes occur and I have mentioned that there is a common hormonal pattern which is seen with low EA including low insulin, elevated cortisol (a stress hormone discussed in the next chapter), low leptin, low levels of thyroid hormone (T3), and a decrease in the levels of a hormone called Insulin-Like Growth Factor -1(IGF-1). This impacts on all aspects of a woman's physiology but here I want to focus on metabolic rate. In amenorrhea (and to a lesser degree the other stages of menstrual cycle dysfunction), T3 levels can be a significant reduced, with up to 17-20% decrease in basal metabolic rate (BMR) compared to normally cycling women. I'd note that this drop is also seen in lean women without amenorrhea along with dieting males and primarily represents the adaptations to dieting per se (50,51). For comparison, BMR can be reduced up to 30% or more in anorexia, a state which shares many commonalities with amenorrhea (52). Other components of daily energy expenditure have not been measured in as much detail but all of the adaptations seen with dieting in general will be in place. NEAT is likely to decrease to overall fatigue and lethargy.

In terms of training, injury risk may increase (see below) while muscular protein synthesis, muscular strength, endurance, recovery both during and between workouts and training response and competitive ability may all be decreased. In one study of junior elite swimmers, amenorrheic athletes had a 10% drop in performance compared to a 8% improvement in normally cycling women, an 18% difference (52a). Judgement and coordination may be impaired along with an increase in irritability and depression Amenorrheic athletes are at risk for nutrient deficiency, although this is primarily due to the low total food intake and food choices that are often seen. There may also be decreased immune system function along with cardiovascular, gastrointestinal and renal complications.

A relatively unappreciated effect of amenorrhea is an impairment of sleep patterns with depression and lethargy often being seen. Normally melatonin goes up at night and decreases in the morning but in many kinds of depression, melatonin stays elevated throughout the day, causing lethargy while being lowered at night, causing sleeplessness (53,54). Called a phase shift, this is common in people suffering from Seasonal Affective Disorder (SAD) and occurs to some degree during the late luteal phase. It also occurs in amenorrhea due to the changes in reproductive hormones that occur (55,56).

The above negative effects, while significant, pale in comparison to what may be the single largest negative effect of amenorrhea which is the potential for bone mineral density (BMD) loss. Women already have lower BMD than men and only have a limited time to develop peak levels. Roughly 90% of the increase in a woman's BMD occurs by age 18 with the remainder finishing by roughly age 30. From that point on, a slow loss of BMD typically occurs, accelerating at menopause (especially if HRT is not begun). Proper training and nutrition may be able to slow or eliminate this normal age-related loss. If the loss of BMD is excessive, osteoporosis (defined as a BMD 2 standard deviations below normal for age) occurs, predisposing women to falls and fractures. Practically this means that the peak BMD a woman reaches in her youth (between adolescence and age 30) is a huge determinant of her risk for osteoporosis later in life.

With the development of amenorrhea, not only will BMD not increase during critical times of a woman's life, it will actively be lost. The amenorrheic woman may lose 2-5% BMD per year when she would have been gaining 2-3% BMD during the year if she were not amenorrheic meaning she will end up 4-8% below where she should be. So long as the amenorrheic state is maintained, not only is a female potentially losing bone mass permanently, she is limiting the peak BMD she may ever reach with some studies finding that amenorrheic athletes have BMD lower than even sedentary women. This predisposes women involved in sports that involve high impact forces such as running or gymnastics to be at a significantly higher risk for stress fractures in the lower leg (57). Cyclists are at risk for hip stress fractures as well. There is also some indication that the bone lost when amenorrhea develops is irreversible (58). This isn't universal and some degree of "catch-up" may occur if a woman re-established normal menstruation and optimizes her training and nutrition. This reversal, if it occurs, can take years (59,60).

While the optimal approach to limit or eliminate BMD loss is to restore normal menstruation (discussed later in the chapter) and optimize nutrition, a number of pharmacological approaches have been examined or used (61). For years it was felt that the loss of BMD when amenorrhea occurred was due to the reduction in estrogen levels. Logically, replacing estrogen with hormonal birth control (BC) should have helped the problem. While some studies have suggested a benefit, the evidence is considered at best weak that providing synthetic estrogen to amenorrheic women can improve BMD or reduce stress fracture risk. This is due to the importance of other hormones such as leptin, thyroid and IGF-1 that all play a critical role in bone metabolism. Just replacing estrogen isn't enough and the optimal solution to the problem of bone loss is to avoid developing amenorrhea in the first place or reverse it as soon as possible if it does occur.

Progressively Increasing Changes

While amenorrhea is the most extreme situation, all of the above described changes occur in progressive ways with increasing levels of menstrual cycle dysfunction. From luteal phase defect to anovulation to oligomenorrhea to full blown amenorrhea the effects increase with a progressive loss of bone density and worsening of hormonal status and metabolic rate (62). Levels of thyroid hormone progressively decrease as does insulin, leptin and IGF-1 with progressive increases in cortisol and this increases the overall metabolic response that occurs. Overall, all of these adaptations point to an energy conserving/starvation state. I would mention that even if the bone density is not always reversible, there is no evidence that any other aspect of reproductive function is permanently damaged (many female athletes report pregnancies soon after regaining normal menstrual function).

I've summarized changes that occur with progressively increasing menstrual cycle dysfunction below (63). These values are compared to sedentary women which is why even eumenorrhea in active women shows some degree of change. Each minus or plus sign represents a proportionally larger decrease or increase in a given aspect of function with a clear indication of the progressively worsening effects.

Menstrual Cycle	Eumenorrhea	Luteal Phase Deficient			amenorrhea
		Luteal Phase Defect	Anovulatory	Oligomenorrhea*	
	Normal	Appears Normal	Appears Normal	Lengthened (35+days)	Absent
T3 (thyroid)	-		--		---
Metabolic Rate	-		--		---
Leptin	-		--		---
Insulin	No Change		-		--
GH	No Change		-		--
IGF-1	No Change		No Change		--
Cortisol	+		++		+++
Blood Glucose	No Change		No Change		--
LH Pulsatility	-		--		---
Estrogen	-		--		---
Progesterone	-		--		---

* Can be related to pre-existing elevated testosterone levels as well.

(Adapted from Reference 58)

The Female Athlete Triad/Relative Energy Deficiency Syndrome

In the earliest days of research on the topic, a cluster of behaviors was identified that was being seen in female athletes including amenorrhea, eating disorders and a severe loss of bone density. This was rapidly given the name the Female Athlete Triad (somewhat unfortunately abbreviated FAT) or simply "The Triad". The concept of the Triad has been modified over the years in many ways primarily being expanded to include the subclinical versions of the original three factors rather than just the extreme endpoints (64). Essentially, the Triad is now conceptualized as an umbrella (or spectrum disorder) over each of the three primary components, each of which can fall along a spectrum of dysfunction.

In this conceptualization, menstrual cycle function can range from a normal menstrual cycle through the subclinical dysfunctions to oligomenorrhea (again, not PCOS/hyperandrogenism related) with amenorrhea as the final stage. Energy availability ranges from an optimal or sufficient EA through a reduced EA (with or without an eating disorder) finally to a low EA (below the critical threshold of 13.6 cal/lb or 30 cal/kg LBM). Bone density ranges from optimal bone density (for a woman's age) to low bone density (a BMD 1 standard deviation below normal) to full-blown osteoporosis (2 standard deviations below normal). I've shown this schematically below from optimal function to the most extreme end-points of the triad in the chart below.

Returning to the issue of bone density loss, it's important to realize that this is an effectively "silent" component of the triad (65). By this I mean that low EA can generally be identified by comparing activity to food intake and at least some forms of menstrual cycle dysfunction are readily apparent. Without specific testing (i.e. a DEXA scan), a woman may be losing bone without ever being aware of it.

The Female Athlete Triad		
Energy Availability	**Menstrual Function**	**Bone Density**
Optimal/Sufficient	Normal Cycle Function	Optimal for age
Reduced with or without an eating disorder	Luteal phase defect Anovulatory Oligomenorrhea (non PCOS/hyperandrogenic related)	Low Bone density (1SD below normal)
Low (below critical threshold) with or without eating disorder	Amenorrhea	Osteoporosis (2SD below normal)

In the above conceptualization, a woman can fall under the umbrella without showing all three components of the Triad. Even if nothing more than a low EA is present, a risk exists as the components tend to happen sequentially. Chronically low EA can eventually lead to menstrual cycle dysfunction, potentially developing to full-blown amenorrhea and that can occur before there is any meaningful impact on BMD which will occur last and over the longest time frame. The recognition and reversal of a low EA when it is first identified, may prevent the other two components from developing.

Given the primary role of low EA in driving the negative effects which occur, it's been recently suggested that FAT be renamed Relative Energy Deficiency Syndrome or RED-S (66). This is meant to achieve several goals not the least of which is the inclusion of all of the other factors caused by a low EA beyond menstrual cycle dysfunction and BMD loss (note that these are already included in the most current version of the FAT). RED-S is also meant to be more inclusive, including both recreationally exercising women (who may not identify as "athletes") along with men. This has not been without controversy and the original authors of the FAT position stand have pointed out numerous errors in the original RED-S position stand (67). Their greater concern is that changing the name might reduce awareness of the profoundly negative effects that are seen specifically in females relative to men (who rarely suffer the same consequences as women on reproductive function or bone health). The original authors of the RED-S have addressed these issues in an update to their original position stand (68). As this is more of an academic debate, I only mention it here for completeness.

Regardless of the above, the primary message of this chapter is that a chronically low EA, below a critical threshold, can be problematic in ways that extend far past just menstrual cycle disorders or a loss of bone density with the potential to negatively impact almost all aspects of training, health and function. As importantly, when and if menstrual cycle dysfunction, or even the recognition of a low EA, occurs, the goal should be to reverse it as rapidly as possible to prevent the more long-term changes from occurring.

Reversing Menstrual Cycle Dysfunction

In an ideal world, women would avoid menstrual cycle dysfunction, or at least full-blown amenorrhea completely. In the real world, for various reasons ranging from pathological dieting practices to the requirements of some sports, menstrual cycle dysfunction will occur to some degree or another. Given this fact, the rapid reversal of the dysfunction is of primary importance and I want to finish the chapter by looking at how that is best accomplished along with some of the issues that might surround what needs to be done. In many situations, various pharmacological approaches are used (or required) but those are beyond the scope of this book and I want to focus only on the non-pharmacological approaches.

Inasmuch as the fundamental cause of hypothalamically based menstrual dysfunction is a chronically low EA, the cure is as simple as raising EA and maintaining that increase until normal menstrual cycle function resumes (69). In practice this means increasing calorie intake, decreasing activity levels or some combination of the two. This will invariably be accompanied by an increase in body fat and weight but this is a necessary aspect of this approach. It is also one of the primary reasons that female athletes often resist doing it, discussed further below.

Research, either involving a single or small groups of athletes, has typically approached this by increasing daily calorie intake by 250-350 calories per day (many use 360 cacl/day due to the use of a commercial protein/carbohydrate supplement) with a reduction of one day of training per day. The success rates of these interventions in terms of restoring menstrual cycle function has ranged from as little as 18% up to 100%. Typically it is the smaller studies showing the best success rates and this likely represents the amount of control that can be exerted over the subjects. In one study of four women who had lost their cycle for 6-9 months, three began menstruating within 2-6 months (one dropped out) although two did not have ovulatory cycles for several months afterwards (70). In contrast, in another study only 18% of 51 amenorrheic athletes regained their cycle after 5 years. In all cases, the women who gained more total body weight were more likely to resume menstrual cycle function. This likely just represents the fact that the women did increase their food intake/decrease their activity and maintain those changes at an appropriate level for long enough to recover their cycle (71).

In cases where menstruation does not occur within the length of the study, benefits are still found. In one, a runner who had been amenorrheic for 14 months, reporting chronic fatigue and injury was compared to three normally cycling women over 15 weeks as she increased her calories and reduce training (72). Despite not menstruating during the study (she would start 3 months after it ended), she showed a huge 50% drop in cortisol levels with an increase in LH levels a drasticaperformance increase after increasing her EA. In another, 5 amenorrheic and 26 oligomenorrheic females did not begin menstruating during a 3 month intervention although all showed signs of hormonal and metabolic recovery (73). The study was most likely simply too short to see full menstrual cycle recovery. I mentioned earlier in the chapter that there is often a lag time between changes in EA and menstrual cycle dysfunction although the reasons for this are unknown.

There does seem to be a general link between the duration of amenorrhea and the amount of time it takes to resume normal function. In one study, women who had lost their cycle for more than 8-12 months took 6 months to begin menstruating while those who had lost their cycle for less than this only took 1-2 months to restore normal function (74). I'll describe two case studies on physique athletes in Chapter that seem to support this. Looking at the studies as a whole, the amount of time it takes for a woman to regain normalcy can vary from a matter of weeks to up to 3 years and there is no real way to predict how long or not it may take for normal cycle function to resume (75). In the case where a woman has not regained her cycle over a multi-year span, it's possible that there are other causes that need to be addressed medically.

It's important to realize that even when menstruation resumes, the cycle may not be completely normalized for up to one year. In one study, two female athletes who had lost their cycle for either 330 or 23 days were followed for one year (76). The first athlete had her first menstruation after 2.5 months but it was anovulatory. She lost her cycle again due to a decrease in food intake before restoring it again but still showed evidence of luteal phase defect. The second woman took only 23 days to resume ovulatory cycles but still had the occasional anovulatory cycle with evidence of luteal phase defect. Other studies mentioned above found similar results. Just as the system progressively becomes more dysfunctional, it would appear to progressively become normally functional again.

So what determines when or if a woman will regain a normal menstrual cycle. Factors such as the rate/size of calorie increase (to raise EA above the critical level), rate of weight/body fat regain (slightly more weight/fat gain is associated with a faster return of a normal menstrual cycle) and individual factors such as stress, sleep or genetics impact on this. In most studies, the degree of weight gain is a critical factor with women gaining 4.5 lbs (2 kg) or more being the ones who begin menstruating. Given the generally weak relationship between weight, BF% and menstrual cycle function, the weight gain is likely a consequence of the increased EA rather than being the actual cause of recovery.

While the above is certainly simple in principle, it is often less simple in practice. Many female athletes are often extremely resistant to increasing calorie intake, decreasing activity or gaining any amount of body fat even if it is required for their long-term health or performance. In many cases, the athlete will compensate for one change with another, increasing activity to offset calorie increases or training more or harder on other training days to compensate for reducing the number of days they train. Inasmuch as certain psychological profiles or attitudes may be present as causing or at least contributing to FHA, just recommending that calories be increased or activity be decreased may not be sufficient. CBT to alter modes of thinking or coping might very well be what is required or could act as an adjunct to raising EA and decreasing activity (i.e. by reducing preoccupation on food intake or body weight). In the case where an overt or subclinical eating disorders are present, psychological counseling is likely to be a required part of the recovery process (77)

Chapter 13: Stress

While I've mentioned the concept of stress earlier in the book in various contexts, I want to look at it more generally in this chapter in terms of its potential impact on a woman's physiology. Here, as would be expected there are significant gender differences in the stress response and, just as with the issues discussed in the last chapter, has implications for how women can or should approach the goal of dieting (whether in general or to the extremes). Many approaches that might be tolerable for men are, at best, not ideal for women and, at worst, physically damaging to them.

The primary focus of this chapter will be the hormone cortisol, a hormone that I have deliberately saved detailed discussion of until now. First I want to define stress in some meaningful way before looking at what cortisol is and what it does. Unsurprisingly there are significant difference in how women and men respond to stress. This will all provide the background for a discussion of how the types of chronic stresses that are often seen among female athletes, recreational exercisers and dieters can cause problems in the long-term, including one potentially permanent effect.

What is Stress?

Given its importance in human health and physiology, it may be surprising that the concept of stress is not well defined in a biological sense (the term originally came from engineering). Somewhat circularly, stress is sometimes defined as the body's response to a stressor where a stressor is defined as anything that causes stress. As I stated in the last chapter, a slightly more useful definition would be the body's response to anything that tries to push it out of homeostasis, the relatively fixed level of function that it tries to maintain. In this context, there are endless potential stressors such as environmental stress (heat or cold), physiological stress (intense exercise), energetic stress (calorie restriction) or psychological stress (worrying about taxes). Each causes the body to respond in some form or fashion physiologically. Heat will induce sweating while cold will cause shivering, exercise causes a short-term increase in calorie burning and nutrient mobilization, etc.

While many tend to think of stress as nothing but a negative, this is incorrect. Rather, the way that the stress occurs determines whether it has overall positive or negative effects on the body. When stresses are relatively short-lived, occurring and then ending relatively rapidly, the body not only has time to recover but is often stimulated to grow stronger from that stress. Exercise is perhaps the best example of this where a workout or series of workouts stresses some tissue the body (both physically and hormonally) which stimulates the body to adapt (i.e. muscles and bones grow stronger, the heart and enzymes adapt, etc.). This adaptation makes the same workout less stressful in the future   It is only when too much stress occurs for extended periods that problems occur. Here the body never has a chance to recover or rebuild itself and this causes it to eventually break down. I would point readers interested in more details of this topic to the eminently readable <u>Why Zebras Don't get Ulcers</u> by Robert Sapolsky. He explains the ins and outs of the stress system along with providing advice on decreasing stress.

While each type of stress tends to cause a specific physiological response, they also stimulate a more generalized stress response. Surprisingly, extremely different stresses tend to generate a fairly similar stress response. There may be subtle differences in the stress "signature" but the overall effect is identical for the purposes of this book. This explains a point I made in the last chapter which is that every stressor applied to the body ends up adding to the overall stress (or allostatic) load. One stressor may be bad but two stressors is worse than one, three is worse than two, etc. and this is due to each stressor causing the same general physiological and hormonal response. And while other hormones such as adrenaline are involved, the primary hormone of relevance in the context of stress is cortisol.

Cortisol

The hormone cortisol is actually one of several hormones that are grouped under the heading of corticosteroids but I will refer to them all as cortisol for simplicity. Cortisol is released from the adrenal gland which releases many other hormones such as adrenaline, the adrenal androgens such as DHEA and the mineralocorticoids, hormones involved in water balance, such as aldosterone. As with many hormones, the signal to release cortisol comes from the hypothalamus which, via release of Corticotrophin Releasing Hormone (CRH), stimulates the pituitary gland to release adrenocorticotrophic hormone (ACTC) which signals the adrenal gland to release cortisol. The general trigger for this process to occur is, as the name of the title and the previous section suggest, stress.

Cortisol has broad reaching effects in the body and, due to many of its effect, is often thought of as being a bad hormone. This is prevalent in both the athletic community as well as the general public due to endless advertisements claiming that it increases belly fat. But just as the effects of stress can be positive or negative, the effects of cortisol (which really mediate the effects of stress) can also be positive or negative. Simply, acute pulses of cortisol (caused by short term stress) tend to be beneficial while chronically elevated cortisol (caused by long term stress) is not.

In the short-term for example, cortisol works to generally mobilize energy. Fatty acids are released from fat cells, glucose is produced in the liver and even protein breakdown is stimulated. Even this latter effect is adaptive, helping muscle to rebuild and remodel itself in response to that stress. Acutely, cortisol does impair bone growth but this is primarily a way to conserve energy (and when the stress ends, the bone can rebuild). Cortisol pulses helps to form memories which is why people tend to remember acutely stressful events and acts as an anti-inflammatory, explaining its use to treat injuries.

Perhaps confusingly, cortisol acutely impairs immune system function but this too makes sense: the immune system uses a stunning amount of energy and inhibiting it in the short-term helps to provide energy for whatever stressor is being dealt with. Cortisol also impairs the function of the reproductive system; in the short-term this makes perfect sense for the same reasons menstrual cycle dysfunction makes perfect sense when insufficient energy is available. But in the aggregate, all of these effects are extremely beneficial for the body and are part of what helps it to adapt to stress over time (1).

In contrast, when cortisol is elevated chronically, its effects become distinctly negative. Cortisol causes insulin resistance and leptin resistance in the brain, both of which can have negative effects on body weight and body fat regulation. If insulin levels are high when cortisol is chronically elevated, visceral fat storage can be stimulated (hence the claim that cortisol leads to belly fat). With chronic stress, cortisol increases protein breakdown but without the recovery period, tissue never get a chance to repair themselves. In the long-term this causes muscle loss and other bodily damage. Bone production is inhibited continuously and eventually this will cause the loss of bone mineral density (BMD). Memory is impaired and immune system, reproductive function and sex drive are all inhibited as well.

As background for later in the chapter, there is a slightly more complex aspect of cortisol dynamics called feedback inhibition that I need to briefly describe. In general, when levels of a hormone go up, this inhibits further release of the hormone and this is meant to maintain that hormone at a relatively constant level. Relative to cortisol and the HPA, the hypothalamus has cortisol receptors that, when cortisol binds to them, is meant to inhibit the hypothalamus from telling the pituitary gland to have the adrenal gland release more cortisol. If this loop stops working correctly, a huge number of problems can occur. As an example, impaired feedback inhibition of cortisol release is seen in 95% of people with depression. Finally let me mention that cortisol is metabolized extensively in fat cells (especially visceral fat cells). Active cortisol can be converted into inactive cortisone and vice versa and local levels of cortisol may be as important as blood levels in determining many aspects of metabolism (2). The details of this system are unimportant and are only relevant for discussion of some of the hormonal modifiers later in the chapter.

The primary take home of this section is this: acute pulses of cortisol are generally beneficial and important to help the body adapt to stress over time while chronically elevated cortisol levels are bad. As well, while chronically elevated cortisol is extremely damaging to the body, having too little produced is equally bad. At the extremes this shows up in Addison's disease (where the body can't mount a stress response at all) or Cushing's disease (where cortisol is chronically elevated). People with Addison's may pass out simply standing up as their bodies can't raise blood pressure adequately and other stresses simply can't be handled. Cushing's patients are in a state of chronically elevated cortisol with all that implies. While disease states, there are situations that occur in response to stress that share similarities with them.

Cortisol and Bodyweight

While obesity can lead to an overactivated HPA, stress and cortisol also play a major role in the overall control of bodyweight (3). Confusingly, stress may increase or decrease hunger depending on a host of factors including the nature of the stress and the person's psychological profile (discussed below). In the short-term, primarily due to increases in CRH, stress tends to blunt appetite (it may also increase energy expenditure) and this would tend to reduce bodyweight. As expected, chronic stress has the opposite effect. Active thyroid is reduced (lowering metabolic rate) and the leptin/insulin resistance that develops may cause food intake to increase especially from high-sugar/high-fat "comfort foods". Sugar intake reduces cortisol levels which decreases the feeling of stress and people may end up self-medicating their stress in this fashion (4). This can lead to a vicious cycle of stress-eating over time.

Another way that cortisol can impact on body weight by causing water retention (this is in addition to any impact of the menstrual cycle). Due to similarities in structure, cortisol can bind to the same receptor that would normally bind hormones involved in water weight regulation such as aldosterone. While cortisol doesn't bind that strongly, there is up to 10,000 times as much cortisol and the effect can be pronounced. In the extremes of Cushing disease, the condition of chronically elevated cortisol I mentioned, water retention is absolutely enormous. And, to a lesser degree, chronic, dietary, exercise and psychological stress can cause this (starvation edema has been known to occur since the 50's). Falling leptin on a diet allows cortisol to increase further and lowered thyroid levels also cause water retention. This can cause apparent weight loss plateaus and I will discuss this in detail in Chapter 26.

Gender Differences in the Response to Stress

While all stressors cause a relatively similar stress response (hormonally at least), there are gender differences in how the system works. As I mentioned in Chapter 2, there is a slight difference in the hormonal response between women and men (and here I'm talking about more than just cortisol) but I won't detail them here. In general, women and men show similar levels of cortisol in their bloodstream under unstressed conditions and throughout this section I'll only consider how those levels change in response to stress. While it depends on the specific stressor being examined, women show an overall reduced stress response compared to men and this is thought to exist to protect the developing fetus from excessively high cortisol levels (4a). This difference manifests itself in that women and men differ in their propensity for specific stress-related diseases (5). For example, women are far more likely to suffer auto-immune diseases (probably contributing to their higher likelihood of developing Hashimoto's, an autoimmune thyroid disease); contributing to this is the fact that women have a stronger innate immune system than men (6). Women are also about twice as likely to suffer from depression (often related to cortisol) with this risk increasing with age (7). In contrast, men are more likely to have problems with heart disease or infectious disease due to a generally heightened stress response and poorer innate immune system function.

Certainly there are other issues contributing to the above differences in disease risk (i.e. women vs. men's fat patterning) but it does appear that women and men's HPA operate differently (8). Of perhaps more interest is the fact that the stress response system seems to have a different underlying purpose (in an evolutionary sense) in women versus men. Classically the stress response has been thought of as the fight or flight response and certainly this is true when looking at men's overall hormonal and behavioral response to most stressors. In contrast, it's now thought that women's stress response triggers more of a tend and befriend response (9). Tending here refers caring for/protecting children while befriending refers to women's tendency to form social bonds with other women as this decreases their stress levels.

Subjectively, women seem to experience more stress, that is they report things as being more stressful. Women also appear to report stress more frequently although this seems to be mostly due to men reporting stress less frequently overall. For technical reasons related to how cortisol is measured, it's unclear if those subjective reports show up in an increased cortisol response. Of more importance than the subjective reports are the actual changes in cortisol and it's clear that women and men show relatively greater or lesser stress responses compared to one another although this depends heavily on what type of stress is being examined (10). In response to heat and cold stress, for example, women show a larger stress response, releasing more cortisol. While beyond the scope of this book, women also show an increased cortisol release in response to certain drug challenges (i.e. Nalaxone). In other cases, women may release similar amounts or less cortisol compared to men. Discussed more below, women appear to release similar amounts of cortisol in response to exercise and diet.

It's when the topic of psychological stress is examined that the topic becomes more complicated. First and foremost, men have a stress response in anticipation of psychological stressors while women show no increase or even a decrease. This makes some logical sense within the context of what I described above regarding the purpose of the stress response. A man's stress system, oriented towards fight or flight, has to gear up prior to either, raising heart rate and mobilizing fuel for energy. A woman's, oriented towards tending and befriending, has no such need. In terms of the actual stress response to psychological stress, it has been classically believed that women always release less cortisol than men. But this turns out to depend on the type of stress being examined. Specifically, women show a larger stress response than men in response to studies of interpersonal conflict and social rejection while men show a greater response when they have to solve math problems or speak in front of people. This too seems related to the difference in purpose of the stress system. Women would be more likely to find social rejection (an inability to befriend) more stressful while men would find an inability to perform a competitive task more stressful.

There are other gender based differences in cortisol release that can play a role here. One is that, even when women release less cortisol than men, they release it more quickly, causing blood levels to reach a higher peak. Of some importance to the issue of short-term versus long-term stress is that women's bodies clear cortisol from the bloodstream more slowly than men. So however much cortisol is released in women will remain in the bloodstream for a longer period of time.   This makes any absolute type of stress a relatively longer lived stress for a woman than a man. I'd emphasize that word relatively here, it's not as if a woman will maintain a day-long cortisol response to something that a man might only show an hour response to.   But on average, her cortisol levels will remain elevated for a longer duration than his.

Adding to this is the fact that the feedback inhibition loop I described above works more poorly in women than in men (this might contribute to women's double risk for depression).   That is, when cortisol levels are elevated for some reason, women's bodies are generally poorer at preventing further cortisol release. In response to chronic stress, a woman's cortisol levels may continue to rise and rise while a man's generally will not. There are individual differences here as some women are relatively better than others in terms of how well or poorly feedback inhibition works: when their cortisol is elevated, further production is inhibited. But overall women show decreased feedback inhibition compared to men. I'll discuss the implications of this later in the chapter.

Finally, and while not represented by any research that I am aware of, it seems possible that women may face more total overall stress (a higher allostatic load) than men. Whether or not this was true historically, in the modern world women either expect (or are expected) to work or simply have to do so due to the requirements of a two-income household. To that they may have obligations or expectations to take care of the home and children while maintaining personal relationships. Within the context of this book, to that we might add general societal pressures on appearance and thinness for women in both the general public and among female athletes. The latter is even true for those athletes not involved in sports emphasizing thinness often wear revealing outfits with the reality that women of all walks of life are judged on their appearance in a way that men rarely are.   Women are far more likely to show higher levels of dietary restraint than men, and this all adds up to a high allostatic load and effectively pre-stressed psychological profile before diet and/or exercise are added to the situation.

Reproductive Hormones and the Stress Response

It would seem fairly clear that, given the sex based difference in stress response and cortisol release, that there is a biological basis to it. Certainly some of it may be genetic and/or occur during development but, as always, the differences in reproductive hormones are likely to play a role. Let me say up front that this topic gets extremely complicated very quickly as hormones could be having an effect on the hypothalamus, pituitary gland or adrenal gland.   In many cases, effects are seen in more than one place and determining how the system works is no simpler here than in most other situations. Rather than attempting to explain all of the potential places where reproductive hormones might have an impact, I want to focus on the overall pattern of stress response and how it is impacted.

While complex, a general picture has emerged with estrogen and progesterone determining a woman's stress response and androgens/testosterone determining a man's response. The data on testosterone's effects are all over the place and, as they are not really relevant to this book, I won't even try to describe them. Focusing on women, estrogen seems to play a primary role in determining women's greater stress response to at least certain types of stressors. Supporting this is that giving estrogen to men increases their stress response to psychosocial stress to levels similar of that seen in women (11). There is even some indication that it is the lack of estrogen, rather than the presence of testosterone that is responsible for men's generally reduced stress response. This doesn't explain the similar stress response to exercise for both women and men, however. Clearly there are differences in purely psychological and physiological stress so this may not be that surprising even if the mechanisms behind it are not known.

The role of progesterone on the stress response is unclear in terms of whether it has an effect in the first place and what those effects might be. Observationally, women's stress response to exercise is increased during the luteal phase (12). As well, women's response to the types of psychological stress that they generally have a lesser response to (compared to men) is increased to levels similar to that of men during the luteal phase (13).   So progesterone is having some effect although whether it's a direct effect or by blocking the effects of estrogen is unclear. Women's already less responsive feedback inhibition loop is further impaired during the luteal phase compared to the follicular and a general conclusion would be that women's overall stress response will be elevated in during the luteal phase (and possibly in any progesterone-like hormonal state).

The Effects of Hormonal Modifiers

Looking at the other hormonal modifiers, I mentioned in the previous chapter that cortisol levels are elevated in women with menstrual cycle dysfunction and that the increase becomes greater with increasing levels of menstrual cycle dysfunction. In amenorrhea, cortisol may be elevated 10-20% above normal levels but levels can be doubled in women with full blown anorexia (14); this appears to be due to an impaired feedback inhibition loop. Essentially, these women's bodies are no longer able to shut off cortisol release effectively. They also have a larger cortisol response to exercise than women who have not lost their menstrual cycle which only compounds the problem.

Research on hormonal birth control (BC) is somewhat inconclusive. One study cited above found that women using combined birth control had a lower cortisol response to exercise than women in the follicular phase who had a lower response than women in the luteal phase. It appears that the ethinyl estradiol component increases levels of cortisol binding protein in the liver. This means that, even if the same amount of cortisol is released, less free cortisol will be present and the overall effect will be lessened. But not all studies find this, possibly due to differences in study design or the type of BC used. There simply isn't enough research to draw a conclusive picture.

Women with PCOS/elevated testosterone show a hyperactive HPA response to stress and this appears to be due to negative changes in the metabolism of cortisol within fat cells that I mentioned above (15). This altered fat metabolism of cortisol may be part of what is maintaining the hyperandrogenic PCOS woman's increased output of adrenal androgens, further contributing to the problem. Women with more visceral fat (as seen in PCOS and obesity) tend to show an overreactive stress response and this is seen very clearly in the case of women who develop abdominal, but not lower body, obesity (16). The entire system becomes dysregulated due to the accumulation of body fat and the increase in adrenal output is part of what elevates obese women's testosterone levels. This can become a self-perpetuating cycle due to the way that cortisol can impact on bodyweight and food intake.

With aging, the overall stress response in both genders increases but this increase is roughly three times higher in women then in men (17). As always this suggests that the decrease in estrogen, progesterone or both at menopause is responsible. In response to hormone replacement therapy (HRT) while estrogen-only therapy increases the cortisol response to stress, a combination of estrogen and progesterone decreases it (18). Regular exercise also reduces the stress response here (19).

Individual Differences

In addition to the gender differences that exist in response to stress, there are also large individual differences in how people will or will not respond to a stressful situation. Readers may be familiar with the terms Type-A or Type-B personalities and, even if they are not, everyone has known someone who will have an enormous (over)reaction to the smallest of situational stresses while others remain calm in the face of disaster. Even when faced with an identical stress, two people may perceive it differently, showing a completely distinct stress and cortisol response. Adding to this is are differences in how two people may recover from a stressful situation after it has ended. After a given stress, one person may move past it quickly while the other remains stressed out over it hours (or days) later. The latter individual will be chronically over-activating their HPA and generating what amounts to a chronically elevated stress response even if the stress itself was relatively short-term in nature. So consider two people who are in a slow moving line at a store. One may be seething with rage over the speed while another is completely calm about it. Hours later, the first may still be angry about the situation, maintaining an overactive stress and cortisol response long after it was necessary, while the second was barely affected at all.

Effectively, some people show greater stress reactivity compared to others, both reacting more strongly to stress to begin with and possibly maintaining that stress response for longer after the stress has ended (recall that this, along with an inability to cope with daily hassle was found in a group of women suffering psychologically caused amenorrhea). While some of that behavior may be learned, it's clear that there is a also a biological hardwiring during fetal development with high levels of cortisol exposure causing an overactive HPA later in life. In response to any stressor, the stress response will be greater and potentially longer, also predisposing the person to certain stress-related diseases. Even here there is a gender difference with women being more sensitive to this effect (20). That is, when exposed to elevated cortisol levels in utero, women are more likely to develop an overactive HPA later in life (this can also predispose them to certain stress related diseases). While clearly part of a person's underlying biology when it is present, it's equally clear that coping skills to reduce stress can help enormously here (recall that CBT restored menstrual cycle function in psychologically stressed women). While not studied to my knowledge, this could explain why some women show a poorer feedback inhibition loop to stress than others. That is, perhaps a generally overactive HPA is part of why their bodies continue to produce cortisol in response to additional stress (whether real or perceived) when output should be inhibited.

Adding to the above is how a given person perceives a given stressor. So consider something like speaking in front of people (a commonly used stress test as mentioned above). Someone who is outgoing and loves attention might not see it as a stress at all while an an introvert or someone who is terrified of embarrassing themselves might see it as an enormous stress, showing an elevated cortisol response. Similarly, while one person might find a massage calming and stress releasing, someone who is uncomfortable with being touched by a relative stranger might show a tremendous stress response.

While this is most likely to apply to more social or psychological stresses, it could also impact on the stress response to diet or exercise. Physiologically speaking, any specific workout shouldn't have an enormous impact on the stress response seen but there could be a psychological aspect as well with some people perceiving it as more stressful in a psychological sense. This could be related to any number factors including beginners feeling embarrassed about being in a public gym (or one filled with more advanced people). Fear of not knowing how to do a given exercise correctly or that the workout will be beyond them could contribute to this. The same can hold for diet in that, while any similar diet should be broadly physiologically the same, people can perceive how restrictive or difficult it might be Playing into this is the concept I discussed previously and will discuss more below which is dietary restraint. This refers to a general preoccupation (or obsession) on bodyweight and food intake which can cause some women to show elevated cortisol levels even before they begin their diet.   I'll discuss this more below.

I have to think that these individual differences, whether biological or psychological, are contributing to the relative robustness (or fragility) of women's reproductive systems and/or hypothalamic function in some way. Women who may have an overactive HPA, or a psychological profile causing them to be more pre-stressed, who are exposed to more total stress via diet and exercise, who have an excessive cortisol response to stress and/or don't recover from that stress as rapidly will show an exaggerated and chronic stress/cortisol response compared to those women who do not. This combination of underlying physiology and psychological profile only adds to the stressful effects of diet and exercise, discussed next.

The Stress of Dieting

While stress can clearly occur at any time, regardless of the specific goal, I want to look at how stress relates specifically to the dieting and fat loss process. Or more accurately, how the fat loss process itself can generate stress and increase cortisol levels. Just as in the previous chapter, I will be focusing on exercise, diet and psychological stresses in terms of their individual and combined effects. However, while the focus in the last chapter was on menstrual cycle dysfunction per se, here I will focus primarily on cortisol levels (note that there is overlap between these two issues as an increase in cortisol is part of the hormonal profile of menstrual cycle dysfunction).

Exercise and Diet Related Stress

Looking first at exercise, the impact on cortisol is related both to the type and intensity of activity being done. In general, low intensity exercise does not cause a significant stress response unless it is performed for multiple hours at a time. This tends to be uncommon outside of female endurance athletes such as runners or cyclists (who typically consume carbohydrates and fluids during exercise which offsets much of the hormonal response) although there are female dieters who perform hours of aerobic activity per day. As I've mentioned, women do need to perform somewhat more (25-30% or so) aerobic activity to burn the same numbers of calories as a male but many take this to an unhealthy extreme.

In contrast high-intensity exercise, whether aerobic or HIIT, causes a universally large cortisol response regardless of duration and this can cause enormous problems if excessive amounts are done (21). This has been a trend in recent years as dieters have attempted to replace the more traditional lower intensity aerobic activity with nothing but high-intensity activities. While some may get away with this, it's important to realize that even high-performance athletes rarely perform truly high-intensity training more than two to three times per week (and even then only moderate amounts are done). Attempting to do more than this in and of itself will cause a chronic over-activation of the HPA and increase in cortisol and this can burn people out even if they are eating enough. When it is done while dieting and restricting calories, it can be a disaster. I'd note that a single day of rest from training allows cortisol to return to normal levels and this is an importance consideration for those athletes or dieters who are attempting to exercise (especially at high-intensities) on a daily basis.

An additional concern here is that women, in contrast to men, may continue to produce high levels of cortisol during high-intensity exercise even if it is elevated (i.e. due to dieting or psychological stress) to begin with (22). This is due to the relatively less effective feedback inhibition loop I mentioned but is also a place where there is a great deal of individual variability. Specifically, some women will continue to produce cortisol when it is already elevated while others will not. The former type of women may be destroyed by the types of training and dieting approaches that the latter frequently "get away" with. As I described in the last chapter, the effect of large amounts of high-intensity exercise can be magnified if it is started immediately (23). With more progressive and gradual increases in either the amount of intensity of exercise, the body isn't as overstressed and the hypothalamus will become "conditioned", reducing the total stress response as the amount and intensity of training increased (24). Although not well studied, there is some indication that women release less cortisol in response to weight training than men although this depends heavily on the training being done. There's simply no way to draw conclusions at this point.

Moving to dieting, it's clear that the act of dieting or reducing calorie intake acts as a biological/energetic stress and, among all of the other effects, cortisol will go up to help mobilize energy for the body to use. This happens to some degree in response to any calorie deficit with more extreme diets causing a more pronounced activation of the HPA and a greater increase in cortisol levels (25,26). I mentioned above that simply eating can raise cortisol levels although women show a reduced response compared to men (27). This increase in cortisol assuredly helps with utilization of the ingested nutrients.

Whether specific nutrients play a role is currently unclear. Some research suggests that protein is responsible for the cortisol increase while others find that carbohydrates have the greatest impact. This may depend on the individual and their body fat patterning. In one study, women with either traditional fat patterning or more of a central fat patterning (as seen in PCOS, obesity, etc.) were given a high carbohydrate or high protein/high-fat meal (28). The women with the more traditional fat patterning showed the largest cortisol increase to the high-protein/high-fat meal and less to the high carbohydrate meal while the while the women with a more central fat pattern had the largest cortisol response to the high-carbohydrate meal. This is likely relate to differences in insulin sensitivity and matches with the dietary recommendations I will provide in Chapter 19.

As a final component of diet, I want to discuss caffeine intake and its potential impact on cortisol levels. This is important not only because caffeine is arguably the most used drug in the world but because dieters, especially those dieting to the extreme, often consume an enormous amount of caffeine to get through workouts or to try to fight off the diet-induced lethargy. Caffeine does increase cortisol levels with higher intakes of 600 mg/day raising cortisol more than lower intakes of 300 mg/day and can increase the stress response in women to at least some types of stress (29,30).

Psychological Stress

As psychological stress can encompass an enormous amount of different topics, I can't possibly look at them all. Rather, I want to focus on psychological factors that are most relevant to female dieters and athletes in terms of how they might add to the stress of exercise and/or dieting itself. I do want to reiterate that all life stressors, whether related to diet and training or not, are relevant in terms of the total stress seen. A diet or training situation that could readily be handled under one set of conditions can become excessive if other life stresses increase. Problems with interpersonal relationships, a lack of family or friend support, death in the family, work or school stress, etc. all play a role in whether or not a given amount of other stresses can be handled or not. In this vein, individuals experiencing high levels of stress make poorer strength gains and recover more slowly from resistance training (31,32).

For the general dieting or exerciser, this could include self-imposed psychological stress worrying about actually adhering to their program. Dieting and the goal of weight and fat loss can also act as its own type of psychological stressor. Even before true hunger sets in, there is often a feeling of deprivation and the sense that the person is restricted in what they can eat. All of the above can be exacerbated in those women who are unfamiliar with the concept of body composition or issues relating to the scale and daily or weekly fluctuations in weight. Unrealistic expectations about weight loss rates adds to this as dieters feel as if the effort they are putting towards their goal is not generating meaningful results. All of this adds to the already existent psychological stress load.

For athletes of any sort, there may be additional issues contributing. Adherence to training is rarely an issue although performance pressure, anxiety, coping with injuries or interpersonal problems with coaches or teammates (in team sports) can all add to the overall stress load. Physique athletes often have their own set of issues, somewhat unique to their sport. Many attempt to follow an extremely rigid schedule of eating and being unable to follow it can add to their stress levels. In many cases, they will avoid social events, friends and family for no other reason than to adhere to their meal plan. With appearance as the end metric, a perceived lack of progress or not being on schedule to reach their goal in time for competition adds to their stress levels enormously. The final stages of contest dieting can be enormously psychologically stressful as the diet and training program must be maintained in the face of enormous physiological adaptations and fatigue or the feeling that their appearance is not what it needs to be.

In both cases, there can be additional stressors if the dieter or athlete is not supported by their family or friends who may not understand the importance of the diet (or its requirements) or exercise program. They may encourage the individual to skip training sessions or break their diet "just a little bit", etc. At home and tying into my suggestion above that women may face more total stresses in the modern world, female dieters are often tasked with making two or even three meals in some cases: one for themselves, one for their partner and one for their children (if present). In many cases, this may occur after a full day of work and the day's training session and the amount of stress generated can be significant.

In addition to all of the above are two other factors. The first is the cluster of personality traits such as high stress reactivity, poor coping skills, an inability to handle daily hassles, perfectionism and others that contribute to stress and raised cortisol levels and which may cause FHA in and of themselves. The second is the issue of dietary restraint which I have mentioned several times already in the book. More common in women than men, this refers to a situation where someone is chronically concerned with their body weight and overall food intake. This should not be considered synonymous with dieting as it is possible to be concerned with what is being eaten without trying to lose weight. I'd mention again that restraint can be rigid or flexible and here I am focusing only on rigid restraint.

Women with high dietary restraint show an overactive HPA/stress response and elevated cortisol levels to begin with due to their extreme concern over what they eat (33,34). The same high dietary restraint is also related to menstrual cycle dysfunction, lowered bone density, and stress fractures in runners and at least part of this is mediated through elevated cortisol levels (35-37). Somewhat surprisingly, people with high levels of rigid dietary restraint tend to weigh more than those who show lower levels of restraint. This is explained by the fact that restrained eaters are the ones who often overeat in response to various types of stress (38). This is called disinhibition and the degree of disinhibition seen in any given person is highly related to weight gain or weight regain (39).

This is due to the fact that the foods most commonly eaten when people become disinhibited are high-calorie, high-sugar, high-fat comfort foods. This may cause weight gain and this can put the person into a vicious cycle where weight gain due to disinhibition may cause the person to become that much more restrained and focused on their eating. The next stress can cause disinhibition and overeating to occur and you can see how this cycle can become self-perpetuating. Repeated cycles of this cause a gain in body fat and in those women who start gaining abdominal/visceral fat, the stress system becomes that much more over-activated, generating a chronic cortisol response with everything that implies.

All of the above points to the fact that a variety of psychological stresses, ranging from inherent psychological profile to life stress to various potential concerns about eating and training can add to the biological stress and cortisol response to dieting and exercise. What specific stresses are present may depend somewhat on the population being discussed but some stresses are likely to be present . In all cases, the combination of dieting, intense training and psychological stresses will contribute and add up to determine the total amount of stress present and whether or not it overwhelms any given individual.

Stress and Amenorrhea

In the previous chapter, I examined the various causes of menstrual cycle dysfunction with the general conclusion that a low Energy Availability (EA) is the primary cause with other factors such as psychological stress, genetics, reproductive age and possibly BF% modulating that. Focusing only on the first two it's been traditional to separate energetic and psychological stresses in terms of their effect on the reproductive system but this is a mistake (40). The two factors contribute to the overall stress on the system and may interact in complex ways. For example, someone might choose to exercise for stress reduction and end up imposing an energetic stress on their body. Alternately someone might restrict calories, causing them some degree of mental stress over feeling deprived in terms of what they can eat.

At the extreme, Ann Loucks, who developed the EA concept, has suggested that all stress, including psychological stress, is energetic to begin with (41). She contends that even psychological stress is generating a lowered EA state by reducing food intake or increasing energy expenditure. At the other extreme are those that question whether athletic amenorrhea (FHA found specifically in athletes) should be considered an energetic or psychogenic (i.e. psychological) challenge (42). That is, they suggest that the typical cluster of personality traits that is seen in women, coupled with the additional stresses seen in athletes involving training, travel, team dynamics, etc. may be the cause of FHA in these women rather than low EA itself. Given that behavioral therapy can be incredibly effective in restoring menstruation in these women, there seems to be good evidence that this is, or at least can be the case. There are also anecdotal reports of women who restored their EA to sufficient levels while gaining weight and fat who did not resume normal menstruation until they addressed their psychological stresses.

In a practical sense, there will always be some degree of energetic and psychological stress present when someone is seeking fat loss and it will only be a matter of degrees as to which is potentially more or less responsible. This is especially true for a concept that I want to introduce, an extension of the paper on psychogenic stress above, that I call the psychogenically stressed dieter. This refers to the female who is starting with some degree of psychological pre-stress before adding to that with calorie restriction or exercise. This could take many forms. At lesser levels it might simply be generally high-stress reactivity or a poor ability to cope with daily hassles. In the physique sports, and potentially any sport with a component of appearance, narcissism, perfectionism and dependence on external validation is likely to be present. All athletes have to deal with the overall stress of their training, dieting, travel, etc. At the very extreme, overt eating disorders may be present and, even when they are not, subclinical disorders may be. Even if only extremely rigid dieting attitudes are in place, not only does this raise cortisol levels by 10% above normal to begin with, it can actually lead to eating disorders over time (43).

Highly related to this is a relatively "new" eating disorder called orthorexia which would seem to represent the far extreme of rigid eating attitudes. Orthorexia describes an obsessive preoccupation with the relative goodness/healthiness of foods which, contradictorily, may lead them to become less healthy due to the elimination of nutrient dense foods that are deemed unhealthy for some reason. The orthorexic attitude may be best represented by the idea of "clean" eating. This approach to diet is found in the physique community although it has leaked out into the general public and the idea is that some foods (typically unprocessed foods) are clean while others (refined foods) are not. Tying this back into the psychologically stressed dieter, orthorexia has even been linked to both narcissism and perfectionism and I think this explains the high degree of it found in certain subcultures (44).

Like the orthorexic, clean eaters become obsessed about what is or is not a clean food with the words themselves connoting a moralistic or hygiene aspect of eating. And while they may be meticulous about their food intake under certain conditions, they can show an enormous amount of disinhibition: the slightest deviation from clean eating lead to enormous binges which are then followed by an even more intense focus on restriction going forwards (binges may also be dealt with by performing hours of exercise which takes it into the realm of exercise bulimia). These dieters often engage in many other somewhat pathological behaviors such as avoiding social events or interactions for fear that they might break their diet in the most minor way.

The Psychogenically Stressed Dieter

Regardless of the specific cluster of factors present, the psychogenically stressed dieter is one that is starting with high levels of chronic psychological (or life) stress prior to starting their fat loss diet or exercise program. This means that their cortisol levels are elevated to begin with and that, regardless of the diet or exercise approach that they take, they are likely to show a greater stress response to it overall. I have typically referred to this group of women (and make no mistake, it is also seen in male dieters) as being tightly wound and they are often found in online forums using all capitals with exclamation points about their lack of daily or weekly weight loss (or any loss at all). You can almost "hear" the tension and stress in their typing. In my experience, they are often the ones that are drawn to more extreme dietary or exercise approaches to begin with and this is, more often than not, absolutely the worst approach that they could possibly undertake.

This may include very aggressive diets in terms of the degree of calorie restriction (which may or may not be coupled with a very rigid approach to dieting) along with excessive amounts and/or intensities of exercise, often done with no build up or progression (i.e. they will reduce calories to very low levels immediately while starting a multi-hour per day exercise program). Not only does this often take them below the critical EA threshold immediately (with the hormonal and metabolic effects that implies), it compounds their overall stress levels, elevating cortisol enormously and creating a chronic stress situation on both an energetic and psychological level. This creates a perfect storm of problems.

The Cycle of Chronic Stress and Dieting

Even in the case where a female is not psychogenically stressed prior to beginning the diet, any combination of diet and exercise that causes a chronic stress response to occur is a problem due to the constant elevation of cortisol. Here I am not focusing so much on the metabolic or physiological effects but the fact that chronically elevated cortisol, in addition to many other factors, can cause water retention. In addition to causing the person to look puffy or watery, this can serve to mask true weight or fat loss, especially in the short-term (days or weeks). The diet may be working perfectly well (in the sense that fat loss is occurring) but it is not becoming apparent on the scale or in terms of appearance. This may be coupled with not understanding the difference between weight loss and body composition or unrealistic expectations about the amount or rate of losses. Those who expect the losses to occur linearly may be doubly stressed as fat and weight loss tend to occur in stops and starts to begin with (I'll talk about plateaus and other potential causes in Chapter 26). And there can be two potentially detrimental cycles that occur.

The first is that the dieter assumes that they should intensify their efforts. They reduce calories that much further or increase their activity that much more. Rather than helping the situation, it makes it worse. EA drops even further, more metabolic and hormonal adaptations occur, exhaustion and fatigue reduces NEAT or the dieter may become injured (often working through it). Cortisol rises that much more which causes further water retention. Which causes the dieter to work and stress over the lack of results to that much of a greater degree. More and longer stalls means more restriction which prolongs the stall. Eventually a limit is reached and calories can only be reduced so far and activity increased so far.

Either the dieter attempts to maintain this for extended periods, usually in the absence of good results, or they become injured or crack, abandoning the diet and exercise program completely. Their calorie intake will go up, their activity down (eliminating the low EA) while their mental stress over the lack of results may drop. And as frequently as not, this causes body weight to drop and appearance to improve within a few days as the diet and exercise related stress dissipates, cortisol drops and water is lost. At this point the diet is often resumed but, rather than realize that giving their body a break from the diet was good, they return to the same extreme approach, causing the same cluster of problems to occur again.

The second cycle that can occur is almost the opposite of the first but can cause the same type of issue. This cycle is mainly seen in the extremely rigid or orthorexic eater, the type that can become easily disinhibited. They will submit themselves to extreme restriction and high levels of activity to the greatest degree possible but at any sense of a slip-up they will abandon the diet and go on enormous high-calorie, high-fat food binges. In smaller women, this can be sufficient to offset the dietary restriction during the week, slowing or eliminating fat loss. Even when it doesn't, the frequent guilt and shame about having broken the diet leads to even more extreme degrees of restriction which propagates the same cycle of stress and cortisol elevation with repeated cycles of restriction and disinhibition based binge-eating.

Shockingly, it is often impossible to convince women engaging in either of the types of pathological dieting practices to try a different approach, even in the complete absence of results. Better dieting practices and strategies, that I will present throughout this book fall on deaf ears since they go against how these women think fat loss is best achieved. Some of this ties in with the psychological factors that may be present but at least some of it is due to the fact that successful individuals often do get away with these types of approaches. This may be a situation where these women have a less over-reactive HPA or show better feedback inhibition. While not often talked about, there is also the reality of drug use at the elite level with one effect of anabolic steroids being to reduce cortisol signaling. Regardless of the reason, even if extreme diet and training approaches work for some women, they do not seem to work for the majority. Of more importance, if they are not working for any individual woman, they should be changed.

What the above hopefully points to is not only the need for many, if not most women, to take a different approach to dieting, training and fat loss overall but to find ways to decrease their overall stress. In some cases, full-blown therapy may be required but other stress reduction strategies are also useful. Meditation, massage and yoga are all possibilities here with asana yoga having been found to lower cortisol levels (44a). For some years I have "jokingly" suggested that the chronically stressed woman get drunk, stoned or laid. This might depend on whether or not the sex is satisfying but a hot bath, candles, a glass of wine and some personal time might be the best solution here. Ideally avoiding excessive work, life or relationship stress would be a good thing but this isn't always realistic. In the modern world, it's nearly impossible to avoid all forms of stress but the reality is that chronic stress of either a diet, exercise of psychological nature will eventually takes its toll on the body. If dieters or athletes stress the system too hard for too long, very real problems can occur.

When Chronic Stress Goes Wrong

When stress was first conceptualized, three phases were described which were alarm, resistance and exhaustion. Alarm was the initial stress response, resistance the positive adaptation that occurred if recovery were allowed and exhaustion the state if the stress was unrelenting and the body was not able to adapt. Here I am focusing on the exhaustion stage and want to look at two primary hormonal changes that occur. The first I'll mention only briefly which is an elevation of catecholamine (adrenaline/noradrenaline) levels even in the resting state which causes people to feel generally anxious or overstimulated.

The second and far more important change has to do with the levels of cortisol itself which switch from being chronically elevated to being too low, called hypocortisolism. Normally cortisol shows a peak in the morning (this helps people to wake up) with a decrease over the course of the day. When hypocortisolism develops, this pattern is lost with no morning cortisol increase and lower overall levels the rest of the day. In addition the body loses its ability to increase cortisol levels in response to stress, reducing or eliminating their ability to cope with that stress. Conceptually similar to Addison's disease, sometimes called primary adrenal insufficiency, where no stress response can be mounted, this only reduces someone's ability to respond to stress. This is referred to as secondary adrenal insufficiency.

The Consequences of Hypocortisolism

Hypocortisolism has been found to occur in a number of different situations, all of which share the commonality of being related to or caused by chronically high levels of stress. One of these is burnout, due to work stress, which is characterized by physical exhaustion, depression and chronic inflammation. The risk of autoimmune disease may also increase. Burnout has also been related to an increased risk of heart disease, depression and immune system dysfunction (45). Possibly related to burnout are diseases such as Post-Traumatic Stress Disorder (PTSD), fibromyalgia and chronic fatigue syndrome (CFS), all of which can be related to chronic stress and all of which show markedly similar symptoms of fatigue and exhaustion during the day (46). This fatigue is often coupled with sleep impairment, most likely due to the elevations in catecholamine levels (people are exhausted but overstimulated). This sets up a vicious cycle, difficult to break, where stress leads to poor sleep which leads to an inability to cope with stress.

While not studied in the context of dieting itself, athletes may experience similar types of changes which are referred to as overtraining, the consequence of a long-term imbalance between the training being done and overall recovery (i.e. sufficient food intake, sleep, days off). A chronic stress situation, the earliest stages of this imbalance can cause performance to begin to decrease and here another vicious cycle occurs as athletes begin training harder, worsening the problem. If this continues for extended periods, eventually overtraining will occur, marked by lethargy, a depressed immune system, a lack of motivation to train and mood changes such as depression. Muscles may feel chronically heavy or inflamed and athletes in some sports find it impossible to raise their heart rate or perform and this is a clear indication that the body is no longer able to mount a stress response. The specific cause of overtraining is currently unknown but it is clearly a response to chronic stress and represents a type of adrenal insufficiency (47,48).

At the extremes of true overtraining, athletes may take months to fully recover completely and there are anecdotal reports that some athletes never do. Physique competitors or those who have dieted down to low levels of body fat over report symptoms of joint pain, exhaustion and muscular fatigue not only during their diet but for weeks or months after the competition and diet are over. This is especially true if they use many of the common extreme approaches to dieting. In the aftermath, fatigue, lethargy, depression, chronic inflammation, impaired immune system function and a host of others all occur and this comes along with low morning cortisol, low levels of overall cortisol and a general inability to increase cortisol in response to stress.

Adrenal Fatigue or Adrenal Adaptation?

I expect many readers will recall a diagnosis that was popular years ago called adrenal fatigue. Sometimes called adrenal depletion, the idea was that the adrenal glands become fatigue or exhausted from chronic stress. A variety of mechanisms behind it were proposed, the list of side effects was so vague as to apply to everyone and endless supplements were sold with not a single person ever reporting being cured to my knowledge. This is likely due to the fact that adrenal fatigue, as it was popularly conceptualized, does not exist (49). In no way does the adrenal gland or any other part of the HPA become fatigued in the common sense of the word. The concept of adrenal depletion, that the gland was depleted of compounds needed to produce cortisol was equally incorrect as chemical stimulation of the gland cause cortisol to be produced without issue. This meant that any problems were occurring in other parts of the system.

Specifically changes were found to be occurring in the hormonal receptors in the hypothalamus, pituitary and adrenal gland. At the level of the hypothalamus, the feedback inhibition loop becomes hypersensitive such that even small amounts of cortisol inhibit the release of any more. The pituitary gland may also become resistant to the stimulating effects of the hypothalamus. Both of these lead to reduced cortisol levels both at rest and in response to stress but this does not indicate that any part of the system is either fatigued or depleted. Rather the system has adapted generating what is better conceptualized as adaptive hypocortisolism (50). While these changes clearly have many negative effects, it is still positive in the sense that it is meant to protect the body from the ravages of chronic stress and elevated cortisol (51).

Treating and Preventing Hypocortisolism

Whether or not the reduction in cortisol is seen as a positive adaptation or negative consequence, the fact is that the effects can be profoundly negative for both health and function. This is worsened by the fact that there are at least some indication that the problems are permanent. Perhaps more accurately, I am not aware of any research showing that the effects reverse themselves. As I mentioned above, I'm unaware of anyone ever actually being cured of "adrenal fatigue". Certainly much of what was recommended in this regard such as reducing stress, reducing the amount and intensity of exercise along with ensuring adequate nutrient and a healthy diet was good advice but the situation never seemed to reverse in any meaningful time frame. In the extreme versions of hypocortisolism such as PTSD, fibromyalgia and chronic fatigue, only treatment is available and, so far as I can tell, there's no reason to expect the adaptive hypocortisolism in response to chronic stress to be any different.

The typical first line of treatment is to use synthetic cortisol (i.e. hydrocortisone). The goal here is to raise levels of cortisol to where they should be at specific times of the day to improve energy, mood, etc. This generally requires dosing multiple times per day and determining an optimal intake requires multiple cortisol measurements. Generally 4 or more are taken through the day either by blood or saliva sample. The only non-medication treatment I'm aware of that has been studied is DHEA, one of the adrenal androgens (that I will discuss more in Chapter 24). Another common change in hormone levels is a shift in the ratio of DHEA (the active form) and DHEA-S (the inactive form) and supplementation is aimed at normalizing that ratio. Studies have found that a dose of 25-50 mg of DHEA taken in the morning helps to alleviate at least some of the symptoms of hypocortisolism (52). However, as an androgen, DHEA can also cause many of the side effects seen in women with elevated testosterone such as oily skin, acne, increased body hair, etc. Ideally, testing of DHEA levels should be done so that a proper dose can be determined.

Beyond those two treatments, adaptive hypocortisolism appears to be irreversible and this means that preventing it from occurring in the first place should be the goal. In the most general sense, this means doing one's best to avoid the chronically high stress levels that are so common in the modern world. If possible, this can be combined with other approaches that reduce stress. Within the context of this book, this would mean avoiding pathological dieting practices. This includes extreme calorie deficits unless they are modified in ways I will describe later in the book. Avoiding both excessive amounts of training along with not attempting to perform too much high-intensity training is also important. In all cases, the amount of exercise should be raised gradually to give the body time to adapt. Understanding that weight and fat loss is rarely linear, the limitations of body weight, the potential for water retention to cause short-term plateaus is equally important. If a great deal of psychogenic stress is present, the above becomes even more important. In some situations, therapy may be required.

Even if all of the above is avoided, problems can still begin, especially for the Category 1 dieter going to the extremes of low BF%. Dieters must be on the alert for the first signs of problems. A constant muscular inflammation (the arms and legs may feel "heavy"), a reduction in the motivation to train, a decrease in performance itself, extreme fatigue or low blood pressure upon standing or a constant need to consume caffeine simply to maintain function are all signs that problems may be starting. Certainly there are times when athletes or dieters on a time scale must work through this but often it takes no more than a few days of reduced training with increased calories to reverse the problem. Ignoring the problem, as so many do, simply digs the hole deeper until the system shuts down, possibly permanently. If caught in the earliest stages of development, it is eminently reversible.

Finally, for the majority of women, there are objectively ways to go about the process of dieting and fat loss in terms of how the diet is set up, nutrient intake, specific dietary strategies, the implementation of exercise, etc. These can both avoid the issues above as well as address all of the specific physiological issues I described earlier in this book. Because while there are many issues that women have to contend with, they can be addressed or even fixed. That discussion will start with the next chapter.

Chapter 14: Fixing the Problems

In the previous 13 chapters of this book, I have covered a large amount of information which should make it clear that women's physiologies are distinct from men's in a number of ways related to fat loss, fat gain and altering body composition. While potentially disheartening, I would not have bothered to cover that information or write this book if there were not solutions to these issues. Some of those have already been addressed (i.e. the chapters on body composition should hopefully point out potential pitfalls with focusing on short-term changes in scale weight only) and I won't repeat those here. The specifics of diet set up, nutrient intake, etc. will be covered in detail in later chapters and will not be discussed either.

Rather, in this chapter I want to look at solutions to the major physiological issues. A variety of different topics will be discussed including avoiding excessive fat gain (primarily important for women who are already lean), making gradual versus extreme changes, the Pre-diet phase, moderate versus aggressive dieting approaches, limiting hormonal disruption and enhancing fat loss. Many of my suggestions likely will seem counterintuitive or illogical compared to how women think dieting and fat loss should be approached. However, hopefully at this point it's clear that many of those approaches, whether chosen by or recommended to women, are not only ineffective but potentially damaging. Seemingly illogical or not, these strategies described are meant to take a woman's specific physiology into account and work with it rather than against it, something that must be done for any approach aimed at women (1). Much of the information in this chapter will be aimed primarily at Category 1 women (recall that leaner/normal weight women have far more problems overall) although much of it will apply to all women.

Limiting Excessive Fat Gains

In the most general sense, the ideal way to "fix" the problems that women have in terms of fat loss would be to avoid gaining fat in the first place. This would not only eliminate the need to diet to begin with (except for those women who reduce their body fat to very low levels) but also avoid the problems that come along with fat gain such as increased lower body fat or fat cell number. While theoretically ideal clearly this isn't particularly useful advice to women who have already gained some amount of body fat already. For them this section only becomes particularly relevant after they have first lost fat to begin with.

Primarily here I want to focus on those athletic populations that spend at least some part of their year attempting to gain strength/power or increase their muscle size. Since this is best accomplished by combining proper training with as slight calorie surplus, it's common for at least some amount of fat to be gained. In addition to the many other reasons to avoid fat gain, as those groups usually need to reduce their body fat percentage (BF%) for appearance or performance reasons (or to make a weight class) it's important to avoid excessive fat gains. For those athletes who will eventually need to reduce their body fat to very low levels, keeping BF% at reasonable levels enormously reduces dieting time (discussed in Chapter 25). I'd mention that the above tends to not be terribly relevant for endurance athletes as, outside of injuries, it's rare for them to gain excessive amounts of body fat to begin with and they rarely target large scale gains in weight or muscle for their sport (rowing and swimming are potential exceptions).

For athletes, certainly the risk of excessive fat gain is lessened by the large amount of training that is being done. Exercise, has what is called a partitioning effect, meaning that incoming nutrients tend to be stored within the muscle instead of in fat cells. High intensity exercise such as resistance training or interval training tends to have an even greater impact in this regard as they deplete carbohydrate stored within the muscle itself. The body prioritizes refilling muscular fuel stores before it stores extra calories as fat and this alone helps to avoid excessive fat gain. But this does not make it impossible as a large enough calorie excess can still cause fat gain even large amounts of training is being done.

Even with reasonable surpluses, it's rare to make significant gains in strength, power or muscle mass without some amount of fat gain. The key here is to simply keep the total amount gained limited. This is accomplished by avoiding excessive calorie surpluses or intakes. Muscle mass, strength power and all other aspects of fitness improve relatively slowly and cannot be forced by eating more food. Any excess calorie intake beyond what is required for optimal results simply results an excessive gain in fat which must be lost at some later date (2). While this is true for both women and men, women's lower absolute rates of gain mean that an even smaller surplus in calories will be required. So while a man might be able to gain 2 lbs per month of muscle, a woman will be doing well to gain half of that (a hyperandrogenic PCOS woman might gain slightly more). As I'll show later in the book, one pound of muscle per month requires perhaps 100 calories per day over maintenance. Putting this into perspective, a recent book aimed at women recommended 500 calories per day over maintenance, an intake guaranteed to result in excessive fat gain.

In addition to limiting overall calorie surpluses, I'd remind readers that high-calorie/high-fat meals can cause direct fat storage in the thighs, fat that will be more difficult to lose later on. Whether an athlete or not, avoiding this is important for all women. Certainly this can be difficult in the modern world where many social and life events revolve around not only food in general but those types high-calories/high-fat In that situation where a woman knows that she will likely be eating these types of foods, either the total amount should be limited or offset by slight reductions in food intake the rest of the day. Performing an intense workout that day also helps to ensure that incoming calories are shuttled into muscle rather than fat.

In addition to keeping a relatively tight control over calorie intake, I would recommend that female athletes (especially those who must diet to the middle of my Category 1 or lower for their sport) never allow their BF% to go above 24% (27% via DEXA). At this point, additional body fat gains are more likely to result in lower body fat gain and possibly increased fat cell number, making future dieting efforts more problematic. The exception to this would be women in sports where excess BF% is not a concern and/or there is no need to diet down. This would include superheavy weight powerlifting, Olympic lifting and some of the throwing events. For all other athletes. as soon as BF% has reached the top of my Category 1, body weight should be stabilized before a short diet is performed to reduce BF% to below that level.

The goal here should be to lose only the gained body fat and the combination of proper training and sufficient protein makes this a relatively trivial task. As too low of a BF% makes gaining muscle, strength and power difficult, women should go no lower than 20-22% during this mini-cut. In practice, this means that females trying to gain strength, power or muscle will gradually gain weight (with some fat gain) until they hit 24% body fat, stabilize their weight, diet down briefly to 20-22%, stabilize, gain back up to 24%, etc. Over time, this will allow a gradual increase in performance or muscle mass while avoiding excessive fat gain. It also puts the individual in a good starting place to begin a diet when necessary.

Making Moderate vs. Extreme Changes

In the chapters on menstrual cycle dysfunction and stress, I looked at how both the combination of extreme calorie deficits and/or excessive amounts or intensity of exercise can cause problems in women, especially if they are not gradually built-up to over time. Cortisol levels may skyrocket (and this is worsened in the psychogenically stressed dieter who is so often drawn to the extremes), energy availability (EA) may drop below the critical threshold immediately and hormonal issues can start within as few as 5 days. This leads into a fairly general principle in terms of the overall benefit of making moderate versus extreme changes. This applies to the initiation of the diet, how it is applied and how changes should be made during the diet as fat loss slows (this will be discussed in detail in Chapter 27 rather than here).

Once again, the above primarily applies to the Category 1 and possibly Category 2 dieter while the Category 3 dieter tends to have less overall problems physiologically. However, there can be adherence issues with extreme approaches even in that group. For example, someone coming from a relatively sedentary background who attempts to engage in a large amount of exercise may be too sore, too exhausted or too miserable to continue. At the same time, the Category 3 female with a large amount of fat to lose may find than the results from a more moderate approach are too slow to be rewarding or motivating. A balance between results and adherence must be struck here. The changes here tend to come through diet more than exercise and an extreme approach can be appropriate if implemented correctly.

In that vein, the above is not universal for any Category dieter and there may be places where an extreme/aggressive approach may be appropriate. I will address these later in the book but they tend to revolve around relatively short-term diets where the goal is to lose a maximal amount of fat in a 2-4 week span before moving back to either a more moderate diet or maintenance. For example, the Category 1 female who is in a muscle or strength gaining phase may wish to do a short diet to reduce their BF% before returning to maintenance and then resuming their gaining phase. This tends to be in very specific situations and it only for fairly short-term use. This general principle of making more moderate changes really applies to long-term diets or fat loss programs and, with almost no exception, will starting at an extreme level or making extreme changes be anything but detrimental.

The Pre-Diet Phase

Moving from the fairly general information above to practical application, I want to start by discussing what I will call The Pre-Diet Phase (a similar concept to be used during active dieting will be discussed later in the book). This is a lead-in phase to the formal diet and is structured to allow women to avoid the stresses and physiological shock that can occur when they do too much too soon. The specifics of how the Pre-Diet Phase will be implemented depends on the specific situation and I want to look at each.

The Beginning Exerciser/General Dieter

I'm going to group these two categories together since there tends to be overlap in the groups. Recall that this group can technically consist of women in any of the three categories and this does impact on how the Pre-Diet Phase should be implemented. For those women who are only looking to improve their general health and fitness (and not targeting fat loss), the Pre-Diet Phase is really more of a Pre-Training phase: a period of 4-8 weeks of gradually increasing exercise training should be done here and I cannot overemphasize the word gradual. Doing too much too soon can cause injury and burn-out in all beginners and long-term adherence tends to be superior when a more gradual approach is taken.

If fat loss is the goal, different Categories of dieters will need to take different approaches. Since they don't need to worry about menstrual cycle disruption (and are often limited in the amount of exercise they can realistically perform to begin with), the Category 2/3 dieter can technically begin their diet at the same time as they begin their exercise program. In contrast, the normally cycling Category 1 non-exercising women does have to worry about causing menstrual cycle disruption along with the other problems I've discussed. In this case, a more typical Pre-Diet phase where exercise is gradually brought in (especially resistance training to limit lean body mass loss) with either no change in calorie intake or at most one of the smaller deficits/slower rates of loss I will discuss in Chapter 17 should be done.

The Serious Trainee

The serious trainee is my terminology for someone who is engaged in a large amount of exercise, typically some mixture of weight training, aerobic and/or HIIT work, but who does not compete in any specific activity. Typically their goals tend to revolve around maintaining their current fitness and/or appearance although specific fat loss may be a goal. Since the serious trainee is typically already performing fairly large amounts of aerobic/HIIT work to begin with, a true Pre-Diet phase is rarely needed. At most calories might be brought to maintenance for 1-2 weeks before beginning the diet.

The Physique Athlete

Since it represents a transition from the off-season focus on gaining muscle mass, the Pre-Diet phase can just as easily be described or conceptualized as Post-Off Season phase. It simply acts as a period between the two phases where the focus is shifting from one goal to the other. In old school bodybuilding practices, this was called a hardening phase and it was meant to represent a period of time when the athlete started to tighten up their diet, perhaps adjust their training and start shifting from gaining muscle to losing fat. Regardless of how it is conceptualized, the goal is the same: to act as a transition phase into dieting.

For several reasons, the Pre-Diet phase is arguably the most important for the physique athlete prior to beginning their contest preparation diet. One is that they are (or should) be starting in Category 1 which puts them at the greatest risk for problems to begin with. This is coupled with the need to diet down low to levels of BF% ranging from 10-12% for physique and bodybuilding to perhaps 16-18% for bikini athletes. Finally is the fact that the physique training is unique in that the off-season training generally consists almost exclusively of work in the weight room while the contest diet includes at least some amount of aerobic and/or HIIT work. This combination of factors makes it critical that they introduce that kind of work somewhat gradually to avoid generating a low EA state or overstressing their body. I would mention that this isn't universal and some physique athletes perform aerobic/HIIT work to one degree or another year round. The Pre-Diet phase is still important here but will be implemented slightly differently.

The Pre-Diet Phase will last anywhere from 2-4 weeks for the physique athlete depending on the situation. For those physique athletes who have been performing some amount of aerobic or HIIT work in the off-season, the phase only needs to be 2 weeks as the amount of exercise can be increased somewhat without problem. In contrast, for those physique athletes who have been performing zero aerobic work in their off-season, a minimum of 4 weeks should be used. In the first week, perhaps 3-4 total sessions of low intensity aerobic work lasting 20-30 minutes would be appropriate and this could be increased slightly in the second week. Any HIIT would be introduced in the second or third week of the Pre-Diet phase.

For all physique dieters, calorie intake should be brought down to predicted maintenance levels with any changes to macronutrient intake being made here (specific recommendations will be given in Chapter 19). For the most part this shouldn't have any real impact on body composition although body weight may go down slightly if carbohydrate intake is reduced. The type and amount of weight training may or may not be changed during this phase and I will discuss training for fat loss briefly in Chapters 28 and 29 and in great detail in Volume 2. If any type of metabolic or depletion training (marked by high repetitions and short rest intervals) will be used, it should be brought in gradually over the length of the Pre-Diet phase.

A final consideration for the length of the Pre-Diet phase applies only to the normally cycling woman. As I will discuss in a later chapter, starting a fat loss diet in the follicular phase is generally superior to starting it in the luteal phase. Depending on the exact starting date of the pre-contest diet itself, the Pre-Diet phase can be adjusted in length to ensure that this occurs. For example, an athlete who in the late follicular phase who's pre-contest diet will be starting on day 1 of the next follicular phase would adjust the Pre-Diet phase to be 3 weeks in length so that it ends just as the actual diet is starting.

Other Performance Athletes

Since they are typically already performing a moderate or large amount of total training, a true Pre-Diet Phase is unlikely to be necessary for most performance athletes. Training is typically gradually increased from throughout the year from the start of the season so doing too much activity too soon is generally less of an issue. If calorie intake has been above maintenance prior to beginning the diet, they should be brought to maintenance for at least 1-2 weeks to make the transition. One possible exception to the above is the pure strength/power athlete who is doing little to no aerobic conditioning. If any will be included to facilitate fat loss, it must be brought in gradually and kept at a low intensity to avoid impairing strength and performance. Brisk walking is often the best choice and 20-30 minutes done 3-4 times per week in the first week is more than sufficient. This can be increased gradually to the target level of aerobic activity for the diet but this must be done progressively and slowly.

The Template

I've provided a sample template for the Pre-Diet phase for a beginning exerciser/dieter along with a physique athlete (this would be appropriate for a strength/power athlete as well) in the chart below (other athlete's training is too variable to give meaningful examples). While I have indicated this relative to the normal menstrual cycle, the template will apply to women with any of the hormonal modifiers as well. As I mentioned above, based on their needs, the physique athlete might use a 2-4 week cycle while beginners would use at least 4 weeks and might even double that to 8 weeks to allow for a gradual build-up.

Please note that the days of training are only for illustration and readers can adjust them as needed. Many physique athletes train more than 4 days per week or may prefer to do cardiovascular work on days off while beginners, who are typically doing shorter workouts may want to do both weights and aerobic work in the same workout for time efficiency reasons. Regardless of the goal training schedule, I do recommend at least one day off per week (or at extremely low intensities if exercise must be done) to allow for stress to dissipate. Certainly, Category 1 dieters at the end of an extended diet where 7 days per week of some type of training may be done but that frequency of training should be avoided for as long as possible to avoid overstressing the system.

Day	1	2	3	4	5	6	7	8	9	10	11	12	13	14	15	16	17	18	19	20	21	22	23	24	25	26	27	28
Phase	Early Follicular							Late Follicular							Early Luteal							Late Luteal						
Note	Menses (3-5 days)						Ovulation															PMS (4-7 days)						
Physique Weights	T	T		T	T	T		T	T		T	T	T		T	T		T	T	T		T	T		T	T	T	
Cardiovascular	L		L		L	L		L		L		L	L		L		L		H	L		L		L		H	L	
Diet	M	M	M	M	M	M	M	M	M	M	M	M	M	M	M	M	M	M	M	M	M	M	M	M	M	M	M	M
Beginner Weights	T		(T)		T			T		(T)		T			T		(T)		T			T		(T)		T		
Cardiovascular	L		L		L			L		L		L			L	L		L	L			L	L		L	L		
Diet	M	M	M	M	M	M	M	M	M	M	M	M	M	M	M	M	M	M	M	M	M	M	M	M	M	M	M	M

T=Training, L=Low Intensity, H=HIIT, M=Maintenance Calories

I've indicated 5 total weight training sessions for the physique athlete and this is most likely to be some sort of split routine or body part training. Low intensity aerobic work is performed on four days per week during the first two weeks of the cycle with one session being replaced with a HIIT workout in Weeks 3 and 4. For the beginner, weight training should be performed a minimum of twice per week with a third session, indicated by (T), being optional. Low-intensity aerobic work should be performed a minimum of three times per week and this could be increased to four per week if desired. Diet should be set at maintenance although a small or moderate calorie deficit (see Chapter 17) would be appropriate. As I mentioned above, concepts similar to the Pre-Diet phase will be described later in this book (for example, the Full Diet Break in Chapter 21) with the same basic goal in mind: to provide a transition from one phase of eating and training to another while minimizing the stress that occurs in response to the change.

Moderate versus Aggressive Diet Approaches

In addition to how a diet is initiated, there is the issue of what specific type of approach is followed. Here I am focusing on the size of the calorie deficit that is created through a combination of diet and/or exercise. While I will be defining three difference deficits in Chapter 17, I will only compare a moderate to aggressive deficit in the following section to illustrate the point. The issue is the potential for an aggressive approach to fat loss taking a female dieter below the critical EA threshold immediately at the start of the diet and causing immediate hormonal adaptation (once again this is primarily an issue for the Category 1 female). At the same time, aggressive approaches have the potential to generate faster fat loss and, as mentioned above, may be appropriate if implemented properly or with certain modifications.

To begin to look at this issue, let me first estimate the potential fat losses that might be achieved for moderate versus aggressive diets. In the chart below I've defined moderate and aggressive diets in terms of the weekly goal weight loss (as a percentage of bodyweight) for each category and shown how that translates into theoretical real-world changes. In it I am assuming 100% fat loss and a 3,500 calorie per pound of fat value to calculate the daily deficit required. So for the Category 1 woman at 150 lbs, a moderate fat loss goal is 0.5-0.75% of her current weight of 150 lbs, or 0.75-1.2 lbs/week. Those values were multiplied by 3,500 to get the weekly deficit and divided by 7 to get the average daily deficit.

Category	Moderate	Rate of Loss	Daily Deficit	Aggressive	Rate of Loss	Daily Deficit
1 (150 lbs)	0.5-0.75%	0.75-1.2 lbs/wk	375-600	1%+	1.5 lbs+/wk	750
2 (200 lbs)	1%	2 lbs/wk	1000	1.5%+	3+ lbs/wk	1500
3 (250 lbs)	1.5%	3.75 lbs/wk	~1900	2%+	5 lbs/wk	2500

While the rates of fat loss clearly increase from the moderate to the aggressive deficit, this requires that a very large daily deficit be created. In some cases, the size of the deficit cannot realistically be achieved to begin with but the specifics of the dieter's Category, their training program and goals all interact with whether or not an aggressive approach can even be considered. Let me first look at some of the potential pros and cons of moderate versus aggressive dieting before coming back to examine when an aggressive approach might be most appropriate overall.

Dieting and Fat Loss Efficiency

One potential issue with aggressive dietary approaches is that they may be somewhat less efficient than more moderate approaches in that the amount of real world fat loss occurs may not be in proportion to the extremity of the diet or how much energy is being expended. That is, the fat loss results predicted above are only the calculated values but the changes in metabolic rate that occur will reduce them. And due to the realities of an extreme diet, it's possible that those changes will happen even faster and to a greater degree than would otherwise be expected. Fatigue from low calories may cause NEAT to go down, any exercise being done may suffer in terms of the amount or intensity, etc., reducing calorie expenditure There is also the fact that once the critical EA threshold is crossed, thyroid hormones and metabolic rate may start to decrease within 5 days, slowing fat loss below predicted levels. Earlier studies had actually made this observation finding that there was an optimal calorie level for fat loss above which thyroid hormones were not as impacted (3). I'd note that this can be offset to a great degree with the modifications I will discuss later in the chapter. As well, even if the predicted fat loss rates are not reached, fat loss will still occur more quickly with an aggressive approach and this may allow the diet to end sooner than it otherwise would. This allows calories to be raised and the hormonal adaptations to reverse themselves.

Effects on Performance and Training

Relevant only to athletes or the serious trainee (beginners will make gains from training almost regardless of the diet), is the potential impact of the dietary deficit on exercise performance, recovery and progress. There is little to no doubt that more aggressive approach to fat loss will impact negatively on an athlete's ability to train or recover effectively although some of this can be at least ameliorated by modifications I will describe later in the chapter. Very little direct research in athletes exists on this although a recent study has examined it in detail. In it, highly trained female and male athletes in a variety of sports (all of whom were near the bottom of my Category 2 in terms of BF%) aimed for either a weekly weight loss of 0.7% or 1.4% of current weight with the goal of losing a total of 5% of their starting weight (4). To achieve this, the fast group used a larger daily deficit (30% vs. 20% below maintenance) but ended up reaching their goal roughly twice as quickly as the slower group.

While neither group actually achieved their full weight loss goals, the slow group actually ended up losing more total body fat than the fast group, probably due to dieting for a longer period. This ties in with my efficiency comments above, the fast group had to diet harder but didn't achieve even equal results. While not measured in this study unfortunately, it's likely that the metabolic rate adaptations occurred more quickly and/or to a greater degree in the fast group, decreasing the effective deficit that was in place. The dieters might also have broken their diet more frequently due to hunger. Unfortunately, the study did not divide the results by gender so it's impossible to know if the women's results differed from the men's.

The study made several other important observations of relevance. The first is that the slower fat loss group improved their performance in a number of different sports specific tests while the fast fat loss group did not (presumably due to an inability to recover optimally). Additionally, the women (but not the men) in the slow group gained a small amount of muscle in their upper body. This was due to the women being involved in sports that do not traditionally weight train the upper body and it was lost a year later (5). The study points out that a more moderate dieting approach may allow fitness and performance to improve. At the same time, by reaching their goals faster, the aggressive group might have made similar or better results by being able to return to normal non-dieting training sooner. I will discuss this further below.

Issues Specific To Category 1 Dieters and Extended Diets

As I mentioned above, many of the issues in this chapter are primarily relevant to the Category 1 dieter as they are at the greatest risk for hormonal and other metabolic disruptions. Adding to this is the practical issue that generating the deficits required for an aggressive approach can be much more problematic. The Category 2 or 3 dieter's higher maintenance requirements and food intake often makes larger scale reductions in food intake more realistic. In contrast, the smaller Category 1 female may have to reduce her food intake so enormously that she is left eating almost nothing or have to increase her daily activity to unrealistically high levels. At best, it can be done for relatively short periods of time if at all.

None of which changes the fact that many Category 1 dieters often do try to move directly into fairly aggressive deficits at the outset of trying to lose significant amounts of fat over an extended time period. They might reduce food intake significantly, increase activity significantly or some combination of the two. And in addition to every other problem associated with this in terms of crossing the critical EA threshold and raising cortisol levels, this approach invariably causes major problems later in the diet. As bodyweight and body fat go down and other metabolic adaptations occur, they start to plateau and fat loss slows. But due to the already significant changes that were made early on, they end up having to reduce food intake to extremely low level, increase activity to truly extreme levels or both. In contrast, the dieter who takes an initially moderate approach avoids these problems, or at least avoids them for longer and is able to make smaller, more reasonable adjustments throughout the duration of the diet.

To demonstrate the difference in approaches, I want to consider two women who represent the sample dieter I will use throughout this book. She is starting at 150 lbs and 22% body fat which gives her 117 lbs of LBM and 33 pounds of fat and has a maintenance calorie intake of 2150 calories at the start of her diet. Dieter 1 will use an aggressive approach, creating an initial 800 calorie per day deficit while Dieter 2 will use a more moderate 400 calorie per day deficit. At 150 pounds, unless they use a fairly high intensity of aerobic activity. they will burn about 5 calories/minute during low-intensity aerobic activity. At that intensity level, unless dieter 2 wants to perform more than 60 minutes per day of aerobic activity, she will be limited to a maximum of 300 calories per day from exercise and will have to reduce her food intake by 500 calories to 2150 calories/day. In contrast, the second dieter can easily do half aerobic activity (40 minutes to burn 200 calories) and half from her diet; she is now eating 1950 calories per day. This summary is shown below.

Dieter	1 (Aggressive)	2 (Moderate)
TDEE (calories)	2150	2150
Goal Deficit (cal/day)	800	400
EA (cal/day)	1350	1750
EA (cal/lb LBM)	11.5 cal/lb LBM	15 cal/lb LBM
EA (cal/kg LBM)	25.3 cal/kg LBM	33 cal/kg LBM
Total Aerobics (min)	60	40
Caloric Intake (cal/day)	1650	1950

On top of having a much more difficult overall diet, Dieter 1's EA immediately drops below the critical threshold of 13. 6 cal/lb LBM (30 cal/kg LBM) meaning that some degree of hormonal disruption will occur within 5 days. In contrast, Dieter 2 remains above the threshold at 15 cal/lb LBM (33 cal/kg LBM) and should have no issues in this regards. Certainly Dieter 1 is likely to lose a greater amount of fat during the first month of dieting but she may also be a a slight risk of losing more LBM. As I've mentioned, women lose less LBM than men in general but as body fat percentage goes down, as much as 7% or more of the total weight loss may come from LBM in women (6). Again, the combination of proper resistance training and protein can avoid almost all LBM loss and I will discuss several case studies in Chapter 34 where female physique athletes dieted to the lowest levels of women's BF% with no loss.

Another potential issue here is that Dieter 1 may be at greater risk for breaking her diet as this becomes more common with more extreme dietary deficits (7). It's not uncommon for women to lose less fat trying to diet in a more aggressive way for this reason alone and they find that more moderate approaches are more effective for purely adherence reasons. Once again I'd note that the psychogenically stressed dieter who is following an extreme approach often starts to retain water due to elevated cortisol levels and the lack of apparent results causes them to make their diet even more extreme. To keep this discussion less complicated, I'll assume that neither of these occurs, that the dieter adheres to their diet perfectly and makes no more changes due to cortisol mediated water retention causing an apparent stall.

At some point in the diet, metabolic rate adaptations will occur, reducing the net deficit and rate of fat loss and the dieter will need to make adjustments. To keep things simple, I will assume that neither dieter experiences any muscle loss and both have 117 lbs of LBM. Due to her fat loss and metabolic rate adaptations Dieter 1's TDEE has decreased by 400 calories per day, cutting her daily deficit in half. She wants to resume her previous rate of fat loss and will attempt to increase the deficit back to 800 calories. Unless she wants to perform more than an hour of aerobic activity (and realistically this will burn less than the original 300 calories), the entire change has to come from food intake. This will mean reducing her food intake by 400 calories to 1250 calories. In contrast, let's assume that Dieter 2's deficit has also been cut in half from 400 to 200 calories per day. To resume her original fat loss rate means generating an additional 200 calories per day deficit. To accomplish this she could add 20 minutes per day of aerobic training (bringing her to a total of an hour) to burn roughly 100 extra calories while reducing her food intake by another 100 calories, taking her to 1850 calories/day. This summary appears below.

Dieter	1 (Aggressive)	2 (Moderate)
TDEE (calories)	1750	1950
Goal Deficit (cal/day)	800	400
EA (cal/day)	1350	1750
EA (cal/lb LBM)	8.1	13.2
EA (cal/kg LBM)	17.8	29
Total Aerobics (min)	60	60
Caloric Intake (cal/day)	1250	1850

At 1250 calories per day, Dieter 1 has has reached what are sometimes called poverty macros online, representing an extremely low daily calorie intake that doesn't allow much food to be eaten. On top of being generally miserable, this can drastically increase the chance of breaking the diet simply due to extreme hunger. Increased fatigue is also likely at this calorie level which may reduce energy expenditure further Her EA, which crossed the critical threshold at the beginning of the diet has dropped further to a low 8.1 cal/lb LBM (17.8 cal/lb LBM), ensuring further hormonal disruption. She is likely suffering from some degree of subclinical menstrual cycle disturbance and it is possible that she has already developed amenorrhea. In contrast, Dieter 2 has only now moved up to an hour of activity (and the gradual increase means less stress to the body since she didn't jump straight into an hour per day) and is still eating a fairly large amount of food at 1850 calories. Her hunger should be controllable with a low risk of breaking her diet. As well, Dieter 2's EA has just now barely crossed the critical EA threshold at 13.2 cal/lb LBM (29 cal/kg LBM). This will start to cause hormonal disruption but it has been delayed by a full month.

And it should be fairly clear that the problem will simply confound itself as the diet progresses. Even if Dieter 1 is losing fat at a proportionally faster rate, the level of adaptations occurring will be making that fat loss far less than predicted. More to the point, every time she has to further adjust the diet, her problems increase. By the time her TDEE has fallen by even 200 calories more from the above, she is in an almost impossible situation. If she is still unable to increase her aerobic activity, she will have to reduce her food intake to a low 1050 calories per day. She may or will be increasing her activity but the problems still compound with every further adjustment. It's not uncommon to hear of smaller Category 1 females attempting to diet on 900 calories per day while performing 2 or more hours of aerobic per day and this can often be traced to starting the diet too aggressively for an extended diet (this often occurs when the diet is started too late). Menstrual cycle disruption or amenorrhea is almost guaranteed at this point and, even if the diet is sustained (perhaps survived is the better word), the physiological and psychological damage can be pronounced both during and after. This can include bone mineral density loss during the along with the potential for adaptive hypocortisolism. As often as not, dieters who take this approach break before they reach their goal, often rebounding in their eating and body fat while abandoning exercise.

In contrast, that same 200 calorie reduction in food intake for Dieter 2 still allows 1650 calories per day to be eaten, a stark difference. Certainly later in the diet, Dieter 2 may end up with a relatively low calorie intake possibly combined with high levels of activity (along with hormonal and/or menstrual cycle dysfunction) but this is just a consequence of dieting to the lower limits of BF% and is unavoidable to some degree. More relevant to this discussions is that Dieter 2 avoids these issues for longer by taking a more moderate approach. She will have to start her diet earlier to be able to take such an approach (and I will discuss how to estimate dieting time in Chapter 25) but this is the better approach overall.

When is Aggressive Dieting Appropriate?

As I mentioned above, and despite their apparent drawbacks, aggressive dieting approaches can be appropriate in some situations. One very real situation is in larger Category 2 or 3 dieters with a significant amount of fat loss to lose. Someone carrying 100 pounds of fat for example (i.e. 40% body fat at 250 lbs) is conceivably looking at up to a year or more of dieting at a loss of only 1-2 pounds per week. Certainly fat loss should be looked at as a long-term process but a slow rate of fat loss may be too disheartening for this person to stick with. In this situation, an initial aggressive approach, even if it is only for a short period of time (i.e. 4-6 weeks) to kick off a less aggressive diet may be completely appropriate.

Quite in fact, faster initial rates of weight loss have been shown to predict better, rather than worse, long-term success (8). Some of this may be due to people who lose weight more easily being but it may also be due to such approaches teaching people that they tolerate eating less than they think (some actually report less hunger on very low calories). It's even been suggested that complete fasting may be the "ultimate weight loss approach" and provide both better short- and long-term results (9). The premise is that, by learning that they can eat nothing for short periods of time, dieters may be able to insert the occasional fasting day whenever they feel their weight increasing. Although I would not generally recommend complete fasting in most cases, I will discuss some modified forms of fasting in Chapter 23.

The success of aggressive weight loss diets is predicated on them being set up around whole foods, including exercise and focusing on long-term behavior change. My own **Rapid Fat Loss** diet is based around sufficient protein, vegetables and healthy fats which provides maximal fat loss with all essential nutrients. It is based around eating whole foods meaning that moving to a less aggressive approach simply means adding foods back to the base diet. It also includes exercise (primarily weight training). In contrast, aggressive diets based around pre-made meals or nothing but liquid shakes (or worse yet, the absurd broth or cabbage soup types of diets) fail miserably. They do nothing to reteach long-term eating habits and never include exercise or any focus on long-term changes. Any approach to fat loss, whether moderate or aggressive, must focus on building long-term eating and activity habits to have any chance of succeeding.

Moving to the Category 1 dieter, there are times when an aggressive diet may be appropriate. One is when the dieter only needs to lose a relatively small amount of fat to begin with and wants to lose it as rapidly as possible. This could certainly be a non-athlete or non-training woman who only wants to lose a few pounds but I'll mainly focus on the athlete who needs to reduce their BF% slightly and wants to do it quickly. This could be a physique competitor in a size gaining phase who needs to reduce their body fat slightly between gaining cycles or even a strength/power athlete who needs to keep their body weight or BF % within a certain range for their weight class. Here, an aggressive 2-4 week diet (often called a mini-cut) can be appropriate and allow them to return to training more rapidly than a slower more extended diet. In both situations, training has to be reduced rather significantly and the athlete must accept that no gains will be made. But this may be an acceptable compromise so that the diet can end sooner and normal non-dieting training can resume. Other performance athletes may not find this approach feasible as they may not be able to reduce their training to the degree necessary.

The biggest issue for the Category 1 female when using short aggressive diets has to do with crossing the critical EA threshold and the hormonal and menstrual cycle dysfunction that can occur. As I showed above, this will occur more or less immediately with an extremely aggressive approach although it will still eventually occur with a moderate approach as the diet continues. This is a very real problem but I've mentioned multiple times that such diets can be modified to limit or eliminate the problems associated with it. This modification is a dietary strategy that, while completely counterintuitive to how most conceptualize of dieting, addresses many of the other issues inherent to not only aggressive dieting but dieting per se. That strategy is discussed next.

Limiting and/or Reversing Hormonal and Menstrual Cycle Disruption

I'm not sure it's possible to identify the worst issue facing women in terms of dieting and fat loss but the negative effects that occur when a chronic low EA state is generated is probably close to the top. Crossing the critical threshold itself initiates the myriad adaptations hormonally and metabolically and this can occur in as few as 5-7 days. Maintained for the long-term, this can lead to a reduced metabolic rate, menstrual cycle dysfunction and potentially permanent bone density loss. As I've mentioned, in an ideal world, no woman would cross this threshold to reach her fat loss goal. In reality, whether it's by conscious choice, due to poor dieting practices or using an aggressive deficit, or necessity, due to the realities of dieting to extremely low BF% levels, it is extremely likely to occur. This leads to the solution.

In the discussion of the studies done to date, which recall were short-term, invariably the low EA state was maintained for the length of the study. In the discussions I've presented regarding the topic, I have made the same assumption, that the change to calorie intake or activity which generates the low EA state is made and maintained. Or that any changes to the diet are made to maintain the original deficit which, as above, serves to further lower EA. Of course, in the real world, outside of when dieters break their diet or become disinhibited this is usually what is happening. Once athletes or dieters generate a low EA state, they typically maintain that for the long-term, generating all of the problems that I have described.

But fundamentally there is no reason that this has to be the case. That is, despite how many conceptualize dieting or are instructed to diet, there is no reason that calories cannot vary from day to day or even be brought from below to above the critical EA threshold. Athletes in the physique community have used a similar strategy, typically called calorie or carb cycling, for years and I will discuss these types of patterns in Chapter 23. For now I just want to look at the fundamental strategy and how it has the potential to reverse or at least limit some of the hormonal adaptations to a low EA state.

Because it turns out that the basic "solution" to the problem of a low EA state is to reverse it for some time period. By that, I mean that calories are increased, activity reduced, or both so as to bring EA back above the critical threshold or to (or sometimes above) maintenance levels. In the short-term at least, this can reduce or even reverse the hormonal adaptations that are occurring. While this would seem to primarily be important to those women who are normally cycling, keep in mind that the other hormonal adaptations to thyroid hormone, cortisol, etc. occur in all women who cross the critical EA threshold. This makes it relevant to all Category 1 females (though it may still have benefits in Category 2 and 3). Despite this approach being counterintuitive or even detrimental to the fat loss process, it is not only profoundly effective but critical to avoiding or at least limiting the problems that occur.

This approach has not been studied extensively although a handful of studies do point to its effectiveness. In one, obese women were first dieted aggressively for 4 weeks before having their calories/carbohydrate intake gradually raised for one week. While they were still technically in a dietary deficit, their leptin levels started to increase, indicating hormonal recovery, while fat loss continued (10). In a study of males in the military, recruits were put through a severe multi-stress environment consisting of severe calorie restriction, enormous amounts of activity and sleep deprivation. This generated a tremendous loss of body fat but there were severe hormonal changes including lowered thyroid and IGF-1, a drop in reproductive hormones (testosterone fell to castrate levels) and a dramatic increase in cortisol levels. A single week of raised calories, even in the face of no change in activity caused all of those hormonal changes to reverse themselves (11). While limited, these studies support the idea that relatively long term increases in calorie levels can reverse the hormonal adaptations to dieting/low EA and I will discuss this topic further in Chapter 20. But what about shorter time periods of increased calories?

In animal models, even one large meal can reverse the adaptations to low EA but animals also respond to changes in diet much more rapidly due to their shorter lifespan and faster metabolisms. One meal for a mouse or rat might be the equivalent of a day or more of eating for a human. Regardless, based on this data Ann Loucks, who had first identified the importance of EA and the critical threshold, examined whether a single day of extreme overfeeding could reverse those changes (12). First she exposed women to an extremely low EA for 5 days during which the standard set of hormonal adaptations occurred. The women were then fed 4100 calories (35 cal/lb or 77 cal/kg or roughly double most people's maintenance) over 24 hours. Surprisingly, this had no impact on reversing the adaptations to a low EA. Related to this, a second study made a fairly accidental observation. In it women were first fasted completely for 3 days, coincidentally this generated about the same net calorie deficit as the first 5 day study. Despite the shorter time frame, the same hormonal adaptations all occurred (13). While not actually looking at the topic of refeeding, the women were then brought back to maintenance calories for 2 days. When hormones were re-tested, they had all reversed. LH pulsatility increased to normal, T3 increased, cortisol decreased, etc.

When combined, these two studies suggest that a single day of increased calorie intake following 5 days of low EA cannot reverse the adaptations no matter how many calories are eaten. In contrast, following a similar energetic stress in terms of the total calorie deficit, two days of eating at even maintenance is able to do this. While unstudied to my knowledge, it is possible (and anecdotally this seems to be effective) that a single day of raised calories used more frequently might be able to reverse those adaptations. That is, while one day following 5 days of low EA cannot reverse the adaptations, perhaps one day following 2-3 days of low EA could. Recall from an earlier chapter that there appears to be a delay of 3-4 days between the decrease in leptin levels and when the brain "senses" the change and starts to adapt. If leptin levels were reversed to normal or near normal at the day 3 mark rather than the 5 day mark, this might be able to delay the changes. Even if a single day is not having a major hormonal effect, it has other potential benefits that I will discuss in Chapter 21. I will also provide specific schedule for how to implement this strategy at different stages of a diet later in this book.

Limited data or not, the above hopefully makes it clear that this completely counterintuitive dieting strategy of raising calories to maintenance or above during a diet is absolutely critical to avoiding or at least slowing the adaptations that occur to low EA in terms of hormones or menstrual cycle dysfunction. LH pulsatility can be normalized, T3 goes up and, if nothing else, the increase in calories will reduce cortisol levels. This can not only help to avoid cortisol mediated water retention (many find that their body weight goes down the day after raising calories) but it helps to ensure that a relentless level of chronic stress does not lead to adaptive hypocortisolism in the long run.

Enhancing Fat Loss

In multiple chapters throughout this book, I have looked in some detail at why women both tend to gain fat more easily while losing it with (generally) greater difficulty compared to men. This included the metabolism of nutrients during and after a meal as well as during and after exercise coupled with differences in body composition and a biology that tends to defend against and adapt to fat loss more strongly than men. This inherent biology combines with the dietary and exercise approaches that women tend to be drawn to (or have recommended to them) which only exacerbates the problem. This includes the issues I discussed above in terms of combining extremely aggressive dietary deficits and exercise but this is not where the problems end in many cases.

Specifically women tend to target fat loss with large amounts of aerobic activity, frequently done at a low intensity. If weight training is performed it tends to be done in a terribly ineffective way, using only very light weights and high repetitions. This is combined with a diet containing excessive carbohydrates and often inadequate amounts of dietary protein and/or fat. But these choices combine with a woman's inherent biology to generate suboptimal results. About the only place this isn't seen is in the physique community (who may still use too aggressive of an approach) or strength/power athletes (both of whom combine high protein intakes with proper weight training) which may explain their better results.

As I discussed in Chapter 10, while women's bodies use a larger percentage of fat for fuel during aerobic exercise, a larger proportion of that comes from fat stored within the muscle (Intra-Muscular Triglyceride of IMTG) with relatively little of it coming from body fat to begin with (women also burn less total fat due to burning less total calories even if the percentage of fat burned is higher). Women's bodies also use less glycogen and rely more heavily on blood glucose during exercise. Essentially their bodies spare both body fat and muscle glycogen during certain types of exercise. Additionally, women's bodies shift back to using less fat and more carbohydrate for fuel the rest of the day. While what is burned during exercise would logically have the largest impact on fat loss, it is actually the calories and nutrients used during the other 23 hours of the day that are important. In contrast, men use less fat for fuel during exercise, relying more heavily on stored muscle carbohydrate, while burning more fat the rest of the day. Since it is the other hours of the day that are important, this contribute to men's generally greater loss of fat.

It is a general truism that the the body in general and muscle in specific burns the fuel for energy that is present in the largest quantities (it's slightly more complicated than this but I don't want to get into the details). A muscle that is full of carbohydrate tends to use more carbohydrate for fuel (a muscle full of IMTG will use IMTG for fuel) which means that less fat is used for energy. This works in reverse, if muscle glycogen and/or IMTG is depleted with intense exercise (and/or dietary changes), both lean and obese individuals will shift to using more fat for fuel at all times (14,15). For years, I have recommended the combination of diet and specific exercise to deplete muscle glycogen/IMTG and generate this effect.

This fact explains part of the gender difference in nutrient metabolism following aerobic exercise. Men, by depleting their muscle glycogen more effectively during exercise use more fat for fuel the rest of the day while women, who deplete their muscle glycogen less effectively do not. Supporting this idea, a recent study found that men who performed aerobic exercise after eating a meal used more carbohydrate during exercise, depleted their muscle glycogen levels to a greater degree and used even more fat for fuel the rest of the day compared to men who performed the aerobic work fasted (16). It's questionable if this will work for women since they tend to rely on blood glucose more than muscle glycogen to begin with and I'm not sure if eating would cause muscle glycogen to be used to a greater degree. It's also been shown recently that women (of varying BF%) lose the same amount of body fat whether they perform aerobic exercise faster or after having eaten (17).

But I think the above explains two major observations that have been made. The first is why women who only perform low intensity aerobic activity (often combined with poor dietary choices) often have disappointing fat loss results. Despite using relatively more fat for fuel, they are using less fat at all other times points of the day. This is in addition to all of the other problems that can occur when women perform excessive exercise in terms of a low EA state, hormonal and metabolic adaptations, etc. The second observation is that when women replace at least some of their endless low-intensity aerobic activity with some amount of High-Intensity Interval Training (HIIT) or properly done weight training, the impact is often enormous in terms of their ability to lose body fat and improve their body composition. I want to look at why as this leads to a way to enhance women's use of body fat for fuel.

HIIT

In Chapter 4 I described High-Intensity Interval Training (HIIT or simply interval training), referring to a type of workout alternating time periods (typically 30-90 seconds) at near maximal intensity with time periods of roughly the same duration of low-intensity exercise. While traditionally used by athletes, HIIT became popular when some research suggested that the fat loss might be greater compared to traditional aerobic activity. There was also a great deal of interest in HIIT for improving general fitness as it was often more time efficient than traditional aerobic exercise while generating similar or the same results.

While the overall effects on fat loss were greatly overstated, there is no doubt that many women found that adding at least some to their training drastically improved their body composition and fat loss and I think that there are several reasons for this. One is that women appear to get a more potent muscle building stimulus from HIIT compared to men (18). HIIT may also increase the amounts of the calorie burning beige/brown fat that I described in Chapter 5 (19). The hormonal response may also play a role here. HIIT raises Growth Hormone (GH) levels, which helps to mobilize fat, to a greater degree in women than men (20). Levels of ANP, the hormone that may sidestep the normal problems with stubborn fat mobilization, go up to a greater degree in women than men as well (21). HIIT causes a larger increase in adrenaline and noradrenaline compared to low-intensity aerobic activity and this has been shown to cause greater lower body fat loss (21a). I wrote about this years ago in my original Stubborn Fat Solution and two of the protocols utilized HIIT for this reason. Women using these protocols reported enormous improvement in their ability to lose lower body fat and I have reproduced them in Appendix 1 of this book.

Of as much importance within the context of this chapter is that HIIT, like most high-intensity exercise, is fueled primarily by carbohydrate and specifically muscle glycogen (IMTG may also contribute during the rest interval). Even here there is a gender difference: in response to one 30 second sprint, for example, women deplete less glycogen in Type I/slow-twitch but equal amounts in Type II/fast twitch muscle fibers (22). There are a number of reasons for this that I will detail in Volume 2 but it has been shown repeatedly that women generate less fatigue and recover more quickly than men in response to certain types of exercise (23). Practically this means that optimizing HIIT for women's fat loss goals will require slightly longer intervals of 45-60 seconds while using shorter rest intervals of 45-60 seconds than men. Women may also benefit from doing slightly more total intervals than men to ensure the same degree of glycogen depletion, enhancing the use of fat for fuel for the remainder of the day.

I want to make it clear the above is in no way meant to suggest that women should replace all of their traditional aerobic activity with HIIT. Many misguided dieters attempted this within the context of a low-calorie diet and other training and it exhausted them and I will discuss this in more detail in Chapter 27 and 28. Rather, it is meant to point out that replacing at least some of a woman's traditional low- or moderate-intensity training with HIIT can have profoundly beneficial effects on fat loss.

Weight Training

While HIIT alone can have potential benefits for women's fat loss efforts and body composition changes, perhaps nothing is as singularly effective as properly performed weight training. By properly here I mean using weights that are challenging to lift and which will actually have benefits in terms of increasing strength or muscle size. An additional, and equally important benefit, is the effect such training has on bone mineral density, either to stimulate it's gain or prevent it's loss. What is defined as challenging will depend on the trainee and the specific type of training being done and I will discuss the specifics of this somewhat in Chapter 27 and in far more detail in Volume 2. This type of proper weight training is in contrast to the type of training that many women do (or are recommended to do) which is to use very light weights, often for a very large number of repetitions. This is typically done to "tone" or for fear of "becoming bulky". As I previously discussed, being "toned" is a function of building some amount of muscle mass and losing fat while becoming muscularly bulky is simply not a fear for most women due to their lower levels of testosterone. At most, the PCOS woman with hyperandrogenism or subclinically hyperandrogenic woman may build muscle slightly more quickly but even this is only in a relative sense.

Invariably when a woman who is only performing enormous amounts of aerobic exercise introduces this type of lifting, or switches from the fairly common ineffective types of training to this type of training, the effects are almost magical. Shape and appearance improve drastically, fat loss frequently occurs and/or becomes easier and this is true even if much less aerobic exercise than previously is being done. Done properly, no single type of exercise has as large of an impact on a woman's health, bone density, body composition or appearance. And I think that there are a number of reasons, some indirect and some direct, that weight training has this effect.

Indirectly, women who start to engage in more productive forms of weight training often stop performing excessive aerobic activity. Some women eliminate it completely although I think this is a bit of a shift to an opposite extreme in many cases. Regardless, even reducing cardio from the often excessive levels seen has a number of positive benefits in its own right. One is that it may allow a woman who has also reduced her calorie intake by too much to go above the critical EA threshold. Contradictorily this may allow her hormonal status to improve and allow some of the metabolic rate adaptations to dissipate. Due to less overall fatigue, she might also find that her NEAT increases and this may potentially add up to an increased energy expenditure despite doing less activity. Anecdotally, many women report being able to eat more calories while doing less activity, while still staying lean or even losing body fat, when they cut out excessive aerobic activity. Additionally, the often chronically elevated cortisol levels will be allowed to drop which has more positive effects. Certainly weight training can raise cortisol but, overall, it seems to have less of an impact here than aerobic exercise.

More directly, there are other potential benefits to weight training although one of the most commonly made claims is likely not one of them. That is the supposed increase in resting metabolic rate that occurs with weight training, a topic I discussed in some detail in Chapter 7. Short of extreme changes in muscle mass, which can take years, the impact is simply minuscule over most realistic time frames. Even the average weight training workout doesn't burn a tremendous number of calories although the major effect of trying to build muscle will come from here. Over time it adds up but the numbers aren't huge.

Given that hormonal response to weight training is fairly short-lived and even the calorie burning effect is small, I suspect that there is another primary reason why weight training has the impact on fat loss and body composition that it does. Like HIIT, the high-intensity nature of proper weight training means that muscle glycogen is the primary fuel. In men at least, multiple sets of weight training deplete both muscle glycogen and IMTG although it takes a fairly large number of sets to have a major effect (24). There's no reason to think that this won't occur in women as well although one odd study suggested that women did not deplete glycogen to the same degree as men (25). However it used three sets of 50 repetitions (more like an endurance test) with a 10' rest which allows for too much recovery and isn't representative of the types of weight training I am describing (26). Studies using more typical resistance training workouts clearly show that, unlike aerobic training, women use more fat for fuel following resistance training workouts, suggesting greater glycogen depletion during the workout (27,28).

Hormonally, weight training does have an effect at least similar to HIIT in that it mobilizes fat from fat cells and high-intensity weight training has been shown to have similar benefits in terms of lower body fat loss (29). I'd note that fat cannot actually be used to fuel weight training and it is most likely used to provide energy during the recovery between sets or after the workout. This hormonal response does depend on the type of weight training being done with relatively higher repetitions (15-20 per set) and shorter rest intervals having a larger impact than lower repetitions and longer rest intervals. In this sense it is not dissimilar from HIIT although, unlike HIIT, weight training can be used to target all muscles in the body (most traditional ways of performing HIIT work only the legs).

The Impact of Diet

Regardless of the exact mechanism, the fact of the matter is that women who decrease their often excessive amount of aerobic activity or replace the often ineffective types of weight training they are doing with more intense and effective types of training, their body composition tends to improve drastically. While purely anecdotal, women can be found online who talk about having spent a year or more doing the cardio grind (i.e. hours of aerobic training per week) who switch to proper weight training and who have an almost overnight transformation, experiencing all of the effects I described above. And while much of this is due to the effects of the training (or changes in training) I think there is another potential factor which has to do with diet and how it interacts with both a woman's biology and her exercise program.

For reasons ranging from biological preference (recall that women tend to prefer carbohydrates and fats) to simply misleading information or misguided ideas about the optimal diet, it's not uncommon to see women eating excessive carbohydrates while attempting to reduce protein and dietary fat to extremely low levels. Not only is this unhealthy in many ways, it combines with the traditional low-intensity aerobic heavy fat loss approach to cause more problems. The exercise itself is burning very little fat to begin with along with not depleting muscle glycogen effectively. Combined with a chronically elevated carbohydrate intake, muscle glycogen remains high and women's bodies end up burning carbohydrates for the majority of the day.

Invariably when women start to incorporate higher intensity exercise, and this is especially true for weight training, large scale changes to the diet are often made (this is due to the general dietary beliefs present in the weight training subculture). Protein and dietary fat intake are often increased with a moderation or reduction in total carbohydrate intake. That change alone has been shown to increase the use of fat for fuel after a meal (30,31). But it also interacts with the change in training that is occurring simultaneously. By depleting muscle glycogen with either HIIT or proper weight training and not refilling it with excessive carbohydrate intake, a woman's overall metabolism shifts to using proportionally more fat for fuel at all times of the day. As much as I find the phrase trite and often misused or misleading, to put it in the common parlance, a woman becomes a "fat burning machine".

Before starting the discussion of diet and dieting itself, I want to make the final comment that I think the above explains at least part of the gender difference that is sometimes seen in fat loss. For both biological and cultural reasons, men often prefer protein and dietary fat over carbohydrates (men love low-carb diets since they get to eat meat and fat at every meal) along with being drawn to weight training when they want to "get in shape". Essentially, men tend to inherently pick the combination of diet and activity that is often superior for fat loss overall. In contrast, women tend to overemphasize carbohydrates, again for both biological and cultural reasons, and tend towards excessive aerobic activity which often ends up limiting their overall fat loss.

In reversing that, performing more high-intensity activity (especially weight training) along with moderating their carbohydrate intake, women's bodies shift at least partially to a metabolism that is more like men's in terms of what fuel is being used during the day. As it is the rest of the day that has the largest impact on total fuel use (i.e. the total amount of fat burned) this helps women to lose fat more effectively overall. Physique athletes have always used a combination of resistance training and increased protein intakes (often with reduced carbohydrate intakes) and I think it is no coincidence that they have traditionally had some of the best success with altering body composition overall.

Chapter 15: Introduction to Dieting

Having detailed the basic problems that women face in terms of both gaining and losing fat, along with a number of general fixes, I will spend the remainder of the book looking at the myriad issues that go into setting up what I consider to be an optimal diet or nutrition program. This includes a large number of topics including determining goal calorie intakes, the nutrient composition (both in terms of amounts and food choices) of the diet, around workout nutrition, meal frequency and patterning and many others. These recommendations are likely to differ from some fairly official recommendations that have been made but most of those are either years out of date or were never meant to apply to dieters or athletes to begin with. In contrast, I will be basing my recommendations on the most current research along with including information from studies done explicitly in dieting or athletic populations.

These recommendations will also likely run counter to much of what women choose (or are recommended) to do but the reality is that much of this is either ineffective or outright damaging in terms of menstrual cycle dysfunction, bone health, iron or thyroid status. That is in addition to the tremendous amount of information, especially for athletes, that was developed or researched on men. As I've noted and will continue to reiterate, while many of the generalities may hold, the specifics frequently do not as women face issues and have concerns that men never will. Before looking into those issues in detail in the next chapters I want to examine some basic concepts first. Since it is the more common goal, it applies mostly to general eating or dieting per se although much of it also applies to other goals such as athletes seeking to gain muscle or improve athletic performance.

Different Needs for Different Goals

While many eating or diet plans take a one size fits all approach, this is flawed. The type of approach taken must interact with a woman's overall goals and needs and this is why I discussed them in some detail in Chapter 4. In the most general, sense, as a woman's goals become more extreme, so will her need to pay attention to details. For example, the Category 3 female may need nothing more than a basic exercise program along with some minor changes to her overall dietary patterns to improve her health. If her goal is explicit fat loss, she may need to pay somewhat more attention but small changes will tend to generate large results in this situation. At a slightly greater extreme, the serious exerciser looking to change her overall body composition significantly will have to pay much more attention to her overall training program and diet. Finally, the Category 1 female trying to diet to the lowest limits of female body fat percentage (BF%) without muscle loss, performance loss or enormous health consequences will have to pay meticulous attention to every aspect of her training and diet. She has the additional factor of trying to balance creating a calorie deficit to generate fat loss while adequately supporting her training and achieving both of these simultaneously is often impossible due to her relatively lowered calorie intake.

I bring this up as the following chapters will be presenting a fairly large information some of which can be fairly complex. Estimations of calorie requirements can get fairly complicated and many of the calculations of nutrient intake require body composition measurement to determine how much lean body mass (LBM) a woman has for example. Once issues of meal patterning and frequency, around workout nutrition, etc. are added in there can be a tremendous amount of information to process and implement. And in many cases it is either not necessary or may be detrimental in that it overwhelms someone trying to make basic changes by giving them far too much to worry about (which can create stress in its own right). And while some people do seem to do better, regardless of goal, with approaches filled with details, I am of the general opinion that they should be avoided until they are necessary. For those women who want to avoid the details until needed, it may be better to use one of the many popular diets already in existence to get started (or simply make some basic changes from my recommendations) and I want to look at this first.

The Pros and Cons of Popular Diets

Although it's common to criticize or dismiss all commercial approaches to dieting (and certainly many are atrocious), I think it's better to look at their potential pros and cons, strengths and limitations. Certainly most of these diets do take a fairly one sized fits all approach to diet. At the same time, since they tend to be aimed at a fairly narrow population, the generally overweight individual, this isn't an enormous problem in and of itself. Clearly they aren't set up to support the serious trainee or athletes but I have seen very few of those types of diets claiming that they are meant for those populations anymore than books aimed at athletes claim to be aimed at the general dieter.

Looking at pros and cons in specific, on the one hand, diets with relatively simple rules about food intake often generate better adherence and work as well if not better than more complex approaches, especially in the early stages of behavior change (1).   These tend to revolve around what can or cannot be eaten or, more recently, when foods can be eaten and are all geared towards getting someone to eat less without realizing it. Given the number of choices that we are faced with on a day-to-day basis, these types of diets remove the need to make yet one more choice in the day regarding food intake and this can reduce the psychological stress inherent to dieting. I would note in this regard that even athletic dieters often reach a place where their meals are relatively standardized in terms of what they contain and this is fundamentally similar in that they don't have to make numerous choices throughout the day.

This assumes that the specific dietary approach meets certain nutritional requirements to begin with. Many commonly made nutritional recommendations that are made, both in terms of overall diet structure and food choices can drastically impact on a woman's overall health along with her menstrual cycle, often in a very negative way.   Contradictorily, many diets that are often held up as healthy frequently are not. In the worst case they may be actively detrimental to a woman's health. Recall for example that vegetarian dietary patterns may be associated with menstrual cycle dysfunction in their own right under certain conditions. Any commercial diet chosen should at least meet the general guidelines for nutrient and food intake that I will present in the following chapters.

If there is a major con to many popular dietary approaches it is that they often exist as nothing more than short-term diets. They usually do little more than cycle water weight off the body while doing nothing to improve actual body composition or generating any long-term behavior changes that can possibly be maintained in the long-term. These are the classic "fad" diets and there are endless versions of them. Juice fasts, all soup diets, only eating a single food every day, a popular fad diet decades ago was based around grapefruit and coffee. There are no shortages of this and any minor finding in obesity research that might be beneficial will rapidly be turned into a quick-fix diet of one sort or another.

Endless versions of these can be found in the types of magazines found at the grocery store checkout counter or online. They all make absurd and impossible promises that never occur to begin with and wouldn't be sustainable if they were. Claims that some specific food will ramp up thyroid metabolism or that avoiding some food will do the same by releasing toxins from fat cells can be found weekly. The same types of media frequently provide equally poor advice about exercise.   Claims that nothing more than walking can melt off the pounds or that lifting weights in some specific way will cause spot reduction in women's lower bodies, etc. I imagine most readers of this book have seen this type of information and many have probably tried them at one time or another. The types of dietary or health advice given by celebrity trainers and television shows is usually just as awful. With so few exceptions, the information provided doesn't work, has never worked and can't possibly work. Which isn't to say that all commercial or popular diet and exercise advice is inherently terrible. Just most of it. Other approaches and sources of information do exist that, at least sometimes, provides a decent approach to weight and fat loss and I want to look at a few of them. Once again I'd primarily suggest that any reader considering one of the following approaches compare it at least generally to my recommendations in the next chapters; so long as it is close to my recommendations, it should be sufficient.

Fitness Magazines

For decades now, there have been speciality fitness magazines that provide information on both exercise and diet/fat loss. With the growth of the Internet there are even more that exist only digitally. Certainly some of the information presented in this type of media can be quite good but an equal amount of is terrible. Much of the dietary advice is either based on males and even the female oriented information is often based on extremely rigid/orthorexic approaches to eating (i.e. clean eating). Many fitness magazines double as outlets to sell endless dietary supplements, most of which are garbage (Supplements are discussed in Chapter 24). I can't comment specifically on any individual magazine or source and once again will recommend readers compare any advice or program being given against the information in this book. So long as it is close to my recommendations in terms of either the dietary or exercise advice, it will be fine even if some minor details differ.

Commercial Diet Programs

For decades, there have been numerous commercial diet programs available with their quality varying enormously from absolutely terrible to fairly good. Perhaps surprisingly, so called medical quick weight loss clinics are often some of the worst approaches imaginable.   They typically use extremely low calorie diets, which is not a problem in and of itself, which are based around nothing but liquid shakes, which does nothing to retrain long-term eating habits. Usually they sell the liquid products being used. Most of these programs seem to advocate against exercise and I strongly feel that this is done to allow more LBM loss which generates faster total weight loss. Some use other approaches, either injections of ineffective drugs (i.e. the HCG diet) or require the purchase of expensive supplements. Other commercial diet programs are similar if not as extreme. One popular program in the US (which I will not name) uses a low-calorie diet that is solely built around their own pre-packaged (and often expensive) foods. While this may be excellent for control and convenience, it does nothing to retrain long-term eating habits. As soon as the person abandons the program or doesn't want to pay for the foods, they have no way to sustain the dietary changes.

In contrast, there are programs that are quite good and avoid many of the pitfalls listed above. In the US, Weight Watchers is one of the better programs in my opinion. They seem to keep up with changing research and improve their overall program with new developments in the field of obesity treatment. They provide generally good dietary advice including at least semi-individualized dietary approaches as well. As importantly, weekly meetings provide a community for social support (which ties into many women's psychological needs), accountability with weekly weigh ins (though this could be an issue for women with major body weight swings due to the menstrual cycle) along with other factors that have been found to improve both short- and long-term results. Perhaps most importantly, while they offer prepackaged foods for convenience, the system works with whole foods as well and this gives the potential for dieters to make long-term changes to their actual dietary intake by learning how to eat to adhere to the program.

In the most general sense, any commercial weight loss program should be based around primarily whole foods rather than meal replacements or pre-packaged foods. Certainly some types of meal-replacement products can be beneficial if used in moderation (this is discussed in Chapter 20) but they must be combined with a change in long-term eating habits. If they are used, it should be in addition to rather than in place of other dietary changes. There should be an exercise component included and approaches to long-term behavior change must be part and parcel of the program. Any commercial program lacking those components should be avoided as they have little to no chance of generating long-term results.

Popular Diet Books

Finally, let me look at popular diet books. Thousands have been published over the decades and while some of them are good, the grand majority of them are patently absurd (perhaps my favorite was one arguing that cold drinks were the cause of obesity). Historically, most have ignored any distinction between body weight and body fat (or even addressed body composition at all) although this is changing in recent years. In many cases, this is probably deliberate as rapid water weight losses in the first few days of many types of diets (especially carbohydrate restricted diets) make it look as if the diet has some metabolic advantage or is working more effectively than it is.

These types of books, even the good ones, are generally written in the same fashion and some of the messages they give can lead dieters down a dangerous path. They usually start out by saying that calories don't matter, that calorie restricted diets don't work in the long term before proceeding to demonize some single nutrient as the cause of obesity (in rarer cases the lack of a certain nutrient may be blamed). This could be dietary fat, sugar or carbohydrates in general. In recent years, High-Fructose Corn Syrup (HFCS) has been blamed as the cause of obesity. The book will argue that by removing the nutrient, weight/fat loss will occur easily without hunger or calorie restriction. A hundred of more pages will be devoted to selling this concept to the reader, interspersed with endless success stories (failures are never mentioned). Food lists and recipes round out the book.

What books like this cleverly leave out is that the nutrient they are demonizing invariably contributes a large number of calories to the body in the first place. And that by removing that food, calorie intake is always automatically decreased. Dietary fat is very calorie dense (9 calories per gram) and when people reduce their fat intake, they generally eat fewer calories. Sugar is similar, providing a large number of calories without being terribly filling and people who remove sugar from their diet almost can't help but eat less. Since carbohydrates typically make up 60% of the day's calories, any diet that removes them makes it nearly impossible not to eat less. Other dietary approaches such as clean eating or paleo type dietary patterns revolve around removing highly processed foods; since those foods invariably contain a lot of calories, people end up eating less. A current trend with these types of diets is to increase protein or fiber intake, both of which tend to increase fullness and cause people to automatically eat less and this is an approach I wholeheartedly endorse. Regardless of the specific approach, all these diet books are doing is convincing the reader that they don't have to restrict calorie intake before tricking them into doing it.

Certainly, it's an effective trick and getting people to eat less without feeling as if they are dieting is in no way a bad thing. It tends to remove a lot of the inherent psychological stress that is inherent to dieting and feeling as if someone has to "eat less" (most of these diet books tell dieters that they can eat as much as they want of the allowed foods) and that's hard to argue against. As well, these types of approaches provide what are called "bright line boundaries" in drug and alcohol addiction research. This is a boundary that simply can't be crossed (i.e. an alcoholic will set up a bright line boundary and not enter a bar) by the dieter and eliminates them having to make a choice or even consider the temptation. If a specific food, especially if it is one that is easily overeaten, is completely off limits, adherence may be better.

While the above approach can be enormously beneficial in the short term, there are a number of problems that tend to crop up in the longer term. One has to do with food cravings and the general fact that dieters tend to crave the foods that are made off limits. In one telling study, women were placed on identical low-calorie diets one of which allowed bread to be eaten and the other did not (2). The women who were allowed to eat bread showed better compliance to the dietary recommendations along with showing a much lower drop out rate from the diet (6% vs. 21% dropout rate). While this doesn't mean that short-term elimination of problem foods can't be useful, it does point to the fact that, in the long-term, such approaches may be more likely to fail. Women who are normally cycling have the added potential issue of food cravings during the luteal phase of the cycle which could cause problems if those craved foods are off-limits in the current diet. There are solutions to this issue, ways to include most if not all foods on a diet while still adhering to it in the long term and I will discuss this more below and in later chapters.

However, there is another potentially larger problem that this type of dietary approach (really the way that the diet books present them) generates and that has to do with changes in food intake over time. Certainly most diets of this type cause people to eat less initially and lose weight and fat. But this doesn't last forever for a number of reasons and eventually weight/fat losses slow or stop. The first are the metabolic adaptations that occur in response to dieting and fat loss that I detailed in Chapter 9. Energy expenditure is decreasing while hunger and appetite are increasing and food intake often goes up. This is especially true when the diet book has told them to eat as much as they wish of the allowed foods.

Compounding this is the fact that, any time a given diet becomes popular, companies will rush concentrated, high-calorie versions of the diet approved foods to market. In the 80's, when low-fat diets were the craze, there were endless low- or non-fat foods that had just as many calories as the foods people had been eating before. In some cases, the low-fat version managed to have more calories than the full-fat version. Currently there are low-carbohydrate approved diet bars and snacks (at one point there were low-carb jelly beans and cookies) that have just as many calories, and often more fat, than normal versions of the food. The same holds true for the paleo diet and highly processed paleo food bars are available which provide a tremendous number of calories in a small package. As often as not, these products are actually nutritionally inferior to other foods that don't fit the structure of the diet in the first place. They may be as high if not higher in calories while having poorer macronutrient ratios.

The above two factors come together with the primary message of most diet books which is that calories don't matter and calorie restriction isn't necessary. People fall into an easy trap of thinking that diet-approved foods can be eaten without limit. Quite in fact, people frequently justify eating more of the diet approved foods. In the 80's, it was found that dieters allowed themselves to eat more of a yogurt that they thought was non-fat compared to the higher-fat version. Low-carb dieters often deliberately add huge amounts of dietary fat to their meals and paleo dieters will eat handful after handful of paleo-approved foods such as calorie dense nuts. And these three factors, the combination of metabolic adaptation with high calorie "diet-approved food" and a mindset that calories don't matter come together to derail the diet. Calorie intake is increasing while energy expenditure is decreasing and progress grinds to a halt.

And this leads to the single largest problem with the message that these types of diet approaches send. Having been told from the outset that calories don't count or need to be restricted so long as the rules are followed, dieters will steadfastly refuse to accept that the reason they are no longer losing weight or fat is due to their calorie intake being too high or that it needs to be reduced or even monitored. Any online diet support forum will have endless threads and discussions where people are looking for every possible reason they are no longer losing except for the one that actually matters: total calorie intake.

Ultimately, these diets can be very beneficial but only so long as their limitations and realities are accepted. While they may work stunningly in the early stages, as fat loss slows, the dieter will have to pay more attention to the overall details of their diet, possibly moving to a more calculated or monitored diet. Before looking at that in the next chapter, I want to look in detail at a topic I have brought up several times in this book which has to do with dietary restraint, disinhibition and rigid vs. flexible dieting attitudes.

Restraint, Disinhibition and Dieting Attitudes

When I talked about stress, I mentioned the concepts of restraint and disinhibition and want to briefly address them again here. Dietary restraint generally describes a concern with overall food intake and may also include deliberately restricting food intake to either generate fat loss or avoid fat gain/regain after a diet. A fairly large body of research has identified potential negatives of having high dietary restraint and I mentioned many of those in Chapter 13. At the same time, in the modern environment, the reality is that a majority of people have to exert at least some degree of restraint over their food intake to avoid gaining weight. As well, losing weight and fat will always require some degree of dietary restraint. This is a problem as restraint is often coupled with disinhibition, the loss of control over food intake in response to various types of stress. This can often set up a cycle alternating between high degrees of restriction/restraint and disinhibition that causes weight gain or diet failure.

However, this situation isn't universal with researchers having identified a subgroup of people who show high degrees of dietary restraint without falling prey to disinhibition. They also show both greater short-term and long-term success in their fat loss goals. This has led researchers to differentiate between those individuals with flexible restraint and rigid restraint with the former representing those people who do not become disinhibited (3). This distinction has led to the concept of rigid and flexible eating attitudes. The distinction between the two is critical as rigid restraint (or rigid approaches to dieting) represent one of the single most damaging approaches to fat loss that can be present. I will provide some specific flexible eating strategies in Chapter 21 and only want to examine the concepts in general here.

Rigid Eating Attitudes

In the most general sense rigid eating attitudes are characterized by a very black and white, good and bad, almost moral approach to eating. People with rigid eating attitudes (or rigid restraint) take an all or nothing approach to their diet where it is seen as either perfect or broken. One way that the rigid eater perceives their diet as broken is if they have eaten even slightly over their predetermined goal for the day. If the day's goal calorie intake is 1600 calories and the rigid eater goes over that to any degree, the day is seen as a failure. In other cases, the rigid eater may have a set of food "rules" that they are attempting to follow. These rules tend to revolve around what foods are or aren't healthy or clean or, at a fundamental level, morally good to eat. Eating the smallest amount of a disallowed foods mean that the diet is ruined.

In both cases, what ultimately represents a fairly irrelevant deviation from the day's diet in the big scheme may turn into an enormous problem as the eater becomes disinhibited and overeats a tremendous number of calories. The dieter who ate 200 calories over their day's goal or a small amount of a disallowed food has done no real harm to their diet or fat loss goals. If their rigid eating attitudes now cause them to eat hundreds or thousands of calories due to disinhibition, they now have. It is relatively trivial to find stories of Category 1 dieters (usually in the physique community) who are attempting to eat perfectly clean and who, after consuming the smallest amount of an unclean food, go on day-long binges. If the diet is not abandoned completely, the dieter often attempts to be even more rigidly restrained following the binge, maintaining or even worsening the cycle.

I've mentioned that women are more likely to show dietary restraint in general and if that restraint is rigid, they might potentially have even larger problems than men. Due to the pressures towards thinness and appearance, dieting often becomes part of a woman's identity (4). Combined with rigid eating attitudes, this may lead to a linkage between their eating patterns and sense of self-worth (this is common among rigid eaters and in orthorexia especially). Eating good foods or adhering to their diet makes them a good person and vice versa with dieting failures becoming synonymous with personal failure. While not studied to my knowledge, this is likely to be even more true if other psychological traits such as perfectionism are present. The perfectionist can never be satisfied with their achievements. If they are reached, they will be redefined as having been too low; if they are not, they will try that much harder.

While it would seem that rigid eating attitudes might generate better overall results, the opposite turns out to be true. Individuals with rigid dietary eating attitudes tend to be heavier, exhibit more mental stress about their diets and are more prone to food binges (5). They also show a near constant focus on their food intake which is part of the mental stress that is present (6). At the extremes, rigid dieting practices are associated with the development of overt eating disorders (EDs) even in lean women (7). This becomes even more problematic given the already increased incidence of EDs in women in general and athletes in certain sports specifically. Certainly some amount of restraint is required for fat loss to occur or to even avoid fat gain in the modern world but it is abundantly clear that rigid restraint tends to cause far more harm than good.

Flexible Eating Attitudes

Contrasting the above are flexible eating attitudes which represent a more graduated or gray approach to eating and this represents several different factors. One is that foods are not seen in a good or bad in an absolute sense but existing on a continuum in terms of their effects on health or calorie intake. They may be deliberately included in the diet in controlled amounts, an approach I will discuss briefly in Chapter 19 and in detail in Chapter 21. Even if they are not deliberately included in the diet, small deviations are seen as nothing but and can either be compensated for at a later point or ignored completely. This goes hand in hand with the realization that small deviations in calorie intake from the goal can be adjusted for with slight changes the next day or throughout the week. Slight is the key word here and trying to compensate for one or two hundred extra calories eaten one day with an hour of hard aerobics the next is equally damaging. Rather, if 200 calories more than the goal were eaten on one day, someone might eat 200 calories less on the next day or perform perhaps 20-30 minute of extra activity. Or they could eat 100 calories less on the next 2 days and perform 10-15 minutes of extra activity. In at least some situations, setting weekly goals can be better than daily goals and this means that calories can be saved up during the week to leave more room for a special event when the person knows that they are going to eat more than usual.

In the same way that rigid dieting is associated with higher body weights, more mental stress and binge eating episodes, individuals with higher degrees of flexible restraint show less frequent and severe binge eating, a lower calorie intake and a greater chance of weight loss than those with rigid restraint (8). The adoption of flexible dieting attitudes is also one of the major predictors of long-term fat loss success (9). In studies of restraint and disinhibition, those with higher degrees of flexible restraint are the ones who do not show disinhibition in response to what those with rigid restraint see as a violation of their diet. Once the realization has been made that one's daily diet and/or food choices are not a black/white, either/or situation, the stress over slight deviations disappears and so do the negative consequences.

Why Is a Flexible Approach to Eating Superior?

While there is still some criticism of flexible eating concepts (usually from those subgroups determined to defend their own often rigid dietary extremism and/or orthorexia), the research is extremely clear that it is a superior approach to the typical rigid approaches that are so often used or advocated and I think it's useful to look at some of the reasons why this is the case. Perhaps the biggest benefit to adopting or least understanding flexible eating attitudes is that it breaks people out of the mindset that there are foods that are good or bad in the absolute sense when it comes to their health or goals or that they are good or bad for eating them. This isn't to say that all foods are equivalent but rather that they fall on a continuum in terms of their effects on fullness, nutrient density, etc. This also means that no single food is so inherently bad that it represents (or can even potentially cause) a complete failure of the diet or dieter or that the diet should be abandoned. Of course making good food choices (in both type and amount) is better than not in the big picture. It is when this idea become absolute about which foods are good or bad that it reaches a pathological extreme. Even here, very large amounts of "healthy" foods can be far more detrimental than a so-called unhealthy food eaten in controlled and moderated amounts.

Once it's realized that there are no magical diet foods that are required for fat loss (or foods that instantly ruin a diet), much of the mental stress of dieting itself is removed. That same recognition also helps to eliminate the idea that eating the smallest amount of a specific forbidden or unclean food means that the day's dietary intake should be abandoned completely. Along with that is the realization that small calorie deviations in either direction are meaningless in the short-term. Fat loss or even long-term maintenance is a long-term process and has to be seen as such. As I mentioned above, someone who has created a significant daily deficit who eats slightly more than their goal has made no significant impact on anything. The extra 100-200 calories above the day's goal are meaningless overall. When the dieter eats 1000 extra calories due to disinhibition, that is no longer the case. For a small Category 1female dieter, that binge eating episode absolutely can set their diet back significantly.

Perhaps one of the largest issues that tend to derail changes in eating habits are food cravings and this is true both when actively dieting or simply trying to maintain a current body weight or body fat percentage (10). Cravings occur for a variety of reasons including simply being exposed to tasty foods. Recall from Chapter 9 that fat loss and dieting increases a person's attention to these kinds of foods in the first place. Women, especially those who are normally cycling, have the additional factor of their menstrual cycle and the changes that occur during the luteal (and especially the late luteal phase) to contend with. The simple act of having to restrict food intake can cause cravings and there is a tendency for the off-limit foods to be particularly craved (the women who couldn't eat bread in the study above specifically craved bread).

Rigid dietary approaches or attitudes that make certain foods completely off limits make this worse as they make the off limit food that much more desirable. In contrast, the knowledge that that food can be included to one degree or another, albeit in generally limited quantities, can help to eliminate those cravings. The idea of never being able to eat a certain food is suddenly replaced with the knowledge that it might be included at some point. Psychologically, the difference between never being able to eat a specific food and occasionally being able to eat it occasionally is absolutely enormous. This idea and approach can be applied to the idea of dieting and calorie restriction itself where the diet itself is stopped briefly. I discussed this in terms of reversing hormonal and menstrual cycle dysfunction in the last chapter and will look at specific approaches in Chapters 21 and 23 that are expand on this.

The Importance of Control

That brings me to what I think is perhaps the most important benefit of flexible eating attitudes and especially the flexible eating strategies I will discuss in Chapter 21. That benefit is control. In many if not most situations, deviations from a diet are due to a loss of control. The person is hungry and eats more than their daily goal or is tempted by a tasty food and eats it, breaking their own personal set of diet rules in terms of the foods or amounts that they are allowed to eat. For the rigid eater, this causes them to feel as if they have failed the diet or are inherently a failure for their inability to adhere. This leads to disinhibition and overeating acutely or abandonment of the diet entirely. Even if it is not due to a lack of personal control, deviations from the diet almost always occur in an unplanned fashion. Dieters become frustrated with their lack of results especially as the effort of dieting is becoming more difficult. Sometimes life just gets in the way with a holiday or vacation making the dieter feel as if they can't stick to their diet.

As often as not, this causes the dieter to simply give up, returning to their previous eating habits and regaining all the weight and sometimes more. When and if they decided to diet again, they may try to be even more rigid and restrictive which then fails, causing weight regain and sets up the same restraint/disinhibition cycle I described above but on a longer time scale. Dieters end up either being on a diet or not being on a diet and there is no middle ground to be had. I should mention that the same can occur with exercise programs where people who have been regularly exercising end up missing one or more workouts and, having decided that everything has been lost, abandon their program completely.

But none of the above fundamentally has to be the case and adopting more flexible eating attitudes is a key to this realization. As I described above, in the most general sense, flexible eating attitudes help people to recognize that small deviations aren't that important or can be compensated for. That is, just because someone can't adhere to their dietary goals for a few days after having dieted successfully for 3 months doesn't matter since it's impossible to regain significant body fat or weight in that time frame. The diet can simply be resumed after that time period. But this can be taken a step further by not only accepting that unplanned dietary deviations are irrelevant but also by planning those deviations and making them an inherent part of the diet. Now, rather than a food being technically off limits but acceptable within the concept of flexible eating attitudes, it is actually included explicitly within the overall plan.

This concept is actually demonstrated by a study done years ago where the researchers completely failed to achieve their goal but ended up making a brilliant observation (11). Their goal was to examine what happens when dieters go off their diets. Dieters (mostly women) were either placed on a diet for 14 straight weeks or instructed to go off their diet with some dieters taking a 2 week break after every 3 weeks of dieting and others taking a 6 week break after week 7. The researchers wanted to see how much weight was regained, why and how it was regained and why the subjects did or did not resume the diet. And here the study failed spectacularly as none of those things actually happened. The subjects experienced no major weight regain during the break, were able to return to dieting without difficulty and all three groups lost roughly the same total amount of weight (just over 15 pounds).

So what happened, why didn't the subjects regain weight or fail to resume dieting? In my opinion, it is because rather than seeing the 2 or 6 week break as having failed on their diet, they saw it as part of the overall program which changed the psychological impact of the break completely. Rather than seeing it as a personal failure to adhere to the diet, they were just doing what they had been prescribed/planned to do. A similar difference would be seen in the dieter who deliberately plans to raise their calories to maintenance to offset hormonal adaptations (as discussed in the last chapter) rather than having calories go up due to disinhibition or a binge eating episode. Put more simply, planned deviations from an eating plan allow the person to be in control of their diet rather than the diet being in control of them and this has been shown to be one of the best way to adhere to that plan over time (12). Certainly it goes against how most conceptualize dieting (or how it is recommended) but for many it is a far better approach.

There are a number of different way that planned deviations might be allowed or accommodated within a flexible eating framework. As I said above, many will simply brush off small deviations and/or compensate for them at a later time. For many who are resistant or simply new to the concept of flexible eating or dieting, I find that what I paradoxically call Structured Flexible Eating is often useful. These represent specific approaches to flexible eating that, while flexible, still have some specific rules and this can be a good transition in the early stages. I will describe these strategies in detail in Chapter 21.

When Should a Woman Start a Fat Loss Diet?

As a final general dieting concept, I want to address the question of when a woman should start her fat loss diet. Certainly most start their diets on a Monday (giving them a last chance to overindulge on the weekends) and there are considerations for those dieters who must reach a certain BF% by a given date but, beyond that, does it really matter on what week or month a diet starts? For the normally cycling woman, the answer is yes. Readers may recall from Chapter 2 that a woman's hunger and appetite is generally lowered during the follicular phase and lowest immediately prior to ovulation. This is reversed as hunger and cravings go up during the luteal phase with the late-luteal phase being the worst. Logically, it makes the most sense to start a diet after menstruation starts when hunger is lowest and the dieter is most likely to be successful to gain some positive momentum (13). This can be contrasted to attempting to start a fat loss diet in the luteal phase where the greatest difficulties in adherence will be encountered, possibly harming long-term adherence.

For those women who must reach a goal BF% by a certain date, this means determining the predicted length of the diet (discussed in Chapter 25) and then adjusting the start date based on where in the cycle it falls. In some cases this may require starting the diet two weeks earlier than otherwise planned so that it will synchronize with the follicular phase; in others there may be no other option but to start during the luteal phase. The possible need to include the Pre-Diet phase and this adds another factor to consider in determining the start of the diet. For a 2-week Pre-Diet phase, it could easily be placed during the luteal phase so that the diet itself can be started during the next follicular phase; a 4-week Pre-Diet phase would have to start in the follicular phase for the fat loss diet itself to start in the follicular phase as well. I've shown this below.

	Follicular Phase	Luteal Phase	Follicular Phase
Diet		2-week Pre-Diet Phase	Begin Diet
	4-Week Pre Diet Phase		Begin Diet

The above will not apply to any women with hormonal modifiers with the possible exception of women on some types of birth control with a withdrawal week. Since estrogen rebounds during this week, hunger may be relatively more controlled relative to the other three weeks of use and that would make the withdrawal week the best time to start the diet. For all other women, when the diet itself starts will be of little consequence beyond meeting the person's individual needs.

Chapter 16: Determining Maintenance Calories

The first step in setting up a calculated diet for any goal is to determine, or at least estimate, maintenance calorie requirements. This is the number of calories that should ideally maintain both body weight and body composition without change and it is from here that any changes will be made to achieve different goals. I say ideally as there can be situations where body weight is relatively stable but body composition may change for the better or worse (i.e. some types of birth control can cause a slight gain of body fat and loss of muscle despite no weight change). I've referred to this value as Total Daily Energy Expenditure (TDEE) earlier in the book and will do so here.

As discussed previously in the book, TDEE is made up of four components which are resting metabolic rate (RMR), the thermic effect of food (TEF), the thermic effect of activity (TEA, formal exercise) and Non-Exercise Activity Thermogenesis (NEAT). RMR is related mostly to lean body mass (LBM) but can be estimated with total weight while TEF is usually taken as 10% of total calorie intake. The calorie burn from TEA can vary massively and NEAT is incredibly difficult to estimate at this point.

It's crucial to understand that any estimate of TDEE is only that, an estimate. Even with complicated equations, there is some variability between any two individuals at an identical weight and body composition with the greatest variation, outside of people performing a large amount of formal exercise, coming from variations in NEAT. While it's certainly possible to estimate good starting values for TDEE, real world changes in body composition will indicate if that starting point is correct or needs to be adjusted. It's equally important to remember that TDEE can change in both directions in response to dieting or overeating. For this reason it's better to think of it as a range than a fixed value.

All components of TDEE adapt downwards in response to dieting and fat loss while they can be reversed or even increased in response to overeating and weight or fat gain. Women who have been on low calories for extended periods of time frequently report that their weight and body composition remains relatively stable even as they begin to increase their calorie intake. This is invariably due to changes in NEAT, coming above the critical EA threshold which may allow some degree of hormonal recovery, etc. Athletes often find that they can train more intensely which means that their TEA goes up along with those increasing calories.

There are a number of ways that maintenance calories can be estimated and I will look at two different approaches, one of which I think is potentially problematic, especially for women. I'll also present a slightly more complicated but, in my opinion more accurate method of estimating maintenance. While I won't discuss them in detail, some of the new activity trackers may also be useful in obtaining a better estimate of TDEE as well.

Tracking Calorie Intake and Bodyweight Method

Used for years, one of the simplest approaches to estimating TDEE is to track bodyweight (and again I'd recommend a 7-day rolling average) and calorie intake for some period of time. Generally two weeks is taken as the minimum time frame due to daily variations and the assumption is that, if body weight is stable over this time period, the current calorie intake is equal to TDEE. That is, if someone gained weight over this time period, presumably their calorie intake exceeded TDEE and if they lost weight, their calorie intake was below their actual TDEE. In premise this approach makes a good deal of sense and determines an actual calorie intake level rather than trying to estimate it but I think there are some problems with it.

The primary one is that it requires calories to be tracked accurately. This entails measuring and writing down all food and drink that is consumed This is not necessarily a bad thing and, as I will describe in a later chapter, is one of the most information exercises any person can go through to learn what real world portion sizes and calorie values are. At the same time, it can be a bit of a pain in the butt and, outside of the Category 1 dieter, may be overkill in the beginning. For the woman adopting a simpler diet approach it would be excessive. Those women are usually not setting calorie intakes to begin with.

Even for the Category 1 dieter, this approach may be problematic. First and foremost is that weight isn't the same as body composition although the odds of any significant changes in body composition occurring over this time period are slim so that's really a non-issue. The normally cycling female have the additional issue of menstrual cycle related water weight changes. A woman tracking during the first two weeks of the cycle can't get an accurate idea of whether or not she has gained, maintained or lost weight when her weight may swing wildly due to water retention. She could track for a full month and compare similar weeks of the cycle and this would be reasonably valid. Women with a hormonal modifier won't have this issue for the most part but in most cases, I recommend the next method.

Calculation Method

Although more complex than the previous method, I think that using a calculation based method to determine or at least estimate TDEE/maintenance calories is generally more appropriate. This is especially true for the normally cycling female who may not be able to use the above method due to shifts in her water weight every week. With this method, TDEE is calculated by estimating the four components of TDEE and then adding them together. While there are more complex methods that can be used (that I feel are generally unnecessary), the method I will present will be to first estimate RMR which will be increased by an activity multiplier based on both both activities of daily living (NEAT) and formal exercise (TEA). Since it is generally small, TEF is often ignored completely but I will factor it into the activity multipliers. As well, the NEAT value will only include overall daily activity as the unconscious part of NEAT (fidgeting, etc.) cannot be estimated in any meaningful way.

Traditionally a single multiplier has been used based on overall or average activity levels during the week but I find this problematic. Most people's activity is not identical every day of the week and their work days may look very different than their non-work days. Athletes have the added issue of their training often varying significantly from day to day (some sports have training sessions that are more alike than not but this is not universal). An endurance athlete who used the same multiplier every day but who did 4 hours of training one day and only 1 hour the next would be vastly mis-estimating their true calorie requirements, making it impossible to match their nutritional needs. Practically this means that any day of the week might have it's own multiplier (and resulting TDEE) although most will probably end up with only a handful of different values for different types of training days.

Women, as usual, have their own specific issues related to maintenance calories. The first is that their energy expenditure for all components of TDEE are roughly 10% below those of men. As discussed in Chapter 10, most of this is related to differences in body composition (1). This difference is also reflected in the calculations below and no further adjustments have to be made. There can also be slight adjustments to TDEE based on the hormonal modifier present and detail-oriented readers may wish to apply those. Do remember that all of these calculations are only estimates at best; no matter how close to TDEE they come, they may still have to be adjusted over time.

Estimating RMR

The first step in calculating TDEE is to estimate RMR, the number of calories that the body burns at complete rest. There are endless equations that have been developed over the years that range from simple to very complicated. Since they all tend to give results within a few hundred calories of one another, I prefer to use the simpler equations. For the most part, RMR equations have only been based around body weight (often including age, height, gender and others) but given the importance of LBM in determining RMR, these tend to become increasingly inaccurate for women with a very high or very low BF%.

For example, a commonly used equation for women is to multiply bodyweight by 10 cal/lb (22 cal/kg). While this is accurate within a certain range of BF%, it becomes progressively more inaccurate as BF% goes up. For this reason, I prefer equations that take body composition into account and am presenting a simple one that I derived myself from other, more complex, equations. It requires body weight and some estimation of BF% so that the total amount of LBM can be calculated. I've shown the calculation for two women of different body composition below.

> RMR = (12 calories * LBM in pounds) + (2 calories *fat mass in pounds) or
> RMR = (26.4 calories * LBM in kg) + (4.4 calories * fat mass in kg)
> **Example 1**
> Female at 150 lbs, 22% body fat with 117 lbs LBM and 30 lbs of fat
> RMR = 150 lbs * 10 cal/lb = 1500 calories
> RMR = (12*117) + (2*30) = 1404 + 60 = 1464 calories or 9.8 cal/lb
> **Example 2**
> Female at 250 lbs, 50% body fat with 125 lbs LBM and 125 lbs of fat
> RMR = 250 lbs * 10 cal/lb = 2500 calories
> RMR = (12*125) + (2*125) = 1750 calories or 7 cal/lb

You can see from the above calculations that while the 10 cal/lb value is very accurate for the leaner woman it drastically over-estimates the woman with a high BF% with the actual value for RMR dropping from 10 cal/lb to 7 cal/lb. For women who don't want to perform the above math, the following chart can be used to estimate RMR from just bodyweight. Some estimate of BF% is still required but the values under each BF% can be multiplied by total body weight to estimate RMR.

BF%	20	25	30	35	40	45	50
RMR (cal/lb)	10.0	9.5	9.0	8.5	8.0	7.5	7.0
RMR (cal/kg)	22	21	20	19	17.5	16.5	15.5

To use the chart, bodyweight is multiplied by the RMR value underneath the appropriate BF% value. The sample female at 150 lbs and 22% body fat would have an estimated RMR of 150 lbs * ~9.7 (halfway between the 9.5 and 10.0 values for 20 and 25% body fat) or 1455 calories which is effectively identical to the value I showed above. The 250 lb/50% body fat female would multiply her weight of 250 by 7 to get an RMR of 1750, identical to the value calculated with the first equation. This value for RMR will be modified by the activity multipliers, described next.

Activity Multipliers

If someone did nothing more than lay in bed all day, their TDEE would be equal to their RMR. Since most do not, this value will be increased based on the level of activity being done. Traditionally, activity multipliers have combined both TEA and NEAT but I find it more useful to split them up for better accuracy. This approach also makes it easier to take into account changes in each when activity levels are varying from day to day. Certainly only needing a single multiplier for every day would be simpler but this tends to be unrealistic unless someone's daily activity is extremely consistent.

Daily Activity (NEAT)

Since not everybody is involved in formal exercise but everyone (unless they are completely bedridden) performs at least some amount of daily activity, I will start with an estimation of that multiplier. In the modern world, someone's activity may range from completely sedentary to requiring extremely high levels of activity is their job or lifestyle is very labor intensive. For this reason, RMR multipliers from 1.2 to 1.9 are usually considered to be realistic with 2.5 times RMR being the maximum energy expenditure that can be sustained for extended periods (athletes may surpass this for short periods due to their incredibly high TEA values). For most people a realistic NEAT multiplier will be 1.4-1.7. In the chart below, I've shown multipliers for different activity levels and their general descriptions.

Activity Level	Description	RMR Multiplier
Sedentary	Sitting, talking, reading, watching TV	1.3-1.4
Light	Office work with moderate walking	1.4-1.5
Moderate	Busy lifestyle w/ lots of walking	1.6-1.7
High	Construction, hard labor	1.7-1.9

If no formal exercise is being performed, RMR can simply be multiplied by the value above to get the estimated TDEE. If our 150 pound female with a maintenance of 1455 calories had a sedentary lifestyle, she would use a multiplier of 1.3 to get a maintenance of 1890-2040 calories (1455 * 1.3 or 1.4). If she were moderately to highly active, she would use the 1.7 multiplier to get an estimated TDEE of 2475 calories/day (1455 calories/day * 1.7). If formal exercise is being done, it will have to be added to the above value. I will also provide a chart later in the chapter that will simplify all of the calculations.

When using the above chart, I strongly encourage readers to be realistic about their daily activity levels. Someone who sits in front of a computer most of the day and does little else will be somewhere between sedentary and light activity even if they feel that is too low or dislike the relatively low TDEE value that is estimates. Someone on their feet all day will be in the moderate category and few will achieve the highest values unless they are moving continuously or working a very labor intensive job. While many older estimates put most people's multiplier closer to 1.7, I feel that changes in the modern world have made this too high for many people. Practically I would generally suggest erring on the side of too low of a multiplier than too high. Calories always need to be adjusted based on real world changes and it's better to be eating slightly too few and having to increase due to weight loss than the converse under most circumstances.

Exercise Energy Expenditure (TEA)

Once the daily activity multiplier has been determined, the calorie expenditure from formal exercise, if it is being done, will need to be added to determine TDEE. The number of calories burned during exercise can vary enormously depending on the type, amount and intensity of the exercise done. In many forms of exercise, bodyweight also plays a role with larger bodies burning more calories. This is often offset by heavier individuals often being limited in the amount of exercise that they can perform. To put this into perspective, a relative beginner or untrained individual may burn only 200-300 calories in an hour of exercise (although this will increase as fitness improves) while a highly trained endurance athlete might burn up 650-900+ calories per hour and double or triple that for an extremely long duration workout.

Observationally, female athletes report calorie intakes ranging from 15-23 cal/lb (33-50.6 cal/kg), representing a 1.5-2.3 RMR multiplier, depending on the sport and amount of training being done (2,3). Weight lifters tend to be towards the lower end of the range, high-intensity and team sports fall somewhere in the middle and only endurance athletes achieve the highest values due to the amount of training that they do. Due to difficulties in measuring actual energy expenditure, the above values are based on reported food intakes. As many female athletes undereat relative to their actual energy expenditure, it's possible and somewhat likely that actual values for true energy expenditure are somewhat higher. However, the American College of Sports Medicine (ACSM) position stand on the topic recommends a BMR multiplier of 1.7-2.3 (~ 17-23 cal/lb or 37.4-50.6 cal/kg) from moderate to heavy training and this is right in range of the reported calorie intakes (4). I'd note that these values are roughly 10% what is seen or recommended for male athletes in keeping with the differences in body composition, etc. As well, these values are for hard training athletes only. Recreational exercisers will not achieve all but the lowest of those values.

Readers may see that the above values overlap with the general daily activity and some of this is due to the above representing total daily calorie expenditures rather than exercise alone. However, there is often an inverse relationship between the amount of exercise being done and other daily activities. The busier someone is, the less time or energy they have to put into exercise and athletes doing a large amount of training are often less active at other times of the day due to fatigue or simply recovering after a hard workout (in the case where a hard training athlete may be working many hours at a labor intensive job, their TDEE can skyrocket). A woman with a 1.9 multiplier for her daily activity is unlikely to do much exercise on that day and surpass a 2.3 multiplier. On a day off from work, when her daily activity is much lower, she might be able to fit in a much larger amount of exercise. Conceivably she could have similar activity multipliers for each, just accomplished through a different pathway: NEAT versus TEA.

In the chart below, I've listed some general types of exercise along with their rough calorie burn per pound/kg per hour of activity. If 2 cal/lb is listed, a 150 lb woman would burn 150 calories in 30 minutes, 300 calories in an hour and 450 calories over 90 minutes. I've grouped the activities by intensity although more complete lists can be found online. In many cases, the values shown in those lists will be higher than what I have shown below. This is because I have factored out what a woman would burn doing no exercise at all. If someone would have burned 60 calories/hour sitting and burns 300 calories/hour during exercise, they have actually only burned 240 extra calories per day. This not only gives a more realistic indication of actual calorie expenditure from exercise but is the value that should be used to estimate energy availability (EA) if those calculations are being made.

Activity	Examples	Per Hour of Activity	Multiplier
Low Intensity Aerobic (130 HR or lower)	Brisk walking, slow cycling (<13 mph)	1.5 cal/lb (3.3 cal/kg) 2 cal/lb (4.4 cal/kg)	0.15 0.2
Medium Intensity Aerobic (130-150 HR)	Swimming, jogging cycling (13-15mph)	2-3 cal/lb (4.4-6.6 cal/kg)	0.2-0.3
High Intensity Aerobic (160-180 HR)	Cycling (17-18mph), running (6' mile)	3-4 cal/lb (6.6-8.8 cal/kg)	0.3-0.4
Highly Trained Athletes	Cycling (18+mph), running (8' mile or faster)	5-8 cal/lb (10.5-17.6 cal/kg)	0.5-0.8
Weight Training	Recreational Physique/PL/OL	1 cal/lb (2.2 cal/kg) 2 cal/lb (4.4 cal/kg)	0.1 0.2
Team Sports (variable)	Volleyball Basketball Soccer	1-2 cal/lb (2.2-4.4 cal/kg) 3.75 cal/lb (8.25 cal/kg) 6 cal/min (13.2 cal/kg)	0.1-0.2 0.375 0.6

While calculating actual calorie burn from exercise is important (especially to estimate EA), from the standpoint of determining TDEE, the fourth column is most important. Here I have put exercise energy expenditures in terms of an activity multiplier by dividing the value by 10. So 2 cal/lb/hour becomes a 0.2 RMR multiplier which should be added to the activity multiplier from above. This value is per hour and must be adjusted if more or less than an hour of exercise. A 90 minute workout would become a 0.3 multiplier (0.2 * 1.5) and a 30 minute workout would become a 0.1 multiplier (0.2/2). A female with an activity multiplier of 1.4 (sedentary) who performed an hour of physique weight training would add 0.2 to get a total multiplier of 1.6 times her RMR. If she added an additional hour of low intensity aerobic training she would add an additional 0.2 for a total multiplier of 1.8 and that times her RMR would represent her TDEE. If she were an endurance athlete and performed 2 hours of medium intensity aerobic she would add 0.4-0.6 to her original 1.4 multiplier to get a final multiplier of 1.8-2.0 times RMR.

It should be clear that the energy expenditure for a given type of exercise can vary widely from extremely low to extremely high depending primarily on the intensity. Brisk walking burns fairly few calories and a 160 pound woman walking for 30 minutes would burn only 120 calories. Done three times per week this is a mere 360 calories burned. In contrast a 130 lb endurance athlete performing 4 hours of low to moderate intensity cycling could burn up to 1600 calories (130 pounds * 3 cal/lb/hour * 4 hours).

Estimating TDEE

With RMR, NEAT and TEA calculated or estimated, TDEE can be determined. There are two ways of doing although both will generate identical values. The first is to calculate RMR (using the equation I provided above), then multiply that by the general daily activity factor. Finally the number of calories burned during activity would be added to get the TDEE. This requires a bit of math but is needed to do an EA calculation. The second method is to determine the total daily multiplier and use the chart below.

BF%	RMR	1.2	1.3	1.4	1.5	1.6	1.7	1.8	1.9	2.0	2.1	2.2	2.3
20	10.0	12.0	13.0	14.0	15.0	16.0	17.0	18.0	19.0	20.0	21.0	22.0	23.0
25	9.5	11.4	12.4	13.3	14.3	15.2	16.2	17.1	18.1	19.0	20.0	20.9	21.9
30	9.0	10.8	11.7	12.6	13.5	14.4	15.3	16.2	17.1	18.0	18.9	19.8	20.7
35	8.5	10.2	11.1	11.9	12.8	13.6	14.5	15.3	16.2	17	17.9	18.7	19.6
40	8.0	9.6	10.4	11.2	12.0	12.8	13.6	14.4	15.2	16	16.8	17.6	18.4
45	7.5	9.0	9.8	10.5	11.3	12	12.8	13.5	14.3	15	15.8	16.5	17.3
50	7.0	8.4	9.1	9.8	10.5	11.2	11.9	12.6	13.3	14.0	14.7	15.4	16.1

To use the chart, an estimate of BF% will be required and will be cross referenced with the total activity multiplier on the top column as determined above to get the actual daily multiplier. Bodyweight will be multiplied by that value to get TDEE. A 150 lb female with 22% body fat, a daily activity multiplier of 1.4 who performs an hour of physique training which adds 0.2 for a total 1.6 multiplier. Using the above chart, she is partway between two values and she would use roughly 15.8 cal/lb. She would then multiply 150 lbs by 15.8 cal/lb to get a TDEE of 2370 calories. The calculation method generates nearly identical values. First she would take her calculated RMR of 1455 calories and multiply that by 1.4 to get 2037 calories. She will burn roughly 375 calories (150 lbs * 0.25 cal/lb/hour) during weight training and added to 2037, her TDEE would be 2400 which is within 30 calories of the value that the simpler method produces. If a 250 lb female with 50% body fat had an activity multiplier of 1.4 (moderately active) and added an hour of low intensity aerobic exercise (0.2 multiplier), she would use the 1.6 multiplier under 50% body fat and multiply her body weight by 11.2. Her TDEE would be 250 lbs * 11.2 cal/lb = 2800 cal/day. Again this is only an estimate that will be adjusted as needed.

Variable Activity Weeks

The simpler method I presented, using the chart to determine the bodyweight multiplier has an added advantage in that it makes calculating TDEE for different days of the week much easier. All that needs to be done is to determine the total activity multiplier for any given day to get the TDEE in cal/lb from the above chart which is then multiplied by body weight. So imagine a 130 lb female with 25% body fat. She has a lightly active job during the week but is more sedentary on the weekend. In addition she performs 6 one hour physique workouts per week with Sunday as a day off.

	Monday	Tuesday	Wednesday	Thursday	Friday	Saturday	Sunday
Activity Multiplier	1.4	1.4	1.4	1.4	1.4	1.3	1.3
Exercise Multiplier	0.25	0.25	0.25	0.25	0.25	0.25	0
Total Multiplier	1.6	1.6	1.6	1.6	1.6	1.5	1.3
BW Multiplier	15.2	15.2	15.2	15.2	15.2	14.3	12.4
TDEE (cal/day)	1975	1975	1975	1975	1975	1860	1600

In this example, TDEE doesn't really vary much with an ~400 calorie difference from highest to lowest. This tends to be common for physique athletes and some strength/power sports.

As another example, consider a female cyclist who weighs 140 lbs at 20% body fat and who has a highly variable training schedule. She performs an hour of low intensity cycling on Monday and Friday, a hard hour on Wednesday and does a 4 hour ride on Saturday and a 2 hour ride on Sunday.

	Monday	Tuesday	Wednesday	Thursday	Friday	Saturday	Sunday
Activity Multiplier	1.4	1.4	1.4	1.4	1.4	1.3	1.3
Exercise Multiplier	0.2	0	0.4	0	0.2	0.8	0.4
Total Multiplier	1.6	1.4	1.8	1.4	1.6	2.1	1.7
BW Multiplier	16	14	18	14	16	21	17
TDEE (cal/day)	2240	1960	2500	1960	2240	2940	2380

TDEE is far more variable here and can vary 1000 calories from the highest to lowest days.

Hormonal Modifier Adjustments to TDEE

While the above covers the overall estimation of TDEE, women have an additional potential factor to take into account which is the impact of hormonal modifiers on daily energy expenditure. Most of the values I will present are generally small and only high-level athletes who must match their calorie intake closely to their expenditure or the smaller Category 1 dieter should probably worry about them. Other women may choose to use them but their impact is small relative to daily activity and exercise. Since I listed the changes in metabolic rate due to hormonal modifiers in a previous chapter, I will only recap them.

During the luteal phase, the normally cycling woman may see a 2.5-11% increase in RMR, amounting to 100-300 calories. I'll use a mid range value of 5% or about 150 calories. A similar increase occurs in response to some types of birth control and I'll use the same value. In PCOS/obesity, TEF is decreased by about 50% due to insulin resistance which might amount to 100-150 calories. As I described in Chapter 12, there is a progressive impact of menstrual cycle dysfunction on metabolic rate with amenorrheic women having a TDEE up to 20% below normally cycling women. I'll use 15% below. Women who are menopausal and on HRT will show a reduction in RMR of about 4 calories per year or 40 calories per decade. In contrast, postmenopausal women who forego HRT may see a 14 cal/year (140 cal/decade) drop. I've shown the potential impact for a 150 lb woman with a TDEE of ~2250 calories and assumed 10 years post menopause for that adjustment in the chart below.

Hormonal Modifier	TDEE (cal/day)	Adjustment	Calories	Adjusted TDEE
Luteal Phase/Birth Control	2250	+2.5-11%	+55-250	2300-2500 cal/day (2350*)
PCOS/Category 3	2250	TEF - 5%	~100	2075 cal/day
Amenorrhea	2250	- 15%	-337	1910 cal/day
Menopause w/o HRT	2250	-14 cal/year	-143	2032 cal/day
Menopause w/HRT	2250	-~4 cal/year	-40	2132 cal/day

*2350 represents a 5% increase over baseline as an average value

With the exception of amenorrhea, most of the changes are quite small and within daily variability in food intake. Outside of extreme dieting situations they can generally be ignored.

Chapter 17: Adjusting Daily Calories

Having estimated total daily energy expenditure (TDEE) and the number of daily calories that would be needed to meet that energy expenditure, the next step is to whether or not calories will be adjusted, in what direction and by how much. In some cases, this will be due to unwanted changes in weight (up or down) although it's more common to deliberately raise or lower calories to achieve one of several goals. The three I will focus on are maintenance, gaining muscle/fitness, and losing fat.

Maintenance is clearly just that and may occur when someone is either happy with their current weight and body composition or have finished a diet and want to stabilize at that new weight. Calories are often increased when the goals are gaining muscle mass, strength/power or improve athletic performance but there are other situations where this may be done. One is at the end of an extreme Category 1 diet where the achieved level of leanness is not meant to be sustained in the long-term and I will address this in detail in Chapter 33. There is also the occasional situation where someone is underweight for one reason or another. Often this is associated with an overt eating disorder which is beyond the scope of this book.

Perhaps the most common adjustment to maintenance calories is to decrease them. While this may be done to avoid unwanted (often age-related) weight gain, the more common goal is explicit fat loss or altering body composition. As this is the more common goal and has more complexity to it in terms of determining how much fat needs to be lost, the size of the deficit to be used, etc. I will spend proportionally more time on it.

Maintaining Current Weight and Body Composition

If someone's current goal is maintenance of their current weight or body composition, there should be no need to adjust the estimate of TDEE and maintenance calories unless body weight or fat are changing. Whether they are going up or down, this simply means that the estimated value for maintenance calories was not correct in the first place. It may also mean that the person is not eating what they think they are and this is extremely common. Generally speaking, people underestimate how much they are actually eating although I've mentioned that many hard-training female athletes may fail to eat enough to meet their energy expenditures. In this case, the problem is not necessarily with the estimation of TDEE but rather with the actual amount of food being eaten.

But in the case where someone is accurately tracking their caloric intake and is eating the amount that they think, changes in body composition from maintenance mean that the TDEE estimation should be adjusted. If body weight and body fat are moving upwards the estimated maintenance calories should be adjusted downwards. Let me reiterate that small day to day changes are meaningless and it is only long-term changes measured over weeks or months that are relevant. Cutting calories because body weight spikes by a few pounds overnight or during a specific week of the menstrual cycle should never be done. If bodyweight and body fat are going down and this is not the explicit goal, the estimate for maintenance calories should be raised and/or the actual caloric intake should be measured to see if it is too low.

In general, I wouldn't suggest making more than 10% or so changes to the estimated TDEE at a time. So a woman with an estimated TDEE of 2400 calories per day who was gaining fat should adjust her maintenance estimate downwards by roughly 200-240 calories. If she were losing fat and that wasn't the goal she should raise her calories by the same 200-240 calories. That level would be maintained for several weeks and adjustments made again as necessary. Eventually true TDEE will be determined and achieved.

Muscle, Strength and Performance Gains

While many women will seek to improve their body composition by gaining small amounts of muscle while losing fat, this doesn't generally require any major changes to energy intake and deliberately increasing calorie intake (unless it is very low to begin with) is usually not necessary. This changes in the situation where the serious recreational trainee or competitive athlete is seeking significant improvements in muscle, strength/power or performance (i.e. improved aerobic performance or speed). While this obviously requires a proper training program, these goals will always happen more effectively when calorie intake is at least slightly above maintenance levels. I want to emphasize the word slightly as the rate at which most women will improve their muscle mass, strength/power or any other aspect of performance is relatively low in an absolute sense. I say absolute as women are generally found to make the same relative improvement as men in response to training. A woman lifting 50 pounds and a man lifting 100 may both improve by 10% but the changes will be 5 and 10 pounds respectively. Their relative improvements are identical but her absolute improvements are less due to her lower starting point.

While a slight calorie surplus is required, I'd reiterate that any excess calorie intake beyond the level necessary to support maximal rates of improvement will simply lead to an accelerate increase in body fat. Outside of those athletes such as throwers, superheavy weight Olympic lifters/powerlifters for whom this is not an issue, excessive fat gain should be avoided to as great a degree as possible. I discussed the reasons in Chapter 14 including the potential for making new fat cells in the lower body along with the need for many athletes to have to reduce their body fat percentage (BF%) at some point. Excess body fat gained while trying to improve performance is fat that has to be dieted off eventually. Many physique and strength/power athletes find out the hard way that attempting to "bulk up" by consuming enormous numbers of calories does little to improve their performance/muscle mass but leads to excessive fat gains.

To optimize gains in strength, muscle mass or performance while limiting total fat gain, I'd suggest perhaps 5-10% over maintenance for most women. A woman with a TDEE of 2400 calories per day would increase them by 120-240 calories per day and even that might only be appropriate on her hardest training days. For most realistic daily energy expenditures, this 5-10% will likely be in the realm of 100-300 calories unless activity and energy expenditure is simply enormous. This is typically restricted to endurance athletes in heavy training but the surplus needed to support endurance training adaptations is not very large to begin with. As a general rule, a 200-300 cal/day surplus would be the maximum necessary to maximize LBM gains while minimizing fat gain (1).

Realistic Rates of Weight Gain

To look at this a little bit more accurately it's useful to look at some realistic rates of weight/LBM gain. I'm focusing on muscle gain here as there is more research, along with anecdotal observations, on realistic rates of muscle gain than other fitness components in natural athletes. Given the high energetic cost of building muscle, the surplus required here is likely to represent the maximum required to improve any other aspect of fitness. The book "The Muscle and Strength Nutrition Pyramid" by Eric Helms, Andy Morgan and Andrea Valdez presented a chart on recommended rates of weight gain that I have adjusted based on the differences in LBM between women and men.

Year of Training	Rate of Monthly Weight Gain
1	0.85-1.25% of current bodyweight
2	0.4-0.85% of current bodyweight
3	Up to 0.4% of current bodyweight

Adapted from "The Muscle and Strength Nutrition Pyramid" by Helms, Morgan and Valdez.

Here the chart is referring to total bodyweight instead of LBM. So a woman who weighed 120 pounds and who was targeting a 0.85% increase would aim for almost exactly one pound of total weight gained per month (120 lbs * 0.0085 = 1.02 lbs). This will not all be muscle as some small gain in body fat is nearly unavoidable and a ratio of 75% muscle to 25% fat will be be assumed. So this one pound of weight gain should result in 0.75 lbs of LBM and 0.25 lbs of fat gained. If instead she targeted the 1.25%, her monthly weight gain would be 1.5 pounds and 75% or 1.1 pounds should be LBM although fat gain will increase to 0.4 lbs Since this approach is based on percentages, heavier women have the potential to gain weight faster while lighter women will gain weight more slowly. This can become a problem for lighter women as the rate of gain is lower than the accuracy of most measuring devices. Anything less than one pound per month will be difficult to track accurately and it may take several months of consistent training to determine if LBM is being gained. Any faster rate will simply result in excessive fat gain.

Once the goal weight gain has been determined, this can be used to determine how much of a monthly surplus will be required to achieve it. Readers may recall that it takes ~2600 calories to gain one pound of LBM. But as some of the total weight gained will be from fat, the actual value will be higher than this. Practically it's easiest to use assume 3,500 calories per pound of total weight gain. The 120 pound female targeting 1 lb/month would therefore need 3,500 calories per month over her maintenance. Her weekly surplus would be just under 900 (3500/30 days) calories which would give just over 130 calories per day (900/7) over maintenance to maximize her gains. If she were targeting 1.5 pounds per month, her monthly surplus would increase to 5,250 calories with a weekly surplus of 1300 calories and a daily surplus of just under 200 calories/day. A larger female at 150 lbs targeting a 1.25% gain would be gaining 1.85 lbs/month. This would require a 6550 calorie monthly surplus or a 1650 calorie/weekly surplus which is a 235 calorie daily surplus. In all cases, the values fall right in the 100-300 calorie range I provided above.

For reasons I will discuss in a later chapter, it is often beneficial to place the surplus on training days with slightly fewer calories on non-training days. A woman performing 4 workouts per week would take the 900 calorie weekly surplus and divide by 4 to get 225 calories which would be the surplus on her training days. With 5 workouts per week, each day would have a 180 calorie surplus. In the chart below, I've shown the predicted weight gain, monthly, weekly and daily calorie surplus for women of different weights aiming for different rates of weight gain. Women who cluster the surplus onto training days should divide the weekly surplus by the number of workouts/week rather than by 7 to get a daily surplus.

Weight	0.4%	Monthly	Weekly	Daily	0.85%	Monthly	Weekly	Daily	1.25%	Monthly	Weekly
100	0.4	1400	350	50	0.85	2975	744	106	1.25	4375	1094
110	0.44	1540	385	55	0.94	3273	818	117	1.38	4813	1203
120	0.48	1680	420	60	1.02	3570	893	128	1.5	5250	1313
130	0.52	1820	455	65	1.11	3868	967	138	1.63	5688	1422
140	0.56	1960	490	70	1.19	4165	1041	149	1.75	6125	1531
150	0.6	2100	525	75	1.28	4463	1116	159	1.88	6563	1641
150	0.6	2100	525	75	1.28	4463	1116	159	1.88	6563	1641
160	0.64	2240	560	80	1.36	4760	1190	170	2	7000	1750

You can see from the chart that the rough estimate of 5-10% above TDEE or roughly 100-300 calories per day is fairly accurate although some of this depends on whether or not the surplus is provided every day of the week or only on training days (which roughly double the surplus on those days). Even here, for a training week with 4-5 workouts per week, the daily surpluses rarely exceed that value. Consider the 160 lb female targeting 1.25% weekly weight gain. Her weekly surplus is 1750 calories which, across 5 workouts per week is still only 350 calories above maintenance. The primary message, regardless of the exact application is that women never need more than the most moderate of calorie surpluses to support maximal rates of muscle growth or adaptation to their training. Any excess will simply result in fat gain.

Effect of Hormonal Modifiers

Looking at hormonal modifiers, the use of hormonal birth control (BC) won't enormously impact on the above values for calorie surplus although, as I'll discuss in Volume 2, some types may impair muscle growth slightly. Women who have lost their menstrual cycle should be raising calories to eliminate the low EA to begin with and I will talk about how calories should be raised following an extreme diet in a later chapter. Women with the hyperandrogenic type of PCOS or subclinical hyperandrogenism tend to gain muscle more easily although the rate is still slow relatively speaking. At most the values above might be increased by 50% and she would be the most likely to achieve the highest levels of bodyweight increase (i.e. 1.25% in the first year, 0.85% in the second year and possibly more than 0.4% in the third). So the rough increase might be 7.5-15% over maintenance or 200-400 calories per day maximum. With age, the rate of muscle gains slows significantly and the peri/postmenopausal women is unlikely to need a large surplus of calories to support muscle growth and I'd recommend the lower rates of weight gain and relatively smaller deficits (10% maximum over maintenance).

Fat Loss: Introduction

As I've mentioned throughout the book, fat loss will only occur is there is a long-term imbalance between calorie intake and calorie expenditure. This causes the body to mobilize stored fuel for energy (or adapt metabolically). However, unlike muscle and performance gain, where the rate of gain (and surpluses needed) are relatively fixed, the rate of fat loss can vary from slow to moderate to fast depending on the approach taken and the dieter's needs or situation. This makes the overall discussion of adjusting calorie levels for fat loss more complicated and I will be spending much more time discussing the factors that go into setting the calorie deficit both in general and specific terms.

Exercise vs. Diet

The first general issue I want to address is whether the calorie deficit will be created through increased energy expenditure or decreased calorie intake. In one sense, there is no real difference in how the daily deficit is created. Whether food intake is decreased by 500 calories per day, activity is increased by 500 calories per day or calories are decreased by 250 calories and activity increased by 250 calories, the same 500 calorie per day deficit is created. However, this is clearly untrue in both a physiological and practical sense and there may be differences in the way that metabolic rate changes, whether LBM is lost (or gained), where the fat is lost from, how hunger changes along with dietary adherence for one approach compared to the other. So let me look at each, starting with energy expenditure.

In premise at least TDEE could be increased through any of the four components I have described in this book. In practice, this is not true. RMR can be increased by gaining weight or overeating but, by definition, that is not what fat loss entails. I've mentioned that adding muscle has insignificant effects on raising RMR. RMR can be increased slightly (by perhaps 5% per day) through the use of specific supplements and I will discuss this in Chapter 24. There are drugs that can also accomplish this but these will not be discussed in this book. TEF is equally resistant to increase. Eating more food would raise it slightly but, once again, this runs contrary to the act of dieting (conceivably one might eat more and exercise more but this would only raise TEF slightly). Although the impact is small, replacing carbohydrate or fat with protein will raise TEF but it takes fairly large-scale changes to have a significant effect. This leaves NEAT and TEA as the only potential ways to increase TDEE.

Despite the general focus on formal exercise that has existed for decades, many researchers feel that increasing NEAT represents the best approach to the obesity issue/losing fat. This is due to the fact that the calorie expenditure from increasing NEAT often exceeds what can be done by most during formal exercise and it accomplishes this without feeling like exercise. As I showed in a previous chapter, a 1 cal/min increase in energy expenditure over a 6-8 hour work day might burn an additional 360-480 calories, equivalent to an hour of moderately intense exercise. This does require modifications to the work space which is not always possible, meaning that increases in NEAT may have to occur from increases in other daily activities. This takes conscious attention and effort to moving more during the day and, as I mentioned earlier, this can be facilitated with activity monitors or a step counter.

That leaves formal exercise as the more common approach to increasing energy expenditure and there are many reasons to consider increasing exercise as the sole, or at least partial, way that a calorie deficit is created. For the normally cycling woman, recall that LH pulsatility is slightly less impacted by increasing exercise than decreasing food intake, probably due to maintaining carbohydrate availability to the brain. Do keep in mind that those studies compared exercise only to diet only and nobody has looked to see if the combination of the two has the same or a different effect. Regardless of the mechanism, exercise would appear to send less of a signal of low energy availability (EA) to the brain than calorie restriction alone. Similarly, leptin levels and pulsatility are also changed to a lesser degree with exercise versus diet alone (2). This effect along would be enough to make exercise at least part of how the deficit is created, at least for the normally cycling woman, but there are other potential benefits for all women. As I've detailed many of these previously, I will only recap them here.

In a general sense at least, while dieting invariably increases hunger, exercise either has no effect or may decrease it (3). I'd reiterate that this tends to be highly variable depending on the type, amount, and intensity of exercise along with the dieter's BF% (and this interacts with their diet). There is also the huge individual variability in the increase in hunger with exercise with women being more variable than men (4). Of critical important is that exercise helps to limit the loss of LBM and it is clear that resistance training is superior to aerobic exercise (5). Additionally, by sparing LBM loss, exercise ensures that the proportion of total weight being lost from fat is maximized. This is especially true for visceral fat which is an issue for women with PCOS/subclinical hyperandrogenism or Category 3 dieters. Here aerobic activity is superior to diet alone for reducing visceral fat while strength training appears to have little effect (6,7).

Aerobic exercise may also be superior to diet alone for losing subcutaneous body fat although it must be done at least 3-4 times per week to have an impact (8). I mentioned in an earlier chapter that resistance training has been found to improve lower body fat loss, probably due to the hormonal response. Combining aerobic exercise and strength training is generally superior to doing one or the other since they tend to have different effects and purposes (9). If a dieter finds themselves in a situation where they can only choose one type of exercise, resistance training should be the first choice. In this vein, a recent study found that the combination of resistance training and diet even without aerobic exercise generated optimal results in terms of both fat loss and LBM gains (10).

With all of the above said, I'd mention again that exercise alone tends to be fairly ineffective for weight or fat loss unless fairly large amounts can be done. This is generally only possible for people who are already fairly fit or highly trained with beginners having a limited ability to burn many calories initially.

This can be increased over time and readers may remember the study I discussed in Chapter 11 where women worked up to burning 400 or 600 calories per day over 5 months, losing significant fat. In this situation, some amount of calorie restriction will be required with the combination of diet and exercise always being superior to either used in isolation (11). Even when exercise itself has no major impact on the total weight or fat loss seen from diet, it has a profound impact on long-term weight maintenance (12,13).

All of which points to the fact that, ideally, exercise should be used to create at least part of the deficit whenever possible. Keep in mind that activity, whether NEAT or formal exercise was included in the TDEE estimates in the last chapter so here I am mainly talking about increased amounts of exercise over the current level. For someone not currently on an exercise program, this will mean an increase over zero whereas for already active individuals, this will represent an increase over their baseline levels. For those individuals, depending on their current exercise program, there is often a limit to how much additional exercise can be done. A physique or strength/power athlete performing 4-5 weight training sessions only may be able to gradually add a fairly significant amount of aerobic activity while an endurance athlete already performing 15-20 hours of activity has a very limited ability to add more to their training load. In the situation where the amount of activity that can be added is limited or cannot generate the necessary deficit, some degree of calorie reduction will be required. In some cases this may represent the majority deficit, in others only a part of it.

How to Set the Deficit

With the understanding that the daily deficit for fat loss will generally be created through some combination of exercise and diet (with the relative proportions varying depending on the specifics of the situation), I want to next look at how the daily deficit should be determined. Let me note that while I will simply use the word deficit going forwards, this is within the context of the previous section: whether diet alone, exercise alone or a combination is used is irrelevant so far as the actual deficit itself is concerned. So if I suggest at some point that a 400 calorie/day deficit would be created, this could come from a 400 calorie food reduction, 400 calorie increase in activity or some combination of the two (i.e. 200 calorie foods reduction plus 200 calorie exercise increase). Since they are still in altogether too common use, let me first look at two approaches that should not be used to set the deficit.

Perhaps the oldest and worst ways of setting calorie levels for fat loss is to use some absolute calorie intake level without any consideration of body weight or activity levels. Common recommendations are 1200 calories per day for women (1500-1800 calories per day for men) or occasionally lower in some cases (Very Low Calorie Diets or VLCD may contain 400-800 calories per day for example). Exercise is generally not included with this type of approach and the above really represents the daily caloric intake rather than the deficit per se. While commonly used, this problem is ultimately flawed as it does not take factors such as body weight, BF% or activity levels into account. Certainly it was typically aimed at the general overweight or obese individual but I still think it is far too general of a recommendation to be used.

Perhaps the most common approach to setting a daily deficit is to use a basic mathematical approach to fat loss based on the old 3,500 calories per pound rule of thumb which I discussed is not entirely correct. With this approach, the dieter decides how much weight they want to lose per week and multiplies that by 3,500 to get the necessarily weekly deficit (daily deficit is determined by dividing by 7). If they want to lose 1 lb/week, they have to set a weekly deficit of 3,500 calories. This is usually divided across the week for a 500 calorie deficit per day. If they want a 2 lb/week loss, that's a 7,000 total deficit or 1,000 calories per day. Ignoring all of the issues I mentioned regarding this type of approach in a previous chapter, there is a larger one which is that the same absolute daily deficit can be profoundly different for two people with different body composition, activity levels and TDEE.

Consider a 150 lb female has a TDEE of 2250 calories per day and another at 250 lbs has a TDEE of 3000 calories per day. Applying a 500 calorie per day deficit represents a 22% reduction in TDEE for the first woman but only a 17% for the second. A 1000 calorie per day deficit is 44% for the first dieter but only 33% for the second. And this larger relative deficit could very well cause more problems for the 150 lb female in terms of the metabolic adaptations or potential to take her below the critical Energy Availability (EA) threshold. Assuming only food restriction is used to generate the deficit, a 500 calorie per day food reduction would also be a significantly larger reduction in her total food intake, potentially making hunger and adherence a problem (to expend 500 calories from activity would require a large scale increase in her current levels). In contrast, the larger female is eating more total food and will have less hunger problems reducing her food intake by that much simply because she is eating more to begin with. She also doesn't have to worry about the EA threshold to begin with.

The above dynamic is identical to what is seen when comparing a relatively lighter woman to a relatively heavier man; here it is simply applied to two women at different weights and BF%. A larger female at a higher BF% can (and probably should) lose fat more quickly (necessitating or simply allowing a larger deficit) than a smaller female. But the problems described point to the solution being to set either the daily deficit or the weekly weight/fat loss targets as a percentage of the dieter's starting point. I want to describe two methods in this chapter although both generate effectively the same end result.

Setting the Deficit as a Percentage of TDEE

The method I have traditionally used and recommended is to set the daily deficit as some percentage of the current TDEE. So consider the two women above who both apply create a 20% deficit to their TDEE. At 2225 calories per day, the first woman will have a daily deficit of 450 calories per day (2225 calories/day * 0.20) while the second will have a daily deficit of 600 calories per day (3000 cal/day * 0.20). The absolute deficit is higher in the second case but the relative deficit is identical. To match the fat loss of the second dieter, the first would have to create a 27% deficit (2225 * 0.27 = 600 calories), identical to the fact that smaller women have to perform more total exercise to match the calorie expenditure of (generally larger) men. In using this method, it is common to define small, medium/moderate and large/aggressive deficits which correspond to a 10-20%, 25-30% and 40% or higher deficit relatively to TDEE. Each deficit has its own pros and cons and I want to look at each briefly.

Small deficits tend to require the smallest changes to lifestyle and relatively small reductions in food intake or increases in activity will be required to create it (even an untrained individual will be able to create at least some of the total deficit with activity). The Category 1 woman is almost assured of not crossing the critical EA threshold as well. For women in Category 2 or 3 this can be useful in that relatively small, qualitative changes in the diet (i.e. switching from juice or soda to water or Diet drinks) may be all that is required to reduce calories by the desired amount. For some people at least, small changes are more likely to be adopted although this is not universal. One recent study did find that aiming for a smaller (10%) rather than moderate (30%) deficit actually led to better results in at least some dieters (14). In this case, the dieters aiming for the smaller deficit ending up creating a larger one overall while those aiming for the larger deficit showed worse long-term adherence to the diet.

The biggest disadvantage to the small deficit is the relative slow rate of fat loss that will occur. Unless someone has an enormous TDEE, a 10-20% deficit simply will not be that large. Certainly a slow rate of fat loss is often superior for lean Category 1 women, especially near the end of the diet, but the Category 2 or 3 female may find that slow rates of fat loss disappointing, compromising adherence. One very real problem with the small deficit is that even small mistakes in food intake or measurement can severely reduce or even eliminate the deficit. Consider a small Category 1 female who is targeting a 200 day reduction in food intake and a 200 calorie increase in activity. If she eats even 100 calories over her goal by mistake, her deficit is significantly reduced and her already slow fat loss will be even slower.

The medium/moderate deficit is arguably the one that is most commonly recommended and for good reason. First, it generates more fat loss than the small deficit while only requiring moderately larger changes to diet or activity. For example the smaller dieter with a 2250 calorie TDEE above would have to increase her daily deficit from 450 cal/day on the small deficit to 560-675 cal/day on a moderate deficit. This doesn't require an enormously larger amounts of food restriction or increase in activity levels. Certainly an untrained individual may be unlikely to generate more than a small portion of the total deficit from activity but the highly trained individual can probably generate a significant amount, decreasing the need to reduce calories.

Hormonally, a 30% deficit is about the largest that might allow a woman to remain above the critical EA threshold and even here she may cross it slightly which can cause menstrual cycle dysfunction down the road. This level of deficit is generally not so large as to compromise an athlete's training. Both of these issues are readily addressed by ensuring that calories are raised to maintenance with a sufficient frequency. The Category 2 and 3 dieters may find that this approach strikes a perfect balance between the slower fat loss of the small deficit and the extreme nature of the large deficit.

Finally is the large or aggressive deficit, generally referring to a 40-50% or greater deficit from TDEE (in some new dietary approaches I will discuss in Chapter 23, some days may have a deficit of 75% below maintenance). For the female above with a 2250 calorie TDEE, this would mean a 900-1125 calorie/day or greater deficit (or nearly 1700 calories at 75% below maintenance). Perhaps the biggest potential benefit of this size deficit is that it has the potential to generate the largest and fastest fat losses possible. But there are a number of potential cons as well. First, recall from Chapter 14 that aggressive dietary approaches may be less efficient in the sense that the actual fat loss does not increase in proportion to the deficit due to faster and/or larger rates of metabolic adaptation. Of primary importance is that the large deficit requires enormous changes in lifestyle.

Since only the most highly trained athletes would even have the potential to create such a large deficit from activity (and even here that would mean adding a staggering amount to their current level), those changes will have to come almost exclusively from the diet. This usually means removing all or nearly all of the carbohydrate and fat from the diet leaving mostly protein and some fibrous vegetables (my own Rapid Fat Loss Handbook is designed around this approach). This is not inherently a problem and so long as such diets are based around whole foods, they can be very effective both for fat loss and to retrain/create a good baseline of proper nutrition. This can be particularly useful for the Category 2/3 dieter assuming that the diet can be adhered to. Frequently, the best approach is to use an aggressive deficit initially before adding food back to the diet and moving to a moderate/medium deficit for the longer term.

For the Category 1 or highly active female, there are a number of other potential cons to an aggressive approach. One is that the Category 1 female will absolutely and immediately go below the critical EA threshold with this type of approach. This can at least be addressed by modifying the diet and raising calories frequently enough. As well, training will invariably suffer and/or have to be significantly reduced during the diet. In this situation, the best use of the aggressive deficit is a short 2-4 week diet to achieve a rapid fat loss before returning to normal eating and training.

Determining Realistic Weekly Rates of Weight/Fat Loss

A second approach to setting the deficit is to set target weekly weight/fat loss as a percentage of the dieter's initial total body weight (in this case LBM is not used). This is conceptually identical to setting calorie surpluses based on goal weight gain and allows the required deficit to be calculated in reverse. While any percentage of current weight could be used as a goal, 0.5%, 1.0% and 1.5% tend to be the most commonly used. Certainly there is no reason that intermediate values such as 0.75% or 1.25% could not be selected. This percentage is multiplied by the current body weight to determine the weekly goal weight loss and this is then multiplied by 3,500 calories per pound to determine the weekly and daily deficits (for women it is generally safe to assume that most if not all of the weight loss is coming from fat).

So consider the two women above who both target a weekly loss of 0.5% of their weight. This yields a 0.75 lb/week weight loss for the 150 lb female (150 lbs * 0.05 = 0.75 lbs), requiring a weekly deficit of 2625 calories (0.75 lbs * 3500 = 2625) which can be divided by 7 to get a 375 calorie per day deficit. The 250 lb female will also target a 0.5% weight loss which will be 1.4 lbs per week, requiring a 4800 calorie per week deficit or roughly 680 calories per day. Note that these values are very close to the 375 and 600 cal/day deficits that the 20%/small deficit above generated.

I've shown predicted weekly weight losses in pounds along with the weekly and daily deficits for women of different body weights. The numbers listed under the percentages are weekly weight/fat losses while the values under weekly and daily are the calorie deficits needed. Roughly speaking, the 0.5% level corresponds to the small deficit, 1.0% to the medium deficit and 1.5% the large deficit.

Weight	0.5%	Weekly	Daily	1.0%	Weekly	Daily	1.5%	Weekly	Daily
120	0.6	2100	300	1.2	4200	600	1.8	6300	900
130	0.65	2275	325	1.3	4550	650	1.95	6825	975
140	0.7	2450	350	1.4	4900	700	2.1	7350	1050
150	0.75	2625	375	1.5	5250	750	2.25	7875	1125
160	0.8	2800	400	1.6	5600	800	2.4	8400	1200
170	0.85	2975	425	1.7	5950	850	2.55	8925	1275
180	0.9	3150	450	1.8	6300	900	2.7	9450	1350
190	0.95	3325	475	1.9	6650	950	2.85	9975	1425
200	1	3500	500	2	7000	1000	3	10500	1500
250	1.25	4375	625	2.5	8750	1250	3.75	13125	1875
300	1.5	5250	750	3	10500	1500	4.5	15750	2250

By looking at this chart, it becomes clear that the old idea of a 1-2 lb per week weight/fat loss being a reasonable goal only holds in specific situations. A smaller Category 1 female targeting the 0.5% value for fat loss will be losing less than 1 pound of fat per week while a heavier Category 3 female using the 1.5% value might be losing 3-4 pounds per week or more. This fact alone should hopefully demonstrate why any approach to setting a deficit or goal must take into account the person in question. Heavier women with a higher BF% can lose far more quickly than smaller women with a lower BF%. As with percentage based deficit, which of the above weekly targets is appropriate depends on the specific situation being discussed. The amount of fat that needs to be lost, the dieter's Category, whether or not a time frame to reach a certain goal is present, the length of the diet and other all factor in to what rate of fat loss is most appropriate. So let me next look at how specific populations can or should set their fat loss goals.

Let me finish by addressing what may seem like a contradiction in this chapter. When I discussed poor methods of setting the deficit, I described the approach of selecting a weekly weight loss goal (i.e. 1-2 lbs) and calculating the deficit based on math. Conceptually this may seem similar to the above approach where weekly weight loss goals are calculated and the deficit determined by the same math. While it is similar, the difference is that the weight loss goals are based on current bodyweight rather than some fixed value. For a 130 lb female to target a 2 lb/week weight loss will create a diet or exercise program that will be nearly impossible to achieve in most cases. If that same dieter uses a percentage of their current weight, they will determine a realistic weekly weight loss goal for their individual needs. The same holds true for heavier women and the point is that using some absolute deficit of 500 cal/day or absolute weight loss goal does not take the individual into account. Using a percentage deficit or percentage weight loss goal does.

Chapter 18: Goal Setting

Having looked at how calories should be adjusted from the estimated maintenance, I want to move to the topic of goal setting. By this, I am not referring to the general goals that I discussed in Chapter 4 but how best to determine the desired or required amount of change in body weight, body fat or muscle mass to reach that general goal. While I will look at gaining lean body mass (LBM) first, primarily in terms of what represents realistic goals for total amounts of LBM, the majority of the chapter will be focused on dieting and fat loss since that tends to be a more common goal and has more specifics to consider. Setting goals for dieting is extremely population specific and I will be looking at a number of factors for each group. A primary issue is how much total weight/fat loss is desired or required to reach a certain goal. Additional factors include whether or not there is a specific time constraint on reaching that goal. I will also look at how the menstrual cycle (for normally cycling women) may or may not impact the end goal. I'll also make suggestions for what degree of deficit might be most appropriate in a given situation.

General Goal Setting

While an individual's goals can be set in many different ways, perhaps the best way is to apply the acronym SMART. This refers to goals being Specific, Measurable, Achievable, Relevant and Time Based. Specific means exactly that, a goal of losing 20 lbs of fat, gaining 5 lbs of muscle or lifting weights three times per week is specific while losing weight, getting bigger or being more active is not. Measurable means that progress (or lack thereof) towards the goal can be tracked and this is part of why the goal has to be specific in the first place. If the current fat loss goal is 20 lbs and only 10 lbs have been lost, the dieter knows that they are only half way to their goal. Achievable means that the person should have some chance of actually reaching that goal although in some cases unrealistic goals may actually be superior (similarly very low goals may not be motivating enough to pursue). Achievability also ties in with the issue of time discussed below.

Relevant means that the goals are relevant to the person's interests and abilities. Someone who sets a goal to be an elite distance runner but who only has the time to run three times per week is setting a goal that is not relevant to their abilities (nor is it achievable). Time based refers to the fact that setting a time frame to reach a goal helps to keep the individual focused on what they are trying to accomplish. Someone who sets out to lose 10 lbs of fat with no time frame has no reason to remain focused on their goal or what is needed to achieve it. In contrast, if they set a three month limit on reaching that goal, they will be much more likely to do so. Any time based goal that is set must actually be achievable. Expecting to lose 50 lbs of fat or gain 10 lbs of muscle in 3 months is unrealistic no matter what the person does.

In this regard, it is often useful to set multiple goals for different durations of time. This includes short-term (1 month), medium-term (several month), and long-term (one year) goals. Realistically achievable goals can be set for each time frame and this not only helps the person to maintain focus but breaks up what may seem like impossible (or impossibly far away) goals into more reasonable blocks. A long-term goal of 50 lbs fat loss in a year can be broken two six-month goals of 25 lbs and 12 one month goals of merely 4 lbs fat loss. While the 50 lb goal may seem overwhelming or impossible, the 4 pound monthly short-term goals are more reasonable and likely to be achieved. Finally, some recommend setting dream goals, the ultimate goal that might finally be reached assuming everything goes right. The dream goal might or might not actually be realistically achievable but, as I'll discuss more below, can often help to keep individuals focused over the longer term. What the dream goal might be will be population specific. For someone seeking fat loss, it might be the final weight or BF% they wish to hit. For an athlete, it might be competing at the national or world level. For the physique athlete it might be reaching nationals.

Gaining LBM

While the goal of gaining (or at least maintaining) LBM is an important one for all women, many readers of this book may only be interested in gaining relatively small amounts without huge consideration for the total amount that is or has been gained. The combination of proper resistance training with some basic changes in diet generally accomplishes this without difficulty or attention to many specifics. For that reason, this section will be aimed at those women who are deliberately trying to gain muscle. This could be the serious trainee simply trying to improve appearance, the physique athlete looking to optimize their physique for competition or the performance athlete attempting to gain muscle for performance reasons. In some cases, this might represent a relatively small amounts of muscle gain while in others, the goal might be to gain the maximum amount of muscle possible.

Since it will vary so much depending on a female's goal, I cannot provide recommendations on how much muscle should ideally be gained. Rather, I want to focus on two more inter-related issues which are the maximum amount of muscle that can be gained along with the speed with which it might be gained (this is required to determine the size of the surplus). I addressed the second in the last chapter in terms of monthly goal weight increases relative to the number of years of proper training but this interacts with maximum potential. The further a woman is from her maximum the faster she can gain and vice versa.

So what is the maximum amount of LBM (here I am talking about total LBM, not just muscle) that a woman might carry? A variety of studies have examined this in different types of athletes, finding LBM in the realm of of 125-140 pounds (56.8-63.6 kg) for women weighing between 144 and 165 lb (1,2). None of these studies were on competitive bodybuilders, who's aim is to maximize muscle mass, and it's conceivable that higher levels of LBM would be seen given that the sport is geared towards maximizing muscle size. One study compared female powerlifters to bodybuilders, finding that the powerlifters had 119 lbs (54kg) and the bodybuilders 108 lbs (49 kg) of LBM (3). Another compared female bodybuilders to athletic females, finding that the bodybuilders had 119 lbs LBM (54kg) while the athletic females only carried 99 lbs (45 kg) of LBM (4). Given the nature of the sports, it is somewhat surprising that the powerlifters and bodybuilders in these two studies have LBM levels below those seen in other sports.

I have no real explanation for this although the lower LBM values are from relatively older studies while the higher values are from more recent work. A larger talent pool along with better training and nutrition might be contributing to these results. In that vein, looking at online competition results, a recent Natural Superheavyweight female bodybuilding world champion weighed 130 lbs (59 kg) on the day of her competition. Assuming she competed at 10% body fat, that would put her at 13 lbs of fat and 117 lbs of LBM (identical to this book's sample dieter). Bodybuilders are typically somewhat dehydrated on the day of a competition and, if she lost some LBM during her diet, her off season LBM might be as high as 125-130 pounds (56.8-59kg), similar to the other values above.

In general, taller and/or heavier women may be able to carry more LBM. In a study referenced above on elite athletes, an LBM of 154 lbs (70 kg) was recorded in a 200 lb (90 kg) athlete who was most likely a superheavyweight weightlifter or thrower (some of this LBM represents increased water, glycogen and connective tissue). Height is also a factor and tends to show a relatively strong relationship with the total amount of LBM that is seen in female athletes. One early study comparing female and male bodybuilders found that the females had a 1.73 lbs/inch (0.31 kg/cm) ratio of LBM to height (5). So a 5'5" (65 inch/167 cm) female might realistically carry 114 lbs of LBM, well below the values listed above. Another study, looking at athletes from different sports found an average value for female athletes of 1.51-1.84 lb/inch (0.27-0.33 kg/cm) of LBM (6). It also identified several extreme outliers, six women exceeding 132 lbs (60kg) of LBM with one reaching 180 lbs (82.1 kg) of LBM at a bodyweight of 215 lbs (98 kg) at a height of 6'2" (188 cm). This yielded a value of 2.45 lb/inch (0.44 kg/cm) of LBM which they suggested as a theoretical maximum value for female athletes. This was actually close to values for the lighter males and I have to see it as an outlier (or an indication of steroid use) rather than any sort of realistic goal.

Height	Inches	1.51 lb/inch	Weight (lbs)	1.67 lb/inch	Weight (lbs)	1.84 lb/inch	Weight (lbs)
5'0"	60	90.5	116	100	128.5	110.5	141.5
5'1"	61	92	118	102	130.5	112	144
5'2"	62	93.5	120	103.5	132.5	114	146
5'3"	63	95	122	105	135	116	148
5'4"	64	96.5	124	107	137	118	151
5'5"	65	98	126	108.5	139	119.5	154
5'6"	66	100	129	110	141.5	123	158
5'7"	67	101	130	112	143.5	123	158
5'8"	68	103	131.5	113.5	145.5	125.1	160
5'9"	69	104	133.5	115	148	127	163
5'10"	70	105.5	135.5	117	150	129	165
5'11"	71	107	137.5	118.5	152	130.5	167.5
6'0"	72	109	139.5	120	154	132.5	170

Divide height in cm by 2.54 to get inches, divide LBM/weight by 2.2 to get kg

With that in mind, I have calculated the potential amounts of LBM that women of different heights might carry based on the more realistic values in the chart above. To put this in more real world terms, I've also shown what their total bodyweight would be assuming 22% body fat. Simply to make the point, using the theoretical maximum value, a 5'7" woman would have 164 lbs LBM, 41 lbs more than the high average value above and simply an unrealistic goal for almost all women. A current top professional female bodybuilder competes with 141-149 lbs LBM at 5'7" and this is a sport marked by steroid abuse.

At any given height it's fairly clear that women may vary significantly in the maximum amount of LBM that they might realistically be able to carry. This is going to be related to genetics and overall hormone levels with women having elevated levels of testosterone being far more likely to be at the higher levels of LBM relative to their height than those without. This is consistent with the finding that women with PCOS/hyperandrogenism are found in large percentages of high level sport, their hormones giving them a competition advantage. To the above maximum values, I would add that most women will be very close to their genetic limits after perhaps 3-4 years of proper training. Beyond that point, gains in muscle mass will be slow to the point of being almost insignificant.

All of this information can be used to determine how much more potential muscle mass might be gained going forwards and it's important to be realistic here in terms of what is possible. The 1.84 lb/inch value for maximum muscle mass is likely to hold for the majority of women and some will not even reach that level. A woman who has been training properly for 2-3 years who is between the first and second columns above may have the potential to achieve the second column with another year or two of intense training but she will be unlikely to come close to the third column. In contrast, a woman who has surpassed the second column by her second year of proper training is likely to reach or at least get close to the third column in terms of her maximum LBM. This can be used to determine what level of surplus should actually be used. If a trainee determines that she only has the potential to gain 5 more pounds of LBM, she might target as little as 1/2 pound of LBM per month during a gaining phase. Alternately she could look at the number of years she has been properly training and aim for a percentage bodyweight increase per month. In either case the surplus would be calculated as per the last chapter.

The General Dieter

Moving to dieting and fat loss, let me first look at the general dieter. While this can technically include women in any category (recall the population of inactive Category 1 females), it's arguably more common to find Category 2-3 women in this group. Typically, the general dieter tends to focus only on weight loss although I hope that the earlier chapters of this book have shown that body composition/BF% are more important. I would note that, in Category 2 and 3 especially, weight and fat loss tend to be synonymous so long as the very early rapid weight loss is ignored. The risk of LBM/muscle mass loss in this population is essentially zero so long as a basic exercise program and proper diet is in place meaning that a 5 lb weight loss will most likely represent a 5 lbs fat loss (if some amount of LBM is gained, total fat loss will exceed weight loss). As I've mentioned this may not be the case for the Category 1 female here.

In at least a general sense, the goal of weight/fat loss in this group tends to be aimed at improving appearance more than health although this in't universal. For example, the Category 3/PCOS woman may desire fat loss to improve fertility or overall health. As I've mentioned previously, even moderate fat losses of 5-10% of current body weight can have significant effects here. Quite in fact, this 5-10% weight/fat loss goal is often held up as a good goal for most weight loss efforts, primarily due to the fact that losses greater than this are often poorly maintained in the long-term. Putting this in perspective, a 5-10% total fat loss would represent 12.5-25 lbs for a 250 lb Category 3 woman, 10-20 lbs for a 200 lb Category 2 woman and 7.5-15 lbs for a 150 lb Category 1 woman and this will have clinically meaningful benefits on health. But will those levels be sufficient or satisfying for most women?

Research on this topic typically find that women both expect and desire significantly greater losses than the 5-10% above. They also tend to have unrealistic expectation about the ease with which they will achieve those losses (most information on diet does not help here as it promises rapid, easy and enormous weight losses). In one study, nearly half of women expressed unrealistic weight loss goals that were 50% above medically recommended levels of 10-20% of current body weight (8). That is, the women expected a total weight loss of 15-30% of their current weight. In another, women had a goal weight that was 32% below their current weight, stating that a 55 lb (25kg) weight loss would be acceptable while a 37.5 lb (17kg) weight loss would be disappointing (9). After 48 weeks of dieting, 47% of the women had failed to reach even their disappointing weight loss goal. Almost universally dieters set unrealistic weight loss goals and, unsurprisingly, women are more likely to do so than men (10).

And while this would logically suggest that setting more moderate weight loss goals is superior to setting unrealistic goal, this isn't necessarily the case with several studies suggesting that women who set larger weight loss goals experience more success. In one study, obese women who set weight loss goals of 20-30% of their current weight (60-90 lbs for a 300 lb woman) had no worse results than women who set more moderate goal (11). Quite in fact, and contrary to what you might expect, the women who set the highest dream goals (goals that were higher than even the long-term goals) lost more weight after 18 months compared to those with lower dream goals. Presumably, setting a higher goal kept them more focused on their efforts over time. This may not be universal and individual readers may find that unrealistic goals are demoralizing due to dissatisfaction with slow progress towards them.

Since long-term and dream goals can sometimes be a bit overwhelming to dieters, I suggest setting additional short- or medium-term goals which represent a portion of the long-term goal. An ultimate dream-goal that might take multiple years could be broken into a long-term goal of a year which could be broken into multiple medium-term goals of 4-6 months duration which could be further broken into short-term goals of 1-2 months. Repeated achievement of the shorter terms goals not only brings the dieter closer to their medium-, long-term and dream goals but helps to build confidence and what is called self-efficacy, the belief that something can be accomplished.

As most of the research on this topic is done on overweight or obese women, I want to look at goal setting relative to diet Category. Since there is a general relationship with this and starting body weight, setting any goal in absolute or even percentage terms will be inappropriate. A Category 1 dieter can't target a 30 lb loss or 30% reduction in their current weight although this might be more than appropriate for a heavier Category 3 female. By the same token, a 10% weight loss goal for a Category 3 woman who weighs 250 pound (114kg) only represents 25 pounds (11.4 kg). While clinically meaningful and more easily sustained in the long-term, this is unlikely to be satisfying. In general, I would probably recommend the following as long-term goals for each Category. In the chart below, I've shown the dieter's weight/Category and BF% (using relatively representative numbers) along with a goal percentage loss, the total fat loss that will be required and the ending BF% when that loss is achieved.

Weight	BF%	Cat	Long-Term	Total Fat Loss	End Weight	End BF%
130	24%	1	5%	7.5 lbs	122.5 lbs	19%
180	35%	2	15%	27 lbs	144 lbs	24%
250	45%	3	20%	50 lbs	200 lbs	31%

As you can see, with even a relatively small 5% goal, the Category 1 female will achieve a body fat level of 19% and anything more than this would take her to a BF% that is either undesirable in terms of appearance or impossible to maintain. As body weight and Category go up, the percentage and absolute losses will both potentially increase. In all cases, the losses I have calculated will have meaningful health and appearance effects with the Category 2 woman reaching the top of Category 1 and the Category 3 female achieving Category 2 if the above goals are met. Dream goals for Category 2 and 3 can potentially be higher and might be as high as 20% (36 lbs fat loss) and 30% for the Category 3 female (75 lbs) with the understanding that it may or may not be met.

Ignoring the dream goal for a moment, that long-term goal would be broken down into one or more short-term goals. I say one or more as heavier individuals might or might not be able to reach their goals in one single dieting phase. As the amount of fat loss being targeted goes up, this becomes progressively more and more difficult in both a psychological and physiological sense. For a 250 woman to lose even 50 pounds (23 kg) is likely to take at least one year if not longer (in one study I mentioned above, women achieved a 35 lb/16 kg loss in 48 weeks). It's both impossible to think in those terms or to diet continuously for that long without a break for both psychological and physiological reasons.

I mentioned the use of breaks in Chapter 14 and will discuss it in more detail in Chapter 21 and will recommend breaks at varying frequencies depending on Category. A Category 3 dieter might realistically diet for 4-6 months without needing a break (thought they might choose to take one sooner) while a Category 2 female might diet for 2-4 months before a break. The Category 1 female might only take a break every 2 months and that might be more than sufficient to achieve the relatively small losses required. The long-term goal would simply be divided up by the number of dieting blocks with the understanding that weekly fat loss will be slower later in the diet as the body adapts.

To put all of the above information together, I've shown some potential short-term, long-term and dream goals in the chart below (medium-term goals are not shown and simply represent a series of short-term goals strung together) to expand on the chart above. The values meant to be representative only of how dream goals might be broken into long-, medium- and short-term goals. For each, I've shown the total weight loss achieved along with the ending weight. Long-term goals are roughly 2-3 months for Category 1, 6 months for Category 2 and, 12 months for Category 3. Due to the relatively low losses required, medium-term goals wouldn't apply for Category 1 and the duration here corresponds to the amount of time between diet breaks which are roughly 2 months for Category 2 and 4 months for Category 3. Short-term goals represent monthly goals. I am also assuming a roughly 1% goal weight loss per month in each case.

Cat	Weight	Dream	Wt Loss	End Weight	Long	Weight	Med.	Weight	Short	Weight
1	130 lbs	7.5-10%	10-13 lbs	~120 lbs	5 lbs	125 lbs	N/A	N/A	3 lbs	127 lbs
2	180 lbs	15-20%	27-36 lbs	153 lbs	15 lbs	165 lbs	7.5 lbs*	172.5 lbs	7. 5 lbs	176 lbs
3	250 lbs	30%+	75 lbs	175 lbs	40 lbs	210 lbs	20 lbs*	230 lbs	10 lbs	210

While the above can be useful, I would more often recommend that the general dieter at most set goals and then focus primarily on the process. Fat loss always occurs more slowly than predicted (or desired) and while time based goals are better than non-time based goals, expecting exact targets to be hit without fail can be more problematic than not. This is especially true if falling short of the desired goal causes the dieter to give up completely. Dieting and fat loss is a process and focusing on that process tends to work better than focusing only on the end goal. At the same time, not having somewhat of a specific goal can be equally detrimental and finding a balance will be the key. Outside of the potential for the normally cycling dieter to have water weight shifts that may throw off measurements of body weight, there are generally no issues to be considered. Only the Category 1 dieter would be at risk for issues related to a low EA state but their generally low goal fat losses should prevent any major problems from occurring.

So far as choosing the deficit size/goal weekly weight loss, technically any of the three levels (0.5%,1.0% or 1.5% per week) could be used in this situation. If exercise is being done, it is unlikely to be so intensive as to be harmed excessively by hard dieting and, realistically, reaching their weight/fat loss goals is a bigger priority than maintaining exercise performance for this group. Certainly for the Category 1 woman a 1.5% weekly weight loss goal will be difficult to achieve even if most women try to diet that way. For very short time spans of perhaps 2-4 weeks it can be effective and will likely get her to her goal but it should not be used for longer than this. Resistance training must be part of this approach or the Category 1 woman is likely to lose so much LBM that she will rebound to a higher BF%. Overall, for Category 1 women, the 0.5% or 1.0% goals are probably more appropriate overall.

As the Category 2 women will generally have more total weight and fat to lose, the 0.5% weekly loss may be too slow. The 1.0% level or possibly the 1.5% per week level to start the diet would be appropriate here. If 1.5% is used initially to generate rapid fat losses, it could be changed to a 1% weekly weight loss goal after the medium-term goal is reached. For the Category 3 woman, the degree of fat loss required and the realistic duration of dieting involved would tend to make the 0.5% level inappropriate due to slow rates of fat loss. The 1.0% level would provide a nice balance of rate of fat loss and difficulty but using a 6-8 week block at 1.5% before moving to a more moderate 1.0% can be very effective.

In terms of menstrual cycle effects, the general lack of a time constraint on reaching the dieting goal in this population makes issues with water weight shifts, etc. mostly inconsequential. The normally cycling woman must simply realize that changes in water weight need to be taken into account in terms of tracking progress. It is also beneficial for the normally cycling woman to try to start her diet during the follicular phase when hunger and appetite is best controlled to give the best chance for success early on.

All Other Dieters: Introduction

While it would be ideal if the general dieter focused on changes in BF% and body composition, this may represent an unnecessary level of detail in the initial stages, especially since weight and fat loss will be more or less identical. In contrast, all other dieters must focus primarily if not exclusively on their BF% rather than their weight per se. I say primarily here as athletes in sports with weight classes will have to reach a specific target weight as well. More than just focusing on the changes in BF% (i.e. lose 3% body fat), it's more common to have a goal BF% (i.e. 18%) that is either simply desired or required by the sport. This makes it necessary to determine the total fat/weight loss that will be required to reach that goal.

Before looking at that calculation, I want to make a few comment about goal setting for athletes or the serious trainee. Because just as the general dieter often sets unrealistic goals in terms of the amount or rate of weight loss that will occur, athletes often set similarly unrealistic goals. This can take many forms but one of the most common is to vastly overestimate the amount of fat loss that can be lost or, perhaps more importantly, how quickly it can be lost (men invariably overestimate the amount of muscle that they can gain and how quickly it can be gained). More specifically, both athletes and the serious trainee tend to have exaggerated ideas about how much fat can be lost in a reasonable amount of time. Women in Category 1 expect to drop to the lowest limits of female BF% in only 12 weeks when, realistically, it might take twice that amount of time. A Category 2 female would require a year of strict dieting to reach those same lower limits although she might expect or hope to reach it in half that time or less.

As a general rule here, I would suggest that female dieters should not aim to drop more than one half to a full category in any single diet before taking a relatively extended break to maintain tha new BF% level. The woman at 35% body fat (high Category 2) might set a goal of 30% (middle Category 2) while the woman at 30% might set 25% as her intermediate goal. This would be reached before taking a break before continuing to diet as desired. This doesn't hold for the woman in Category 1 who is trying to diet to the lowest levels of female BF%. This goal almost always has a specific time frame and it is not feasible to diet down halfway before taking an extended break. Rather, this group will perform one single extended diet punctuated by short breaks until the goal is attained.

Determining Total Fat Loss for Athletes

Once the goal BF% level has been determined, and more specific values will be given below for different situations, it will be necessary to calculate the total amount of weight/fat loss required to reach that from the current BF%. The first step is to use the calculation at the end of Chapter 5 to determine the total amount of fat and LBM present. This is done by multiplying body weight by BF% as a decimal (i.e. 24% becomes 0.24) to get the total amount of fat and subtracting this value from total weight to get LBM. For the book's sample dieter at 150 lbs/22% body fat, this yields 33 lbs of fat and 117 lbs of LBM. The LBM value will now be used to determine her target weight and fat loss to reach her goal.

To perform the goal weight/fat loss calculation, first the goal BF% should be converted to a decimal and then subtracted from one (i.e. 24% is converted to 0.24 which is subtracted from 1 to get 0.76). The total amount of LBM will be divided by this value and this will determine the goal weight that must be achieved. The target weight is then subtracted from the current weight to determine the total fat loss required. I've shown the values that LBM should be divided by for different values of BF% in the chart below. Other values can be calculated.

Goal BF%	10	12	15	18	20	25	30
Divide LBM by	0.9	0.88	0.85	0.82	0.8	0.75	0.7

Using those values, I've shown how the sample dieter with 117 lbs of LBM would calculate her goal weight and total weight loss to reach 12% body fat.

Step 1: Determine Goal Bodyweight
Divide LBM by 1 minus the BF% as a decimal.
117 lbs LBM/0.88 = 133 lbs
Step 2: Determine Goal Weight Loss
Subtract goal weight from current weight
150 lbs - 133 lbs = 17 lbs total weight loss

The above calculation assumes 100% fat loss which may or may not be a safe assumption. In general, as BF% decreases, there is a greater risk for LBM loss but recall that women are at less risk than men in this regard. Several case studies that I will discuss in Chapter 34 found that Category 1 women were able to diet to low BF% levels with essentially zero LBM loss by combining resistance training with sufficient dietary protein. Even so, adding 10% to the target weight loss to account for potential LBM losses may be beneficial to ensure that sufficient total fat is lost. This entails multiplying the goal weight loss by 1.1 yielding slightly under 19 lbs (17 * 1.1 = 18.7 lbs) of total weight loss. Subtracted from 150 lbs, this would put her at 131 lbs at 12% body fat, 115 lbs of LBM and 16 lbs of fat. For the Category 2/3 woman, fat loss should almost always be 100% of total weight loss and no adjustment will be needed.

The Serious Trainee

As I described in an earlier chapter, I use the term serious recreational trainee to describe any woman involved in a moderate to high amount of training including proper resistance and/or aerobic/HIIT training but who is not interested or planning to compete in any sort of sport. Generally, the serious trainee will be found in Category 1 or 2 although it's not impossible that a woman in Category 3 might be in this group. Most in this group will have moved past focusing only on bodyweight with body composition and appearance being the larger priorities. Goals may include adding some amount of muscle mass but will tend to be focused on achieving a goal BF% or, more frequently, a visual appearance that corresponds to a given BF%. The woman seeking to be generally lean and fit but with some muscularity (to appear "toned") might target 22-24% or so as a goal BF%. Many wish to go lower but, in many cases, the goal BF% is unsustainable in the long-term. As a general rule, I'd suggest a BF% goal of no lower than 18% as sustainable and healthy (in terms of avoiding a low EA situation or menstrual cycle/hormonal problems).

With a target BF% between 18% and 24%, goal weight losses in this group will be determined by dividing LBM by a value between 0.82 (for 18%) and 0.76 (for 24%). A female at 135 lbs and 22% body fat (30 lbs fat and 105 lbs LBM) who wants to reach 18% body fat will divide her LBM by 0.82 and her goal weight will be 128 lbs. This will require a total 7 lbs fat loss (135 lbs - 128 lbs) which might be adjusted upwards by 10% (to roughly 8 lbs total weight loss) to account for potential LBM losses. A 160 lb female at 30% body fat with 48 lbs of fat and 112 lbs of LBM who wants to reach 24% would divide her LBM by 0.76 for a target weight of 147 lbs. This will require a 13 lb fat loss and LBM loss is unlikely to be significant if resistance training is performed with a sufficient protein intake.

Unlike competitive athletes, discussed in the next sections, the serious trainee rarely has any explicit time constraints on when they must reach their goals. There can be exceptions, some gyms will run weight loss competitions (where unfortunately, the focus is on bodyweight only) and there are often physique transformation contests which allow some time frame such as 12 weeks to make the largest changes possible. In many cases, any time constraint is set by the trainee themselves, attempting to reach a certain goal prior to a vacation or swimsuit season or what have you. Even outside of those situations, time bound goals may help to keep the dieter focused and should usually be set regardless of the specific situation. This of course assumes that the goal being set is achievable in the first place and the serious trainee is as likely to set an unrealistic goal as the general dieting public.

This makes it useful to look at what might be a realistic goal to set and here I'll be assuming a 12 week time frame. Referring back to the chart on page 169, a 0.5% weekly weight loss goal will have women in this group losing roughly 3/4 lb per week (slightly less for very light women and slightly more for heavier women) and the majority of this will be from fat. Over 12 weeks this allows for a maximum of about 9 lbs of total fat loss although it will be slightly lower than this due to metabolic adaptation. At this rate, the first dieter above (seeking a 7-8 lb loss) should achieve or get very close to her goal at this rate of fat loss while the second dieter (requiring 13 lbs of fat loss) will not. To use this weekly rate of weight loss, she would need at least 16-18 weeks of total dieting or will need to adjust her goal downwards.

If the goal weekly weight loss is increased to 1% per week, the average weekly loss will double to 1.5 lbs per week and ~15 lbs of fat could theoretically be lost in 12 weeks (again, it will be somewhat lower than this). This would allow the first dieter to reach her fat loss goal in 6-8 weeks of the 12 week diet allowing for several weeks to gain a small amount of muscle mass. She might diet for 4 weeks, switch to gaining muscle (aiming for perhaps 1 lb total weight gain) for 4 weeks and then finish dieting for 4 weeks. Alternately she could start her diet later or end it sooner and simply maintain. The second female would need to use at least this size deficit to have a chance of reaching her 13 lb fat loss goal in 12 weeks. For the serious trainee, a 1.5% weekly weight loss goal could be used but only for a short period of time. On average it will yield a roughly 2 lb/week loss and this would get the first dieter to or very close to her goal in only 4 weeks (which is about the longest she could use such an approach). The second dieter might reach hers in only 7-8 weeks or so and this would be possible given that she is in Category 2.

As with the general dieter, the general lack of an explicit time frame to reach the dieting goal makes menstrual cycle effects less problematic. Certainly a diet that ends in the late-follicular or late-luteal phase may make visual comparisons problematic due to water retention but unless the dieter is doing some type of body transformation contest this should be of minimal importance. For those women this could be a problem and having her first measurements take place in one part of the cycle while the end measurements are taken in a different part may be unfair. In terms of winning, having the initial measurements taken in the late luteal-phase and the ending in the early follicular would give the biggest difference in total weight loss. Ideally the diet should start in the early follicular phase when hunger and appetite is best controlled.

Performance Athletes

While I separated performance athletes into different categories such as strength/power, high-intensity performance, mixed and endurance I will discuss them all together here (weight-class athletes are discussed below). In the most general sense, athletes in this group do not have to reach any specific BF% (in the sense that physique athletes or those seeking appearance goals). However, most sports do tend to have fairly standard/optimal BF% levels and it is often beneficial to reduce BF% or weight from a performance standpoint. Excess body fat (or muscle) is dead weight that either slows the athlete or increases the amount of energy that is required to propel them through space. There are also sports such as ballet, gymnastics or figure skating that have an aesthetic component and where women carrying excess fat or muscle may be judged downward because of that. As I've mentioned, even outside of those sports, the reality is that women are almost always under intense social pressure for their appearance. Many if not most sports involve wearing tight uniforms during competition and, regardless of sport, this puts a female athlete's appearance at the forefront. Quite in fact, it's not uncommon for sports commentators to focus on a female athlete's appearance rather than her performance, something that would be unheard of towards a male.

Which isn't to say that being lighter and/or leaner is always superior from an athletic (or any other) standpoint and there are cases of athletes (both female and male) performing at the top level above what is often considered the ideal level. While reducing BF% to optimal levels often improves performance, reducing below those levels can harm performance due to the need to chronically restrict energy intake, engage in excessive amounts of exercise, etc. Training can't be adequately supported, injury risk may increase, menstrual cycle and other hormonal dysfunction may occur, muscle may be lost, etc. Targeting or trying to reach a specific BF% at the expense of performance is a mistake, albeit one that too many athletes make. Based on various studies in both collegiate and Olympic athletes, I've presented some representative values for BF% (based on older, non-DEXA methods) for different sports below.

Sport	BF%	1-BF%
Distance Running	10-15%	0.9-0.85
Cycling	15-20%	0.85-0.9
Swimming	14-24%	0.86-0.76
Triathlon	10-15%	0.9-0.85
Sprinters	12-20%	0.88-0.8
Soccer	13-18%	0.87-0.82
Volleyball	16-25%	0.84-0.75
Basketball	20-27%	0.8-0.73

One thing to note from the chart is that there is a significant variability in BF% between sports and this reflects the difference in their overall requirements. As well, readers should note that variance even within the same sport, hopefully pointing out that not only is lower not necessarily better but that there is no singular BF% goal in this case. The above should be used as a starting point with female athletes targeting an optimal BF% range where they achieve their optimal performance. If losing more fat causes performance to decrease significantly, that fat should be regained immediately with the athlete now knowing what their individual optimal BF% is for their sport.

Determining the total amount of fat loss required for performance athlete is done by dividing the athlete's LBM by the chosen range of values from the above. Say a female runner at 130 lbs and 18% body fat (106.5 lbs LBM) wants to reach between 10-15% body. To reach 15%, her goal weight would be 125.5 lbs requiring a mere 4.5 lbs of fat loss. If she lost a pound or two of muscle/LBM, that might increase to 5.5-6.5 lbs putting her at 123.5-124.5 lbs bodyweight. To reach 10%, she would need to achieve a final weight of 118 lbs requiring a 12 pound fat loss. With a slight LBM loss, that might increase to 13-14 pounds. The same calculation will hold for any performance athlete although, in sports where the average BF% is higher, many athletes will need to diet minimally at all.

The performance athlete both does and does not have a time constraint in terms of reaching their dieting goals and this is due to most sports having a relatively long competition season, often lasting many months. Early competitions are often used more as hard workouts (often called "tune-ups") or to identify weaknesses while there are more important competitions that are being targeted at various points during the year. Since top form doesn't have to be reached at the very beginning of the season, the athlete has the option of finishing the diet during the early stages of the competition season, reaching their ideal BF% and bodyweight for the most important competitions. At the same time, as training intensity is often increasing at this point, dieting for too long can be equally problematic. In general, I would recommend that most performance athletes lose at least the majority of fat that they need to lose during the earlier parts of their preparation period when training volume is usually at its highest and the smallest changes to diet will need to be made to generate fat loss. At most, the final month of dieting might continue into the competition season but the athlete should plan on reaching their goal long before any major competitions occur. This will allow food intake to be increased to maintain the current BF% and support training.

In this vein, I'd emphasize the need to avoid excessive fat gains during the off-season or, really, any time of the year (injuries excepted as eating sufficiently is critical to recovery). If there is generally a problem time it is during the off-season, the roughly 2-4 week period following the competition season where training may be eliminated or at least severely reduced. If food intake is not controlled during this time period, significant fat gain can can occur and this can require a significant amount of dieting time to remove. especially for those athletes who may need to reduce their BF% to very low levels for competition. A distance runner who wants to be at 12% body fat for their competition season who gains too much fat may need months of dieting to get to that level, time where training may be impaired due to the need to restrict calories. In contrast, basketball players who compete at a BF% of 24-30% may simply maintain that level year round.

This is not to say that athletes who compete at the lower levels of BF% should attempt to maintain that low level year round as this has the potential to compromise training and health, especially if some degree of menstrual cycle or hormonal dysfunction is present. I will talk about ending the diet and how to regain fat after dieting to very low levels of BF% in Chapter 33 but here I will make the general recommendation for performance athletes to go no more than ~5% above their target weight (for their goal BF%) with a minimum of 18% body fat (this should allow a sufficient EA to maintain normal hormonal functioning). If a female distance runner has dropped from 135 pounds/22% body fat to 123 pounds and 15% body fat, she should attempt to keep her weight/BF% at ~129 lbs and 18% body fat. When she needs to get back into peak racing shape, she will only need to lose 6 pounds to reach her goals.

For the performance athlete, the 0.5% or 1.0% weight loss per week goals will generally be the most appropriate with the choice depending on the context. Those athletes who are dieting to 15% or higher body fat can use the 1.0% per week deficit while those going below 15% will need to switch the to the smaller 0.5% deficit beyond that point. I would remind readers of the research discussed previously where athletes on a smaller deficit were able to make performance gains compared to those on a larger deficit and some athletes may wish to use the 0.5% weekly weight loss goal regardless of their final BF% goal. This can result in extended dieting times depending on how much fat needs to be lost (estimating dieting times will be discussed in Chapter 25). In general an aggressive deficit targeting 1.5% weekly weight loss should be avoided unless they are being used as a short-term (2-4 weeks) approach to reduce BF% as rapidly as possible. Training must be cut back significantly for this to work and, if this is not possible (or the athlete refuses to do so), aggressive deficits should be avoided.

There are several potential issues related to the menstrual cycle that performance athletes may run into. The first is related to the impact of water related weight gain to harm performance. For many athletes, even a small increase in water weight during the late-follicular/luteal phase can be problematic as it will increase the energy required to move their body. Runners and cyclists are especially sensitive to this although all athletes who have to move their bodies across gravity can be affected negatively. There are dietary strategies such as decreasing sodium and increasing potassium that may be beneficial here but athletes must avoid the urge to dehydrate themselves under most circumstances as this has the potential to harm performance significantly.

There is also the potential for a woman's performance to vary through the menstrual cycle although this effect tends to be highly individual with some women showing enormous variations from week to week and others showing little to none (endurance sports seem to show less variation than strength/power sports). At best there are some general patterns but, even here, world records have been set by women in every week of the menstrual cycle. Female athletes and/or their coaches will have to be their own best scientists in this situation, tracking their training performance during different weeks of the cycle to determine not only what variations are present but which weeks are relatively worse or better. Not only can this be used to adjust training (i.e. more and/or more intense training when performance is increased and less when it is reduced) but it can give some indication of whether any given competition will fall during a particularly good or bad performance week.

Unfortunately, this information may not be that useful as athletes often have little control over when their major competitions fall during their own personal cycle. At best recreational athletes or those women only targeting one or two major competitions (i.e. a specific half- or full marathon) might pick an event on a specific date but this is usually outside of the athlete's control. If a qualifying competition or championship falls on a week in which a given woman typically has poor performance, she is basically out of luck. Hormonal birth control has commonly been used to both regulate and control the cycle for high-level female athletes but this can have its own share of drawbacks including the ability to limit a woman's response to training. This topic will be discussed in detail in Volume 2.

Weight Class Athletes

While the majority of performance athletes will be attempting to achieve a given body weight/BF% to optimize performance, there are certain sports which have weight classes. This includes such sports as Olympic lifting, powerlifting and women's strongman competitions along with boxing, mixed martial arts and many other combat sports. Unique among the endurance sports, rowing has both a lightweight and heavyweight class. The number of classes that may be found in a given sport varies enormously, rowing has only two, powerlifting and Olympic lifting have 7, and women's boxing has 10. The specific weight class limits also frequently vary between sports although the differences are not usually enormous.

Weight classes are defined by specific cutoff points that the athlete has to achieve and exist in an attempt to equalize the competition by only allowing women of similar weights to compete against one another. In these sports, the athlete will be weighed, typically either 2 or 24 hours before their competition. When the athlete is weighed, they must be at or below the weight class cutoff to "make weight" and be placed in that class. If they don't make weight, they will be placed in the next higher class and may have to compete against significantly heavier women. Some sports also have an unlimited class where athletes of any bodyweight in excess of the cutoff will compete against one another. For example, the International Powerlifting Federation has an 184.8 lb+ (84kg+) class which means that all women in excess of that weight will compete against one another. Whether she is 185 lbs or 285 lbs, she will be in that class.

While making weight is critical for athletes in this group, BF% is still important. At any given body weight, a woman with a lower BF% will carry more LBM and muscle and is likely to be more competitive compared to a woman with a higher BF% and less LBM. Which isn't to say that women should attempt to achieve the lowest possible BF% as the dieting necessary may harm performance. Quite in fact, in many weight class sports, women tend to compete at a fairly moderate BF% range. I've provided representative BF% values for different weight class sports along with value to divide LBM by for the calculations.

Sport	BF%	1-BF%
Rowing	12-18%*	.88-.82
Combat Sports (boxing, MMA)	Mid-teens or lower	.85-.90
Olympic lifting/Powerlifting	18-22%*	.88-.82
Women's Strongman	18-22%*	.88-.82

*There is currently a lower limit of 12% for rowing and superheavy weight lifters in PL/OL and women's strongman often carry a much higher amount of BF% since they have no weight limit.

In the simplest sense, setting dieting goals for weight class athletes would mean determining the target/ending weight for the athlete when they have reached their target or optimal BF% and seeing if that will achieve the desired body weight. So assume that two female powerlifters are both attempting to make the 139 lb weight class. The first is 150 lbs/24% body fat with 114 lbs LBM and wants to reach 18% body fat. Dividing 114 lbs by 0.82 will give her a target weight of roughly 139 lbs and a fat loss of 11 lbs. The second is 155 lbs/24% body fat with an LBM of 118 lbs and also wants to reach 18%. Dividing 118 lbs by 0.82 yields an ending weight of 144 lbs and a fat loss of 11 lbs. As they both have a goal of 139 lbs, the first lifter will make weight while the second will be five pounds over.

While this would suggest that the second lifter will have to compete in the next higher weight class, there is another consideration which is that weight class athletes can temporarily and rapidly reduce their bodyweight to achieve their target weight for the weigh-in before attempting to regain the lost weight before they have to compete. How much weight can realistically be lost this way depends primarily on when the weigh-in falls relative to the competition. For sports with a 2 hour weigh in, no more than 3-5% of body weight can realistically be lost without harming performance (and some may still see a drop) as there is insufficient time to replace all of the lost weight. In contrast, sports with a 24 hour weigh-in may allow athletes to lose as much as 8-10% of their current weight as there is time to regain it before the competition. As that much weight loss tends to involve extremely aggressive approaches for both the weight loss and regain it will not be discussed in this book. Instead, I will only focus on relatively moderate amounts of rapid weight loss as would be appropriate for sports with a 2-hour weigh-in period (the same moderate weight loss can be used for 24 hour weigh-ins as well).

Traditionally there have been a number of relatively dangerous approaches to rapid weight loss such as vomiting or laxatives but these are not recommended and will not be discussed. Rather, there are a number of well-researched and relatively safe and controlled methods of rapidly reducing weight worth considering that revolve around short-term changes in food intake, activity and fluid intake (12). Each strategy has its pros and cons and I will be addressing them sequentially in terms of those that are likely to have the largest overall impact on body weight with the least impact on performance.

Perhaps the easiest, and the one that is least likely to harm performance is to adopt a low-residue/low-fiber diet in the 2-4 days before weigh-in. By allowing undigested food to pass through the gastrointestinal tract during that time, up to ~2 lbs/1kg can be lost and this may be enough to get the athlete where they need to be in terms of their body weight. This entails eating mostly proteins and fat with little to no fiber or vegetables. It's important here to maintain calorie intake, usually by increasing dietary fats, since the explicit point is to avoid a a calorie deficit. Focusing on very calorie dense foods on the last day before the weigh-in is also beneficial. At this point, the calorie value of the food is less important than the actual weight of the food and eating 200 grams of peanut butter will have less of an impact than eating 450 grams (1 pound) of lettuce despite the peanut butter having enormously more calories.

If the above strategy is insufficient to make weight, another worth considering is restricting carbohydrates to very low levels, generally 50 grams per day or less (i.e. a ketogenic diet) while increasing dietary fats. In conjunction with exercise, this can lead to a loss of body water that might be 1-2% of current body weight or perhaps 1-4 lbs (0.5-2 kg) of additional weight depending on the athlete's current body weight. This will deplete muscle glycogen levels which may or may not impact on performance depending on the sport. Pure strength/power sports such as Olympic lifting or powerlifting are unlikely to be affected since glycogen is not a primary energy source for them. In contrast, sports such as rowing or combat sports are likely to be due to the importance of muscle glycogen as an energy source. A 2-hour weigh-in does not allow for enough glycogen to be resynthesized within the muscle to offset this.

If the above strategies are insufficient to get the athlete into their weight class, they will have to engage in some amount of deliberate dehydration and this may allow for an additional 3% of body weight to be lost without harming performance. Some athletes will still see a performance drop at this level of dehydration but anything more than this level will either harm performance or require aggressive rehydration strategies that cause other problems (13). In a practical sense, it is best for most women to aim for a 3% or less dehydration unless it is absolutely necessary. If more than 5% dehydration will be required to reach the weight class, it would be ideal to lose more total fat instead. If that is not possible, the athlete will have to target the higher weight class. Women can calculate this 3% weight loss by multiplying their current weight by 3% (0.03) but this yields a value of 3.5-6 lbs (1.5-2.7 kg) of bodyweight for women weighing from 120-200 pounds. Adding the 1-2 lbs of weight lost from a low-residue diet will raise this to 4.5-8 lbs (2-3.6 kg) total weight loss. The second powerlifter above who ended her diet at 144 lbs could use these strategies to reduce her body weight by ~4 lbs from dehydration plus 1-2 lbs from food intake for a total of 5-6 lbs bodyweight, putting her at 138-139 lbs and into the lower weight class.

Dehydration can be accomplished through a number of different methods with each having a greater or lesser potential to harm performance. Simple water restriction, primarily on the day prior to the weigh-in will help to reduce bodyweight slightly due to urination and this effect is increased if sodium intake is reduced. A mild herbal diuretic in the 1-2 days before the weigh-in can also be useful. For women who regularly drink, a half or full glass of wine the night before a weigh-in will also cause some dehydration. Water and/or sodium loading can also be used. Here water/sodium intake is increased for 3 days before being decreased and this causes the body to flush out water. Finally there is sweating and this can be accomplished in a number of ways. Active sweating entails light exercise such as brisk walking in a hot environment (i.e. no fans) or with extra clothing and this should be done on the day prior to the weigh-in. Active sweating harms performance less than passive sweating such as sitting in a sauna (dry sauna is better than moist sauna). Even sleeping in hotter than normal conditions (i.e. no fans, more blankets) the night before weigh in can cause extra water loss. The details of this are beyond the scope of this book although many online guides exist that show a typical schedule.

Although dehydration might be ideally avoided and can absolutely harm performance when taken to extremes, there are reasons for weight-class athletes to consider it regardless of their situation. The first is that it may allow an athlete to enter a lower weight class where they may be more competitive. If the 155lb female above would be more competitive at 139, she could diet and dehydrate down to that level. Additionally, any weight that can be lost via dehydration/etc. is weight that doesn't have to be lost via active dieting. This means shortened dieting times and/or smaller required deficits which yields less risk of performance loss. For strength/power athletes, lifters in any given weight class are ranked by bodyweight. If two lifters make the same weight, the lighter lifter wins. So even within any given weight class, there may be a reason to reduce bodyweight below the required level. Let me make it clear that all of the above only matters for those weight class athletes who have a chance of winning to begin with. Any woman competing in her first weight class event should worry about gaining competition experience competing at their current weight while ignoring weight classes or dehydration issues completely.

The above information can be used in one more way which is to determine if an athlete even has the potential to make a given weight class. This can be done by first taking the weight class cutoff and adding roughly 4.5-6 lbs to account for body weight manipulation (a more complicated calculation would be to add 3-5% to the weight class limit for dehydration and then an additional 1-2 lbs for the low-residue diet). Say a woman was targeting the 124.5 lb (57kg) weight class. First she would add 4.5-6 lbs to this value to get 129-130.5 lbs and this is the final weight she would have to reach via dieting. To determine if this is realistic, she could first determine her ending bodyweight as above for her goal BF%. If she were currently 140 lbs and 22% body fat with 109 lbs of LBM, a BF% of 18% would put her at 133 lbs and she would not be able to make the weight class without deliberately losing muscle or dehydrating herself much more severely. If instead she dieted to 15-16% body fat, her target weight would be 128-129 lbs and she would just make weight. This assumes that she could maintain her training and compete effectively at that BF%. In many cases, a woman's target weight class will simply be unrealistic without excessive fat losses (and/or muscle loss) and aggressive dehydration . Unless she has some very good reason such as setting national or world records she should target the higher weight class.

With the possible exception of rowing, where athletes have a fairly long competition season, most weight-class athletes tend to compete relatively infrequently while targeting one or more specific competitions in a year. If they do not reach their weight class goal, they will have to compete in a higher weight class and this has several implications. The first is that, while it's common for many weight-class athletes (especially in the strength/power sports) to train at a higher body weight and BF% than they compete at, they must keep both in check or it will take repeated extreme diets to reach their goal weight class. Second is the fact that weight class athletes must begin reducing their BF% and body weight early enough to reach their goal. Ideally the final week should only be used for any rapid weight loss methods and the diet should end prior to that. For any weight-class athlete who is competing frequently, and who may be dropping weight for competition before regaining it, body weight must never get more than 3% above their weight class cutoff (14). An athlete competing at 129.5 should ideally not go above 133.5 lbs between competitions.

So far as choosing a dietary deficit, for extended diets, most athletes in this group will be able to use the 1% weekly weight loss goal unless they need to drop below perhaps 18% body fat, at which point they should use the 0.5% goal. If they do not have a large amount of fat to lose, the 0.5% weekly goal can be used regardless and this may have less of an impact on training and performance. That said, some weight class athletes such as strength/power athletes have anecdotally reported that shorter more aggressive diets seem to harm their performance less than longer more extended diets. So long as training is reduced, a 1.5% weekly weight loss can be attempted for relatively short periods of no more than 2-4 weeks and this will allow them to resume normal fed training sooner. So long as it will take them to 3% or less of their weight class goal, a short aggressive diet ending a few weeks prior to the competition might be ideal.

Just as with other performance athletes, weight-class athletes face two primary issues associated with the menstrual cycle. The first is the variations in performance that may (or may not) be present as described above and which may cause problems if a competition falls on a week when the athlete performs more poorly. Perhaps as if not more important are the shifts in water weight that may occur during the cycle. This is enough of a problem for performance athletes to begin with but is profoundly problematic here as it could prevent an athlete from being able to make her weight class at all (or without much more aggressive dehydration strategies). It would only take a few pounds of extra water weight during the late-follicular or late-luteal phase to cause a severe problem for a weight-class athlete who is already on the edge of not making weight. Hormonal birth control offers one option here as it can be used to control the cycle but it has other issues with certain types potentially impairing optimal strength and muscle mass gains (discussed in detail in Volume 2). This leaves other nutritional options that I have mentioned previously including lowering sodium and increasing potassium to help ameliorate the water retention. Mild herbal diuretics, as mentioned above, may be required here and the athlete may have to target a 5% dehydration level to reach their goal. While this is certainly problematic, I'd note that the water being lost is technically "extra" water that has been gained during the cycle and this may not as negatively impact on performance. Even so the potential for problems always exists with dehydration and if the athlete simply cannot make weight they will either have to compete in a heavier weight class or target another competition.

Physique Athletes

As described previously, physique athletes represent those women who will be competing in bodybuilding, physique, figure or bikini competition. While it's not unheard of for women in Category 2 to wish to diet down to competition levels, this is far from optimal and going forwards I will only consider Category 1 women to be in this group. As with the serious trainee, the physique athlete will have a relatively specific BF% that is required to be competitive in their division but this requires somewhat of a warning. Ultimately, the physique sports are judged on appearance and this should always take precedence over any specific BF% or number. As I discussed in Chapter 6, all body fat estimation methods have some amount of error and a caliper or DEXA measurement might indicate that someone had reached their goal BF% when their leanness was not yet at the required levels visually. Similarly, any given BF% measurement might indicate that the trainee is above their goal BF% when visual assessment based on previous competition or their coach shows them to be where they need to be. In this case, chasing down some arbitrary number is both useless and potentially damaging in terms of either health or appearance.

This is not to say that using BF% estimate or goals is useless as there must be some way of estimating how much total fat loss will be required to reach the competition goal. These numbers must simply be tempered by visual assessment. This is compounded by the physique competitor having the additional factor of having a strict time frame or a specific competition date by which they must meet their goals (I'd note again that many competitors will do more than one competition in a season in the modern era). If they have not reached their goal in time, they have either missed their opportunity to compete or must choose a later competition. Due to this strict time frame, it is critical to estimate the necessary dieting time which requires having at least a rough idea of how much total weight/fat needs to be lost to begin with.

In the chart below, I've shown the different physique categories along with the approximate goal BF% and the LBM divider that would be used. Please note that the BF% values are based on non-DEXA methods and those competitors using DEXA would add roughly 3% to the below values.

Category	BF%	1-BF%
Bodybuilding	10-12%	0.9-0.88
Physique	10-12%	0.9-0.88
Figure	10-15%	0.9-0.85
Bikini	13-20%	0.17-0.8

The values for bodybuilding and physique represent the lower limits of female BF% with the primary difference between the categories being the amount of muscularity that the competitor has developed. Both figure and bikini competition have a relatively large range due to the often changing judging criteria from year to year. Sometimes being too lean, dry or hard can hurt a competitor and other times it is expected. Competitors will need to look at previous competitions within the federation and category they are in to determine what level of leanness may be required to be competitive but the above will be generally correct.

Determining the total amount of weight/fat loss required is done as for the serious trainee with LBM being divided by the appropriate value above to determine the target weight. Once again I'll use this book's sample dieter who is starting at 150 lbs/22% body fat with 33 lbs of fat and 117 lbs of LBM. If she were competing in bodybuilding or physique and wished to reach 12% body fat, she would divided 117 lbs by 0.88 to get a target weight of 133 lbs and a total fat loss of 17 lbs. If she wanted to factor in potential muscle loss, she would add 10% or just under 2 lbs of this and her total weight loss would be 19 lbs with an end weight of 131 lbs (she may weight less than this on competition day due to dehydration). If instead she was competing in women's figure and was targeting 15% body fat, she would divide 117 lbs by 0.85 to get a target weight of 137.5 lbs and a total fat loss of 12.5 lbs. This could be increased by 10% for a total weight loss of ~14.5 lbs and a final weight of 136.5 lbs.

In addition to having specific BF%/visual requirements, some physique federations also have weight classes (some use height classes but this is not relevant here). The specific weight divisions vary by federation and different contests may have different numbers of weight classes ranging from 2-4. In the case of a 2 weight class event, the divisions might be under 125 lbs and over 125 lbs meaning that all women under 125 lbs will compete each other and vice versa. In this situation, not only does the physique competitor have to reach their target leanness but they have to achieve a specific body weight. In some cases, this body weight will be realistically achievable and in others it will not with the above calculation giving a first indication of whether or not the competitor has a chance of reaching it to begin with. So long as the target weight is under the weight class cutoff there is no problem but, even if it is slightly above it may be possible to reach the lower weight class. This can be done through various strategies (discussed under weight class athletes) and allows the fat loss goal to be roughly 3% above the weight class cutoff. That is, so long as the dieter ends up no more than 3% above, they may make the lighter weight class.

To determine what weight this will be requires that the weight class limit by multiplied by 1.03 which will increase it by 3% respectively. To have a chance of reaching a 125 lb weight class would mean an ending dieting weight of no more than 129 lbs (125 lbs * 1.03 = 129 lbs). If the sample dieter above only reaches 12% body fat she will be between 131-133 lbs and her chance of making a 125 lb weight class will be unlikely without drastic and potentially dangerous dehydration strategies. She could also deliberately allow some muscle loss during her diet. This is a worthwhile consideration when a competitor is just slightly above the weight cutoff for the lower class. She may be better off losing 1-2 pounds of muscle and coming in at the top of the lighter class rather facing women much heavier and muscular than her.

Moving to the topic of choosing a dietary deficit, most physique competitors will be able to start with the 1% weekly weight loss goal early in their preparation. For those physique competitors targeting a BF% no lower than 15% (i.e. some figure and bikini competitors) the 1% goal can be used from the start to end of the diet. Once a body fat percentage of 15% has been reached and dieters are attempting to get even leaner and the various dieting adaptations are becoming more pronounced, moving to the 0.5% weekly weight loss goal would be more suitable. This actually runs counter to the common pattern which is to start moderately and end by becoming more aggressive with the diet but makes more sense physiologically. Early in the diet the overall adaptations hormonally, metabolically, etc. are not as pronounced and faster rates of fat loss are more feasible without danger. As the dieter reaches the sub-15% body fat level and the body is fighting back more and more (and menstrual cycle/hormonal dysfunction becomes more problematic), a more gradual approach is the best choice.

As I discussed in Chapter 17, the 1.5% weekly weight loss goal is generally inappropriate for extended diets and this is absolutely true in this case. However, there are two situations where it might have some use. The first is when a competitor has begun their contest preparation too late or has fallen behind their fat loss schedule for some reason. Inserting a 2-week aggressive deficit diet targeting 1.5% weight loss may be appropriate before moving back to the previous deficit level to attempt to get the competitor back on schedule. This isn't ideal and, anecdotally at least, seems to work more poorly on female than male competitors overall.

If more than 2 weeks of aggressive dieting will be required, the competitor should pick a second competition at a later date (the first can be used to test peak week strategies). Perhaps the more common use of the 1.5% per week fat loss is for a short diet (often called a mini-cut) during the off-season. At least some fat gain is common when athletes are gaining muscle and, given the importance of starting a diet at a sufficiently low BF%, short, aggressive diets can be used to keep BF% in check. It also allows fully fueled training to resume sooner. This should be limited to 2-4 weeks maximum and training must be severely reduced or the athlete is highly likely to burn out or overtrain.

The major issue regarding the menstrual cycle has to do with water retention although the impact of this depends on the specific physique category a woman is competing in. Bodybuilding, physique and to a lesser degree fitness/figure expect the competitor to be somewhat dried out and various strategies have been used over the years in an attempt to ensure that the muscles are visually full with little excess water underneath the skin. A competitor who's contest fell in the late-follicular or late-luteal phase is at risk for menstrual cycle related water retention to harm their appearance. A light herbal diuretic can help to offset this problem and this should be tested prior to the contest. I'd note that, in many cases this will be offset by the reality that female physique competitors may have become amenorrheic to begin with, removing the cyclical changes in water weight that would otherwise occur and this might be seen as a small benefit to amenorrhea in this circumstance.

Chapter 19: Calculating Nutrient Requirements

Having determined the goal calorie level, whether maintenance, a slight surplus or deficit based on goals, the next aspect of diet setup will be to determine the specific amounts of protein, carbohydrates and fats that will make up the daily diet (specific food sources will be discussed in Chapter 20). While alcohol can certainly be included in the diet, I won't be discussing it explicitly in this chapter or including it in any of the calculations.

As with other topics in this book, it's becoming abundantly clear that there are differences in women's metabolism or requirements for specific nutrients and the idea of sex-specific nutrition is becoming more well accepted and studied (1). These differences must be taken into account and both this and the next chapter will be geared towards setting up what I consider an optimal diet relative to a woman's needs and specific situation (i.e. general health, sport performance, etc.)

In this chapter, I will show readers how to calculate specific protein, carbohydrate and fat intakes based on their goal calorie intake, body weight, BF%/diet Category and lean body mass (LBM). As I discussed in Chapter 15, this level of precision will not be necessary for all readers but I will also give some general intake numbers for different situations. I'd recommend that even those women who are using a non-calculated type of diet look at the information in this chapter so that they can compare whatever diet they are intending to use to what is optimal. So long as the values are close, the diet being chosen will be sufficient. Before looking at those specifics, I want to look at a few other topics first.

A Comment on Precision

While the calculations in this chapter will give recommendations for each nutrient to the gram, I want to emphasize that this is not clinical nutrition and that achieving those exact numbers is not necessary. Rather, nutrient intakes should be considered as a range where some amount of variation around the recommended value is acceptable. Even single days when nutrient intake falls short of the desired value are not particularly important although multiple days with large scale deviations can eventually cause problems. Dieters in different situations will find that their need for precision varies. The general dieter or athlete in the off-season simply needs to get within a reasonable range of their macronutrient goals and a 5-10% variance in either direction might be more than acceptable. In contrast, the lean Category 1 dieter attempting to reach 10-12% body fat must attempt to achieve near perfection in their daily numbers with only a few gram variance from their goals.

The Menstrual Cycle, Hormonal Modifiers and Diet

As I discussed in detail in Chapter 2, the menstrual cycle is arguably the defining difference in physiology between women and men with the cyclical changes in estrogen and progesterone causing large scale changes in factors such as insulin sensitivity, nutrient utilization, metabolic rate, hunger and others across the cycle. And while it has not traditionally been done except for a recent study that I will discuss at the end of this chapter, working within those changes is a key aspect of designing an optimal diet. In a practical sense, this means that two different diets, one geared towards follicular phase physiology and the other geared towards luteal phase physiology will need to be set up.

Briefly recapping the changes that occur: during the follicular phase, appetite and hunger are well controlled (with the greatest effect in the few days before ovulation), insulin sensitivity is high and a woman's body will use proportionally more carbohydrate than fat for fuel. In contrast, during the luteal phase, hunger and appetite are higher (and cravings may manifest themselves, especially in late luteal phase), metabolic rate is slightly increased, insulin sensitivity is reduced and a woman's body will use proportionally more fat for fuel. She is also at risk for fat storage if her calorie intake is too high.

As protein requirements appear to be minimally impacted across the menstrual cycle it will remain constant in both phases with the primary changes occurring in carbohydrate and fat intake. During the follicular phase, the diet should be higher in carbohydrates but lower in dietary fat (without going so low as to cause problems with menstrual cycle function or adherence) while the luteal phase diet should be relatively lower in carbohydrates and higher in fat (this helps with fullness). While I won't include this in the calculations, the normally cycling woman could technically increase her calorie intake slightly in the luteal phase to leverage the increase in metabolic rate that occurs. This would allow a slight increase in food intake including the possibility of an increase intake of typically craved foods and I will address this briefly at the end of the chapter and again in Chapter 21.

To take into account hormonal changes, the normally cycling female will need to calculate out both the follicular and luteal phase diets for optimal results but women with one of the hormonal modifiers discussed in Chapter 3 may not need to to this. As discussed in that chapter, the modifiers tend to put women in one of several hormone-like states which will create either an effective follicular or luteal phase physiology. This determines whether she needs to set up only one or both dietary phases. I've summarized those modifiers below and indicated the dominant hormone or hormones along with which phase diet will or will not have to be set up (amenorrhea will be discussed in Chapter 32). Yes indicates that that phase diet should be set up while No indicates that it will not be necessary.

Situation	Hormonal State	Follicular Phase Diet	Luteal Phase Diet
Normally Cycling	2 wks Estrogen, 2 wks Progesterone	Yes	Yes
Amenorrheic	Discussed in Chapter 32		
PCOS/Hyperandrogenism Category 1 and active	Testosterone but Insulin Sensitive	Yes	No
PCOS/Hyperandrogenism Category 2/3 or inactive	Testosterone but Insulin Resistant	No	Yes
Birth Control (1st,2nd gen.)*	Progesterone*	No	Yes
Birth Control (3rd,4th gen.)	Estrogen	Yes	No
Category 3	Testosterone	No	Yes
Early Peri-Menopause	Estrogen	Yes	No
Late Peri-Menopause	Testosterone	No	Yes
Post-Menopause w/o HRT	Testosterone	No	Yes
Post-Menopause w/HRT	Estrogen	Yes	Yes
Hysterectomy with HRT	Estrogen	Yes	No

*Women using birth control with a withdrawal week will have one estrogen-like/follicular phase week each month.

While the normally cycling female would need to set up both the follicular and luteal phase diets, the woman with PCOS/hyperandrogenism would only need to set up the follicular or luteal phase diet depending on their Category/activity level and the Cat 3 female would only use the luteal phase diet, etc.

Sports Specific Nutrition

In Chapter 4 I looked at different types of exercise and goals including putting various sports into different general categories. As I expect many readers of this book to be female athletes, prior to showing general diet set up I want to make a few comments about sports specific nutrition. For years it's been quite common for all sports, regardless of type, goal or focus to be given nearly identical nutritional recommendations (usually coming from research on endurance athletes) in terms of dietary protein, carbohydrates and fats with many still doing this. This is nonsensical for many reasons not the least of which being that different types of sports burn different numbers of calories from different types of fuels and have different overall goals in terms of gaining muscle mass, strength or power versus endurance.

In general, the endurance athlete has the highest calorie and carbohydrate requirements along with relatively lowered protein requirements (but still higher than many realize). In contrast, strength/power athletes burn fewer calories in training and their carbohydrate requirements tend to be lowered with a relatively higher protein requirement. Physique athletes are similar but have higher carbohydrate requirements due to the nature of their training. High-intensity performance sports can vary but tend to be closer to the strength/power/physique athletes than not. Mixed sports tend to be about halfway between the two extremes in terms of their calorie, carbohydrate and protein requirements. Due to the way I recommend setting up the diet, these issues will tend to take care of themselves for the most part.

Diet Set Up Parameters

To show how the diet(s) should be set up, I will be using the sample dieter from earlier in this book, a Category 1 female at 150 lbs and 22% body fat who has 117 lbs of LBM and a maintenance calorie intake of 16.6 cal/lb or 2370 calories per day. Her goal is fat loss and she will be targeting a 1% weekly weight loss or 1.5 lbs, requiring a 750 cal/day deficit. She will generate this by increasing her aerobic activity by 375 cal/day (~40 minutes) and decreasing her food intake by 375 calories/day to 2000 calories. As noted above, I will not increase her maintenance during the luteal phase although this could be done if desired.

For the calculations, I will be using the standard calorie values (called the Atwater factors) of 4 calories/gram for protein and carbohydrates and 9 calories/gram for dietary fat. For completeness, alcohol has 7 calories/gram and fiber is usually given 1.5-2 calories/gram although I will not discuss alcohol or make a distinction between starchy and fibrous carbohydrates calorie wise. Do note that the calorie value for any given food can vary slightly from these numbers but the difference is usually small and in a typical diet will tend to cancel out. As described in a previous chapter, while the body is not a bomb calorimeter in terms of the calorie yield, factors such as digestion and metabolism are factored into the above values. The above values are not perfect or without limitations but they do work when applied consistently.

Dietary Protein

The word protein comes from the Greek word "proteos" meaning primary and that alone should indicate the extreme importance that it has to proper nutrition. While the body can technically survive without dietary carbohydrates or fats for fairly extended periods, a lack of dietary protein will lead to the loss of muscle and organ tissue eventually resulting in death. For other reasons as well, I simply cannot overstate the importance of eating sufficient dietary protein and I say with no exaggeration that if women only internalize a single idea from this book, it should be that one. Strictly speaking, the body doesn't have a requirement for dietary protein but rather the amino acids (AAs, of which there are roughly 20 that occur in foods and many others are made in the body) and nitrogen (which I won't discuss further). Of the 20 AAs found in food, roughly half are considered essential, meaning that they must be obtained from the diet. The other half are considered inessential, indicating that the body can make them. Since effectively all dietary proteins contain all the AAs, both essential and inessential in some proportion along with nitrogen, this is more of a semantic distinction than anything of actual relevance. That said, athletes do often take isolated AAs (i.e. leucine or the BCAAs) for one reason or another.

Dietary protein has a fairly endless number of crucial roles in the body but most of them can be considered structural, meaning that they are used to build other parts of the body. Skeletal muscle, which is about 25% total protein is one, internal organs are another. Skin, hair and fingernails are also made of protein, hence the practice of consuming gelatin, a protein high in the AAs that are used to make them to improve their quality. A number of hormones, called peptide (AAs are also called peptides) hormones are also synthesized from protein including insulin, IGF-1 and growth hormone (GH). Under certain circumstances such as dieting or exercise, amino acids can also be used to produce energy, first being converted to glucose or ketones (despite often made claims, protein is essentially never converted to fat).

Debates over both adequate or optimal protein intakes have been going on for decades (or longer) and show no signs of stopping. Many continue to argue that excess protein is either unnecessary or directly harmful and there are long-held myths about protein intake regarding its impact on health that I will address below. The current DRI (Daily Recommended Intake) in the US for protein is roughly 0.35 g/lb (0.8 g/kg) although there is increasing evidence that up to double this amount (0.55-0.7 g/lb or 1.2-1.6 g/kg) may be a more appropriate value for overall health (2). This is potentially even more true for older individuals and women approaching or who have passed menopause require higher amounts of protein to stave off age-related muscle loss (3). While many continue to state that active individuals or athletes need no more protein than the DRI, it's been known for decades that this is untrue and that protein intakes above the DRI are necessary to optimize the adaptations to training (3a).

Looking at weight and fat loss in general, eating insufficient dietary protein may cause people to over eat in general (presumably the body increases hunger in an attempt to get sufficient protein), contributing to obesity in the modern world (4). Protein has long been known to be the most hunger-blunting and filling of the three macronutrients and one reason that currently popular "high-protein" diets are successful is that they control hunger more effectively. Dietary protein also helps to stabilize blood sugar while dieting, avoiding energy swings and rebound hunger. When calorie intake is decreased, as with dieting, protein is more likely to be used for energy, leaving less for structural purposes. In a sense, this creates a "protein deficiency" which causes the body to break down tissue such as skeletal muscle to obtain the protein it needs for other purposes. Increasing protein intake while dieting is critical in its own right and combined with resistance training, this works to spare LBM loss. This becomes especially true as dieters get leaner and the chance of LBM loss increases and the Category 1 female dieter will have the highest protein requirements to spare LBM (5). After a fat loss diet has ended, higher protein intakes have been shown to not only help prevent weight regain but, especially when resistance training is being done, to cause more of any weight that is regained to be from LBM (6). Finally, the combination of sufficient protein intake with proper resistance training has the additive effect of improving body composition (7,8).

Myths and Misconceptions about Protein

Let me look next at the myriad number of myths and misconceptions that surround the supposed "risks" of excessive protein intake (excessive is rarely defined here but many would consider it to be any intake above the DRI). Perhaps the most pervasive is that excessive dietary protein has potentially negative effects such as being hard on the kidneys but this represents a reversal of what is actually happening. Specifically, individuals with compromised kidney function have to reduce their protein intake and this got turned around to suggest that protein harmed the kidneys (9). Quite in fact, increased dietary protein intake may actually improve kidney function and there is no evidence that a high-protein intake has any effect unless there is a pre-existing condition. There has never been a case of kidney damage linked to protein intake and studies using providing amounts to athletes show no negative effects (10). It's also often stated that a high protein intake is harmful to bone health but this is only true if insufficient calcium/Vitamin D along with fruits and vegetables are being consumed. When those nutrients are consumed in adequate amounts, a higher protein intake actually improves bone density (11).

An extremely common and completely misguided idea is that high-protein diets automatically imply a high-fat intake. While this is arguably true in the general public consuming the modern diet, the simple fact is that there are fairly endless numbers of lean or almost non-fat protein sources available including skinless chicken, tuna and other low-fat fishes, pork tenderloin and even very low fat cuts of red meat (many cheeses have more fat). It is relatively trivial to eat a high-protein diet that is low in fat (athletes have done it for decades) and there is the simple fact that women need adequate dietary fat to begin with for optimal health and menstrual cycle function. I should mention a relatively recent study suggesting that meat intake, especially processed meats, increased the risk of colon cancer as this is being used as more evidence against a high meat intake. Not only was the impact small to begin with, the reality is that the rest of the diet cannot be ignored. In the modern Western diet, high meat intakes are typically associated with a low fruit and vegetable intake and it is the lack of fruits and vegetables that are more to blame than the presence of meat itself (12). It should be obvious that both meat and fruits/vegetables can be eaten in the same diet and, quite in fact, they should be. Lean red meat has been shown to improve health and meat actually contains many cancer preventing nutrients (13,14).

Women and Dietary Protein

I am going into a perhaps excessive discussion of dietary protein here as I find it all to common for females to consume too little protein on a day-to-day basis (the exception here are athletes in the strength/power or physique sports). Some of this is assuredly due to the gender differences in food preferences I discussed earlier in the book where women tend to prefer carbohydrates and fats while men prefer protein and fats. Many women report simply not having a "taste" for protein foods, especially meats which may be biologically based or related to the types of foods they ate when younger.

In addition, women often seem to actively avoid protein (or at least specific types of proteins) for any number of reasons. A common one is an attempt to reduce dietary fat intake to extremely low levels (or the fear that excess protein will be stored as fat) but I'd reiterate that there are plenty of low-fat protein sources available. Endurance athletes especially tend to drastically overemphasize carbohydrates at the expense of both protein and fat, often for similar reasons. Another is often out of fear of either health risks or the fear of excess muscle gain (which I'd note doesn't occur in women to begin with). This may also be a response to the many official sources which continue to (incorrectly) state that more protein than the DRI is harmful.

I am harping on the topic of dietary protein due to the critical importance of women to eat sufficient amounts daily. This is necessary to optimize their general health, well being, training results and especially fat loss (recall from Chapter 14 what happens as women switch out some of their often excessive carbohydrate intake for proteins and fats in terms of shifting their body to using fat for fuel). The amounts I will suggest will seem high compared to many other recommendations and often seem daunting to women who are not used to eating much dietary protein (in the next chapter I will show how easy it is to achieve those amounts). Even those women who find that they don't have much of a taste for protein find that their taste buds change over time. After experiencing the often profound changes in their hunger and appetite, energy levels and body composition that are occurring, getting them to eat sufficient protein is rarely a problem. As stated above, if there is a single nutritional concept that women get from this book, it is the need for sufficient protein. The other important concept is the need for proper resistance training and the combination of the two is truly the key for women to optimize health and body composition.

While the negative claims about protein are mostly false, there is one potential negative of high protein intakes in a woman's diet although this is more of a practical issue than anything related to health.

This has to do with a topic I've discussed previously in this book which is that, due to their relatively lower calorie intakes, women often have trouble fitting sufficient amounts of all of the nutrients into their diet on any given day. As calories go down and protein goes up, this leaves less room for both dietary carbohydrates and fats. Since dietary fat needs to be set at a certain level (especially for the normally cycling female), dietary carbohydrate intake may have to be significantly lowered. While not an issue for the general dieter or serious trainee, for athletes this can cause their training to be compromised.

As I've mentioned previously this points to the need for nutritional periodization of some sort for women where nutrient intake is being varied (either acutely or in the long-term) to ensure that their needs are met. Acutely, raising calories to maintenance with sufficient frequency is one approach to this, refilling muscle glycogen in addition to its other benefits. In the longer term, an athlete can alternate phases where the goal is to gain muscle/strength/fitness (with raised calories and carbohydrates) with phases where the goal is explicit fat loss (where diet and/or training may be modified)

To ensure that sufficient protein is being consumed, I almost always set up diets by setting protein intake first. As I noted above, the recommendations I will make are likely to be much higher than most females have seen recommended (with the possible exceptions of strength/power or physique athletes) but this simply reflects out of date recommendations that don't take into account modern research. Due to the nearly insignificant change in protein requirements from the follicular to luteal phase, I will use a single value for both. As well, regardless of hormonal modifier, all women should use these values.

What Determines Protein Requirements?

There are several factors that go into the determination of protein requirements. One is the type of training or exercise being done as extra protein is needed to support muscle repair and resynthesis following training. Resistance training has higher requirements than endurance training and athletes performing both should use the higher values recommended for resistance training. I'd note that trainees doing relatively moderate amounts of exercise are unlikely to have massively increased protein requirements. Only those athletes performing 60-90 minutes or more of intense training multiple time per week will realistically have increased protein needs (and they should eat at that level every day).

As always, gender plays a role and some have suggested that women require 25% less protein than men (15). Since most protein recommendations are made relative to total body weight, a portion of this represents the differences in body composition. However, differences in exercise metabolism, lowered use of protein during endurance exercise and reduced rates of muscle growth also contribute to this. More recent research suggests that women's protein requirements may only be 15% (or less) than men's and my recommendations below will reflect that (16,17).

A major factor in protein requirements, often ignored, is total calorie intake. DRI values and most recommendations are made in the context of a maintenance calorie intake but it has been known for years that protein needs change with changing calorie intakes. For reasons discussed above, when calorie intake is reduced, protein requirements will increase and my protein recommendations during dieting will be higher for this reason. Given the number of women who chronically restrict their food intake, protein requirements are likely to be higher almost by default. However, to maximize the results seen from training, I will actually recommend slightly higher protein intakes than during dieting. Even if this is somewhat unnecessary, the higher protein intake will better control hunger and help the athlete to avoid excessive gains in BF% when they are eating above their maintenance levels.

A major factor impacting on protein requirements is the individuals BF%/Category with women with a higher BF%/in a higher diet category having lower protein requirements. The Category 1 female will have the highest requirements/recommendations with the Category 2 woman requiring slightly less and the Category 3 the least. This isn't to say that higher protein intakes may not be chosen, especially when dieting, to control hunger and the values I will present should be considered more of minimums than anything else. Women can eat more protein than this if desired but they shouldn't eat less.

Two factors that can also impact on protein requirements are the type and timing of protein eaten. While all major dietary proteins contain all of the AAs, they are not identical in their AA composition or ratios. In general, animals source proteins tends to have better AA profiles than vegetable source proteins. Animal source proteins are also absorbed and utilized by the body more effectively. Women eating a majority of vegetable source proteins may have even higher protein recommendations than indicated below. Protein timing refers to when protein is eaten either during the day or relative to workouts (before, during and after) and this may have an impact on protein requirements due to changes in how the protein being eaten is being used by the body. I will discuss this in more detail in Chapters 22 and 23.

Protein Recommendations

In the chart below, I've provided protein recommendations for three different situations: maintenance, dieting, and muscle/strength gain which refers to the level of calorie intake. Maintenance is eating to match the current TDEE while dieting is eating below that level to generate fat loss. Gaining/max. represents optimal intake levels for athletes looking to improve strength, power, muscle mass or some other aspect of fitness and here any athlete involved in heavy weight training should use the higher value while those only performing endurance training should use the lower value. This value also represents the maximum intake level under dieting conditions.

Under both maintenance and dieting, the letters I, A and W stand for inactive, aerobic exercise only and weight training respectively. Inactive means that no exercise beyond daily activities of living are being performed, aerobic for anyone performing only aerobic/HIIT exercise and W for anyone performing any type of resistance training. If both resistance training and aerobic exercise is being done, the higher value should be used. As I mentioned above, the increased protein requirements from exercise applies primarily to those individuals performing 60-90 minutes or more of intense training freqently. For women seeking general fitness and health, the inactive protein intakes may be used if desired though I'd reiterate that higher protein intakes often confer other benefits such as better hunger and appetite control. Keeping with the idea of sports-specific nutrition mentioned at the beginning of the chapter, athletes should choose their protein multiplier based on the primary focus of their training. Physique, pure strength/power athletes and high-intensity performance athletes should use the W value while mixed/team sports and endurance athletes (who rarely have maximal gains in muscle or strength as a goal) will be fine with the A levels.

	Maintenance			Dieting			Gaining/Max
	I	A	W	I	A	W	
Category 1	0.7	0.8	0.9	0.9	1	1.1-1.2	1.2-1.4
Category 2	0.6	0.7	0.8	0.8	0.9	0.9-1.0	1.0-1.2
Category 3	0.5	0.6	0.7	0.7	0.8	0.8-0.9	0.9-1.0

*All values are in g/lb of lean body mass (LBM)

The values above should be multiplied by LBM in pounds (to convert to g/kg, multiply the values by 2.2) rather than total bodyweight due to the fact that body fat has no real protein requirement. Using total body weight to set protein can give unrealistic values for heavier women carrying more BF% unless the values are adjusted downwards to take this into account. In that vein, the values above are higher than what is seen in some research as I have normalized the common values for the average BF% of the women studied (i.e. 1 g/lb bodyweight becomes 1.2 g/lb LBM for women at 20% body fat). This allows women in any category to accurately calculate their protein requirements. Let me restate that the above values should be considered minimums as much as anything else. Women with lower protein requirements often find that increasing their intake above those levels is beneficial in terms of hunger, appetite, energy, mood, etc.

To put the above numbers into a more real world perspective, I've calculated some representative protein requirements for women (all of whom are dieting) in different categories performing different types of activities. The Category 1 dieter is the sample dieter I've been using throughout this book and the others were chosen simply to be representative examples.

Weight	BF%	LBM	Activity	Protein Intake	Grams Protein
150	22% (Cat 1)	117	Weights	1.2 g/lb LBM	140 g/day
250	35% (Cat 2)	162.5	Aerobic	0.9 g/lb LBM	146 g/day
300	45% (Cat 3)	165	Inactive	0.7 g/lb LBM	115 g/day

Once protein requirements have been determined, the grams per day should be multiplied by 4 cal/g to determine the total calories per day from protein and this will be necessary to calculate the rest of the diet. I've shown this for the sample dieter below. This amount should be eaten daily.

> 140 grams protein * 4 cal/g = 560 calories/day from protein.

To ensure that minimum values are met, the next step in diet set up is determining fat intake.

Dietary Fat and Cholesterol

Since they tend to be so linked in people's minds, I will talk about dietary fat (the triglycerides I have discussed in previous chapters) and cholesterol together. While many tend to use the terms interchangeable, they are distinct chemical compounds. Dietary fats or triglycerides (TGs) consist of three fatty acids bound to a glycerol molecule while cholesterol is a steroid molecule which is actually used to synthesize hormones such as testosterone, estrogen, progesterone and others along with being part of the cell membrane. Cholesterol is found only in animal foods (including low-fat foods) although the body makes significant amounts in the liver. Traditionally concerns over cholesterol have come out of worry over the role of blood cholesterol on cardiovascular and other diseases. But while there is a small percentage of people who seem to be sensitive to dietary cholesterol intake itself, for most it is a non-issue with the type/amount of dietary fat eaten being the bigger issue (if there is a link it is due to some high-cholesterol foods also being in high in fat). As I consider cholesterol intake fairly irrelevant in the big picture, I won't discuss it further or provide intake recommendations, focusing instead on dietary fat/TG.

Dietary fats are identical in structure to the fat stored within fat cells and muscle (as IMTG) and are most commonly separated into categories called saturated, monounsaturated and polyunsaturated fats (this refers to their chemical structure). I will discuss this in more detail in the next chapter and will only mention here that there are two essential fatty acids (EFAs) which are required for optimal health and which must be obtained from the diet (they will be discussed in detail in the next chapter and Chapter 24). None of the other dietary fats are essential and, strictly speaking, so long as the small EFA requirement were met, someone could eat no other fat without problem.

Dietary fats have a number of roles in the body including being part of the cell membrane and modulating cholesterol production in the liver, inflammation and others (the EFAs are especially important in this process). However, arguably the primary role of dietary fat in the body is to provide energy, either to the body after a meal, or by being stored in fat cells or muscle for later use. In this role it is more efficient than carbohydrate or fat. As discussed in Chapter 5, this is due to its caloric density, yielding 9 calories per gram (compared to 4 for protein or carbohydrate) and being stored with very little water. This makes dietary fat very calorie dense, that is it contains a large number of calories in a relatively small amount of food volume. A single tablespoon of oil contains 14 grams of fat and just under 140 calories, the same amount found in a 4.5 oz (127 g) chicken breast, a very large apple or a large amount of vegetables. Foods high in fat, whether protein and fat or carbohydrate and fat also tend to contain a lot of calories in a small space which makes it relatively easy to over consume them. Adding to this, dietary fat does not send a strong short-term fullness signal and is often found in highly tasty, easily overeaten foods.

Dietary fat is also the nutrient most efficiently stored as fat (and, as discussed in Chapter 10, moreso in woman than in men) although carbohydrate intake also plays a role in fat gain. This has led to a general suggestion or idea that, by limiting fat intake, fat gain will be reduced. This is true to a limited degree in that reductions in dietary fat tend to reduce total calorie intake but excess carbohydrate intake can also lead to fat gain. More to the point, many women, athletes or not attempt to reduce dietary fat to extremely low levels and this can cause a number of potential problems. Very low-fat diets (20-25% or less calories from fat) are often unsatisfying to dieters with more moderate fat diets providing better short- and long-term adherence, even when weight and fat loss are identical (18,19). Dietary fat gives foods a certain mouth-feel (improving texture) and, while it doesn't blunt hunger in the short-term, often keeps dieters fuller between meals. This is even more pronounced with a higher fiber intake and, combined with the hunger blunting effects of protein, may explain the relative success of those types of diets for many people.

In athletic populations, it's just as common to see female athletes attempting to reduce dietary fat to the lowest levels possible, often below 15% of total calories or less. Many factors contribute to including misconceptions about the health risks of dietary fat or, more usually, the fear that dietary fat will cause fat gain (or conversely that eliminating dietary fat will eliminate fat gain). While dietary fat certainly can and does contribute to fat gain, the fact is that carbohydrates can also cause fat gain just as effectively in the long run (20). As well, due to their high levels of activity, the potential health issues that can accompany high fat intakes simply aren't relevant to athletes. A lean female athlete who is highly active isn't in the same situation as an inactive women carrying a large amount of body fat.

There are number of potential problems associated with reducing dietary fat intake to extremely low levels. One is that it may make it more difficult to meet daily energy requirements for athletes in hard training which can cause a low energy availability (EA) with all of the problems that may cause. I discussed previously that fat intakes below 20% of total calories might independently contribute to menstrual cycle dysfunction but they also have the potential to impair immune system function or limit

IMTG storage in athletes (21). While depleting IMTG may be valuable for fat loss as discussed in Chapter 14, this can both harm endurance performance along with making physique athletes look somewhat smaller muscularly. Limited research suggests that low dietary fat intakes can increase the risk of stress-fractures as well although it's unclear why this would occur (22). Most likely it is due to very low fat intakes preventing athletes from eating enough calories or getting enough essential nutrients, especially micronutrients. In one study, female endurance athletes who raised their fat intake from 17% to 31% or 42% of total calories came closer to achieving sufficient calorie intake, improved their overall micronutrient intake and improved their endurance performance significantly (23). While I wouldn't recommend a 42% fat intake, my point is that very low fat intakes are problematic and should generally be avoided. There are exceptions, of course, situations where fat intake must be taken to very low levels but these should be purely short-term situations with moderate fat intakes being resumed afterwards.

Fat Intake Recommendations

Given the importance of sufficient dietary fat in a woman's diet, I recommend determining dietary fat intake after protein and this means that carbohydrates intake will be determined last. Due to changes in nutrient metabolism that occur during the menstrual cycle, dietary fat is also the first nutrient for which two values will be calculated, one for the follicular phase and one for the luteal phase (I will also provide a minimum fat intake). In the follicular phase, when insulin sensitivity is high and carbohydrates are being used for fuel, dietary fat will be set at moderate intake levels. In contrast, during the luteal phase, a slight degree of insulin resistance develops and setting dietary fat slightly higher while reducing dietary carbohydrates will be better. The normally cycling woman will need to calculate both while women with a hormonal modifier should use the chart presented earlier to determine which value is appropriate.

While it's clear that both extremely high and extremely low intakes of dietary fat are problematic, determining what might be an optimal level is somewhat problematic. Most of the studies looking at women's hormones tend to compare extremes of intake such as 20% to 40% total fat intake but this gives no indication of what might happen at intermediate levels in terms of when problems either start or are eliminated. This also has to be weighed against other issues such as ensuring that there are sufficient carbohydrates in the diet to sustain training and it can become quite a balancing act.

Splitting the middle of those two extremes and taking into account the physiological changes that occur during the phases, I will recommend a dietary fat intake of 25% of total calories in the follicular phase and 35% in the luteal phase. That latter value, going up to even 40% of total calorie intake has been recommended as optimal for the treatment of insulin resistance/PCOS, supporting it's benefit in the relatively more insulin resistant luteal phase (24,25). As an absolute minimum dietary fat intake I will use a value of 0.25 g/lb (0.55 g/kg) body weight although only Category 1 females near the end of an extreme diet will need to consider approaching this, primarily to keep carbohydrate intake high enough (extremely aggressive diets may also reduce fat below this level for short periods of time). Readers used to dieting on extremely low fat intakes may find these intakes to be high or be concerned with health risks (or slowed fat loss) but these concerns are unfounded. These values will hold across all categories and types of activity and women with higher calorie intakes will be eating more total grams of fat.

The calculation for dietary fat intake is slightly different than for protein and there are two steps to it. The first is to multiply calorie intake by either 0.25 (25%) or 0.35 (35%) which provides the number of calories of fat being eaten per day. This value is then divided by 9 calories/gram to get the total grams of fat to be eaten. The minimum fat intake in grams is determined by multiplying total bodyweight by 0.25 g/lb (0.55 g/kg). I've shown these calculations below for the Category 1 sample dieter eating 2000 calories per day. I've also shown the absolute minimum intake level based on 0.25 g/lb total body weight.

Follicular Phase Fat Intake
2000 calories * 0.25 = 500 calories per day from fat
500 calories / 9 calories/gram = 56 grams of fat per day
Luteal Phase Fat Intake
2000 calories * 0.35 = 700 calories per day from fat
700 calories / 9 calories/gram = 78 grams of fat per day
Minimum Fat Intake
150 lbs * 0.25 g/lb = 38 grams of fat per day

In the chart below, I've shown the same values for the Category 1 female above along with two representative women in Category 2 and 3 with different daily calorie intakes and dietary deficits.

Weight	BF%	Maintenance	Deficit	Cal/day	Follicular (25%)	Luteal (35%)	Minimum (0.25 g/lb)
150	22% (Cat 1)	2250 calories (15 cal/lb)	20%	2000	56 g/day	78 g/day	38 g/day
250	35% (Cat 2)	3125 calories (12.5 cal/lb)	30%	2185	61 g/day	85 g/day	63 g/day
350	45%(Cat 3)	3850 calories (11 cal/lb)	40%	2310	64 g/day	90 g/day	87 g/day

In the case of the Category 1 dieter, both the follicular and luteal intake levels are well above the minimum but this might potentially change as calorie intake is reduced. The Category 2 and 3 female are unlikely to ever reach a point (unless they are doing a very extreme diet) where total fat intake is below the minimum cutoff level. Before moving on to carbohydrates, the diet set up so far for the Category 1 female has protein providing 560 calories per day with dietary fat providing either 500 or 700 calories per day for the luteal and follicular phase respectively. These values will be needed to determine the amount of carbohydrate being eaten in each phase, determined next.

Carbohydrates

Dietary carbohydrates is a bit of an umbrella term which refers to several broad categories of foods including sugars, starches (i.e. breads, grains, pasta), vegetables and fruits. While similar, they are not identical and I will talk about them somewhat separately in terms of how much of the diet they should make up. All digestible carbohydrates (excluding fiber) are made from the same simple sugars which are glucose (aka dextrose, blood sugar), fructose (fruit sugar), and galactose (milk sugar). These are often called monosaccharides ("mono" = one, "saccharide" = sugar). These combine into two sugar molecules called disaccharides ("di" = two) which are sucrose (aka table sugar, glucose + fructose), lactose (glucose + galactose) and maltose (glucose + glucose). I will discuss high-fructose corn syrup (HFCS) in the next chapter; for now realize it is effectively identical to sucrose as it is roughly half glucose and half fructose.

Starches are very long chains (often thousands of molecules) of glucose bonded together; in the body these same long chains are called glycogen and are stored in the muscle or liver. All digestible carbohydrates contain roughly 4 calories per gram and during digestion they are broken down to simple sugars for absorption with only glucose and fructose actually entering the bloodstream. The only real difference here is in how long it takes for this to occur. Fructose is almost exclusively stored in the liver as glycogen (which will be broken down to maintain blood glucose when needed) while glucose is used to directly raise blood glucose or is stored in muscle as glycogen for use by that muscle. While technically the body can convert carbohydrates to fat, this only occurs with extremely high daily intakes (~700-900 grams of carbohydrates) and this pathway can generally be ignored. Any impact of carbohydrate intake on fat gain is due to carbohydrates increasing the body's reliance on glucose for fuel. This decreases the amount of fat burned after a meal or during the day so that any dietary fat is stored in fat cells.

Fiber, while typically considered a carbohydrate is structurally very different and made up of a variety of different compounds that I won't detail. Rather, fiber can be more easily divided into soluble fibers (which mix in water) and insoluble fibers (which do not). Both play important roles but soluble fibers can be metabolized in the stomach by gut bacteria, producing short-chain fatty acids. These have critically important health effects but also provide roughly 1.5-2 calories per gram to the body. Many foods containing fiber, such as vegetables, also typically contain some digestible carbohydrate as well. Fruits contain a mix of disaccharides and simple sugars with some (usually small) amount of fiber.

While carbohydrates have a few structural roles in the body, their primary purpose is to provide energy. There is always a small amount of glucose in the bloodstream and, as mentioned, both liver and muscle store glycogen for later use if it is not needed immediately. Fat cells use a small amount of glucose to produce glycerol, the backbone for TG's and there are even small stores of glycogen in the brain. While most tissues will prefer to use carbohydrates for energy if they are available (the heart is an exception, using fatty acids exclusively), most can also switch to using fatty acids for fuel if they aren't. The brain can't use fatty acids and this has led to the belief that it can only use glucose but this is untrue as ketones, a by-product of fat metabolism in the liver, can be used by the brain

Skeletal muscle is a primary user of carbohydrate (both as glucose and via stored glycogen) both at rest and during exercise with the proportions of carbohydrates being used depending on the type and intensity of the exercise being done. Generally, lower intensity exercise relies more on fat and less on carbohydrates with more carbohydrates being burned as the intensity increases (very high-intensity exercise can only be fueled by carbohydrate). I'd refer readers back to Chapter 10 for the specifics of how women's bodies use fuel (both in general and compared to men).

Carbohydrate Requirements

Given the many roles of carbohydrates in the body and the general emphasis that most dietary recommendations have placed on them, it may surprise some readers to realize that strictly speaking carbohydrates are not an essential nutrient and the actual requirement for them under normal conditions is zero. This is due to the facts that the body can switch to using fat for energy (or ketones in the case of the brain) along with being able to make glucose out of other nutrients such as amino acids (from protein), lactate and glycerol. This amount the body can make isn't unlimited but will cover the body's basic needs. I am no way recommending zero carbohydrates as the default diet and am simply discussing the underlying physiology of carbohydrate requirements.

When carbohydrates are restricted to 80-120 grams of carbohydrate per day or lower (and most research uses 50 g/day), a state of nutritional ketosis (not to be confused with the ketoacidosis that occurs in Type I diabetes) will develop where ketones build up in the bloodstream to provide the brain with fuel. Fatty acid levels also increase providing energy to most other tissues. This 80-120 g/day value is unrelated to bodyweight and represents the amount of glucose used by the brain (women are typically at the lower end of this range due to their smaller body size). In a practical sense, this level of carbohydrate intake represents a cutoff point with any diet containing less than that being a ketogenic or very-low carbohydrate (VLC) diet. In many cases, this type of diet is also high in dietary fat and this may be referred to as a low-carbohydrate high-fat (LCHF) diets.

While the body does not strictly require carbohydrates for basic functions, this is not necessarily the case for exercise. At low intensities of aerobic activity (roughly 120-130 heart rate or lower, what I will call LISS in Chapter 28), carbohydrate needs are minimal and this is probably more true for women due to their higher reliance on fat than men. However, as exercise intensity increases, the requirement for carbohydrate also increases and fat cannot fuel exercise above a certain aerobic intensity or for HIIT or resistance training. For trainees performing relatively moderate amounts of this type of activity, carbohydrate requirements may still be relatively modest but athletes on lowered (or low) carbohydrate diets will eventually deplete their muscle glycogen stores (which recall may improve fat loss), harming performance. Only athletes in those handful of sports done at low intensities (perhaps race walking and ultra-endurance events) might be able to sustain performance on such a diet and we might say that carbohydrates are conditionally required for anyone performing high-intensity exercise.

So how many carbohydrates might female athletes require? For decades it was common to give relatively identical (and high) recommendations, most of which came from research on endurance athletes, for all athletes but it's now recognized that actual carbohydrate requirements depend enormously on the type and amount of activity being done. Looking at endurance athletes, low-intensity training may require no more than 1.3-2.2 g/lb (3-5 g/kg) of carbohydrate and, as noted above, women might need slightly less than this. In contrast, an athlete involved in 4-5 hours per day of training (only seen at the highest levels) might need 3.5-5.5 g/lb (8-12 g/kg) of carbohydrates with other amounts/intensities of training falling in-between those extremes.

Other sports have different (generally lower) carbohydrate requirements which is related to the type of training being done along with the overall goals. This also impacts on calorie and protein requirements. For pure strength/power athletes such as physique athletes, Olympic lifters and powerlifters recommended values are in the realm of 1.5-3 g/lb (3-6.5 g/kg). Physique athletes are likely to be at the higher end due to the nature of their training, based around more total training and higher repetitions, while more pure strength/power athletes, who typically use lower repetitions, are likely to be towards the lower end (26). It is interesting to note that, empirically, bodybuilders have long recommended a carbohydrate intake of 1-3 g/lb (2.2-6.6 g//kg) which is right in line with those recommendations. High-intensity performance sports such a sprinting, middle distance running, track cycling tend to have slightly higher carbohydrate requirements ranging from 2.5-5.5 g/lb (6-12 g/kg) with women generally falling at the lower end (27). Team sports are much harder to predict due to the variation inherent in the sports in this category but intakes of 2-3 g/lb (5-7 g/kg) should be appropriate (28).

When fat loss is the goal and calories have to be restricted with increased protein, the above goals are unlikely to be met on a consistent basis, especially for female athletes as there simply isn't room for all of the required nutrients. A compromise level of 1.8 g/lb (4 g/kg) of carbohydrate has been suggested in this situation (29) In some cases, intakes may fall below this to as little as 1 g/lb (2.2 g/kg). Eventually this will cause muscle glycogen to be depleted, impairing performance but this is offset by regular increase in calories to maintenance which increases carbohydrate intake. I've provided a chart below summarizing the different carbohydrate values below along with daily intake levels for our sample 150 lb female dieter.

	Carbohydrate Recommendations	Carb Intake
Minimum Requirements	Zero grams per day	0 g/day
Cutoff for Ketogenic Diet	~80-120 g/day	80-120 g/day or lower
Fat loss	1.8 g/lb (4 g/kg) or lower	270 g/day or lower
Strength/Power/Physique	1.5-3 g/lb (3-6.5 g/kg)	225-450 g/day
High-Intensity Performance	3.5-5.5 g/lb (6-12 g/kg)	525-825 g/day
Mixed/Team Sports	2-3 g/lb (5-7 g/kg)	300-450 g/day
Endurance Sports		
Light: Low Intensity/Technical	1.3-2.2 g/lb (3-5 g/kg)	195-330 g/day
Moderate: 1 hour/day	2.2-3 g/lb (5-7 g/kg)	330-450 g/day
High: 1-3 hours/day	2.7-4.5 g/lb (6-10 g/kg)	405-675 g/day
Very High: 4-5 hours/day	3.6-5.5 g/lb (8-12 g/kg)	540-825 g/day

All values are relative to total bodyweight rather than LBM.

Carbohydrate Intake Recommendations

Having looked at the issue of carbohydrate requirements, including those for athletes, I want to move to the final step of diet set up which is calculating daily carbohydrate intake. In contrast to the other nutrients which were calculated relative to LBM or calorie intake, carbohydrate intake has to be calculated as the difference between total calorie intake and the calories coming from protein and fat. This is done by subtracting the calories from protein and fat from the calorie goal and then determining carbohydrate intake in reverse. This means that, as protein and fat intake are basically fixed, carbohydrate intake will go up with increasing calorie intake/expenditure and vice versa. Practically this means that under some conditions, especially dieting, carbohydrate intake levels may fall below the recommended optimal levels. In some extremes, typically smaller Category 1 females at the ends of an extreme diet, they may approach or fall below the 80-120 grams per day cutoff for a VLC diet and I will address this below.

There are two steps to calculating daily carbohydrate intake and, as was the case with dietary fat, the follicular and luteal phase diets will have different amounts (dieters who are only calculating one or the other diets will only have a single calculation). The first step is to subtract the calories from protein from the day's total calories; this determines the calories left for fat and carbohydrate. Our sample dieter is eating 2000 calories and 140 grams (560 calories) of protein and I've shown the calculation below.

2000 calories total - 560 calories from protein = 1440 calories

Her fat intake was calculated to be 56 grams (500 calories) of fat during the follicular phase and 78 grams (700 calories|) of fat in the luteal phase. These values should each be subtracted from the 1400 calories to determine the number of calories from carbohydrate in each phase. That calorie value is then divided by four calories per gram to get the total grams of carbohydrate. I've shown the calculation below.

Follicular phase
1440 calories - 500 calories = 940 calories from carbohydrate
940 calories / 4 cal/g = 235 g carbohydrates/day
Luteal phase
1440 calories - 700 calories = 740 calories from carbohydrate
740 calories from carbohydrate / 4 cal/g = 185 g carbohydrate/day

The Sample Diet

Putting the above together, the sample female physique athlete dieter, once again at 150 lbs/22% body fat (117 lbs of LBM) will therefore have the following diets set up for each phase of the menstrual cycle.

	Follicular Phase	Luteal Phase
Calories	2000	2000
Protein	140 g/day	140 g/day
Carbs	235 g/day	185 g/day
Fat	56 g/day	78 g/day

I'd note that her carbohydrate intake values come out to 1.5 g/lb in the follicular phase and 1.2 g/lb in luteal phase which is broadly consistent with values that physique athletes have used for years. While certainly lower than the 1.8 g/lb (4 g/kg) value I described above, physique athletes rarely perform the amounts of training seen in the Olympic level athletes that value is recommended for. A physique athlete might be performing 60-90 minutes of intense weight training per day while a high level athlete may perform 2-4 hours and their calorie and carbohydrate requirements will vary accordingly. While the luteal phase diet carbohydrate intake is relatively low, it is at least approaching the cutoff for a VLC diet and,may cross that threshold later in the diet. For that reason I want to look at VLC diets in some detail next.

Very Low-Carb, High Fat/Low-Carb and Ketogenic Diets`

While the above calculations will give most readers of this book at least moderate carbohydrate intake recommendations, there may be situations where smaller female dieters (especially if their activity is not high) end up below the threshold for a VLC diet (~80-120 grams of carbohydrates per day) or others where a dieter deliberately chooses to lower carbohydrates to that level (i.e. PCOS/Category 3). This latter situation would typically be the woman with severe PCOS or obesity related insulin resistance for whom such diets are often profoundly beneficial. For those reasons, I want to look again at the topic of very-low carbohydrate/high-fat/low carbohydrate diets in more detail.

While 80-120 g/day is the physiological cutoff for the development of nutritional ketosis, both popular diets and research studies typically define the diet as containing 50 grams of digestible carbohydrate per day. In general, these diets also tend to be higher in fat (since the day's calories have to come from somewhere and only so much protein can be eaten) but this is not universal. It is more than possible to do a very-low carbohydrate/very-low fat diet where the diet consists of almost purely protein (with some vegetables and essential fats). This is generally called a Protein Sparing Modified Fast or PSMF. While frequently surrounded by a combination of controversy, criticism, zealotry and misconceptions, VLC diets have both pros and cons that I want to examine.

Perhaps the largest disadvantage of VLC diets is that many go through a roughly 3 week phase of feeling very fatigued as they adapt to the diet. This can be limited by ensuring sufficient intakes of sodium, potassium, magnesium and calcium, all of which are excreted in larger amounts. Even with sufficient mineral intake, many still feel bad for those few weeks as the brain shifts to using ketones for fuel. Along with mineral losses comes significant water loss which can cause some amount of dehydration along with causing a rapid drop in body weight. This is one of the reasons people think that such diets have a metabolic advantage and why dieters like them so much: losing several pounds of body weight in only a few days is very rewarding. Some women also experience depression on such diets as brain levels of serotonin drop. In contrast, others report feeling nearly euphoric with stable blood sugar and energy levels throughout the day. This is highly individual and my experience is that anyone following a ketogenic diet who hasn't started to feel better by week 3 probably isn't going to and the diet should be abandoned.

Overall, people with insulin resistance seem to be the ones who feel best on ketogenic diets, at least after the adaptation period (and I mentioned earlier that lowered carbs/higher fat is already a better approach in this case). Women in Category 3 who are inactive and/or who have PCOS related insulin resistance often respond very positively to VLC diets. Even in the absence of weight/fat loss, health parameters usually improve and often these diets are found to be at least slightly superior for weight and fat loss, mostly due to better adherence (30). I'd add that a VLC diet combined with a reduction in goitrogenic foods was found to reduce the thyroid antibodies seen in the autoimmune Hashimoto's thyroiditis (30a). Whether this would be effective for other autoimmune conditions is unknown but, as women are more likely to experience Hashimoto's, a VLC diet could be worthwhile consideration.

While most of the benefits on hunger and appetite is most likely due to an increased protein intake (this tends to happen automatically on such diets which is another benefit), there are other potential causes. Stable blood sugar is one of them as falling blood sugar can stimulate hunger. The presence of ketones in the bloodstream may also be having some benefit. Perhaps the largest effect is that, for many people, carbohydrate foods may act as triggers and cause a loss of control and overeating. As these foods have to be eliminated on VLC diets, this is avoided. However, as I mentioned in Chapter 15, the removal of broad categories or even specific foods can cause adherence issues over time as cravings increase.

This can be addressed later in the diet by finding ways to include those foods (strategies are discussed in Chapter 21) and often women's taste for them decrease as taste buds change (requiring about 4-6 weeks). I should note before continuing that, even in insulin resistant women, studies frequently find that high-carbohydrate/low-fat diets can be effective but only so long as they are based primarily around unrefined/high-fiber carbohydrates. In my experience, these aren't the types of foods most people on higher-carbohydrate diets tend to eat and I feel that reducing total carbohydrate intake is usually superior.

I'd note that, in contrast to the above, women with good insulin sensitivity, including leaner women (including the lean PCOS woman) or those who are highly active often feel terrible on very low-carbohydrate intakes. They don't ever seem to fully adapt to the diet and simply do poorly on them. Which isn't to say that VLC intakes cannot still have benefits in this population. Four days of very-low carbohydrate intake (20% of total calories which would be right at 100 grams per day for our sample female at 2000 calories per day) has been shown to naturally inhibit the alpha-2 receptors in the hips and thighs which will make mobilizing fat easier (31). For the Category 1 female dieting to the low extremes, this can be beneficial and I'll examine this and other strategies to target stubborn fat in Appendix 1.

But this raises two other problems in this group. The first is the potential, admittedly based on limited data, for VLC/ketogenic diets to impair menstrual cycle function in the normally cycling Category 1 dieter. If that same woman is highly active, a chronic low-carbohydrate intake will eventually lead to her muscles becoming depleted of glycogen. Once again, while this is beneficial for fat loss in the short term it will eventually harm high-intensity exercise performance in the long-term. The above problems can be addressed by using what is called a Cyclical Ketogenic Diet (CKD). This is a cyclical approach to dieting where 3-4 days of a VLC intake are alternated with 1-3 days of increased carbohydrate intake. This generates the benefits of the VLC intake on alpha-2 receptor inhibition and fat loss while refilling muscle glycogen and helping to offset menstrual cycle dysfunction issues. This isn't to say that a CKD should be the first choice for a Category 1 female who is dieting but rather to point out that that such diets must be modified in this context. I would mention that smaller Category 1 females may end up fairly close to 100-120 g/day of carbohydrates near the end of an extended diet and, by the time this is combined with increasing calories to maintenance, the diet will be at least similar to a CKD to begin with.

This brings me to the consideration of VLC diets for performance athletes. For decades, researchers have examined the idea of fat adapting athletes, predominantly those involved in the endurance sports (low-carbohydrate diets simply cannot sustain high-intensity exercise). The idea is that, by shifting the body to using more fat as fuel, glycogen will be spared, both improving performance and ensuring that the athlete has the necessary fuel for sprints or hard efforts. Various protocols ranging from multiple weeks of LCHF diets to as few as 5 days have been shown to increase the use of fat for fuel during activity but this has repeatedly failed to improve actual performance. One problem here is that athletes generally report that higher intensity workouts are much more difficult to perform under VLC conditions and in some cases, they cannot be completed. It should be clear that any diet which impairs the ability of an athlete to train effectively will not help performance. In some cases, fat adaptation actually harms performance as the body actually loses the ability to use carbohydrate for fuel during high-intensity efforts such as sprinting. It's now thought that glycogen sparing is really more of glycogen impairing (32). I would also note that most of the research on this topic has been done on males and it's possible that women are even less likely to see a benefit due to their already increased use of fat for fuel. In this sense, male athletes who try to fat adapt themselves are trying to make their physiology more like a woman's.

For athletes involved in more high-intensity training, long-term VLC diets are a mistake as performance will invariably suffer. This can easily be integrated with a fat loss diet with lower carbohydrates on low-intensity training days and increased calorie days synchronize with higher-intensity training days and I will discuss this more in later chapters. It's at least been suggested that VLC diets might be effective for weight loss/control in certain types of strength/power or weight class sports (33). Even here, there are potential issues with dehydration and mineral loss and lean normally cycling women face the issue of menstrual cycle dysfunction.

Returning to Diet Set Up

Regardless of those situations where a woman might choose to follow a VLC diet of some sort, there will be situations where the calculated diet results in carbohydrate intakes that are near the 80-120 g/day cutoff (this is far more likely to occur for the luteal phase diet). For those women who do not want to follow a ketogenic/VLC diet, modifications can be made where dietary fat is reduced slightly and carbohydrates increased. For every gram of fat removed from the diet, 2 grams of carbohydrates could be added as this will be roughly equivalent calorically (i.e. 9 calories for the fat vs. 8 calories for the carbs). A woman who's diet calculations put her at 100 g/day of carbohydrates who wanted to consume 130 g/day could reduce her daily fat intake by 15 grams so long as this does not take her below the minimum cutoff value for dietary fat intake.

The Menstralean Diet Study

For many readers of this book, the above approach to diet set up may seem daunting and unnecessarily complex and, in many situations it probably is. However, for those women looking to optimize their diet and fat loss, I want to emphasize the potential benefits of the above. To do so, I will examine a study that came out in the middle of 2016, long after I had worked out the above based on a woman's fundamental physiology (38). In it 60 overweight women with a bodyweight of roughly 195 lbs/88 kg and a BF% of 29-35% (my Category 2) were assigned to one of two diets. The first was a diet based around the menstrual cycle changes that occur in a woman's physiology (called the Menstralean diet) and the other based on standard Danish government regulations. The Menstralean diet actually had three distinct diets (early follicular differed from late follicular) but I don't see this as necessary. Exercise was varied slightly during the cycle as well but I won't discuss those details here.

The control diet provided 1600 calories per day with a ratio of 15-20% protein, 45-50% carbohydrate and 30% fat throughout and this is consistent with most country's general dietary recommendations. The Menstralean diet provided the same 1600 calories with 30% protein/50% carb/20% fat diet during the follicular phase and 30% protein/40% carb/30% fat during the luteal phase. I've compared these values to the percentages that my calculated diet above yields and it's clear that they are nearly identical.

	My Follicular	Menstralean Follicular	My Luteal	Menstralean Luteal
Protein	28%	30%	29%	30%
Carbohydrate	47%	50%	37%	40%
Fat	25%	20%	35%	30%

In addition to adjusting the diet overall, the Menstralean diet also factored in the change in metabolic rate and food cravings during the luteal phase with calorie intake were raised by 200 calories by allowing the dieters to consume a portion of dark chocolate. While both groups showed a substantial drop out rate, it was lower in the Menstralean dieters (38% vs. 61% drop out). High drop out rates are quite common in diet studies, especially in the control groups so this is not a surprise. It's likely that improved overall results in the Menstralean group probably resulted in improved adherence as well. While both groups lost significant amounts of weight, the most adherent dieters in the menstrual cycle showed the best results, losing 11 lbs (5kg) more total weight with a larger drop in waist circumference compared to the control group. This was likely due to several factors, not the least of which was the increased protein intake in the Menstralean diet. But adjusting the diet to fit the women's physiology in terms of fuel use, cravings, etc. assuredly also played a role.

While this study is certainly preliminary and more work on the topic needs to be done, I find it interesting that the idea of female specific approaches to diet and fat loss (along with the recognition of female specific needs in sports nutrition) is finally being examined. I expect more research on this topic to begin to be done and I'd mention in a related vein that research I will discuss in Volume 2 finds that synchronizing training with menstrual cycle changes improves results. If nothing else, this study points out that matching diet to a woman's changing physiology throughout the cycle or due to any hormonal modifier present improves her overall results. While complex, the above represents a more ideal of setting up a woman's overall diet.

Chapter 20: Nutrient Sources, Electrolytes, Fluids and Diet Products

While getting the proper amounts of each of the macronutrients is important, it's equally critical to ensure that proper food choices are made. All sources of a given nutrient are not identical in terms of how they may impact on health, performance and body composition or how well or poorly certain nutrients within those foods are absorbed, etc. As well, there are a number of common nutritional deficiencies that are seen in general or especially in active females or athletes and this is generally related to food choices or, more specifically, the elimination of certain foods from the diet. While it is possibly to simply use dietary supplements to correct these deficiencies, nutrients from food are almost always more effectively absorbed due to the presence of other nutrients and co-factors in food.

For that reason, I will focus on whole food sources of those nutrients in this chapter, making specific recommendations for types and amounts of proteins, carbohydrates and fats. I'll also address some of the common concerns that tend to surround certain foods in terms of health or body fat. In addition to looking at food sources, I also want to address sodium and potassium intake, general fluid intake as well as some common dieting aids. Outside of a small handful of issues that I will mention as needed, the hormonal modifiers do not impact meaningfully on optimal nutrient intakes or food sources. However, there are some sport-specific considerations due to commonly seen deficiencies among female athletes.

Common Micronutrient Deficiencies

While my focus in this chapter is on food sources of protein, carbohydrates and fats, I do want to look briefly at some specific micronutrient (vitamins and minerals) of particularly importance to women. Many are found to commonly be deficient in women while others are critical for some aspect of health (especially bone health), performance or fat loss. I will mention many of these again in Chapter 24 when I discuss supplements. I will only note here that, ideally nutrients should come from whole foods rather than isolated supplements as they are invariably absorbed more effectively from foods due to the presence of other nutrients and co-factors which are present.

Looking first at female athletes, a number of common nutrient deficiencies are frequently seen in this population including inadequate intakes of B12, iron, zinc, calcium, Vitamin D and magnesium (1,2). Each has their own important functions in the body (often interacting with one another) and I want to look at each of them briefly along with the foods they are generally found in. I'd note that low iron, zinc, calcium and possibly magnesium have been found in patients suffering with fibromyalgia, one of the low cortisol related diseases I mentioned in Chapter 13 (2a). While not studied to my knowledge, I have to wonder if those same deficiencies might not be contributing to adaptive hypocortisolism.

Vitamin B12 is involved in a huge number of physiological processes including red blood cell formation and neurological function. Extreme deficiencies can cause what is called pernicious anemia (which is not the same type of anemia as is caused by iron deficiency), an autoimmune condition that can cause neurological disorders. Vitamin B12 is only found naturally in animal source foods such as meat and dairy foods although B12 fortified vegetarian foods are often available.

Iron is involved in a number of processes important to women not the least of which is red blood cell production (important for endurance and overall performance) and thyroid hormone metabolism with low levels of iron decreasing both. Low iron stores have also been linked to problems with cognitive performance, emotions, quality of life and behavior (2b). Iron deficiency also interacts with most aspects of menstrual cycle dysfunction and FAT/RED-s (2c). Iron status can be defined among different levels with anemia being the most extreme level of iron depletion. Only blood work can determine this.

Iron occurs in food in two forms, heme and non-heme with heme iron being absorbed 10-30% more effectively than non-heme iron. Animal foods contain a mixture of heme and non-heme iron while vegetable source and fortified foods only contain non-heme iron. A number of dietary factors can either increase or decrease the absorption of both kinds of iron. Vitamin C, some types of fermented foods and small proteins found in meat (called the 'meat factor') and alcohol all increase iron absorption and 100 mg of Vitamin C consumed with a meal can increase non-heme iron absorption by roughly 85%. In contrast, phytates found in grains, nuts, seeds, beans and other foods inhibit the absorption of iron (and other minerals). Compounds in tea and coffee inhibit iron absorption as does calcium although the effect is small.

Zinc is involved in numerous physiological processes including the metabolism of protein, carbohydrates and fats. Zinc also plays a role in immune system function. Along with iron, selenium and iodine (found primarily in iodized salt), sufficient zinc is also critical for normal thyroid hormone metabolism (3). Diets low in these nutrients will decrease the level of thyroid hormones, lowering metabolic rate and energy expenditure (low thyroid levels are also one of the most common sources of misdiagnosed depression in women). Zinc, like iron is found in larger amounts in animal source foods and is absorbed more effectively from those foods.

Calcium and Vitamin D are both critical for optimal bone health, both in terms of developing peak bone density in a woman's younger years and limiting or reversing bone density loss as she gets older (4). Calcium has others roles in the body with dairy proteins (discussed below) having a potential role in fat loss and improving body composition. Dairy foods are the primary source of calcium in the diet (dairy food also contain other nutrients such as protein, carbs, sodium and potassium that improve calcium absorption). Calcium is often found in vegetable source foods but the amounts are lower and the calcium is absorbed less efficiently (calcium from dairy is absorbed with 97% efficiency versus 22% from broccoli).

I can't imagine readers of this book haven't heard about Vitamin D in terms of not only it's role in human health (low levels being related to almost any problem you can think of including colon cancer, diabetes risk, depression, autoimmune diseases, PCOS and many others) but the fact that most people are deficient in the modern world. Of relevance to athletes, Vitamin D has a direct role on skeletal muscle with low levels impairing athletic performance (5). Vitamin D is extremely unusual as a vitamin in that, outside of fortified foods, the levels found in most foods are quite low. Rather, Vitamin D is produced in the body in response to direct sun exposure with a lack of sufficient sun exposure being a direct contributor to the deficiencies seen in the modern world. Between working indoors and avoiding the sun due to fear about skin cancer, sun exposure has decreased drastically causing Vitamin D levels to be low (5a).

In addition to calcium and Vitamin D, a number of other nutrients such as Vitamin K, phosphorous, magnesium and others (including iron, zinc, fluoride, protein and fat) are critical for optimal bone health. Vitamin K is found primarily in leafy green vegetables such as broccoli, kale, spinach and turnip greens. Phosphorous is found in foods such as meat, dairy, nuts, beans and cereals (foods typically containing other nutrients that improve bone health). Too much phosphorus combined with insufficient calcium can contribute negatively to bone health and both are important. Magnesium, which is often deficient in the diet (and has numerous other physiological roles) is found in whole-brains, vegetables, nuts and seeds.

While the above was focused more on female athletes, other populations are often found to be deficient in one or more of the above nutrients. In postmenopausal women, for example, sufficient calcium, Vitamin D and Vitamin K is critical for helping to limit the risk of osteoporosis and optimal intakes are rarely seen (6). There are also indications of nutrient deficiencies associated with obesity although it's difficult to determine if this is due to poor food choices per se or changes in how nutrients are being metabolized (7). Women using birth control may be at risk for deficiencies in certain B vitamins (including B12), zinc, selenium, magnesium and Vitamin C and may require more on a daily basis (7a).

Causes of Micronutrient Deficiencies

In the most general sense, micronutrient deficiencies will be related to eating inadequate amounts of foods containing that nutrient or removing it from the diet completely. This means that the specific nutrient deficiency that is seen is likely to be population specific. In the general public, poor overall dietary patterns will be the primary contributor although it would be more likely for deficiencies to be seen in the micronutrients found in fruits and vegetables such as magnesium as mean intake is often high. In contrast, deficiencies in athlete tend to be related to low total energy intake, often inadequate protein intake and, more importantly, the removal of specific protein sources from their diet (discussed further below).

In addition to their dietary choices, there are other reasons athletes might be predisposed to some of the nutrient deficiencies listed above. One is that exercise often increases nutrient requirements over normal levels. Zinc, magnesium, iron and calcium are all lost in sweat during exercise and endurance training can cause a depletion of iron from the body due to increased turnover and the need to make new red blood cells, further increasing requirements requirements. In some sports, red blood cells actually burst during exercise and it's been estimated that athletes may need up to 30-70% more iron than sedentary individuals (8,9). Dieting also causes depletion of the body's iron stores over time (9a). This type of effect, an increase in nutrient requirements in response to training, is likely to be present for most nutrients.

It has traditionally been argued that any increased nutrient requirements due to exercise will be met by increased food intake but there are two assumptions here that are frequently incorrect. The first is that female athletes are consuming enough calories to begin with or that food intake will increase with increasing activity. Clearly many female athletes are doing neither and are chronically restricting their food intake and/or undereating relative to their often high energy requirements. Even when sufficient calories are eaten, women's generally lower food intakes can cause problems. As a singular example, an iron intake of 18 mg/day is recommended for pre-menopausal non-athletes. The typical modern diet contains ~6 mg iron per 1000 calories which means that 3000 calories per day would be required to obtain the necessary amount. That high of a calorie intake would be excessive for all but the most heavily training women and, even there, the up to 70% increase in iron requirements would make it nearly impossible to meet iron requirements. In this case, achieving sufficient iron intake would require increasing the relative proportion of iron in the diet (i.e. 8-10 mg/1000 calories) by consuming foods with a high-iron content daily or with supplementation.

The second assumption regarding nutrient intake for active women is that they are making proper food choices in terms of providing the required nutrients. As mentioned above, this is often not the case with the usual issue being insufficient total protein intake or the avoidance of specific foods. Women have a general tendency to remove many animal source proteins such as red meat and dairy foods which reduces or eliminates the intake of critical nutrients in their most well absorbed form. By their very design, vegetarian or vegan diets can increase the risk of nutrient deficiency for this reason (10). This is due to both a reduced total intake along with the nutrients in question being absorbed more poorly. For example, a lack of heme iron in the diet can raise iron requirements for vegetarians by up to 80%. Even when vegetarian diets provide more total iron in the diet, iron status is still found to be lower. The same holds for zinc where decreased absorption can increase zinc requirements for vegetarian athletes by 50%. I'd note that vegetarian diets are often much higher in nutrients that are found in lower amounts in animal foods and the bigger point is that both animal and vegetable foods should be part of a healthy and/or athletic diet.

Micronutrient Recommendations

I've summarized the recommended intakes of the above nutrients in the chart below for women aged 18 and up along with places where the values may change or there is debate over optimal levels.

Nutrient	Recommended Intake	Best Food Sources
B12	2.4 µg/day	Meat, dairy, fish, fortified vegetarian foods
Iron	18 mg/day 23-30 mg/day (athletes) 32 mg /day (vegetarian) 8 mg/day (menopause)	Red meat, chicken, pork, fortified foods, various vegetable source foods
Zinc	8 mg/day 12 mg/day (vegetarian)	Red meat, chicken, fortified foods, vegetable source foods
Calcium	1000 (1500) mg/day 1000 mg/day (menopause w/HRT) 1500 mg/day (menopause w/o HRT)	Dairy foods, kale, spinach, broccoli
Vitamin D	600 IU/day (15 µg/day)	Sun exposure, fortified foods
Magnesium	320 mg/day	Dark leafy greens, beans, seeds, nuts
Vitamin K	90 µg/day	Broccoli, kale, spinach
Phosphorous	700 mg/day	Meat, milk, cheese

Looking at iron, the recommended daily intake is 18 mg/day (this can vary from country to country) and this may increase to 23-30 mg (a 30-70% increase) for athletes. Due to poorer absorption of non-heme iron, vegetarians and vegans might need 32 mg/day total iron and it's unknown if vegetarian athletes need even more than this due to the impact of exercise itself. Approximately 10-25% of women have a particularly heavy menstrual flow which can increase iron requirements by 1 mg/day while women on birth control may have slightly decreased requirements due to reduced or absent bleeding (10a). With the cessation of menstruation iron requirements drop to 8 mg/day after menopause. For zinc, the recommended intake is 8 mg/day and this may increase to 12 mg/day for vegetarians due to decreased absorption.

Looking at calcium, an intake of 1000-1200 mg/day for pre-menopausal women is recommended. There is some belief that 1500 mg/day may be more appropriate in this situation but this level of intake requires supplementation and there is a great deal of debate over it at the current time. At menopause, women who are on Hormone Replacement Therapy (HRT) only need 1000 mg/day while those women not on HRT require 1500 mg. That level is also appropriate for women with hypothalamic amenorrhea. For Vitamin D there is current controversy over appropriate daily intake levels with many pushing for higher than traditionally recommended levels due to the common occurrence of deficiency.

The Sample Diet

Having looked at the issue of micronutrient deficiencies, let me examine different sources of protein, carbohydrates and fats within the context of the sample diet calculated last chapter.

	Follicular Phase	Luteal Phase
Calories	2000	2000
Protein	140 g/day	140 g/day
Carbs	235 g/day	185 g/day
Fat	56 g/day	78 g/day

Dietary Protein Sources

Given the importance of sufficient protein in the diet (discussed in the last chapter) along with the potential for protein source foods to enormously impact on micronutrient intake, I want to discuss it first. I will only look at whole food proteins here and will save a discussion of protein powders for Chapter 24. Dietary protein is found in a majority of foods with a few exceptions such as pure sugars and pure fats. Realistically most protein in the diet comes from either animal source foods such as dairy, red meat, chicken, pork, fish, etc. along with being found in foods such as beans, nuts and grains. Fruits and vegetables may contain a gram or two per serving but this is rarely worth paying attention to and it is impossible in a practical sense to get sufficient protein in the diet from these foods.

In addition to differences in their micronutrient content, all protein are not equivalent in terms of their amino acid profile, digestibility and how well or poorly they are used by the body for various processes such as muscle growth. Animal source proteins are absorbed with roughly 90-95% efficiency while as little as 80% of some vegetable proteins may be absorbed. Practically this means that more total protein will have to be eaten to meet requirements if the diet contains a large amount of vegetable proteins. This is in addition to the fact that many micronutrients are absorbed more poorly from vegetable source proteins.

Animal proteins are also the most concentrated sources of protein in the sense that they provide the greatest amount of dietary protein in the fewest number of calories (this is not true if the foods are particularly high in fat). Grains and vegetable source proteins always contain significant amounts of carbohydrate and calories and women trying to obtain enough protein from those sources often end up over-consuming both carbohydrates and calories unless their activity levels are very high.

Red Meat: Beef, Lamb, Emu, Bison, Buffalo

I mentioned previously that women often report less of a taste or desire to eat protein foods and that this often manifests in a reduction in animal protein intake and a trend towards vegetarian or vegan dietary approaches. Beyond even that generality is the fact that even women who do regularly consume chicken or fish often remove red meat from their diets (recall from earlier in the book that one study of amenorrheic women found that none of them ate red meat). Some of this is clearly just a general food/taste preference but there are often other factors behind this choice.

One is the frequently seen attempt to reduce dietary fat to extremely low levels combined with the often held belief that red meat is automatically high in dietary fat. While it is absolutely true that many cuts of red meat are extremely fatty (often having equal gram amounts of protein and fat), very lean cuts of red meat are available, often having no more than 4-8 grams of fat per 4 oz (113 g) serving. While often more expensive, even leaner cuts are sometimes available with various types of "game" meats such as bison, buffalo, emu, elk and others being extremely low in fat. I'd note again that the goal of reducing fat to extremely low levels is a mistake in the first place for reasons previously discussed in this book.

One of the second reasons often given for removing red meat from the diet has to do with concerns over health, especially colon cancer risks. There is an element of truth to this although it often has to do with other factors such as the fat content or how that meat is cooked. Charring meat excessively does promote the production of unhealthy chemical compounds while other forms of cooking do not. As important is the person's overall lifestyle. A large consumption of overcooked, fatty meats for someone who is inactive, carrying excess body fat and eating too few fruits and vegetables is far different than someone who is lean, active and choosing leaner red meats along with eating plenty of vegetable foods (10b). Lean red meat has been shown to health benefits, the cancer risks tend to be drastically overstated in terms of the real-world impact it has and red meat actually contains many anti-cancer compounds (11).

While there may be other reasons women remove red meat from their diets, the fact is that this one choice can put them at an increased risk of deficiencies in B12, iron and zinc. Of all the meats that can be eaten, red meat has the highest amount of zinc and iron (with both being absorbed more effectively than from other foods) and is second only to fish in terms of B12. Certainly these nutrients are found in other foods but either the amounts present, absorption or both are decreased. Iron supplementation is always possible but often causes stomach upset or tarry stools. Red meat is also superior to supplements for correcting iron deficiency, most likely due to improved absorption caused by the presence of other nutrients (12). While not technically red meat, I want to mention pork products such as ham, bacon, pork loin here. While pork is often considered synonymous with fattier cuts of meat such as bacon, pork loin is actually an extremely low-fat protein source and, like all meats, contains iron, zinc and B12 in varying amounts. Liver is also one of the best sources of iron with nearly triple the level of red meat.

Fowl: Chicken, Turkey, Duck, etc.

Relatively speaking, fowl of various types seems to be less likely to be removed from the diet than red meat with many women including it fairly regularly based on it's lower fat content or relatively reduced concerns over the problems often attributed to red meat. That said, the fat content of fowl can vary quite significantly. Skinless white chicken is nearly fat free while dark meat or chicken with the skin contains more fat. Methods of cooking can alter the fat content drastically. Grilling may keep fat intake very low while deep-frying can increase the fat content significantly. In terms of micronutrients, chicken is a decent but not fantastic source of iron with anywhere from 1/5th to 1/10th or so the amounts found in red meat. Italso contains the same nutrient that improves iron absorption from other foods. It'z zinc and B12 content is decent but less than red meat and the fattier dark meats have more of all three nutrients than the more commonly eaten white meats.

Eggs

Eggs have had a long and varied history in human nutrition. On the one hand, eggs are one of the highest quality sources of protein available. Whole eggs are a slightly higher quality than egg whites (though both are good) although raw eggs are absorbed very poorly. On the other hand, the high fat and cholesterol content of eggs caused an enormously negative reputation to develop over potential health risks from egg intake. Whether or not eggs are or are not harmful in the diet has flip-flopped over the years with recent research finding that most of this fear is unfounded with eggs containing many health promoting nutrients as well (13). As I mentioned in the last chapter, any concern over dietary cholesterol intake is mostly unfounded and, in any case, when blood cholesterol increases due to increased egg intake, it is the healthier type to begin with. All of the fat and cholesterol in eggs is found in the yolk (which also contains most of the micronutrients) with egg whites being effectively fat free. When dietary fat intake must be reduced or limited, a mixture of one to two whole eggs with egg whites (to increase the protein content of the meal) can provide an optimal compromise in terms of taste, protein quality and fat/calorie content. Eggs are a good source of zinc and B12 but are a very poor source of iron overall.

Dairy Proteins: Milk, Yogurt, Kefir, Cheese and Others

Along with red meat, the removal of dairy foods from the diet is not uncommon although the reasons tend to be population specific. At least some of the reductions in the general public have more to do with milk being replaced by other drinks such as soda or juice than a deliberate desire to consume less dairy specifically. However, there are often other reasons, both good and bad, for women to choose to remove dairy foods from the diet.

One very real reason dairy foods are often eliminated has to do with the inability to digest lactose, the sugar found in milk. Lactose intolerance (and less commonly allergies) exist and certain dairy products can cause gas, bloating and diarrhea. Most who are lactose intolerance can handle yogurt as the active cultures have pre-digested the lactose along with some types of cheeses although milk is usually problematic. Pills containing lactase (the enzyme that breaks down milk sugar) can be taken with foods that cause problems and there are also some lactose-removed foods although they tend to be proportionally much more expensive. Dairy protein powders (discussed in a later chapter) have often had the lactose removed or pre-digested as well. Just as with red meat, dairy foods are often removed from the diet due to the perception of them as a high-fat food. And just as with red-meat, reduced, low- or even non-fat dairy foods are very often available (some of this may be country specific). Let me reiterate that the desire to reduce dietary fat to extremely low levels is misguided to begin with.

While assuredly not the reason for performance athletes, in the physique community milk is often seen as being an unclean food (the reasons for this are unclear but the definition of clean and clean is somewhat vague) or for causing smoothness in an appearance sense. The reasons for this belief are obscure but might be due to the relatively high sodium levels in many dairy foods which would cause women on a low-sodium diet to retain water. This isn't a problem if sodium intake is kept at appropriate levels to begin with (sodium restriction has its own set of issues discussed later in the chapters) and even if there is some truth to this, it only matters on the day of the competition to begin with. Some feel that dairy exacerbates acne problems and this might be one reason to eliminate it from the diet (14).

Like other animal foods, dairy is not only a good source source of very high-quality protein but also contains many critical micronutrients with both zinc and B12 being found in decent amounts. In contrast, the iron content of dairy foods is quite low. Arguably the most important nutrient found in dairy foods is calcium (Vitamin D is often added as well) as it is found not only in large amounts but is absorbed with extremely high efficiency. As noted above, sufficient intake of calcium, along with the other nutrients I listed above is absolutely critical for women's bone health. An insufficient calcium intake earlier in life prevents the development of peak bone density and inadequate intakes at other times of a woman's life can cause bone density loss. That fact alone would be sufficient reason to include dairy proteins but there are many others, many of which aren't as well known.

One is that dairy calcium has been shown to positively impact on body composition, increasing fat loss during a diet (15). This combines with properly performed resistance training to improve body composition in both obese women and female athletes (16,16a). While some of this is due to correcting calcium deficiencies (suggesting that supplementation might have the same effect), dairy proteins seem to be more effective due to the presence of other nutritional compounds which increase their health benefits (17). Dairy proteins are also an extremely high quality protein, containing large amounts of something called Branched-Chain Amino Acids (BCAA) which are important for both muscle growth and preventing lean body mass (LBM) loss on a diet. BCAA help to maintain blood sugar and the slow digesting nature of dairy proteins tends to keep people full which is crucial when dieting for fat loss. Yogurt may have additional benefits here due to the presence of active cultures and acting as a probiotic to improve gut health (17a). Yogurt is lactose free so even lactose intolerant women can consume it. I've shown some representative dairy foods with their calcium content in the chart below.

Food	Serving	Calcium Content
Milk	8 fluid oz (236ml)	300 mg
Yogurt	1 cup (227 g)	350 mg
Greek Yogurt	1 cup (227 g)	225 mg
Cheese	1 slice (21 g)	125 mg

If you recall the recommended intake of 1000 mg/day for women aged 18-50, this would mean 2.5-3 full servings of dairy per day depending on the food being eaten (the 1500 mg/day recommendation would require 4-5 servings). Again, other foods do provide calcium to the diet but often in lower amounts or less absorbable forms. They contribute to calcium intake but are unlikely to provide the required amounts.

Fish

Even women who often eliminate red-meat and/or chicken frequently consume fish which is a high-quality, concentrated protein source. The dietary fat content of fish can vary significantly with warm-water fish being very low in fat and cold-water fish containing more. The fats in cold-water fish are generally of the healthier kind (the essential fatty acids I mentioned are often called fish oils) and the only real issue with the fat content has to do with calorie intake. Athletes tend to gravitate towards the lower-fat fish such as tuna, tilapia and others both for taste reasons and to reduce dietary fat intake. In my experience, the consumption of cold-water fish tends to be somewhat cultural and people who did not grow up eating those foods often don't a taste for them. From a micronutrient standpoint, fish is one of the best sources of B12 and iron and contains decent amounts of zinc; it also seems to be more filling than other proteins. A very real concern with a large fish intake is the potential for excess mercury intake. The mercury content of fish varies enormously and more information can be found here:

http://www.bodyrecomposition.com/nutrition/fish-intake-and-mercury.html/

Legumes: Nuts, Seeds and Beans

While animal source proteins tend to be the most concentrated form of dietary protein in terms of the number of grams of protein per serving, at least moderate amounts of protein are found in foods such as beans, nuts and seeds. As I mentioned above, the digestibility and quality of these foods isn't generally as high as animal source proteins although this isn't a major issue so long as the diet contains sufficient amounts of other high quality proteins as well.

Nuts and seeds contain decent amounts of protein although many are high in fat and most tend to provide a large number of calories in a fairly small volume of food and this can easily lead to eating too many calories. That said, the regular consumption of nuts either doesn't cause weight gain or may even cause a small weight loss. This may be related to the protein content or simply because they are not digested effectively and the calories are excreted. Both are still easily over-consumed and it's common for dieters to eat handful after handful and then report that they are no longer losing weight or fat.

Beans are probably one of the most well-known vegetable source proteins containing decent amounts of protein, fiber, and some carbohydrates. Many are at least decent sources of zinc and calcium although there are also anti-nutrients that can impair the absorption of those same nutrients. Most beans are low in fat with the exceptions of soybeans and chickpeas which contain relatively higher amounts of dietary fat. Beans contain a significant amount of iron although, once again, it is the less well absorbed non-heme iron along with a decent amount of zinc. As a non-animal food, beans contain no B12.

Soy Beans

While soy beans technically fall into the above category, I want to discuss them separately here. My comments will be brief as I will address the topic in detail when I discuss supplements. Soy protein is found in foods such as tofu, tempeh, miso and others. Unlike other beans, soy is a high quality protein in terms of meeting human amino acid requirements. Soy became extremely popular with it was found that women in cultures who ate soy based foods had lower rates of breast cancer than those that didn't. This was linked to the presence of phytoestrogens, plant nutrients that are similar in structure to estrogen and bind to the estrogen receptor. Whether or not its effects are positive or negative depends on the situation and I will look at this in detail in Chapter 24. I will only say here that even in Asian cultures, the total amount of soy protein/phytoestrogens is not large and excess soy can cause problems (not the least of which is impaired uptake of thyroid medication, especially if sodium is low). These foods can be included in a diet but I would suggest limiting their intake to no more than 25-30 grams of soy protein per day.

Grains

Since fruits and vegetables contain such insignificant amounts of protein, I'll finish by discussing grains such as rice, bread, pasta and many others. As with most vegetable source proteins, grains aren't a fantastically high quality protein and are absorbed less effectively than animal proteins. They should still be counted in the daily totals. Depending on the specific food the amounts of zinc and iron can vary and many foods are fortified so it's impossible for me to give average values. The protein content of grains is generally low although protein fortified versions are sometimes available. Trying to obtain large amounts of protein from grains tends to increase calorie intake drastically due to the high carbohydrate content.

Dietary Protein Recommendations

It should be clear from the above that I strongly feel that both red meat and dairy products should be part of an optimal diet for all women with red meat ideally being consumed at least several times weekly to ensure adequate iron intake. Chicken is a decent secondary source of iron and zinc but I still consider red meat to be best. Unless there is a very good reason such as an allergy to avoid dairy products, they should be a regular part of the diet to provide both a high-quality protein along with the most concentrated source of highly absorbed calcium. Dairy foods should be consumed daily and, if multiple servings are consumed they should ideally be split into morning and evening. The other protein sources including both animal and non-animals sources can be eaten as desired by preference, availability and budget.

For illustration, I've listed some common foods along with their average protein content based on a fairly standard serving size in the chart below. It should be clear that animal source foods contain far more protein per serving than any non-vegetable protein and this is in addition to the other difference I've discussed in terms of quality, micronutrient content, etc. As well, inasmuch as women may feel that the protein recommendations in this book are impossibly high, the chart should make it clear that the consumption of even moderate amounts of animal source proteins make them fairly simple to achieve.

Food	Serving	Protein	Food	Serving	Protein
Red Meat	4 oz (113g)	24 g	Whole egg	1	6 g
Chicken(white)	4 oz (113g)	18 g	Egg white	1	3.5 g
Chicken (dark)	4 oz (113g)	21g	Beans (pinto)	113 grams	11 g
Tuna fish	6 oz (158g)	32 g	Grains*	Varies	2-5 g
Yogurt or milk	8 oz (244g)	~8 g	Broccoli	1 cup (91g)	2.5 g
Cheese	1 oz	6.5 g	Apple	Small	<1 g
Kefir	8 oz	11-14 g	Protein Powder	1 Scoop	25-30 g
Greek Yogurt	8 oz	Up to 25 g	Protein Bars	Average size	20-30 g

*The protein content of most grains is highly variable but generally within the range listed.

To put the above into real-world perspective, consider the sample dieter who has a daily protein target of 140 grams per day. If she spreads her total protein intake over four roughly equal meals per day, she will need to eat 35 grams of protein per meal. Some of this protein will come from other foods in her diet but here I will only focus on specific protein sources to show how they could be used to achieve her per meal goals. A single can of tuna fish or 4-5 oz (113-140g) of any meat would provide ~35 grams of protein. A cup of Greek Yogurt along with additional proteins from grains or half a scoop of protein powder or a cup of regular yogurt (8 grams protein) with a scoop of protein powder (25 grams protein) would also achieve this level. A combination of 2 whole eggs (12 grams protein) with 4 egg whites (12 grams of protein) and 1-2 oz of cheese (7-14 grams) would provide 31-38 grams of protein. In contrast, 7 servings of grains would be required to provide the same amount of protein.

Dietary Fat Sources

Similar to dietary proteins, dietary fats are not all the same in terms of their effects on metabolism and health and dietary fat quality is just as critical to the diet as its total quantity. As discussed in the last chapter, I consider dietary cholesterol more or less irrelevant and will not discuss it, primarily focusing on the different types of fatty acids that are found in the diet and their effects on the body. There are four primarily classes of fatty acids, based on their chemical structure that I want to examine: trans-fatty acids, saturated fats, monounsaturated fats and polyunsaturated fats. I will also look at the fat content of some specific foods and how they might fit into the sample diet in a real-world way.

Trans-Fatty Acids TFAs

Trans-fatty acids, which go by other names such as partially hydrogenated vegetable oils, generally refers to man-made fats that are found almost exclusively in processed foods to improve shelf-life (I say generally as there are some naturally occurring TFAs). These fats have a purely negative effect on the body and their intake should be minimized or eliminated to as great a degree as possible.

Saturated Fats (SFA)

Saturated fats refers to a variety of different fatty acids such as palmitic and stearic acid that are found more or less exclusively in animal source foods and which are solid at room temperature. Two exceptions to this are palm kernel and coconut oil (which has quite a cult following) two non-animal sources foods which are high in saturated fats. Of some note, both foods are high in a special type of SFA called medium chain triglycerides (MCTs). MCTs are metabolized differently than most fats, going to the liver after digestion and providing energy more rapidly than other fatty acids.

Of all the fatty acids, SFAs tend to get the most blame for causing negative health effects such as increasing the risk of heart disease. There is both truth and falsehood to this due to the fact that not all SFAs have identical effects in the body. Some have negative effects while others have a positive or no effect (recall that saturated fats may play a role in menstrual cycle function). To equate SFAs with health risks is simply mistaken. This is in addition to the fact that the quantity of SFA being consumed along with the rest of the diet and lifestyle will all contribute to any effects that might or might not be seen. Someone who is inactive, carrying excess body fat, eating few or no fruits and vegetables, high intakes of saturated fats are likely to have negative health effects. In someone who is active, lean, eating plenty of fruits and vegetables, the risk are minimal or absent. Certainly, within the context of this book and its overall recommendations in terms of total fat intake, there is minimal to no risk. So long as this book's fat intake recommendations are met, there should be no issue with either excessive or insufficient SFA intake.

206

Monounsaturated Fats (MUFA)

Monounsaturated fats technically fall under a more general category of unsaturated fats but I will consider them separately from the polyunsaturated fats. Although there are many monounsaturated fats probably the most well known is the fat found in Olive oil, called oleic acid. While not essential for life, the monounsaturated fats either have neutral or positive health effects overall and probably contribute to the health benefits of diets high in them. A frequently unrecognized fact which is that the predominant fats in many 'high-fat' foods (including red meat) are MUFAs. For example, 30% fat ground beef contains 13 grams of fat per 3 oz (84 grams) but over half of that is MUFA. This means that ny diet meeting the fat recommendations in this book will contain mostly MUFA almost by default. If dietary fat is being added explicitly to the diet (i.e. in the luteal phase of the diet or for PCOS), it should generally be from MUFA.

Polyunsaturated Fats (PUFA)

While also falling under the general heading of unsaturated fats, PUFAs are distinct and important enough in their effects to be discussed separately. While there are others, the two major classes of PUFA that I will focus on are referred to as either ω-3/n-3 or ω-6/n-6 fatty acids (this just refers to their chemical structure but isn't important beyond the names). You will also see them called omega-3 or omega-6 fatty acids. These two PUFA, unlike other fatty acids, are essential in that they must be obtained from the diet and I will refer to them going forwards as the essential fatty acids (EFAs). Here things get slightly complicated as there are two parent EFAs, alpha-linolenic acid (ω-3) and linoleic acid (ω-6) which are converted to other compounds in the body with varying efficiencies.

In general, the modern diet tends to contain an excess of ω-6 fatty acids (found in abundance in most vegetable oils) and the body stores a large amount of these fatty acids in fat cells. Unless dietary fat intake is extremely low for long periods of time, it is extremely uncommon to see deficient intakes of ω-6 fatty acids and I won't say much more about them. In contrast, most people consume insufficient or suboptimal amounts of the ω-3 fatty acids and this will be my focus. As noted above, the parent fatty acid of the ω-3 is alpha-linolenic acid and this is converted to other compounds in the body, eventually producing EPA and DHA (the full names are not relevant) which have the primary metabolic effects in the body. Frequently referred to as the fish oils, EPA and DHA are found in fattier/cold-water fish but, outside of groups that eat those foods culturally, intakes of ω-3 in general and EPA/DHA specifically are invariably sub-optimal.

The metabolic effects of fish oils in the body is immense and increasing intake levels to optimal has a stunning number of positive effects (18). Two are a positive effect on both inflammation and immune system function, including a reduction in autoimmune symptoms (19). Large doses of fish oils have recently been shown to help with rheumatoid arthritis (RA, another autoimmune condition) and female athletes with low EPA/DHA intakes show more anxiety while those with higher intakes showing more mental toughness (20,20a). While the effects are relatively small, adequate fish oil intake increases fat loss slightly while impairing fat storage (20b). There are other effects of fish oils and they are almost all positive. This isn't to say that more is better but that ensuring optimal amounts pays enormous dividends.

Unfortunately, achieving this is not always simple. Current recommendations are to consume fatty fish such as salmon several times per week and this is probably superior to taking supplements in terms of improving the body's EPA/DHA status (21). However, in my experience, the consumption of fatty fish tends to be somewhat culturally specific and people who do not grow up eating fatty fish may not have a taste for it and supplements may be the only option to increase fish oil intake. Many years ago, flax oil was commonly recommended as a source of EFA due to its high content of alpha-linolenic acid. However, it is far from optimal due to the fact that the conversion to EPA is poor with the conversion of EPA to DHA being almost zero (21a). Women's bodies are better at producing DHA than men's and this is probably related to the importance of adequate DHA for the development of a child's brain during pregnancy (21b).

For this reason, I do not consider flax oil an ideal source of EFAs and, in the case where someone will not regularly eat fatty fish, a preformed source of fish oils must be found. Capsules are commonly available (containing varying amounts of EPA/DHA) as are liquid products such as Carlson's fish oils which can be used on salads or by people who dislike swallowing pills. Recent years have seen the development of 'high' EPA/FHA eggs and bread but the amounts present tend to be small with the foods being disproportionately expensive compared to buying the regular food and taking a supplement. I recommend that women consume 1.8 grams of combined EPA/DHA per day (women above 160-180 lbs can increase this to 3.0 grams/day) for general health. The amount of fish oils present in cold water fish can vary but salmon, herring, mackerel, anchovies, and sardines tend to contain the most. Salmon contains 1.4-2.2 g of fish oil per 4oz (113 g) serving which would meet the above amounts.

Dietary Fat Recommendations

Strictly speaking, only the EFAs are truly required in the diet overall or on a day-to-day basis but consuming only those fats would result in an incredibly low dietary fat intake which would be problematic in the long-run (this is not a problem for short, aggressive diets). Since consuming excess EFAs is neither recommended nor beneficial (and is potentially problematic), the rest of the day's fat intake will have to come from a mixture of saturated, monounsaturated and ω-6 fatty acids. As any fat intake above the lowest levels will contain sufficient amounts of ω-6 fat, only saturated and monounsaturated fats will be considered and an optimal ratio would be up to 1/3rd of total daily fat coming from saturated fats with the rest coming up from monounsaturated fats (22). Unless a woman has eliminated all animal source foods, her saturated fat intake will tend to take care of itself without any explicit effort on her part. That means that any additional fat that is required will come primarily from the monounsaturated fats. Olive oil can be used on salads and peanut butter is a perennial favorite of dieters.

In the sample diet, dietary fat is 56 grams in the follicular phase and 78 grams per day in the luteal phase. Assuming that fish oil supplements are being used and that the 1.8 g/day intake is coming from six 1 gram fish oil capsules, I have calculated the ratios of SFA and MUFA from the above ratios. Frankly, if women ensure their EFA intake along with sufficient fat intake, dietary fat ratios will work themselves out.

	Follicular Phase	Luteal Phase
Fat	56 g/day	78 g/day
EFA	1.8 g/day (6 g fat)	1.8 g/day (6 g fat)
SFA	16 g/day	24 g/day
MUFA	34 g/day	48 g/day

As I noted in the previous chapter, the above numbers may seem high to those women who are used to reducing dietary fat to the lowest levels possible but they represent perfectly appropriate intake levels. Generally the bigger problem is that dietary fats are incredibly easy to overeat due to their high caloric density. Containing 9 calories/gram, even small amounts of high-fat or pure fat foods can contain a tremendous number of calories and I've shown the fat content of a few representative foods below to show this. For illustration, I've included ground beef ranging from 30% fat to 5% fat (extremely lean) and you can see that the fat and calorie intake various enormously. When the grams of fat and calories do not match up numerically, it is due to the presence of protein or carbohydrates which are not listed.

Food	Serving	Fat (g)	Calories
Any Oil	1 tbsp (16 g)	14	125
Butter	1 tbsp (16 g)	11	100
Peanut Butter	1 tbsp (16 g)	8	95
Whole egg	1	5	70
Ground beef	4 oz (113g)	4-32	152-372

To round out the discussion of dietary fat, I think that even readers who won't be following a calculated or measured type of diet should measure some pure oils or higher fat sauces to see just how little it takes to contribute an enormous amount of fat to the diet. Even when they are being tracked, small misdmeasurement such as packing a tablespoon of peanut butter fuller than it should be can increase the fat and calorie content significantly. I mention peanut butter specifically as it tends to be used as a treat in the physique community but often causes problems when the spoon is slightly overpacked, people lick the bottom, etc. and end up consuming far more calories than they think (this is discussed more in Chapter 26).

Dietary Carbohydrate Sources

Recall from last chapter that, strictly speaking, all digestible carbohydrates are comprised of the same three simple sugars (glucose, fructose, and galactose) either bound to one another or in long chains. As well, after digestion, all digestible carbohydrates regardless of type release glucose and fructose into the bloodstream. While this makes them more alike than not, it is useful in a practical sense to divide carbohydrate foods into the separate categories of simple sugars, fruits, starches and fiber/vegetables.

Simple Sugars

While simple sugars are found in foods such as fruits, they are most commonly associated with candies and other "junk foods" (many of which are also high in fat) and I will focus on those here. Most would tend to classify these foods as "unhealthy" and there is at least some truth to this. Typically foods of this sort are high in calories, low in fiber, and digest quickly without providing much fullness, especially if eaten by themselves. They are frequently devoid of micronutrients although most foods in the modern world are fortified with vitamins and minerals to one degree or another. It would be rare for most to debate the above points but there is often an attitude where these types of foods are considered completely off limits, are unclean, or ruin health or the day's diet at any intake level. This is an extremist approach and represents the types of rigid eating attitudes discussed earlier in this book that cause so many problems. Rather, there are time when such foods can and/or should be worked into the day's eating patterns. Some of this is to avoid rigid wRINF attitudes (and recall the Menstralean study were a portion of dark chocolate was incorporated into the diet during the luteal phase) and I will address strategies aimed at this in Chapter 21. A more specific situation is when calories are eaten around a workout as more easily digestible carbohydrates and proteins are actually superior to avoid gastric upset or promote rapid recovery.

Perhaps the largest misconception or belief about food containing simple sugars is that they can magically cause weight or fat gain or prevent fat loss irrespective of their calorie content. This idea has been around for quite some time but more recently came to light with the hysteria over High-Fructose Corn Sugar (HFCS). Nearly identical to sucrose, HFCS is found in many processed foods including many candies and sugary soda and many have attempted to link its intake to increasing rates of obesity (23). To consider this singular factor misses the point as enormous changes in both the diet and environment have occurred. In recent years, HFCS intake has decreased while obesity continues to rise. Realistically any effects of HFCS had to do with their presence in sugary sodas and the enormous amount of calories that can be consumed this way. In general, liquid calories other than milk, digest very quickly and don't send a fullness signal to the body which results in an increase calorie intake (24). I'd note that people who drink sugary sodas almost invariably have poor diet and activity patterns. To blame HFCS alone is misguided.

Along with the fear of HFCS came a specific concern over fructose as research showed that large intakes could cause a number of metabolic problems. This even led many in the physique community to consider fruit (which is relatively higher in fructose) as off limits on a diet but there are two problems here. The first is that HFCS is only about half fructose to begin with. Large amounts of fructose eaten in isolation cause stomach upset. Few people actually consume it alone and studying it in isolation makes little sense here. As well, whatever amount of fructose was studied would represent twice as many calories as HFCS (or sucrose). That is, 60 grams of isolated fructose would require the intake of 120 grams of HFCS to begin with. Many studies on the topic used ludicrous amounts of fructose, far beyond what anyone could realistically consume (25). One used 300 grams of fructose per day, equivalent to 600 grams of HFCS/sucrose or 2400 calories of pure sugar per day. No one would argue that this amount of sugar is unhealthy but any impact on fat gain would be due to the calorie content rather than any magic effect of the fructose, sucrose, or HFCS per se. Anybody consuming that much pure sugar would be likely to have a terrible diet overall including a high-fat intake. Focusing only on the sugars missed the point completely.

This is not to say that I am recommending that large amounts of sugar in general or HFCS in specific be consumed in large amounts and I generally recommend against consuming liquid calories except for milk, especially while dieting (athletes with high energy requirements may find that liquids make it easier to match their calorie needs). Rather, I am trying to make the point that the absolutist idea that foods containing simple sugars are inherently fattening, prevent fat loss or must be removed from the diet completely is flawed. Certainly they cannot be consumed without limits and current recommendations are that no more than 5% of a day's total calories should come from added sugars, that is sugars added to the diet that are not found naturally, such as those in fruit (26).

For the sample dieter eating 2000 calories per day, this only amounts to 100 calories or 25 grams of added sugars per day which is not a large amount. For women dieting on lowered calories, even that small amount may be problematic in that it can represent a fairly large amount of the day's calorie/carbohydrate intake without providing much fullness. Practically it may be impossible to work such foods into the diet other than very occasionally and they may have to be eliminated for that reason alone (this is fundamentally different than eliminating them due to rigid eating attitudes). This has to be weighed against long-term adherence and I will discuss specific dietary strategies to address this in the next chapter. So far as I am concerned, consuming a small amount of candy in a controlled and planned fashion is better than losing control, bingeing and eating far more.

Fruit

In terms of their carbohydrate content, fruits contain primarily a mixture of both single sugars such as glucose and fructose along with sucrose. Unlike the foods in the above category, fruits also contain at least some fiber (amounts can vary enormously) along with other nutrients. Water makes up a large proportion of fruits which lowers the calorie density (here I am talking about whole fruits and will address fruit juice and dried fruit below). One hundred calories of apple is a far larger amount of food than 100 calories of jelly beans. It would be fairly rare for someone to consider fruit an unhealthy food although you will occasionally come across this idea. In the physique community especially, fruit often has a somewhat odd reputation and is often removed from the diets of lean competitors attempting to reach extremely low levels of body fat and one of two reasons is typically given for this.

The first being a very old claim that fruit somehow slows fat loss (or even causes fat gain) in very lean dieters. This idea is still promoted based on the fact that very high intakes of fructose can cause fat to be made in the liver but it would take an enormous amount of fruit to cause this to occur. Anecdotally at least, more modern physique diet coaches find that women's fat loss improves with fruit intake although the reasons for this are unclear. The second reason ties into the differences in how glucose and fructose are metabolized in the body that I described previously. Since fructose can't be used to refill glycogen stores in muscle, it's sometimes claimed that it is a poor food choice from an exercise performance standpoint, especially when calories are severely low. Thus it is argued that glucose containing foods will be better as they will refill muscle glycogen to better support training. There is at least some slight logic to this but fruit also contains glucose which can be used by muscle and to eliminate fruit for this reasons seems misguided. As well, dietary glucose is used more effectively to refill muscle glycogen when small amounts fructose are consumed as the fructose refills liver glycogen, sparing glucose for muscle.

Practically, many dieters also find that keeping liver glycogen levels higher helps to control appetite when dieting. Specific to women, recall that blood glucose can become unstable during the luteal phase, especially the late luteal phase. Consuming at least some fruit can help to limit this, improving mood, energy and appetite for the normally cycling woman (this is less important for women with other hormonal modifiers). Fruit can obviously be consumed during other parts of the cycle or by any woman as desired.

I'd mention that, contrary to its image as a healthy food, I don't think of fruit juices as a particularly good food source, especially while dieting. It provides no fiber, requires no chewing, digests very quickly, provides little to no fullness and a large glass can have just as many calories as sugary soda. I'd make similar comments for dried fruit. Also seen as healthy, it is extremely calorically dense due to the removal of the water content. One oz (28.4 g) of dried fruit has the same number of calories as a medium (182 g) apple and it's trivially easy to consume hundreds of calories by eating the occasional handful of dried fruit. In general, I don't recommend either food, especially while dieting. For those athletes with a very high energy expenditure, they might be a valuable way of increasing calorie and carbohydrate intake.

Focusing on whole fruit, an average apple or banana weighing 185 grams contains about 95 calories while smaller amounts (134 g) of melon is similar. Other fruits vary slightly but can be looked up online. The fat content of fruit is effectively zero and they have, at most a gram of protein and neither are worth considering in the big scheme of the diet. For women on all but the lowest calorie intakes, at least some amount of fruit can generally be fit into the diet, gaining the benefits described above.

Starches/Grains

The final category of digestible carbohydrates are the grains and starches, sometimes referred to as complex carbohydrates (distinguishing them from the simple sugars). This includes naturally occurring starches such as potatoes/sweet potatoes or refined grains such as bread, pasta, rice, etc. As mentioned in the last chapter, these consist of long chains of glucose molecules (often thousands) strung together and the process of breaking these chains down in the stomach is what makes them digest more slowly than simpler sugars (which require little breakdown).

Most starches consist primarily of carbohydrate with fairly minimal fat with a small amount of protein (roughly 3-5 grams per serving). Nutritionally they are a primary source of the B-vitamins and even the most highly processed grains are typically nutritionally fortified with other vitamins and minerals. The fiber content can vary widely with more processed grains having less fiber than less processed grains although the difference is frequently not large. Many high-fiber grain foods such as high-fiber pasta are often available as well. Many will make distinctions between different types of grains depending on their degree of processing (more highly refined grains generally digest more quickly due to having less fiber content) but I will treat them most or less identically in this section.

Since it has been at the forefront of nutritional fears in recent years, I want to briefly mention gluten, a type of protein found in grains that has been claimed to cause many if not most of the ills in the modern world for those people who are gluten intolerant (with a staggering number of gluten free foods being available). Certainly there is a small percentage of people suffering from celiac disease (marked by severe stomach upset and diarrhea when they consume even tiny amounts of gluten) but the majority claiming gluten intolerance have no such issue. When those individuals are given foods containing gluten without their knowledge, they report zero symptoms (27). The removal of gluten containing foods has also been found to cause nutrient deficiencies to occur (27a). While those with a true intolerance or celiac disease must avoid gluten, for the majority I see no reason to do so.

I've shown some representative starches in the chart below along with their carbohydrate, fiber and calorie content . Protein and fat content are not listed as they tend to be fairly negligible in most starches (although higher protein versions of some foods have also become available).

Food	Serving	Carbs (g)	Fiber (g)	Calories
Bread	2 Slices	28	2	160
Rice	1 cup (158g)	45	0.5	200
Pasta	1 cup (140 g)	43	3	220
Pasta (whole wheat)	2 oz (57g)	37	6	210
Oatmeal	1 cup (234 g)	27	4	158
Sweet Potato*	1 cup (133 g)	27	4	114

*Potatoes are actually vegetables but they are better considered as starches.

It's important to realize that most starches, depending on the degree of processing, are fairly concentrated, providing a large number of calories in a relatively small amount of food. A cup of cooked pasta or rice is a fairly small amount and often unfulfilling due to the low food volume. When eating these foods, many will eat two to three times the typical serving size, doubling or tripling the calorie count with ease. This can be a problem during a diet as concentrated starches can easily use up the day's carbohydrate intake without providing a large amount of food. In contrast, for those athletes with high energy requirements, the concentrated nature of most grains can help them to meet their calorie needs.

Fiber/Vegetables

The term fiber encompasses a variety of different compounds, the details of which aren't important, but can be divided roughly into soluble fiber (which mixes in water and turns into a gel; guar gum is an example) or insoluble fiber (which doesn't). Since vegetables often (but not always) contain large amounts of fiber, the two terms are often used interchangeably and I will do so in this section. Nutritionally, fiber has a number of important roles not the least of which is providing bulk to the diet and slowing digestion, which helps to keep people full. This effect is even more pronounced in meals containing even moderate amounts of fat. Vegetables are also a primary source of many vitamins and minerals along with a class of compounds generally referred to as phytonutrients. These are compounds that, while not essential to human life, often benefit human health. As I mentioned above, while certain nutrients such as Vitamin K and magnesium are absorbed more effectively from vegetable sources, many others such as iron, zinc and calcium are absorbed far more poorly.

On this topic, I do want to mention one specific class of vegetables with potentially profound benefits and importance for women (28). These are the cruciferous vegetables (the name refers to their cross-like physical structure) and includes broccoli, brussel sprouts, cabbage, cauliflower, collard greens, kale and others. While all of these are generally healthy, they are specifically important to women as they may play a role in the prevention of breast (and other types of) cancer. This is thought to be due to the presence of a compound called Di-Indole Methane (DIM) which is converted to Indole-3-Carbinol (I3C) in the stomach. I3C impacts on a small metabolic pathway of 17-beta estradiol resulting in the production of lowered amounts of a "toxic" subtype of estrogen. This only impacts on cancer risk and, despite claims, has no impact on women's fat loss in any form or fashion. While supplements of DIM and I3C are available (and might have some use for those women with a familial risk of breast cancer), the regular consumption of these specific vegetables is likely to be a better choice due the presence of other health promoting (and possibly synergistic) nutrients.

For decades it has been stated or believed that fiber cannot be digested in the human stomach and provides no calories to the body. At the very extreme, some have argued that vegetables are negative calorie foods that take more energy to eat than they provide and many diet plans consider vegeatbles as "free foods" that can be eaten without limit. However, the idea that fiber provides no calorie to the body is not strictly true. While insoluble fibers cannot be digested in the human stomach, soluble fibers can. Rather than providing carbohydrate to the body, the metabolism of soluble fibers generates what are called short-chain fatty acids which appear to have a number of health benefits (28). These provide 1.5-2 calories/g to the body although they should not be counted against the day's carbohydrate intake. I'd note that few vegetables are purely fiber and most contain at least some digestible carbohydrate although the amounts can vary widely. So-called starchy vegetables such as carrots, peas, corn and a few others (beans and potatoes are technically vegetables but I discussed them elsewhere) can contain a decent amount of carbohydrate and calories per serving while most fibrous vegetables contain only small amounts.

There is no doubt that vegetables are relatively more difficult to overeat (hence their classification as a free food on many diets) although the high-fat and high-calorie toppings that are often put on them cause this to stop being the case. And for most women, dieting or otherwise, it would seem odd to put a limit on vegetable intake of any sort. That said, it is not uncommon for smaller Category 1 females to consume so many vegetables during the day, usually in a quest to remain full in the face of extreme hunger, that they end up consuming a significant amount of calories from them. When the daily deficit is small to begin with, this can actually reduce the deficit, slowing fat loss.

I've provided a representative sample of a number of fiber/vegetable foods in the chart below (specific vegetables can be looked up online). All are based on a 1 cup (180g) serving of vegetables.

Food	Carbs (g)	Fiber (g)	Calories
Asparagus	7.5	3.5	40
Broccoli	12	4.5	60
Lettuce	6	3.8	30
Corn	33	3.5	155
Carrots	17	5	75
Peas	25	10	145

While the serving sizes of the above foods is not large, it's clear that vegetables contain generally far fewer calories than grains. However, even this varies significantly with the two starchy vegetables (corn and peas) containing double, triple or more calories than more fibrous vegetables which generally have extremely low calorie contents. This makes the latter excellent for staying full on a diet although they will be ineffective for refilling muscle glycogen stores or supporting training intensity. Regardless of the intake of any other carbohydrates source, vegetables must always be part of the diet.

Carbohydrate Recommendations
For the most part, there aren't any optimal or suggested ratios for the different types of carbohydrates that should be eaten. Rather, the specific amounts of each will depend primarily on the total amount of carbohydrates being eaten in a given day. There is, however. a hierarchy of importance in terms of what carbohydrate must be eaten daily and which should be limited or eliminated if there is no room. Vegetables must always be part of the diet and if one cup of fibrous vegetables were eaten at each of four meals per day, this would only provide 15-20 total grams of carbohydrates. Two cups per meal would provide 30-40 total grams which fulfills the entirely of the daily intake on a very-low carbohydrate diet.

When more carbohydrates are being eaten, it's hard to say if fruits or starches are relatively more important. Fruits tend to provide more food volume and can help to maintain blood sugar and fullness but are not optimal for refilling muscle glycogen or supporting training while starches will do more to support training but may provide less food volume and fullness. Until daily carbohydrate intakes get very low, it is generally possible to eat a combination of the two but, as carbohydrate intake goes lower, a choice may have to be made. Since muscle glycogen can be refilled between workouts when calories are raised to maintenance, relatively more fruits may be preferred at this point. Finally are sugars which should only be included in the diet after the other three types are being consumed. When carbohydrate intake is decreased, they will be the first to be removed, being saved for specific situations such as days at maintenance.

Meal Planning

While I have never included meal plans in any of my books, and will discuss meal frequency and patterning in detail in Chapter 23, I do want to look at how the information in the previous and this chapter might be put together in terms of daily food intake and meal plans. I will also look at how women using both the follicular and luteal phase diets might adjust them in a real-world sense.

Outside of the physique community, which often falls into it's own extremist patterns of eating, a major mistake I have seen many women make is to eat meals that are severely imbalanced in their macronutrient intake. Typically this manifests as meals of nearly pure carbohydrate being eaten and a common pattern would be a bagel for breakfast, pasta (with no meat) for lunch and only the dinner meal having an appreciable amount of protein. These types of all carbohydrate meals invariably cause a blood sugar and energy crash followed by hunger for more high-carbohydrate or sugary snacks. As soon as those women start getting sufficient protein and fat, both in their diet in general, in every meal, their blood sugar and energy stabilizes and they find themselves remaining full between meals in a way that they did not before. This leads to a general rule that every meal should ideally contain some amount of protein, carbohydrates, fats and fiber. The only meaningful exception to this are meals eaten close to training where a combination of protein and carbohydrates is superior, especially before and during the workout.

Now let me look at how a general approach to meal planning would look or the sample dieter. I've reproduced her diet below and shown what her per meal goals would be assuming 4 meals per day.

	Follicular Phase	Per Meal	Luteal Phase	Per Meal
Calories	2000	500	2000	500
Protein	140 g/day	35	140 g/day	35
Carbs	235 g/day	58	185 g/day	45
Fat	56 g/day	14	78 g/day	20

I would generally recommend setting up the day's or meals overall diet in the following order. First, the carbohydrate content would be determined. As noted above, vegetables should always be part of the diet and would be calculated first. After that, fruits will probably come next with starches being last if there is room for them. For those women setting up both a follicular and luteal phase diet, both fruits and starches will usually fit within the follicular phase while they may have to be reduced or eliminated during the luteal phase. Under most dieting circumstances, added sugars may be difficult to include although there are ways of doing so. Meals around workouts should come from rapidly digesting carbohydrates and some amount of sugars could be included here. There are other strategies, discussed in Chapter 21, that will also allow some amount of sugars to be included as desired.

For the sample dieter in the follicular phase, she might plan on 2 cups of fibrous vegetables per meal which will provide 15-20 grams of carbohydrates. To this she could add a half piece of fruit providing 12.5 grams of carbohydrates leaving room for a single serving of a starchy carbohydrate for a total of roughly 60 grams of carbs per meal with a mixture of types. In the luteal phase, this would need to be reduced by 15 grams which would mean cutting the serving of starchy carbohydrate in half or eliminating it entirely and eating a whole piece of fruit instead (meals could vary in their fruit or starch content).

The next step would be to add a protein source and, unless the starchy carbohydrate choice has significant amounts of protein, it can be ignored (if the protein source chosen has carbohydrates in it, the above will have to be adjusted). A goal of 35 grams of protein would require roughly 4-5 oz of any meat almost regardless of type. The other protein sources listed above would also be appropriate and there is little to no difference as to when different proteins are eaten (most preferences tend to be culturally based) so long as my recommendations for both total protein intake and types of proteins are met.

Finally is the fat source and what is required here will depend on the rest of the meal. If a higher fat protein source was chosen, very little additional fat may be required to reach the per meal goals. If the protein source was low in fat, more may need to be added to reach the meal's goals. If this is the case, straight oils such as Olive oil are good choices and peanut butter (which also contains protein and carbohydrate) is a perennial favorite among dieters. During the luteal phase, the increase in fat intake per meal is only 6 grams which is just under one tablespoon (16 g) of any pure fat.

For those women who want help setting up meal plans within the context of this books' recommendations, numerous websites and apps exist that can do just that. One I'd recommend is the site eatthismuch.com which will help set up specific meal plans.

Sodium and Potassium

While I discussed micronutrients earlier in the chapter, I want to address sodium and potassium separately. Both are commonly referred to as electrolytes and are involve in endless processes in the body. Both are found in foods in varying amounts with potassium being found in the largest amounts in plant based foods such as beans and spinach and sodium being naturally found in the largest amounts in animal based foods such as meat, eggs and dairy. Sodium is also added to many processed foods with many, if not most cultures adding salt (sodium chloride) to food to improve its taste. In the modern world salt is a primary source of iodine, a nutrient critical for proper thyroid metabolism.

As with many other nutrients, excessive sodium intakes have been blamed for many modern ills not the least of which is high blood pressure. As with those other nutrients, while excessive sodium intakes may be part of the problem, this has to be considered within the context of overall lifestyle. One important factor here is that the frequently low intake of plant based foods seen in the modern diet frequently leads to insufficient potassium intakes. This is important as it is the relative ratios of sodium to potassium that have the largest impact on overall health (30). The modern diet contains roughly twice as much sodium as potassium while it's thought that a potassium intake 5 times that of sodium is optimal. I would note here that while excessive sodium intakes, above 4 grams per day, can have a negative impact on bone health, this is only the case when calcium and potassium intakes are too low to begin with.

Just as with dietary fat intake, it's not uncommon for women to attempt to reduce sodium intake to the lowest levels possible. While this often revolves around health issues, it is more likely done in an attempt to reduce water retention. Certainly sodium plays a role here (and recall that increased sodium retention is part of the water retention occurring in the late-follicular and luteal phases) but water retention has more to do with changes in daily sodium intake than the absolute intake levels. Someone on a low-sodium diet who eats a large amounts of sodium will retain water and someone on a high-sodium diet will temporarily lose water if they lower sodium intake. But this effect is short-term as the body will adjust hormone levels within about 3 days of either change. If a woman on a low-sodium diet increases her sodium, she will retain water for about 3 days before it is lost as the body regains balance and vice versa (when I talked about weight class athletes in Chapter 18, I talked about how this can be manipulated to flush water out of the system). Potassium intake also impacts on water retention and increasing potassium intake can help to offset the problems of sodium related water retention in the late-follicular or late-luteal phases.

This is all important as extreme restrictions of sodium can cause its own set of problems. While rare, iodine deficiencies can occur when sodium intake is extremely low and this can negatively affect thyroid metabolism (this is compounded by a high soy intake, discussed in Chapter 24). Low sodium intakes also cause the hormone ghrelin to remain higher after a meal, meaning that dieters may be hungrier than if sodium intake were higher (31). In athletic populations, due to the loss of sodium in sweat, requirements are likely to be higher to begin with. During exercise, if too much sodium is lost and/or too much pure water is consumed a dangerous condition called hyponatremia, discussed in the next chapter, can occur. The water retention that occurs in the normally cycling athlete could put female athletes at risk for this an sufficient sodium intake must be ensured, especially during exercise in the heat.

For the general public, the maximum recommended amount of sodium is 1,500 mg/day but this will be higher for hard-training athletes. Unfortunately, it's impossible to provide guidelines as sodium losses can vary enormously (ranging from 115-5000 mg of sodium per liter of sweat) between athletes. I would generally recommend that athletes not restrict their sodium intake, liberally salting their foods while ensuring sufficient potassium intake. This can be facilitated by the use of Lite- or Lo-Salt, a combined sodium and potassium chloride salt tasting identical to normal salt. The ratios in different products can vary from 50% of each to as much as twice the potassium as sodium. It's important to get an iodized form to ensure sufficient intake of iodine. Pure potassium chloride salt is available but very bitter tasting and potassium supplements are limited to 99 mg/day. Lite or Lo-Salt could be used along with high-potassium vegetables while trying to reduce the intake of high-sodium processed foods.

About the only time I would suggest limiting sodium intake would be during the immediate pre-ovulatory and late-luteal phases of the menstrual cycle when water retention can drive women, especially dieting women, crazy. Here, reducing total sodium intake somewhat while ensuring sufficient potassium can help immensely with water retention. Ensuring an intake of 1200 mg/day of calcium adds to the effect (32). Other manipulations to sodium and potassium intake may also be made for physique competitors or weight class athletes in the final week before a competition but these are purely short-term changes to achieve competition goals. In all other situations, I do not recommend an excessive restriction of sodium but, rather, a sufficient intake of potassium.

Some Final Comments About Diets for Women

Before addressing a few other diet related issues, I want to make some final comments on the topic of women and the food choices that they make (or have recommended to them) during dieting. As I have hopefully shown in this and the previous chapter, not only are those choices often suboptimal but, in many cases, they are actively damaging. The irony here is that, those same choices, frequently made in an attempt to improve health or fat loss, often have the exact opposite effect. Insufficient protein intake causes a loss of LBM along with increased hunger while a very low dietary fat intake both reduces long-term diet adherence and can negatively impact on menstrual cycle function. Eliminating red (or all) meat can lead to suboptimal B12, iron and zinc intakes (impairing thyroid function) while removing dairy can cause calcium deficiency, harming both fat loss and bone density. I think you get the idea.

Certainly many of those ideas have been suggested at one point or another to improve health and they may (in a broad sense) in a population consuming excessive amounts of fatty charred red meat, dietary fat, reined grains and sodium on a backdrop of inactivity, excess body fat, high levels of stress combined with eating too few fruits and vegetables. Even in that context, increasing fruit and vegetable intake while moderating the intake of the other components of the diet is usually sufficient with complete elimination rarely being necessary. The largest effect on overall health in this population comes from fat loss itself. For active individuals, almost none of these factors are generally in play to begin with with the combination of regular activity, reduced body fat levels and other dietary components more than offsetting them. Eliminating foods/food categories containing critical nutrients does no good and often causes harm.

Essentially, I feel that what the way that many females approach fat loss and dieting, both in terms of their overall approach and food choices, is more or less the exact opposite of what they should be doing. Red meat should be consumed by women multiple times per week (along with other sources of iron and zinc) with dairy foods consumed multiple times daily. Dietary fat intake should be sufficient (with the right types of fats being chosen), sodium should be sufficient albeit balanced by potassium, etc. Certainly some of those factors are relatively more critical to the normally cycling woman who is losing iron every month or who has a menstrual cycle to lose but even women with the various hormonal modifiers can cause themselves problems if they create a nutritional deficiency through certain foods choices.

Related to that, let me make a few more comments about some currently popular dieting approaches that women often report getting superior results (in terms of health, menstrual cycle function, fertility, etc). Here let me focus on the ketogenic and Paleo diets and why I think they seem to "work" better than other, more commonly used diets. Invariably both diets revolve around a fairly high meat intake which more or less ensures sufficient protein, dietary fat and sodium intake. Dietary carbohydrates are are either severely (ketogenic diet) or moderately (Paleo diet) reduced with the focus being on vegetables and/or fruit intake and starches being reduced if not eliminated. Dairy intake is more variable in both diets depending on the interpretation. But overall both dietary patterns are far closer to what I have recommended both in terms of overall nutrient content and food choices compared to what women so often choose to do.

This isn't to say that I am automatically recommending either approach, here I am just making a point about how certain diet structures (with fairly simple rules) may serve to avoid some of the problems inherent to how some women choose to set up their daily diet. Any diet that effectively mandates sufficient protein from certain sources, sufficient dietary fat, etc. will be effective but that can be accomplished without following sometimes extremely rigid approaches to dieting. Ketogenic diets may not be appropriate for women with a normal menstrual cycle and the limitation on carbohydrate intake can impair training and performance. Even paleo diets may be too low in carbohydrates to sustain large amounts of training and I would argue against the removal of dairy foods (often seen as non-Paleo) is a mistake across the board. Rather than focusing on the specific dietary set up, I would rather readers of this book focus on my broad nutrient and food recommendations in terms of setting up an optimal diet.

Hydration and Fluid Intake

Although not strictly nutritional, an important aspect of the daily diet is maintaining adequate hydration status. Accomplishing this means matching the body's fluid losses (occurring through sweat, urination and other processes) with fluid intake. Here I am including anything that provides fluid or water to the body and I will discuss fluid sources below. Even slight levels of dehydration can have negative effects including decreased exercise and cognitive performance, increased headache (or risk of migraines), worsened skin appearance, diarrhea and others (33). As well, sufficient fluid intake has many potential benefits for dieting and fat loss. Very directly, consuming water or other fluids can decrease hunger by physically filling the stomach which sends a signal of fullness to the brain (34). Maintaining sufficient

215

hydration may also impact positively on hormones involved with fat mobilization (34a). Indirectly, staying hydrated can help to prevent at least some types of water retention, primarily due to its effects on the hormone aldosterone (this will not have an effect on stress and cortisol related water retention).

This raises the question of what a sufficient fluid intake is and this is, unfortunately, an impossible question to answer. For years at least in the US, the suggestion that eight 8oz (236 ml) glasses of water per day are required for normal hydration but this value has no actual basis in anything related to physiology. Others have offered daily fluid intake values based on bodyweight or what have you but this too is problematic. The issue here is that fluid requirements can vary wildly between any two people (this is especially true during exercise), making any general or absolute fluid intake recommendation meaningless.

A common recommendation to assess hydration status is urine color with darker colors (moving from clear to yellow to brown) indicating various degrees of dehydration (note that a high B-vitamin intake can make urine bright yellow). In a related vein, an old rule of thumb is that the average person should have 5 clear urinations per day with at least two of those occurring after workouts (if they are done). Of course, both of these require that urine color be observed which many may not wish to do. Contrary to common belief, thirst ends up being an excellent indicator of hydration status and simply drinking when thirsty will cause most people to drink adequate fluid. An exception to this is older individuals for whom the thirst mechanism may not work as well. The postmenopausal woman may need to drink more fluid than she thinks she needs to ensure adequate hydration. I would note that while maintaining proper hydration is critical, it is possible to overhydrate by drinking too much. I will discuss this more in the next chapter.

Fluid Sources
The body's fluid needs can be met by a fairly large number sources. High-water foods such as fruits and vegetables actually provide a fairly large amount of the body's fluid needs on a daily basis but here I'm going to focus here only on actual fluids/beverages in terms of their impact on hydration status as well as other issues surrounding them. Since all fluids sources ultimately provide water to the body, many tend to consider water itself as the only or best way to ensure hydration. Not only is this an extremist stance, it's incorrect. By itself at least, water is actually inferior for hydration (or rehydration after exercise) to some other beverages due to the lack of sodium and potassium. Both compounds increase fluid retention and it can take 20% or more of plain water to match the hydrating effect of drinks containing them. As well, all fluids, save alcohol which is always dehydrating, end up contributing to the body's hydration status and there is nothing magical about water in this regards.

Coffee and tea are two of the most commonly consumed liquids and there is a common belief that, due to their caffeine content, they cause dehydration. Certainly caffeine is a slight diuretic (causing water loss) but caffeinated drinks always contribute more fluid to the body than is lost due to the caffeine. If an 8oz (236ml) cup of coffee caused 1 oz (30ml) of fluid loss, the body still gains 7oz of fluid (210 ml). The body also rapidly adapts to caffeine consumption and chronic coffee and tea drinkers will see little diuretic effect. Women do lose slightly more water due to caffeine than men although the effect is still fairly small and caffeinated beverages will still contribute positively to a woman's overall hydration status (35).

Fruit juices contain a large amount of water (as does whole fruit) meaning that they can contribute positively to hydration. However, as I mentioned above, I consider them a generally poor food choices as they provide large amounts of simple sugars and can contribute large amounts of calories to the diet easily without being very filling (36). The exception would be for athletes having trouble meeting high calorie requirements or perhaps around training as they can provide both fluid and carbohydrates. As a calorie containing beverage, milk is actually an excellent choice for a number of reasons including the dairy protein and calcium content. As I'll discuss in the next chapter milk is actually more hydrating than either plain water or sports drinks due to its sodium and potassium content. Finally I'd mention sugary sodas. While providing fluid to the body, they also contribute significant numbers of calories as pure sugar with essentially zero nutritional value (at least fruit juice contains micronutrients). I see no place for them in the diet from any standpoint, hydration or otherwise.

Artificially Sweetened Beverages
My brief comments about sugared sodas above bring me to what is a somewhat contention area of nutrition which is the issue of sugar free or artificially sweetened beverages. Here I will include both diet soda and artificially sweetened drinks such as Crystal Light (a drink powder) and I will discuss other artificially sweetened products separately below. The point of these types of products is to provide a similar if not the identical sweet taste of sugars without the calories and most sugar free products contain

zero calories per serving. Various artificial sweeteners exist including saccharin, aspartame, Acelsulfame-K, and sucralose. More recently, Stevia, a natural no calorie sweetener, is starting to appear in commercial products as well. While somewhat unrelated to this topic, Olestra was developed as a fat substitute but had only limited use and has been more or less discontinued.

The majority of artificial sweeteners have been available for decades and since their introduction there has been a variety of concerns over their health effects during that time. More recently, these products have been claimed to promote sugar cravings, increase food intake, cause people to gain weight or that regular soda containing pure sugar is somehow healthier than their calorie free equivalents. First and foremost, there is an enormous amount of safety data available and problems have only been found when absolutely staggering amounts (usually tested in rats) are consumed. For example, it would take 17 cans of aspartame sweetened soda or 175 packets of powder per day to reach maximum intake levels although only 5 cans of soda sweetened with sucralose would achieve this value. Stevia, a natural sweetener currently has no safety data. For all but the most extreme intakes, there are no apparent risks.

The concern with hunger, food intake and obesity is equally misguided. Early studies did find a relationship between diet soda consumption and obesity but this is most likely a reversed relationship where people start using diet products after they gain weight. There is also a psychology where people feel that they can eat more freely if they are consuming diet products. It's been theorized that consuming these types of products might drive cravings for sweets and/or make people hungry but this is not usually the case. Even studies where people report increased hunger from diet products, there is no increase in actual food intake (37). Studies of successful dieters and those who maintain their weight loss in the long-term routinely find that the use of sugar-free products is part of their program (38). Recently, artificially sweetened drinks were found to be superior to plain water both for short-term weight loss and long-term weight maintenance (39). Any theoretical dangers are not occurring in the real world.

The above section is not to say that artificially sweetened drinks are magic and it's important to realize that they do not generally cause weight or fat loss in and of themselves. Rather, they provide a zero-calorie option for people who are thirsty or having sweet cravings which, in the aggregate, is far better than consuming a sugary soda with hundreds of calories. They are in no way required but they can be useful.

Other Fluid Choice Issues
To wrap up the discussion of general fluid intake, I want to address a few other issues. The first has to do with caffeinated beverages, including coffee tea or sodas. While these are often consumed for their taste or to quench thirst, many also drink them purely for their caffeine content. When dieting, they help to stave off hunger, can increase metabolic rate slightly (discussing Chapter 24) and may help to offset the fatigue that occurs, especially in Category 1 females. But this can lead to enormous intakes of caffeine on a daily basis and, as I discussed in Chapter 13, caffeine does raise cortisol. While this isn't a problem in and of itself, excessive intakes of caffeine by psychogenically and physiologically stressed dieters could eventually lead to problems. Looking briefly at hormonal modifiers, caffeine or caffeine containing drinks have been shown to improve insulin sensitivity, reduce body weight and decrease the risk of diabetes and this makes them especially valuable to women with PCOS or obesity related insulin resistance (40). Women using hormonal birth control should be aware that caffeine will stay in their body up to twice as long which might impact sleep if caffeine is consumed too late in the day (41).

Moving to the topic of bone health, it's often claimed that caffeine has a negative impact on bone health but this isn't entirely correct. Caffeine itself has at most a small effect on calcium absorption or excretion and most of the effect of caffeine has to do with caffeinated beverages replacing milk in the diet. It takes a trivial amount of milk to offset the impact of caffeine on calcium excretion and most of the negative impact of caffeine on bone health is seen in populations that consume too little calcium (41a). Similar comments can be made for soda which is often claimed to harm bone health. But most of the effect being due to soda replacing milk in the diet and/or there being inadequate calcium intake overall.

Finally let me make a few comments on alcohol. While providing nothing but empty calories to the body (with the relationship with bodyweight being complex as discussed previously), alcohol does not contribute to fluid intake, acting purely as a diuretic. In terms of overall and bone health, alcohol seems to have positive effects at moderate intake levels (1-2 drinks per day) although this may be due to better overall lifestyle patterns. In postmenopausal women, alcohol simulates the production of estrone which sends a small estrogenic signal, potentially improving bone health (43). At excessive intakes, alcohol is extremely detrimental to bone health, impairing the absorption of critical nutrients such as iron, zinc and calcium. It is also associated with overall poor food and nutrient intakes which compounds the problem.

Other Sugar Free Products

While there are a host of diet related products I only want to focus on a few here starting with some other commonly used sugar-free/artificially sweetened products such as sugar free gum and sweeteners. Rather than the above sweeteners, these types of products tend to use sugar alcohols such as xylitol, erythritol, sorbitol, and mannitol (all carbohydrates with names ending in "ol" are sugar alcohols). Due to their structure, sugar alcohols aren't metabolized in the body like normal dietary carbohydrates but they do provide calories to the body. The specific amounts depends on the sugar alcohol but it is often just as many as regular dietary carbohydrate. While highly individual, large amounts of sugar alcohols can cause severe stomach upset.

Looking at a few specific products, sugar-free gum is commonly sweetened with xylitol. Like sugar free drinks, it is often used by dieters to provide a tiny bit of sweet taste to help deal with sugar cravings. Like sugar-free drinks of varying kinds, gum may help people stick with their diets and avoid eating higher calorie foods. Gum has been shown to decrease appetite and snack intake although, used only by itself, it does nothing to cause weight loss (43,44). It's important to realize that the typical sugar-free gum has about 5 calories per stick and used in excess, this can add up. A person chewing 10-20 sticks of gum per day may add 50-100 calories to the diet although chewing gum itself burns about 10 calories per hour (assuming it is chewed continuously). Some sugar-free drinks powders also contain the same 5 calories per 8 oz (235 ml) serving. Certainly this is much less than the typical sugar-containing versions but, consumed in excess, the calorie content will start to add up.

Another popular product that can often be found are sugar-free toppings which can be added to foods to improve taste without adding as many calories as a normal topping would. Walden Farms is popular with US dieters and uses Splenda in addition to other natural flavors. The same comments made above apply to these types of products. Certainly these may help to improve dietary adherence in some situations and, while not calorie free, are far superior to using the full-calorie versions. Used in excess or without limit, they can contribute more calories to the diet than many realize.

A third sugar-free product worth discussing are the variety of low-carb or low-sugar foods that are typically aimed at low-carbohydrate dieters. By replacing some or all of the normally found carbohydrates with sugar alcohols, these products will often list only the "net" (i.e. digestible) carbohydrate content which is often quite low. In many if not most cases, due to a generally high-fat content, these products tend to have the same, if not more, calories than the normal versions and I see little point to them under most circumstances. For women with PCOS/insulin resistance or who are trying to reduce carbohydrates during the luteal phase, they might have some value but I think it's better to simply reduce total digestible carbohydrate intake overall since these products frequently provide no actual calorie reduction benefit.

Meal Replacement Powders/Bars

Unrelated to the above, a final diet product that may be worth considering are meal replacement products (MRP's). These are typically powders mixed in water or milk containing protein, carbohydrates, sometimes fat and other nutrients that are made to provide a relatively complete "meal" in a convenient form (commercial versions such as Ensure in the US also exist, usually aimed at older individuals who have trouble getting sufficient calories and nutrients). I'd include protein bars here with many modern bars having tastes and texture not dissimilar from candy bars, cookies, or brownies all while providing much better nutritional content. This gives them some amount of potential to help with sweet craving along with providing convenient, quick nutrition. The nutritional content of these products all vary somewhat but some combination of protein, carbohydrate, fat, micronutrients and fiber is usually present. Of some interest, MRPs containing high-fructose corn syrup have been repeatedly shown to help people lose weight which should point out that HFCS has no magic ability to either cause weight gain or prevent weight loss outside of its calorie content (45).

While convenient, these products should never make up the entirety of a day's diet but but women with busy work or life schedules or athletes with heavy training loads and high calorie requirements and limited time can use them as needed to ensure proper nutrient intake throughout the day. I'd generally recommend that no more than 1-2 meals per day be made up of MRP's with the other consisting of solid foods. As with all of the other products I've discussed, these products are in no way required but they may be useful or helpful for meeting nutritional needs.

Chapter 21: Flexible Eating Strategies

In Chapter 15, I looked in general at the conceptual differences between rigid and flexible restraint. I also looked at the reasons why flexible restraint (which I am referring to as flexible eating in this chapter) is superior to the more rigid approaches that are either implicit in many dietary approaches or that dieters impose upon themselves. I also mentioned that flexible eating, in a research sense at least, is more of a general attitude towards eating where small deviations are accepted as normal and either ignored or compensated for. While this probably represents the ideal approach overall, I find that many do better with what I call structured flexible eating strategies. At least in the early stages, these strategies are often less psychologically stressful as they allow the person to maintain somewhat more control. Over time, as people start to realize that their goals are as or even more effectively met by being more flexible, their overall attitude often starts to shift to a more global set of flexible eating attitudes.

In my original book on the topic, I described three structured flexible eating strategies which were the free meal, the refeed, and the full diet break. A fourth approach, called If It Fits Your Macros or IIFYM has been conceptualized and formalized in recent years. Each strategy is used at a different frequency and can be more or less appropriate under certain conditions. Even in hindsight, my own formalized approaches to flexible eating aren't appropriate in all situations and I have made some large-scale changes to them. When I examine the flexible eating strategies, I will work backwards from the least frequently used to the potentially most flexible approach in terms of their purpose, how they can or should be used along with any specific considerations that must be taken into account. Before doing that, let me look at some potential problems with all of the flexible eating approaches I will be discussing.

Problems with Flexible Eating Approaches

It's clear from the research that developing flexible eating attitudes is a huge component of improving long-term success rates for dieting. And as much as I truly think that adopting them has the potential to improve dieter's results by getting people out of a problematic mindset, there can still be problems that crop up that it would be unreasonable to ignore. While I will address specific problems or criticisms of each type of flexible dieting in the appropriate section, I want to address one potentially global issue that applies to all of them. This has to do with the potential for any type of "break" in a diet to throw the person off the diet completely. Certainly this seems to be less of a problem if the break is planned since it causes a psychological shift in how the break is framed (i.e. being seen as part of the diet rather than a personal failure) but that doesn't mean that it can't be a problem for any given individual. Making the mental shift from rigid to flexible dieting strategies takes time and practice and the emotions or issues that crop up when people feel as if they have "gone off their diet" may not go away instantly.

This is arguably more true for the Category 2/3 dieter who is just starting a diet and/or exercise program and who may have long-standing dietary habits that need to be changed before even planned breaks can be taken. The same would hold for that subpopulation of Category 1 females who may not be exercising but still want to "lose weight" and who often go about it with very poor dieting practices. In all three groups, it may be better to adhere more strictly to a new diet (prior to using one of this chapter's strategies) to give new habits time to be more established. Taste buds take 3-6 weeks to adapt to changes in eating and the Pre-Diet phase (which may be 4-8 weeks in some cases) would be a good time to adhere strictly to new dietary changes prior to implementing the various flexible eating approaches I will describe.

For the most part, athletes and the serious trainee (who are typically but not universally low Category 2 or Category 1 dieters) don't have as many issues in this regard. Since their current eating habits are generally extremely well-ingrained (even if they are often sub-optimal) breaks tend to cause far less of a problem with a loss of control over the diet. If there is a problem here, it's getting very rigid dieters past the psychological blocks they may have against using more flexible approaches. My experience is that initial resistance to the ideas dissipate over time as they are implemented. As cravings dissipate with the knowledge that foods can be eaten in a planned and controlled way or with the realization the diet breaks or refeeds improve progress rather than slowing it, most dieters find that their attitudes change.

Which isn't to say that there can't still be problems for any given dieter and some do report that various types of flexible eating approaches cause problems regardless of their category or situation. As a rule of thumb I'd ay that if someone has attempted to use a given flexible dieting approach more than three times without success, it should be abandoned until later in the diet or not used at all. Variations can always be tried and each lack of success should be seen as a learning experience rather than being framed as a failure. Different foods or environments can be used until a workable approach is found.

The Full Diet Break

Building off of the study I described in Chapter 15 on prescribe diet breaks, the Full Diet Break is a period of variable duration where food intake is either not meticulously tracked or adjusted to roughly maintenance calories depending on how it is being used. The duration of the Full Diet Break can vary and I have traditionally recommended 7-14 days or longer with 7 days as the absolute minimum. For dieters on a schedule trying to to reach the lower limits of body fat percentage (BF%) dieting times are already fairly prolonged and 7 days will be the realistic maximum although it will still pay dividends. For dieters with less extreme goals 2 weeks may be better and for the general dieter, the Full Diet Break can be even longer and will be effectively identical to the Pre-Diet Phase I described in Chapter 14.

The full diet break has a number of goals and benefits. Several of these are purely psychological in nature. One is that, since calories can and will be higher during the break, there can be controlled increases in what would typically be non-diet foods. This can be problematic in it's own right (discussed below) but knowing that foods that were either limited or eliminated during active dieting can be included to some degree helps to limit the cravings that may occur during active dieting. This doesn't mean that the person should return to their old eating habits and at least some of the nutritional recommendations in this book must be continued during the full diet break. Eating can be loosened during the break but can't become completely uncontrolled. I will provide more specific recommendations below.

Perhaps the major psychological benefit of this strategy is that it breaks dieting into smaller more manageable chunks. This reduces mental stress as any given period of active dieting is limited in its duration before there will be a break. That is, two six week active dieting phases broken up by a 1-2 week break is far less psychologically overwhelming than 12 weeks of straight dieting. This is even more true for those individuals with a very large amount of fat or weight to lose. A Category 3 dieter who has 50+ pounds of fat to lose may be looking at 1-2 years of dieting to reach their goal. The idea of restricting their food intake or feeling deprived continuously for that long is simply overwhelming and the perceived slow progress to the goal can itself derail the dieter. In contrast, a shorter term dieting phase of 3 months alternated with a 2+ week break is far more manageable. For the general dieter, this fits in with my suggestion to set a long-term goal broken into several smaller short-term goals to begin with.

A potentially enormous benefit of the Full Diet Break is to better handle the life events that often arise during the dieting process. Vacations, holidays, etc. are times when diets are often abandoned as the dieter feels as if they have no control over the situation or their ability to maintain their diet. Deliberately and consciously planning those time periods as a break will help the dieter to still feel psychologically in control of what they are eating and this goes a long way towards keeping food intake under control. The Full Diet Break also allows dieters to practice maintenance eating and exercise strategies. Problems can be identified that might make long-term maintenance more difficult and solutions can be found with the knowledge that active dieting can always be resumed. When problems occur, and by this I would generally mean an excessive weight or fat gain or a loss of food control, they can serve as a learning experience to develop strategies for when actual maintenance is the goal. While people often don't conceptualize it this way, fat loss and long-term maintenance is a skill that must be developed over time.

In addition to the above psychological benefits, there are a number of physiological benefits to the Full Diet Break. A primary one is the reversal/normalization of at least some of the hormonal and metabolic changes I described earlier in this book. Leptin, thyroid, reproductive and other lowered hormones will all increase and cortisol levels will decrease which may reduce water retention and improve appearance (often weight is lost initially during the break when this occurs). For the normally cycling Category 1 female dieter, the improvement in hormone levels with a Full Diet Break will go a long way towards limiting or delaying menstrual cycle dysfunction. This is especially true later in the dieting process when their energy availability (EA) is approaching or has crossed the critical threshold.

All of this adds up to at least a partial reversal of the metabolic adaptations that occur while dieting. The adaptations can't ever be completely reversed (this would require regaining all of the lost body fat) but the overall magnitude of the adaptation is decreased when calories are higher. This allows for a stabilization at the current body weight/BF% and can make fat loss more efficient when the diet is resumed. In fact, a recent study compared dieters who either alternated 2 weeks of dieting with 2 weeks of a Full Diet Break with continuous dieting finding that the intermittent dieters lost more fat, due to a reversal of metabolic adaptations during the break (1). While the study used only men I would expect a similar effect in women as other work, already discussed in this book, has found a similar reversal in both hormones and the metabolic effects of dieting. While I wouldn't recommend a break this often in most cases, it does point out that taking a break often makes fat loss more efficient in the long term, rather than less.

For athletes or the serious trainee, the Full Diet Break has a final benefit which is to rebuild any lost fitness, strength or muscle mass. The increased calorie intake means that recovery will be improved and, so long as calories are increased sufficiently to offset any increase in activity levels, the amount of training can be increased during the break before being adjusted as necessary when active fat loss resumes.

Potential Problems with the Full Diet Break

Outside of the general issue with flexible eating approaches I discussed previously, the biggest potential issue with the full diet break tends to be psychological more than anything else. Eating at maintenance is often somewhat more difficult than explicitly dieting or eating in a surplus. It's a nebulous state to be in and since trainees aren't actively losing fat or making gains (at best they are generally regaining lost fitness) they almost feel as if it's pointless. For that reason many find that the good habits that are present during active dieting or when they are trying to make gains in their training go out the window. They stop eating consistently or focusing on proper nutrition and lose focus and momentum. I'm not entirely sure how to fix this except to entreat readers to think of the Full Diet Break as a part of the diet with its own specific benefits and goals. Practicing maintenance, limiting menstrual cycle dysfunction and reversing the adaptations to dieting are all profound benefits and the break should be seen in that light. Once the benefits have been seen and felt, the feeling of a diet break being time wasted usually disappears.

Due to the increase in calories, weight will almost always go up a little bit due to water and more undigested food in the gut (and women must remember to keep the impact of their menstrual cycle in mind when looking at changes in weight) and staying off the scale for a few days after the diet break is begun is probably a good idea to avoid psychological stress. It is possible to gain true weight or fat if food intake becomes particularly un controlled as well but this will not occur immediately. Even in the study I discussed in Chapter 15, this increase was only a few pounds. For the average dieter, this is fairly irrelevant and should represent at most a small percentage of the weight that has been lost before the break is taken. For dieters on a time schedule to reach their goals, this can be relatively more of a problem since the diet can be set back a number of weeks if significant fat gain occurs, especially for smaller dieters. As this is typically the group that has the most food control to begin with it is rarely an issue.

Setting Up the Full Diet Break

The two components of setting up the diet break are calorie levels and macronutrient content. Ideally calories should be set at maintenance levels and this means matching them to activity levels. If activity increases during the full diet break compared to the active dieting phase, calorie intake must increase as well. To take into account the adaptive component of fat loss (which can vary) I prefer to err on the side of slightly two few calories than too many (though note that even a surplus of a few hundred calories is relatively meaningless overall). In general, I recommend setting calories during the break at the dieters currently estimated maintenance minus 5-10%. Most end up eating slightly more than their target during a Full Diet Break to begin with and this gives a bit of a safety valve if this does happen.

In Chapter 16, the sample dieter was found to have a 16.6 calories per pound multiplier for her Total Daily Energy Expenditure (TDEE). Assuming her activity is approximately the same during the break, this will not have changed. If she has dieted from 150 pounds to 140 pounds prior to her first Full Die Break, this will make her estimated TDEE 2325 calories. This would be adjusted downwards by 5-10% or 110-230 calories to 2000-2100 calories. If her bodyweight had dropped to 130 pounds, her TDEE would be estimated at 2150 calories which would be adjusted downwards by 100-200 calories to 1900-2000 calories.

One question that comes up is how rapidly calories should be raised during the Full Diet Break and some of this depends on the duration of the break. For a 7 day diet break, calories should be brought back to maintenance on the first day of the break for the full effects to occur. For a 14 day diet break, it should take no more than 3 days to reach estimated maintenance or the metabolic and hormonal benefits will be lost. For those using more than a 2 week break, calories can be raised to maintenance even more slowly, over perhaps the first week with increases occurring every 2-3 days. This can help with food control.

That calorie level can be used to recalculate her macronutrient intake based on the numbers in Chapter 19 with a few caveats. One is that carbohydrate intake must be at at least 150 grams per day or more during the diet break. This has to do with the fact that many of the hormones of interest including leptin, thyroid and others only respond to carbohydrate intake in the short-term (recall that carbohydrate availability as much as EA may be important for menstrual cycle function). Given the increase in calorie intake during the Full Diet Break, there should be very few situations where carbohydrate intake does not exceed 150 grams per day. If they do not, fat should be adjusted down and carbohydrates raised.

While athletes and those on a time frame to reach a certain BF% goal will need to be more detail oriented in how they set up their break, not all readers will want to apply that level of detail to their Full Diet Break, preferring to eat in a less detail oriented and relaxed fashion.   So long as the fundamental aspects of proper nutritional intake (i.e. sufficient protein and fruit/vegetable intake) are not abandoned, this is not a problem. Some typically non-allowed diet foods can be eaten during the Full Diet Break but keeping their intake limited will prevent unwanted fat gain from occurring. The frequency of their intake should be limited to a few times per week maximum in limited amounts and ideally under controlled conditions (i.e. dessert at a restaurant).   Beyond that, maintaining a majority of the previous dietary habits will make it easier to return to active dieting after the break is over even if the diet is relatively more relaxed.   Primary among this is ensuring sufficient intake of protein, vegetables and fruit; dietary fat intake should be kept at a moderate level. As the most filling nutrient, ensuring sufficient protein helps to control appetite. As I mentioned previously, a higher protein intake also causes any weight to be regained to be in the form of lean body mass rather than body fat (1a).

Training on a Full Diet Break

Outside of those readers who are not on an exercise program of any sort, at least some amount of training should be maintained on the diet break. Ideally this means the combination of proper resistance training and aerobic/HIIT exercise although resistance training should be given priority if a choice must be made. As I've mentioned, exercise may actually have its greatest benefit for most dieters in weight maintenance (rather than improving fat loss) and there are several reasons for this (2). One is that regular activity can help with appetite control (as discussed in a previous chapter). The calorie expenditure from exercise also helps to offset some of the adaptive component of the metabolic rate decrease that occurs. This allows more calories to be eaten while maintaining energy balance. Proper resistance training also synergizes with sufficient protein intake to increase the proportion of LBM gained if weight is regained.

The above is primarily of relevance to the general dieter or reader seeking general health and fitness and I mentioned that the athlete and serious trainee can actually leverage the Full Diet Break to increase their training volume and intensity to rebuild or regain any lost fitness, strength or muscle mass. Training quality frequently decreases while dieting (although other dietary strategies I will discuss later in the book help to offset this) and that can cause a loss of fitness. Although women are at far less risk for muscle loss than men, the risk increases at the extremes of leanness. Increased training during the diet break can help to regain any lost muscle mass.

Any increase in training volume and intensity should not be enormous (and I'd reiterate that calorie intake must increase to match any increased activity). Dieting itself and training while dieting can already put the serious trainee or athlete at risk for overtraining and drastic increases in training volume, even when calories are increased for a short period of time, can put them even further in the hole when they return to active dieting. Dieters who don't increase their training volume or intensity during the break will have enhanced recovery and this may actually help them to avoid overtraining in the long run.

Frequency of the Full Diet Break

The final consideration for implementing the Full Diet Break is how often it should be scheduled. There are two factors to consider here. The first is the dieter's Category, due to the relative differences in how much or how quickly the body will adapt to dieting. Category 3 dieters need a break less frequently than Category 2 and Category 1 dieters need it the most frequently. I'd mention again that this tend to go against how most conceptualize dieting where the thought process is that they must diet more strictly as they become leaner when the exact opposite is actually true.

Another factor involved in setting the frequency of the diet break is the deficit being used. Since there is relatively greater hormonal and metabolic adaptation the larger the deficit, the Full Diet Break should occur more frequently. An aggressive/large deficit will require a Full Diet Break to be taken the most frequently, a small deficit with the least frequency and a moderate deficit in the middle. Some average recommendations for the frequency of the diet break based on category and deficit size appear below.

Cat	Large (1.5%/wk)	Medium (1%/wk)	Small (0.5%/wk)
1	2-4 wks	6-8 wks	8-10 wks
2	6-8 wks	8-12 wks	12-14 wks
3	10-12 wks	12-16 wks	16-20 wk

You can see in the chart how the numbers scale with both category and deficit. The Category 1 dieter using an aggressive deficit might go no longer than 2-4 weeks without a break while the Category 3 dieter using a moderate deficit might diet for 3-4 months before truly needing one. Clearly, based on the studies I have described, it is more than possible to take breaks more frequently as desired or needed. I would note that if someone finds that they lose dieting momentum or fall back into old habits, they should err on the longer durations of active dieting before taking a break to give the new habits longer to become ingrained.

Scheduling the Full Diet break

With the above time frames in mind, let me finish by looking at how to schedule the diet break as there are a few ways to do it. For the general dieter not on a time schedule, the break can occur as needed. This might coincide with the specific durations I listed above, when a life event necessitates it or when the dieter simply feels that they need a break. Basically, there are no strict scheduling requirements in this situation. There are also times that a diet break might be programmed somewhat intuitively. By this I mean that there often comes a time in a longer-term diet where fatigue, hunger, cravings, etc. start to become a chronic issue (fat loss also often slows down drastically). While subjective, this is a sign that the body is adapting to the diet and this can be a good time to take a diet break This can be a dangerous approach as its easy to think a break is needed far more frequently than it is.

In contrast, for those on a strict time schedule, the planning of the breaks should be somewhat more systematic. Once the dieting time has been estimated (discussed in Chapter 25), one approach would be to insert the diet break at relatively even intervals. For example, over a 24 week diet, a break might be taken at weeks, 6, 16, and 24. The final diet break would coincide with peak week and carb-loading for physique or performance athletes Another approach here would be to perform the diet break slightly less frequently in the early stages of the diet and more frequently towards the end as the body is fighting back harder. The same 24 week diet might have a break at 10 weeks, 18 weeks, and 24 weeks (again coinciding with peak week) meaning that the breaks occur at 10, 8 and 6 weeks respectively.

The Normally Cycling Female

There is a potential issue regarding the full diet break that only applies to the normally cycling female in terms of when she should schedule a diet break. Since it's ideal to start (or in this case resume) a diet during the follicular phase (as discussed at the end of Chapter 15), the full diet break should ideally fall during the luteal phase meaning that a 1-week break would be taken during the late luteal phase while a 2-week break would be started immediately after ovulation. This allows calories to be increased when hunger and cravings are at their highest while dieting is resumed when they are at their lowest.

So let's assume that our Category 1 dieter starts her diet with a medium deficit in the follicular phase. Assuming she has an average 28-day cycle, she will reach her next follicular phase in 4 weeks. Two weeks later she will enter the early luteal phase and, having dieted actively for 6 weeks, could begin a 2-week diet break. She could also diet a 7th week and perform a 1-week diet break in the late luteal phase. If it was early in her diet, she could continue dieting through the second month through the follicular phase. At the start of the luteal phase she would have been dieting actively for 10 weeks and could begin a 2-week break. Or she could diet an 11th week and then take a break. In all cases dieting would resume in the next follicular phase. I've shown this schematically below.

	Month 1				Month 2				Month 3			
Diet Length	Early F	Late F	Early L	Late L	Early F	Late F	Early L	Late L	Early F	Late F	Early L	Late L
6-7 Weeks	Diet	Diet	Diet	Diet	Diet	Diet	Break	Break	Diet	Diet	Diet	Diet
	Diet	Diet	Diet	Diet	Diet	Diet	Diet	Break	Diet	Diet	Diet	Diet
10-11 Weeks	Diet	Diet	Diet	Diet	Diet	Diet	Diet	Diet	Diet	Diet	Break	Break
	Diet	Diet	Diet	Diet	Diet	Diet	Diet	Diet	Diet	Diet	Diet	Break

The same will apply for the Category 2 and 3 dieter although the durations of dieting will be longer before a break is taken. I would mention that if a woman has shown that she can control her food intake and cravings during the luteal phase (and the luteal phase supplements discussed in Chapter 24 may help with this), placing the diet break in the follicular phase and restarting the diet in the luteal phase could potentially leverage the small increase in metabolic rate to increase fat loss. While this effect is relatively small, for those dieters on a tight time schedule, it may be worth considering.

For the normally cycling female, especially in Category 1, a rather major problem does crop up here. It's possible that putting a diet break every 6 weeks may be too frequent or unnecessary, especially earlier in the diet. But waiting 10 weeks may be too long, especially in the latter parts of an extended diet when metabolic adaptations are becoming more significant. The best compromise for this is to only perform a full diet break every 10 weeks during the first half of the diet and then move to a full diet break every 6 weeks in the second half of the diet. This is very individual and past experience can be used (if it exists) to decide on whether or not to take a break sooner or later. I find that many dieters, in the same way that they default to larger deficits and more activity do the same with the frequency of their diet breaks, trying to stretch out their dieting times as much as possible. This is usually just another form of psychological resistance to the idea that interrupting a diet can actually solve more problems than it causes.

This is also a potential concern for Category 2 and 3 dieters as well although the issues may be more psychological than truly physiological (in a hormonal and metabolic rate senses). The longer periods between diet breaks are less likely to cause physiological issues in terms of metabolic adaptation here but may be psychologically more stressful. In this case, it might be best to use the longer durations when the diet is first begun to give new habits time to become ingrained, and then use shorter times between breaks after that point. If past diet experience has taught someone that they tend to abandon their diet after a certain time period (i.e. 3 months), it would be best to proactively plan a diet break prior to that.

For women with any hormonal modifier, the full diet break can start any time within the indicated duration. One exception might be certain types of cyclical birth control (BC) as hunger may change slightly from week to week depending on the type of BC being used (recall that the effect seems to be mostly limited to BC with high dose and/or high potency progestins). If a pattern in hunger is observed, the full diet break should be scheduled to coincide with the time of worst hunger so that the diet resumes when hunger is best controlled as this will give the best chance of success.

Refeeds

The second flexible eating strategy I want to discuss is usually referred to as a refeed although other terms are sometimes used. This described a period of variable duration where calories, and specifically carbohydrates, are raised at some frequency within the course of a diet. Within the context of this book, the refeed is identical to the strategy I described in Chapter 14 of moving calories to maintenance to offset menstrual cycle/hormonal dysfunction. While I have previously written about refeeds lasting 5 hours to 2 days, I no longer consider the 5 hour refeed effective and will only consider 1-2 day refeeds in this chapter.

Like the Full Diet Break above, refeeds have several potential benefits although some of these depend on the duration and frequency of their use. Many of those benefits are psychological and more or less identical to what I described for the diet break. Not only can more total food be eaten but at least some of the typically off-limits high-carbohydrate/treat foods can be consumed in relatively larger (but still controlled) portions. The refeed also breaks up longer periods of continuous dieting into more manageable chunks of time (i.e. 1-2 days of normal eating will occur at some frequency during the diet) before a refeed occurs. As they occur more frequently this benefit is accentuated compared to the Full Diet Break (and I will discuss a related diet strategy called Intermittent Caloric Restriction in Chapter 23).

Physiologically, the refeed serves multiple purposes. One is to refill muscle glycogen to sustain high-intensity exercise. This is particularly important for female athletes as their smaller body size and calorie intakes often makes the goals of losing fat and eating sufficient carbohydrate to support their training mutually exclusive. Refeeds are not only a flexible eating approach but a type of nutritional periodization that allows both goals to be met simultaneously. Of equal importance is that refeeds can at least transiently reverse many of the negative hormonal effects of dieting. With increased carbohydrate intake, leptin will increase as will the conversion of inactive to active thyroid hormone in the liver. Cortisol levels will also decrease, reducing the problems associated with chronic overactivation of the stress system.

The decrease in cortisol often causes body weight to drop (and appearance to improve) a day or two after the refeed due to a reduction in cortisol mediated water retention. It's equally likely that scale weight may increase slightly due to the increased glycogen and water storage and when this occurs, women may feel puffy or bloated which can lead to the belief that the strategy is a mistake or impairing progress towards their goals. This weight invariably drops rapidly but I would suggest that women avoid the scale for 2-3 days following a refeed. Finally, as I discussed in Chapter 14, the increase in calories will reverse the adaptations to a low Energy Availability (EA) in terms of menstrual cycle dysfunction. This is only relevant to the Category 1 normally cycling female but the other hormonal effects are important to all dieters and refeeds still play a critical role in lean women with one of the hormonal modifiers.

It's questionable if there are true changes in metabolic rate or energy expenditure from such short periods of increased calories and what little research exists doesn't support that effect. At the very least any actual increase in any component of energy expenditure is fairly small and short-lived. Rather, refeeds may help to limit the rate and size of decrease that would otherwise occur. This depends on a number of factors such as the size and frequency of the refeed, along with the size of the deficit and how lean the dieter is/how long they have been dieting. I will discuss this more below.

Problems with Refeeds

Just as with the Full Diet Break, there are some potential problems that can occur during a refeed. I already addressed the global issue which is the potential for flexible eating approaches to throw people off of their diets. Refeeds have this issue although, as with the Full Diet Break, they will generally not be needed or used terribly frequently in the most problematic groups such as the Category 2/3 dieter. The subpopulation of female Category 1 dieters who aren't training or exercising are in a uniquely difficult situation in this regard: the risk of menstrual cycle dysfunction, etc. is higher but the potential for the refeed to derail their diet can be just as real. I don't have a good solution for this although the Pre-Diet phase should help somewhat by allowing time to establish better food habits and start an exercise program.

There is another potential problem with the refeed that applies to the low Category 2 or Category 1 athlete that I want to mention. It's not uncommon there for food control to be lost although, so long as the calorie increase comes primarily from carbohydrates, this isn't a big issue. Not only will higher calories have a proportionally larger effect on hormones, in a glycogen depleted state, incoming carbohydrates are stored in muscle while the body continues to use fat for fuel (3). Of more practical importance is that many report that their appetite is drastically increased the day following a refeed compared to before the refeed was done when physiologically the opposite should occur. I'm not entirely sure what causes this and whether it's physiological or psychological. For some dieters, moving into a dieting mode often acts as a mental switch in terms of their food intake and control and it may be that the refeed switches them out of this mode. At least some have reported that ending their refeed with slower digesting carbohydrates and a higher fiber intake seems to stop the problem so there may be something physiological going on.

Outside of that, the major problem with a refeed is how it is often interpreted or conceptualized. For years, the concept of a cheat day, a 24 hour span when anything can be eaten, has existed in some dieting subcultures and this is superficially similar to a 1 day refeed. But they are not identical and I find the idea of a cheat day problematic for two reasons. The first is that the term cheat has a negative connotation (you cheat on a test or your taxes) which I think goes against a major point of flexible dieting which is to break people out of a black/white or good/bad approach to dieting. Flexible dieting strategies should be seen as a positive rather than a negative and, for most, using the term cheat does not accomplish that. Practically, by conceptualizing it as a cheat, some dieters seem to deliberately see how much high-calorie, high-fat food they can eat during that time, often eating themselves to the point of sickness. This is made worse when people abuse the concept of the cheat day, eating from 12:01 am to 11:59pm (one day) and consuming such staggering amounts of calories, sugar and fat that body at is regained and progress is reduced or reversed. This defeats the purpose of the refeed entirely and should be avoided.

Setting up the Refeed

Setting up a basic refeed is exceedingly simple and entails raising calories to at least maintenance levels for that day. If training is being done on the day of a refeed, the calories burned during training should be factored in as well and calories increased as needed to ensure that maintenance levels are reached. If a particularly intense workout is scheduled on that day, I would recommend increasing calories by another 10% over maintenance to ensure optimal recovery. Since the goal is to refill glycogen and improve hormonal status, this increase should come mainly if not exclusively from carbohydrates.

There are occasional exceptions to this rule where both dietary carbohydrates and fats are increased with the goal of refilling both muscle glycogen and intramuscular triglyceride (IMTG) stores for competition purposes. In the physique community this is called junk loading and is only used before competitions in an attempt to increase muscle fullness for appearance reasons. Endurance athletes may also use this strategy before important long-duration (2+ hours) events due to the importance of IMTG as a fuel source. Outside of those exceptions, refeeds should be based around increases in carbohydrate intake while dietary fat intake is kept relatively low. Recommended carbohydrate intake levels per pound of bodyweight for different activity levels appear below and I've shown representative intakes for our sample dieter who is currently at 140 lbs body weight.

Activity Level	Carb Intake	Grams Carbohydrate
Day Off	1.5 g/lb (3.3 g/kg)	210
Light: Low Intensity/Technical	2 g/lb (4.4 g/kg)	280
Moderate: 1 hour/day	2.5-3 g/lb (5.5-6.6 g/kg)	350-420
High: 1-3 hours/day	3-4.5 g/lb (6.6-9.9 g/kg)	420-630
Very High: 4-5 hours/day	4.5-5.5 g/lb (9.9-12 g/kg)	630-770

So far as carbohydrate sources, the majority should come from starches and complex carbohydrates as these are best utilized for refilling muscle glycogen stores. Fruit can be included and will enhance the refilling of muscle glycogen and refeeds are a good time to work high-carbohydrate/lower-fat treats into the day's diet since calorie intake is higher and there is room for them to be included. While some amount of vegetables and fiber should be eaten, the refeed should not be based around high-fiber foods as this can cause enormous stomach upset. Rather more easily/rapidly digested carbs should take priority. As I mentioned above, some dieters find that ending the day with more fiber helps prevent next day hunger.

For physique competitors, the refeed is a good time to test out different types of carbohydrates. Some women seem to bloat with certain carbohydrates but not others and determining personal response to different types of carbohydrates will be useful during peak week before a competition. It's also a good time to make notes about when after the refeed they look their best. Some women will hold water underneath the skin the day after the refeed but 2-3 days later their muscles are full but they look dry. This information can be used during peak week to help time the carb-load. If an athlete looks best 2 days after they finish their carb-load, then they should plan on finishing it 2 days before their contest.

During the refeed, dietary protein should stay at the levels determined in Chapter 19. In general, dietary fat should also remain at the levels set in Chapter 19 although the occasional exceptions I mentioned above such as junk loading/IMTG repletion for endurance performance could see it increase to roughly 1 g/lb (2.2 g/kg). For those dieters on a time schedule, it will be necessary to adjust the other days of the week to take into account the higher calories of the refeed (this is discussed in detail in Chapter 23).

Training and the Refeed

A common question about refeeds is how they should be scheduled relative to training. The answer to this question depends on whether a 1 or 2 day refeed is being done and the dieter's goals. Traditionally I have recommended placing the a single day refeed on a training day with a fairly large amount of the day's calories/carbohydrates after training. This is based on the fact that training improves nutrient uptake into skeletal muscle, increasing the amount of glycogen stored in the trained muscles. Adaptation and recovery for that workout will also be enhanced. In contrast, many find that performing a single day refeed on the day before a heavy workout day (i.e. refeed on Friday for a Saturday workout) improves the quality of that workout since glycogen stores are are already increased prior to the workout, improving performance.

For a 2-day refeed, there are multiple options. Conceivably both refeed days could come on the day of the workouts, enhancing recovery and carbohydrate storage in those muscles. As well, one refeed day could come before a heavy workout day with the second day of the refeed on that workout day, giving the best of both worlds since the quality of the workout will be higher and recovery will be enhanced. In some situations, and this is typically for competition purposes such as the carb-loads used by endurance or physique athletes, the refeed might start after a light workout and then continue with little to no training in preparation for competition. This happens infrequently and I won't discuss it here.

Frequency of the Refeed

While setting up the refeed itself is fairly simple, determining the optimal frequency to perform the refeeds is more complicated due to the number of variables that impact on how long it should be or how frequently it should be done. A primary factor is training and most athletes or serious trainees will be performing at least one 1-day refeed per week for this reason alone. In the case of athletes performing extremely large amounts of training (primarily endurance athletes), two single day refeeds may be necessary simply to sustain performance. I will talk about specific dietary strategies revolving around meal patterning that incorporate this in a later chapter. For those dieters, typically in Category 2/3 (but occasionally in Category 1) who are not involved in large amounts of intense training, refilling muscle glycogen is of little concern and the 1-day refeed will not be required from this standpoint.

In addition to the need to support training, there is also the issue of limiting the hormonal and metabolic changes that occur with dieting. There are two primary factors which contribute to the relative need for and frequency of using refeeds. The first is the dieter's category with the frequency of refeeds decreasing with increasing category. The Category 1 dieter will need to refeed the most frequently and the Category 3 dieter the least. This assumes that the Category 2/3 dieter will be using refeeds to being with and I am no longer convinced that they are appropriate, necessary or ideal for this population. While I have traditionally recommended them too all dieters, I now feel that any potential positives of raising calories in this fashion may be outweighed by the potential to throw the Category 2/3 dieter off of their diet (I will address this issue again in Chapter 23 when I talk about Intermittent Caloric Restriction).

This is especially true in the early stages of making behavior changes although the Category 2/3 dieter would be using refeeds infrequently enough to make this far less of an issue. The existence of other, potentially less problematic, flexible eating approaches also tend to make the refeed less useful and it may be best to ignore this strategy until the amount and intensity of exercise being done has increased to the point that the 1-day refeed is appropriate or required. Regardless, it's probably also best for refeeds to be ignored until after the first Full Diet Break has been performed. Coupled with the Pre-Diet phase, there should be enough time to establish better eating habits, reducing any risks of the refeed derailing the diet.

The size of the dietary deficit also plays a role with the frequency of refeeds increasing from small to moderate to large dietary deficits. The Category 1 female, whether normally cycling or not, who has crossed the critical EA threshold will need to refeed more frequently, both for menstrual cycle and hormonal reasons. While this may occur from the start of a diet is a large/aggressive deficit is used, it will almost always happen towards the end of an extreme diet as she reaches the lower limits of female BF%. For the normally cycling female, refeeds become absolutely critical at this point to delay the development of severe menstrual cycle dysfunction or full-blown amenorrhea.

Finally is the issue of the duration of the refeed being used. As I discussed in Chapter 14, two days appear to be required to reverse the adaptations to a low EA state, at least after 5 days have passed. However, a 1-day refeed might be effective if it is done more frequently. So under low EA conditions, while a 2-day refeed might be required every week, a 1-day refeed done every 3-4 days might be sufficient. There are good theoretical reasons, along with anecdotal evidence, that more frequent but shorter refeeds may be effective and I will discuss this in more detail in Chapter 23.

In the chart below, I've provided some general guidelines for refeeding frequencies for both 1- and 2-day refeeds for different dieting categories and deficit sizes (again using 0.5%, 1.0% and 1.5% weekly weight loss goals). The final column is for the normally cycling woman who has crosses the critical EA threshold as is likely to happen at the end of an extreme diet. I should note for readers of my previous books that the numbers in the chart are slightly different than recommendations I have provided before. This reflects the physiological fact of women's bodies adapting more quickly and to a greater degree than men's, requiring a slightly higher refeed frequency for women.

Cat	0.5% Weekly Loss	1.0% Weekly Loss	1.5% Weekly Loss	Below EA Threshold
1	2 days Every 21 days OR 1 day every 10 days	2 days Every 2 weeks OR 1 day per week	2 days Every Week OR 1 day every 3-4 days	2-3 days Every Week OR 1 day every 3-4 days
2*	2 days Every 7 weeks OR 1 day every 3.5 weeks	2 days Every 4 weeks OR 1 day every 2 weeks	2 days Every 3 weeks OR 1 day every 1.5 weeks	N/A
3*	2 days Every 4 months OR 1 day every 2 months	2 days Every 2.5 months OR 1 day every 7 weeks	2 days Every 6 weeks OR 1 day every 3 weeks	N/A

*If the refeed is used at all

For the serious trainee, all recommendations are in addition to the mandatory 1-day refeed being done. each week to refill muscle glycogen. So the Category 1 dieter using a medium deficit would be performing a 1-day refeed weekly and then perform either an additional 2-day refeed every 2 weeks or an extra 1-day refeed per week. In the latter case this might mean performing a refeed on Wednesday and again on Saturday with 5 total diet days per week. If the 1-day refeed to refill glycogen to sustain training is not being done, the recommendations would be used by themselves. So the Category 3 dieter on a medium deficit would use a 2-day refeed every 14 weeks with no refeeds between period of active dieting. Alternately they could perform a 1-day refeed every 7 weeks. Once again, this assumes that refeeds are being used at all and it may be more beneficial to diet more or less straight through without refeeds until a diet break is taken.

Free Meals

The free meal was the third flexible eating strategy I originally described. As it is the simplest of all of the flexible eating strategies in this chapter, I won't divide this into sub sections. A free meal is nothing but a single meal that contains foods that are otherwise not allowed on someone's diet. Someone on a low-carbohydrate diet might include something higher in carbohydrates while someone on a very low-fat diet would eat something higher in fat and the possibilities are fairly endless in what might be eaten during a free meal. Let me emphasize that I suggest calling this a free meal rather than the commonly used cheat meal and the reasons are exactly the same I recommend thinking of a day's increase in calories as a refeed rather than a cheat day.

Although many will still talk about "resetting their metabolism with a cheat meal", it simply doesn't work this way and a single meal will have no hormonal, metabolic or physiological effects. At best the slightly higher calorie content of the meal might burn a few extra calories via the Thermic Effect of Food. This is not only meaningless in the big scheme but is always far less than the calorie content of the meal. Rather the effects of a free meal are purely psychological to allow the occasional consumption of foods that might otherwise be off limits or allowed in tiny quantities. This helps to avoid the feelings of deprivation and restriction that occur with more rigid approaches to eating and gives at least a small break from the rigors of continuous dieting. The free meal can also allow for slightly more social interaction while dieting since it can be scheduled to go out with friends or family without having to adhere strictly to their diet.

So far as the specifics of the free meal, I recommend that the free meal be eaten out since most are a little bit more restrained than if they are eating at home (i.e. most wouldn't order two desserts when eating out). I do strongly advise against going to any sort of all-you-can eat buffet for the free meal as it is trivially easy to consume several thousand calories without even trying. The huge variety of foods stimulates hunger in it's own right and most foods in such environments are both high-calorie and high-fat which can be disastrous. Similarly, a free meal should consist of a single meal and no more. It doesn't mean having a snack an hour before going out to eat, consuming a huge meal, and then picking up dessert on the way home and calling that a "meal." That's an abuse of the concept and some benefit from limiting the free meal to an hour although causes some to see how much food they can eat in that time period.

Although the point of the free meal is to eat foods not normally included in the diet, I strongly recommend at least focusing on some degree of good nutrition during a free meal. It's often best to start a free meal with lean protein and vegetables as this tends to make people full and then, to that, add a single serving of an off-limit diet food. It also tends to be better to put the free meal in the evening as this facilitates moving back into dieting the next morning. When a free meal is eaten earlier in the day, it's often psychologically difficult to move back into dieting mode for the rest of the day.

Depending on what else is going on with the diet, a free meal would typically be included at most 1-2 times per week. For those not using refeeds, typically the Category 2 or 3 inactive dieter, two free meals per week could conceivably be allowed but they should occur on non-consecutive days. A free meal on Tuesday and Saturday or an equivalent spacing would be appropriate, a free meal on Friday and Saturday would not. While the free meal can conceivably be introduced from the very start of the diet, it has the same potential to throw some dieters off of their diet as refeeds and may not be a good choice until some amount of relatively strict dieting has been done. I'd reiterate that if someone has tried a free meal three times without success, it should be abandoned.

For those dieters who are implementing refeeds, no more than one free meal per week should be allowed and it should be spaced away from the refeed itself. The athlete refeeding on Friday might do a free meal on Monday or Tuesday for example but should not do one on Thursday or Saturday. Since the free meal has no major physiological effect hormonally or in terms of refilling muscle glycogen or IMTG, it doesn't matter when it is done relative to training.

Of all of the flexible eating strategies, the free meal may be the one that many dieters see the least point in including. There are no metabolic or physiological effects, the day's dietary deficit may be reduced somewhat (limiting the rate of fat loss very slightly) and there is always the chance that it will throw the dieter off of their diet or do more harm good. For dieters who feel that this is the case, the free meal can be safely eliminated (though I would caution against doing so out of a rigid dietary mindset that considers the free meal bad or unclean in a moral sense). Additionally, with the development and existence of the next flexible eating strategy, the free meal may be somewhat obsolete or at least unneeded at this point.

If It Fits Your Macros (IIFYM)

The newest flexible eating approach, and the one that was not originally described in my book, has been given the name If It Fits Your Macros or IIFYM and was developed as a reaction to the very rigid types of dieting I described in Chapter 15. This refers to the approach whereby, within some limits (discussed below), any food can be included in or on a diet so long as it fits that day's goal for calories, protein, carbohydrates and fats (i.e. the macronutrients or macros). In many ways IIFYM is the closest to the concepts of flexible dieting/eating as it is discussed in the research in that it represents a way of eating where the day's diet may be modified within the calculated parameters without worry. In the physique community, this typically means clean eating where certain foods must be eaten on a diet or specific foods can inherently stop fat loss or render a diet failed regardless of the quantity eaten. While this type of rigid dieting clearly works (in the sense that many reach competition shape), it fails just as often and many of the most vocal proponents of IIFYM come from this dieting background background.

To understand IIFYN, consider our sample dieter who, at one of her meals might be eating 500 calories with 35 grams of protein, 58 grams of carbohydrates and 14 grams of fat. The typically rigid/clean approach to the meal would be that it must come from certain specific protein sources (usually some type of low-fat white fish or chicken), some type of unrefined carbohydrate with vegetables (typically broccoli) with dietary fat coming some type of acceptable oil (perhaps peanut butter). Any other foods would be considered off limits and their consumption at any level would mean that the day's diet has been ruined. Contrast this to someone practicing IIFYM who, if they felt the urge or need, might replace a portion of their allotted carbs and fat with a treat food containing 16 grams of carbohydrates and 7 grams of fat. The rest of their meal would provide the 35 grams of protein from a lean source, along with 32 grams of carbohydrate (starch and vegetables) and 7 grams of fat from typical diet foods. Since the treat food in no way changes the actual macronutrient composition of the meal, that food fits those days macros.

The above is truly all that IIFYM represents and is meant to be represent. Unfortunately, the concept has either been interpreted or mis-represented in one of two extreme directions. On the one hand are rigid/clean eaters who argue that they actually practice IIFYM since they have daily macronutrient goals which they meet with nothing but clean foods. While this is pedantically true, it misses the entire point of the IIFYM concept which was a reaction to the overly rigid eating patterns that caused so many people to give up on their diet, have excessive binge eating episodes or, at the extreme, develop full-blown eating disorders. While the specific foods chosen vary from person to person, IIFYM is meant at a fundamental level, to represent the idea that an occasional snack, treat or "non-diet" food can be incorporated into the diet without any harm so long as it fits the dieter's macros. At the other extreme, and this is really just the nature of the Internet, are people who have taken (or at least claimed to take) IIFYM to an absurd extreme. Generally to push video views or likes on social media, they claim to follow a diet of nothing more than lean proteins combined with nothing but treat foods making up the remainder of their diet. Often specific foods (Poptarts, a toaster pastry snack, is a common choice) are eaten and this has caused people to get the mistaken impression that an IIFYM approach must contain that specific food.

Related to both are recent online articles asking whether clean eating or IIFYM are superior as if they somehow represent two fundamentally different approaches to eating or dieting. This assuredly comes out of the small vocal minority of extremists who make IIFYM appear to be 25-35% protein with the rest of the diet being treat foods. Ignoring those extremists, the reality is that the majority of people practicing IIFYM, vocal or not, are usually eating a diet that is 80-90% so-called "clean" diet foods with the occasional treat allowed as needed. Those treats may not even occur daily and are just included as often as needed to address cravings. Essentially, a false dichotomy of IIFYM versus clean eating has been created which doesn't exist as it is not an either-or type of situation. IIFYM is simply the explicit understanding and acceptance that no food is inherently good or bad within the context of a diet and that, so long as it is eaten in a controlled fashion, essentially any food can be eaten.

Criticisms of IIFYM

Despite the growing amount of research supporting flexible eating approaches as superior to more rigid approaches, there is still criticism of it in general and of IIFYM specifically. These criticisms tend to come from subgroups of people who are determined to maintain or defend their rigid attitudes and I want to look at them briefly. Perhaps the most amusing is that the occasional and limited inclusion of "treat" foods somehow ruins the diet or, at the extremes, will destroy someone's health (this provides perhaps the clearest example of the rigid/orthorexic attitudes that are so often present). Outside of their general extremeness, there are at least two reasons that the above criticism is incorrect.

The first is that health is not some type of on/off switch where someone is either healthy or they are not. As I've said repeatedly, any food eaten must always be considered within the context of the overall diet and lifestyle and, on the background of someone training regularly and eating predominantly "healthy" foods, there is simply no way a small amount of any food can impact on health in any form or fashion. Even the extension of the argument that such foods are nutrient poor in terms of their vitamin and mineral content, is usually untrue as most foods in the modern world are fortified. Even if this is the case, when such foods only occasionally represent 10% or so of the total daily intake, this is an irrelevancy as the dieter's micronutrient needs will be more than met. Even the idea that the diet will be ruined is absurd. So long as there is a calorie deficit and protein intake is sufficient, fat will be lost.

Perhaps the larger reason that this basic criticism fails completely is that those same individuals voicing the above criticisms about IIFYM often report enormous junk food binges when they break their diet in the smallest way. Many even plan a 24 hour cheat-day once per week which, as I described above, usually devolves into the consumption of absolutely enormous amounts of high-calorie, high-sugar, high-fat foods. In practice, this causes them to eat far more of "junk" or "treat" foods on a weekly basis than all but the most extreme IIFYM'er (who may be having a small treat several times weekly) would be eating. And this occurs while they maintain that their rigid approach to dieting, often alternating between days of extreme deprivation and binge eating, is somehow healthier and/or physiologically or morally superior.

An oft-heard claim in the physique community is that no top competitors have reached stage-ready condition using IIFYM but this is flatly wrong. Even at the professional level, it's been extremely common for physique athletes to allow themselves the occasional treat while dieting although this was rarely as formalized as IIFYM. It's worth mentioning that much of the information about what is being done at the top level is often incorrect or deliberately misleading. I know of one recent female professional who was asked to write an article about her contest prep for an online magazine and her discussion of her use of flexible dieting and IIFYM was outright disallowed as this would contradict the magazine's narrative that all professionals eat clean to get into shape. Of more importance, there are increasing numbers of top natural physique athletes getting into as good or better shape using IIFYM/flexible dieting principles.

This isn't to dismiss the fact that many top physique competitors do reach contest ready levels using rigid/clean eating practices. And this fact is often held up as proof that it works or is how the diet should be structured. First and foremost, nobody involved in IIFYM (including myself) would disagree that clean/rigid eating can and clearly does work for many competitors. At the same time, by definition those who make it to contest shape are the one who are successful. What is ignored is the vast number of competitors who never make it to stage, the ones who tried to diet rigidly and failed, who fell into a binge eating pattern and finally gave up. It's misleading to focus on the successes and ignore the failures.

What's also not talked about is what happens after the contest is over. Coming out of months and months of the most restrictive dieting, there is often a complete loss of control over food intake with some dieters reporting that they are never quite able to get it under control again. Along with this comes a tremendous fat gain and this is invariably related to how restricted they felt during the diet. In contrast, those dieters who use flexible eating principles/IIFYM, avoiding the 4-6 months of continuous deprivation an restriction, almost never report nearly the degree of post-contest eating problems. While short-term results are clearly important, the long-term effects must also be considered.

Problems with IIFYM

While the above criticisms of IIFYM are easily addressed, there are potential problems that are often ignored, especially by those in the IIFYM community. As flexible eating practices and IIFYM have become more popular, many in that community have become just as ideological about it as the clean eaters ever were. Many fall into the trap of thinking that since IIFYM worked for them, it should work and be used by everyone (certainly I agree that flexible attitudes should be adopted but there is no specific strategy that must be utilized in this regard). In my experience, most of the most vocal IIFYM'ers are coming from a background of many years of very rigid eating and this has implications for their often seen success with it. During that time they counted and measured every piece of food, tracked every macronutrient along with their calorie levels ate six small meals per day and followed the standard clean eating template, often for a decade or more. Even if those individuals have never dieted down to the lower limits of BF%, this gives them a background and experience with eating and food that those dieters who are new to flexible dieting in general or IIFYM in specific lack. When the former rigid eater is using flexible eating strategies, they are still extremely well aware of what and how much they are eating. This is true even if they go off of their diet for an entire day. Whether subconsciously or not, they are still aware of their food intake on some level. It may only be calorie levels or they are vaguely tracking their protein intake but they are never completely free of their previous background of meticulous eating. Research has even shown that leaner people activate parts of their brain involved in awareness when they eat while the obese do not (4). The ex-rigid dieter has developed this habit to the extremes.

To assume that someone in Category 2 or 3 without a long background in tracking and measuring their foods or who has a number of long-standing poor eating habits can automatically do the same is mistaken. It can be learned with practice but is rarely present to begin with. Adding to this, there is increasing amounts of research showing that overweight or obese individuals have a reward system that functions differently than in lean individuals with highly palatable foods being potentially more rewarding to begin with (5). Essentially, part of the reason that the obese may become obese is that they find the types of high-calorie/high-sugar foods that are so available (and are usually incorporated with an IIFYM approach) that much more rewarding. There is also indication that at least some aspect of eating (moreso than any specific nutrient) has addictive qualities (6). Women have the additional factors of the menstrual cycle and luteal phase with some types of birth control or other hormonal modifiers altering how her brain responds to eating. And all of this adds up to the same potential problem with IIFYM that I described for all flexible eating strategies in that it has as much potential to throw someone off of their diet (or cause short-term overconsumption of that food) as those other strategies. While possibly an ideal approach to flexible eating in the abstract, it may not be appropriate for all dieters immediately in a practical sense.

Even lean dieters can have trouble with IIFYM, at least with certain foods which may act as a trigger food. This describes specific foods where even the smallest intake tends to cause the person to overeat them. This isn't a universal   Not all dieters, lean or obese, experience this and what food acts as trigger may vary from person to person. Even in the case of IIFYM where, conceptually any food can be eaten, if a trigger food is identified it must be avoided or eliminated. The response to that idea in the IIFYM community tends to illustrate how ideological many have become of late as they have begun to call the elimination of any food from the diet an orthorexic behavior but this is not what the term refers to. The person who tries to implement IIFYM in general and find that it doesn't work for them personally for whatever reason are not demonstrating orthorexic behavior. The orthorexic is eliminating or choosing foods based on an obsession with the healthiness, cleanliness, etc. of a food while the person avoiding a given food or not using IIFYM is making an intelligent dietary choice based on it simply not being effective for them. I hope readers understand this distinction.

There is one very real issue with IIFYM that is specific to smaller and lighter Category 1 (and some Category 2) females, especially near the end of a diet. Frequently calorie intake has been reduced fairly significantly with total food intake and volume being quite low. In the physique community this is often called poverty macros and it's not uncommon for smaller females to be eating only 1200-1400 calories per day. This is not a large amount of food even if completely unrefined and high volume foods are eaten but trying to replace even a small amount of those foods with a calorie dense treat can be practically impossible in terms of keeping the dieter full. In general, it's typically larger males who are the most vocal about IIFYM approaches and, as with so many topics where women and men differ, there is a gender difference here due to the differences in body size, body weight and energy expenditure. Since larger males generally eat more, it's easier for them to include higher energy density foods without the hunger problems a small female might experience. For that small female, IIFYM may simply not be workable in a practical sense. So long as calories are being raised to maintenance at the recommended frequency, this is mostly a non-issue as those days will allow some amount of treat foods to be worked into the diet.

Applying IIFYM

While IIFYM is fairly simply overall, I want to provide more specific guidelines for how it should ideally be applied. Despite some of what is seen online, IIFYM should in no way be taken as an excuse to fill the entire day's dieting with treats. Rather, I would recommend that no more than 5-10% of the day's total calories come from IIFYM type foods (I am avoiding the term junk food as it carries the same negative connotations that flexible attitudes are meant to avoid). On a 2000 calorie diet, that is only 100-200 calories per day maximum and that will go down gradually as the day's calorie intake goes down (at some point, most women will be better off avoiding IIFYM completely for hunger and fullness reasons). This should allow at most one small treat to replace a more traditional diet food. I'd note that IIFYM type eating doesn't have to occur every day. It might but the typical application of IIFYM is to stave off the cravings that occur during the dieting process. Here it is far better to allow a small amount of the craved food deliberately than to lose control and eat far more due to deprivation and guilt.

This brings up another female specific issue which is the potential for IIFYM approaches to help deal with the cravings that so often occur during the luteal phase in the normally cycling woman (this tends to be less of an issue or women with a hormonal modifier). As I discussed in Chapter 2, these are well known to occur in response to changes in serotonin and dopamine levels in the brain with the most commonly craved foods being protein foods, chocolate and sweet/salty foods in general (7). While there are cultural factors involved (i.e. in Spain, women tend to crave savory foods), chocolate tends to be craved specifically at this time. Various reasons for chocolate cravings specifically have been proposed including the magnesium content along with various chemicals found in chocolate that effectively work as self-medication for the changes in mood that so often occur at this time (8). It could also be related to the sugar content as carbohydrates raise both serotonin an dopamine in the brain or something about the aroma and texture of chocolate as well (9). It's been suggested that dark chocolate might be superior to other types due to it's sensory characteristics and I imagine most readers are aware of the health benefits attributed to it. Of some interest, the consumption of small amounts (40 g/day) of dark chocolate has been found to improve the health of the bacteria in the gut and reduce cortisol levels (10). The reduction in cortisol was the most significant in women with higher levels of anxiety to begin with and the psychogenically stressed dieter might benefit even more from this strategy.

Irrespective of the reason for chocolate cravings or the mechanism by which it might help, this is a clear situation where an IIFYM strategy may play a profound role in dietary adherence as it will allow for at least a small amount of the craved food to be eaten during a typically problematic time in the menstrual cycle. This helps to address the craving directly and even the knowledge that the food can be eaten if desired helps to reduce psychological stress. Of course this assumes that there are sufficient calories to allow this to occur in the first place and, as above, this is not always the case. This is at least partially offset by the small increase in metabolic rate during the luteal phase which may range from 100-300 calories per day which makes it slightly easier to include the craved food. The Menstralean diet study I discussed in Chapter 19 did exactly this, allowing a portion of dark chocolate to be eaten daily during the luteal phase of the diet. Obviously if other foods are craved, they would be included in this fashion.

As a final recommendation for the implementation of IIFYM, I would strongly recommend that dieters, whether lean or new to the approach, only purchase the amount of a given treat food that they intend to eat on any given day. This avoids the temptation of eating more than is allowed on a given day although this is not a universal problem (some dieters can keep larger amounts of treat foods in the house without problem). Whatever food will be eaten as part of an IIFYM approach should ideally be bought in the quantity it will be allowed (at least in the US single size portions of snack foods are often available) to be eaten. That often means making a specific trip to the store but this is better overall than eating too much of the food because it is around.

Summary

I want to finish the chapter by briefly summarizing the different flexible eating strategies. The Full Diet Break is a 1-2 week (or occasionally longer) time period where calories should be raised to maintenance. It is used between blocks of active dieting and has both psychological and physiological benefits in terms of allowing more food to be eaten while allowing the metabolic adaptations to dieting to be reversed. It should be used by all dieters. The refeed is a 1-2 day period where calories are raised to maintenance with an increase in carbohydrates. It also psychological benefits in terms of allowing more total food intake, along with the potential for a small amount of non-diet or treat foods, along with physiological benefits related to reversing hormonal adaptations and refilling muscle glycogen to sustain training. The refeed is required for anyone involved in high-intensity training or who are in Category 1 but may not be appropriate for many dieters in the early stages.

The free meal is a single meal, ideally eaten out of the house, where some small amount of non-diet food may be included. The benefits are purely psychological in that craved foods may be included in the diet and many find it to be somewhat superfluous or unnecessary, especially if other flexible eating strategies are being used. Finally is If It Fits Your Macros (IIFYM), the newest flexible eating strategy. IIFYM is based around the idea that a small (5-10% of total calories) of the day's normal diet foods can occasionally be replaced by what are usually considered treat foods so long as the day's calorie and macronutrient goals are met. It can be extremely effective but has problems, especially for smaller women who may not have the calorie budget to replace any high-volume foods with more concentrated calories sources. At the same time it can have special benefit for the normally cycling woman as it allows them to address the cravings that occur in the luteal phase while still adhering to their diet.

Chapter 22: Around Workout Nutrition

I want look next at the topic of around workout nutrition, describing any food, fluids or supplements that are consumed around a workout (clearly this chapter is not relevant to those women who are not exercising). For many years, around workout nutrition (often called peri-workout nutrition) has been thought of as being mandatory for anyone who is working out but this turns out to be untrue in many cases. Even in those situations where around workout nutrition is useful or necessary, it is still the day's overall nutrient intake that is of the greatest importance for health, performance or altering body composition. Proper around workout nutrition may add to a properly set up diet but never replace it.

Even for those women who are currently on an exercise program, around workout nutrition doesn't really become necessary until they are trying to optimize their workouts, competition performance, recovery, or adaptation to training. As well, until workouts of 60-90 minutes of moderate- to high-intensity training (or 2+ hours of low- to moderate-intensity training) are being done, little more than perhaps water will be necessary around a workout (shorter duration or low-intensity workouts require little to no around workout nutrition). These two conditions tend to go hand in hand and only the serious trainee or competitive athlete will find themselves in the situation where around workout nutrition is truly necessary. The beginning exerciser or woman seeking general health simply needn't bother. One exception to this is the peri- or postmenopausal woman who should consume some type of fast acting protein (preferably whey protein, discussed in Chapter 24) following weight training workouts as this is critical to either increase lean body mass (LBM) or limit the normal age related losses that may occur (1).

I will be looking at a fairly large amount of information in this chapter including the goals and nutritional components of around workout nutrition. This will tie in with an examination of the four distinct phases of around workout nutrition that are commonly defined. Due to its current popularity, I will examine the issue of training without eating first. Finally, since the specifics of around workout nutrition can vary from sport to sport and situation to situation, I will look at individual categories of sports

As has typically been the case, a majority of research in this area has been done on male athletes (you may recall from Chapter 1 that one of the first studies identifying a gender difference had to do with with carb-loading in female versus male endurance athletes) although more is finally being done on females to identify potential gender differences. As is typically the case, most of these differences are related to differences in body size and composition along with the generally lower speeds, power outputs, weights lifted, etc. achieved by female athletes although the impact of hormones is always present. There are also a number of female specific issues related to bone health, themoregulation and hydration along with the potential impact of the menstrual cycle or other hormonal modifiers that need to be addressed.

Goals and Components of Around Workout Nutrition

There are several distinct goals of around workout nutrition and, although they overlap, each has its own specific purpose and optimal nutritional intake to support that purpose. Of primary importance is fueling the workout itself to optimize performance and prevent premature fatigue. During exercise, different energetic pathways (which I will not detail) and fuel sources provide energy and, in many cases, fatigue is related to levels of those fuels falling below a certain level. For near maximal intensity, short-duration (10 seconds or less) activities, compounds stored within the muscle called ATP and CP (the names are unimportant) provide energy and once they fall below a certain level, fatigue occurs. Around workout nutrition has no impact on levels of either compound and only the supplement creatine monohydrate (discussed in Chapter 24) can raise levels to any significant degree so I will not discuss it further.

The only other energy sources in the body are protein (technically amino acids), carbohydrates and fats. Protein can technically be used for energy during aerobic exercise but it's contribution is generally extremely small. Women use less protein than men for fuel during aerobic exercise than men and, while protein plays a number of other beneficial roles, fueling exercise is not really one of them. This leaves carbohydrates and fats as the primary energy sources to fuel exercise. Fats can only provide energy during low- and moderate- intensity aerobic activity although it may contribute during the rest period of HIIT or resistance training. Recall that there are two stores of fat in a woman's body which are body fat and Intra-Muscular Triglyceride (IMTG). Even the leanest female athlete might be carrying 42,000 calories of worth of stored body fat, enough to walk or run 420 miles and I've mentioned that IMTG can become depleted with the combination of large amounts of aerobic activity and a very low-fat diet. But for all practical purposes, fat will never be limiting for any single exercise session and consuming fat around workouts has no meaningful impact on performance. There is always more than enough.

This leaves carbohydrates as the primary fuel source of interest. Carbohydrate use during exercise increases as intensity increases and eventually an intensity is reached where only carbohydrate can provide energy rapidly enough to sustain exercise. For aerobic activity this is roughly the maximal exercise intensity that can be maintained for about 60 minutes Exercise done above this intensity (typically HIIT or weight training) uses a tremendous amount of stored carbohydrates. A single 30 second sprint can reduce muscle glycogen by up to 25% while 6-9 sets of weight training can reduce muscle glycogen by 25-40%. Even during maximal sprinting where ATP/CP is a primary fuel, there is some glycogen used for fuel. One six second all out sprint can reduce muscle glycogen by 14% and 10 sprints may reduce it by 36%.

This is important as it has been known for decades that if muscle glycogen (or blood glucose) falls below a certain level, fatigue will occur. Aerobic athletes will "bonk" or hit the wall as an overwhelming sense of fatigue and heaviness in their muscles occurs. This is coupled with an inability to maintain their previous speeds or power outputs (here a woman's greater use of fat for fuel gives them an advantage over men who will use up their glycogen stores more quickly). High intensity athletes will feel similar fatigue an find it more difficult to maintain their speeds during HIIT or performance during moderate repetition weight training. Maximal sprinting or low repetition weight training is often relatively unaffected by glycogen depletion. This is all critical as, in contrast to fat, the stores of carbohydrate in the body are quite limited. Roughly 4.5 g/lb or 10 g/kg of carbohydrate can be stored so a 150 lb female might have a maximum of 680 grams stored. This provides just under 2,800 calories and might sustain 60-90 minutes of maximal aerobic activity. This should be contrasted to the 42,000 calories of fat energy that might be stored which could sustain hour upon hour upon hour of lower intensity exercise. I'd note in this regard that carbohydrate stored within muscle can only be used by that muscle. Even if the upper body muscles contain stored carbohydrate, if the legs become depleted, lower body performance will decline.

For all of the above reasons, a great deal of around workout nutrition revolves around carbohydrate intake to ensure that any given workout is optimally fueled. Protein, fat and fiber can still play a role in the different phases I will discuss but only carbohydrate can meaningfully impact on short-term exercise performance. It does this by not only ensuring that glycogen stored are optimal at the beginning of the workout but by also providing an additional source of energy By providing carbohydrates in food, the body's own muscle glycogen stores are spared, improving performance and delaying fatigue.

A second major goal of around workout nutrition is recovery from the exercise session along with stimulating long-term adaptation to the training to improve fitness. While the focus here has long been on carbohydrates, primarily to ensure that muscle glycogen is refilled, dietary protein is turning out to play a much more important role overall. A large part of the adaptation process is the rebuilding of damaged proteins along with the production of new proteins (i.e. enzymes, mitochondria, skeletal muscle) following training. Only dietary protein can provide the building blocks for this to occur although combining protein with carbohydrates can have additional effects and benefits that I will describe below.

A third goal of around workout nutrition is ensuring optimal hydration before and during training along with rehydrating an athlete following the workout. As I mentioned in Chapter 18, even slight dehydration (2-4% of starting body weight or 3-6 pounds for a 150 lb female) impairs most types of exercise performance, often significantly (2). This is true across nearly all sports and I mentioned that weight class athletes who dehydrate excessively often see their performance decrease. The primary determinant of hydration is fluid intake and this has the additional benefit of helping the athlete to deal with heat stress and overheating during exercise. This is especially important under hot and humid conditions and even moreso during the luteal phase when body temperature is already elevated, increasing her risk for overheating. Women have additional issues with post-workout recovery and cooling, discussed below.

Tying in with fluid intake is sodium and potassium intake, both of which play a large number of roles during exercise. Both are required for proper muscle function although it takes fairly extreme changes to cause an issue here. Of more importance is that sodium and potassium increase the retention of fluids and, as I mentioned already, pure water is not optimal for either hydration or rehydration. While I will examine specifics below, there is some current belief that hydration guidelines for exercise are either excessive or, at the very least don't take individual needs into account (3). Sweat rates can vary enormously between any two individuals and the hydration recommendations that will be too little for one woman may be too much for another (there is also a risk, albeit rare, of severe overhydration). Many now argue that drinking to thirst (while ensuring sufficient sodium/potassium in the diet) is sufficient and this is generally very true. One exception is for very long (2+ hour) training sessions in the heat where thirst may lag behind actual fluid needs and athletes will need to focus more on fluid intake. Thirst mechanisms also become impaired with age and master's female athletes will need to pay more attention to their fluid intake overall.

Phases of Around Workout Nutrition: Introduction

While they overlap, I will divide around workout nutrition into four distinct phases, defined by when they occur relative to the training session. First is the pre-workout meal which will ideally fall from 3-4 hours before the workout. Next is immediate pre-workout nutrition, or a pre-workout snack, which describes anything consumed from 2 hours before up to the start of the workout. During workout nutrition refers to anything consumed during the workout itself and post-workout nutrition is anything eaten following the workout until roughly 2-4 hours later at which time normal eating resumes. Each phase may be relatively more or less required depending on the specific situation although in some situations no specific around workout nutrition may be required (though it may still be beneficial). Each phase has it's own potential optimal nutrient composition depending on the type, duration and intensity of workout.

The nature of endurance training/sports in terms of the sheer amount done means that it generally has the greatest requirement for around workout nutrition. This varies enormously with the type of workout being done: a 30 minute easy run is distinctly different than a four hour bike ride including several sets of intervals within the ride. Other sports and activities tend to have lower requirements for around workout nutrition overall with differences in goals (i.e. endurance vs. strength/power/muscle gain) impacting on the relative importance of carbohydrates or protein. Pure strength/power workouts tend to have the least requirements for around workout nutrition and many high-intensity performance types of workouts such as sprinting are similar. Medium repetition weight training/physique type training has proportionally higher requirements and mixed/team sports can vary fairly significantly. For each phase, I will look at the goal of the phase along with ideal amounts of each nutritional component. I'll also address how this might change for different training situations or goals.

Around Workout Nutrition and Stomach Upset

While there are other practical factors that impact on what ideal around workout nutrition might be that I will discuss below, there is one issue that is of primary relevance to the first three phases. That issue is stomach upset and issues such as belching, vomiting, diarrhea, flatulence, cramping and even gastrointestinal bleeding can all occur during exercise in the first place. Consuming food and drink around training can make the problem worse in susceptible individuals and women are actually more prone to report stomach problems than men to begin.

A major factor is the type of sport in question with running and other activities that cause a lot of body movement (the actual term is "joggling") causing more problems than those such as cycling that don't. Very metabolically stressful workouts such as HIIT and high-intensity aerobic activities tend to cause more problems than lower intensity exercise. Moderate to high-repetition weight training may cause problems although low-repetition or pure/strength power work doesn't seem to be as impacted due to the short duration of the set and relatively long rest-intervals that are used. Other factors such as dehydration, a lack of training and excessive amounts of fat and fiber in those three phases also contribute. Athletes with pre-existing stomach issues such as Irritable Bowel, Crohn's disease or others cause further problems and women actually report these diseases more frequently to begin with (4). The form of the meal, whether it is liquid or solid, tends to play a role in the potential for stomach upset.

To all of the above I'd add that there is often huge individual variation in what types of foods or drinks cause problems in any given trainee. Some can't workout effectively without having eaten something relatively close to workout while others experience stomach upset if they consume anything more than a few hours before training. Since it's impossible to provide recommendations for every eventuality, trainees will have to experiment with different amounts and types of foods along with the timing of those meals to optimize their own around workout nutrition. In the case where trainees seem to get stomach upset from having anything in their stomach (but find that their performance suffers for lack of proper around workout nutrition) it appears that the gut can be "trained" to handle progressively more nutrients over time (5).

The Pre-Workout Meal

While many sports nutrition books will refer to the pre-workout meal as anything eaten from 1-4 hours before a workout, I find it more practical to use it to refer to any food or drink consumed roughly 3-4 hours before a workout. For the most part, this makes it part of the day's normal eating but it also serves the purposes described above in terms of preparing the athlete for the upcoming training session. As I mentioned above, unless the workout consists of 60+ minutes of high-intensity activity or 90-120 minutes or more of moderate intensity activity, there is no need to make this meal anything but one of the day's normal meals. In some cases, trainees may choose to train without eating at all (described below).

For the reasons I discussed above, the pre-workout meal has traditionally focused on carbohydrate and fluid intake although protein, fat and fiber should also be part of the meal (assuming they do not cause stomach upset). A carbohydrate intake of 0.45-1.8 g/lb (1-4 g/kg) is a typical recommendation and this would be 70-270 grams of carbohydrate for the 150 lb sample dieter. This causes an immediate problem as the highest intake recommendations exceed both her follicular and luteal phase carbohydrate intakes of 235 and 156 grams respectively. Mind you, the highest values will only be truly required for the longest or most intense workouts. A 2 hour run or competition or 3-4 hour bike ride might very well require intakes near the higher value but these athletes will also be eating far more to begin with. For less intense or shorter workouts, an intake of 0.22-0.45 g/lb (0.5-1.0 g/kg) should be sufficient, representing 35-70 grams for our sample dieter. Both values fit easily within her daily diet and she might choose to use the lower value during the luteal phase and the higher value during the follicular phase when she is eating more carbs.

Given the potential problems with absolute intake recommendations exceeding the carbohydrate allotment available to a given female (especially if she is dieting), an alternate approach to setting carbohydrate intake levels would be to take the daily allotment and divide it out across the number of meals per day (meal patterning and frequency will be discussed in the next chapter). If the sample dieter were eating 4 primary meals per day, she would end up eating 65 grams at this meal during the follicular phase and 45 grams during the luteal phase which is right in line with the 0.22-0.45 g/lb value above. As there are no specific guidelines for protein, fat or fiber intake, the same approach can be used by simply taking the day's totals and dividing them out across the day's meals. This would mean an intake of 35 grams of protein and either 14 or 20 grams of fat with some amount of fiber. While specific foods are rarely recommended, choosing a dairy food high in calcium (i.e. Greek yogurt or milk) should be considered. Not only is it an excellent source of protein in general, a high dairy calcium intake prior to endurance exercise has been found to eliminate any loss of bone calcium that might occur (5a). Athletes who experience stomach upset during workouts will need to adjust the fat and fiber content (or pick more easily digestible foods) for the meal. The meal may have to be reduced in size if it is eaten only 3 hours before training.

To ensure optimal hydration, a standard recommendation is to consume 0.07-0.1 fluid oz/lb (5-7 ml/kg) of fluid 4 hours before the workout. For the 150 lb/68 kg sample dieter, this would be 10-15 oz/340-475 ml of fluid. If this doesn't make the trainee pee (indicating that they may be slightly dehydrated to begin with), roughly half that amount (5-7.5 oz or 170-248 ml) of additional fluid would be consumed 2 hours before the workout. For most situations, the above is unnecessary and simply drinking to thirst while getting some sodium and potassium in the meal will be sufficient. As mentioned above, under hot and humid conditions, especially for women in the luteal phase, slightly more attention to fluid intake is warranted since this helps to prevent heat stress and improves performance (I will mention an additional hydration strategy below as well).

Outside of the potential for stomach upset there aren't any practical issues for the pre-workout meal. Generally any issue has to do with the trainee working out very early in the morning and not having time to eat 3 or more hours before the workout. I will discuss this situation in the next section.

Immediate Pre-Workout Nutrition

I will define the immediate pre-workout phase (or pre-workout snack) as anything consumed from 2 hours up until the start of the workout. This is really just an extension of the pre-workout meal with the goals of ensuring adequate carbohydrates to fuel exercise and ensuring optimal hydration. Providing amino acids (via protein intake) before workouts also has potential benefits as it may improve the long-term adaptation to training. That said, outside of the hydration issue I mentioned above (consuming fluid if the trainee has not peed) and another I will mention below, in most situations a pre-workout snack will not be required although it may still be beneficial. This is due to the fact that any reasonably sized pre-workout meal (perhaps 300-500 calories) will still be digesting and releasing nutrients into the bloodstream 4 or more hours later, overlapping with all but the longest workouts.

There are two situations that occur when a pre-workout snack may be necessary. One situation is when someone is training intensely early in the morning (i.e. before work or school) and where waking up 3-4 hours before the workout to eat the pre-workout meal would compromise sleep patterns. A second situation is when someone's work or school schedule only allow someone to eat 4-5 hours or more before the workout (i.e. 12 pm lunch before a 6 pm workout). Unless an extremely large meal, taking longer to digest, was eaten at that time, the workout is likely to be compromised due to lowered blood sugar or inadequate hydration. In this situation, a small easily digestible snack containing some carbohydrates, protein and fluid can be extremely beneficial. Fat and fiber tend to cause gastric upset in this situation.

Even in those cases where a pre-workout meal has been eaten prior to training and immediate pre-workout nutrition is not required, there may still be benefits to eating at least protein 1-2 hours before training. Pre-workout nutrients are available during and immediately after a workout (when blood flow to trained muscles is highest) and may be superior for long-term adaptation compared to post-workout nutrients (6). This is probably relatively more important for strength/power and physique athletes looking to maximize their gains although endurance athletes may also benefit from this approach.

For endurance workouts of any sort (including HIIT) a protein intake of 0.1 g/lb (0.22 g/kg) lean body mass (LBM) and anywhere from 2-4 times as much carbohydrate would be appropriate in the pre-workout snack. A female with 110 lbs/50 kg of LBM would consume ~10 grams of protein and 20-40 grams of carbohydrates (120-200 calories total). For strength/power or physique types of workouts, a protein intake of 0.15-0.22 g/lb (0.3-0.5 g/kg) LBM and up to twice as many carbohydrates (depending on preference, training volume and personal tolerance) would be appropriate. The sample female with 117 lbs (53 kg) of LBM would eat 18-25 grams of protein with 18-25 grams of carbohydrates (144-200 calories). Some prefer only to consume protein and this choice should be made based on the amount of carbohydrate available in the diet along with personal preference. While small amounts of fat (no more than 4-7 grams) and fiber (a few grams) are acceptable in the pre-workout snack, this can cause stomach upset and may need to be eliminated. For fluid intake, the same recommendation from above of 0.03-0.05 oz/lb (2.5-3.5 ml/kg) or roughly 5-8 fluid oz (170-240ml) would be appropriate. Drinking to thirst is generally sufficient.

Depending on the athlete's preference, solids, liquids or a mixture of the two can be appropriate for the pre-workout snack. Pure fluid nutrition (i.e. a protein/carb shake) has the benefit of providing hydration along with any protein or carbohydrates which are being consumed but some athletes prefer solid foods in their stomach during training (as above, this is highly individual). The time between the pre-workout snack and the workout impacts on this as well. With two hours between eating and the workout, easily digested solids with some type of fluid for hydration may be preferred while the trainee who must eat within 30-60 minutes of training may prefer fluids if they eat anything at all. Even if no protein or carbohydrate will be consumed within 2 hours of the start of a workout, additional fluid and electrolytes may be beneficial, especially for endurance exercise in hot and humid conditions. Female cyclists who drank 21 fluid ounces (628 ml) of water with ~6 grams of sodium one hour before exercise in hot/humid conditions had a slower increase in heart rate, slower rates of fatigue, improved performance and overall decreased heat strain (7).

The primary practical consideration for the pre-workout snack has to do with the potential for stomach upset that I mentioned already. An additional issue is that some trainees experience a drop in blood sugar when they eat close to training although this doesn't seem to harm performance. In both of these situations, it may be best to eliminate the pre-workout snack entirely and move directly to during workout nutrition.

During Workout Nutrition

During workout nutrition refers to anything consumed during the workout itself. The primary goal of during workout nutrition is to fuel exercise along with limiting the degree of dehydration that occurs. As is typically the case, carbohydrate and fluid intake has been the primary focus for decades although it is becoming more established that small amounts of protein during exercise may provide additional benefits. As with the other phases of around workout nutrition, the nature of the workout to be done impacts enormously on what may or may not be required. Water will be sufficient for short/low-intensity training with carbohydrate and protein requirements going up as the intensity and duration of training increases.

Looking first at carbohydrate intake, recall from above that depletion of muscle glycogen in working muscles and/or a drop in blood glucose is a major cause of fatigue during many types of high-intensity exercise. By providing carbohydrate during training, not only is blood glucose maintained but glycogen is spared as the body uses the ingested carbohydrate instead, delaying fatigue. I say delay here as it is never possible to completely offset the use of glycogen at the highest exercise intensities and eventually it will become depleted. Literally decades of research has examined the issue of what amount and type of carbohydrates may be optimal during exercise and I want to look at those recommendations first.

Perhaps surprisingly, not only are there no gender differences in the amount or type of carbohydrates recommended during exercise but the amounts are not related to body weight. Rather they will be given in absolute terms of grams of carbohydrate per hour. This is due to the fact that the limiting factor for carbohydrate intake is the rate of absorption from the stomach. Not only does this vary insignificantly between women and men but the amount of carbohydrate that can be absorbed from the gut is always lower than the amount being used during exercise (i.e. 240-360 calories/hour can be absorbed compared to 450-1000/hour burned). For this reason, neither body weight nor LBM is relevant to recommended intakes.

Different types of sugars are absorbed and utilized by the body at different rates. Glucose, sucrose and maltodextrins (medium length chains of glucose) are absorbed at about 1 gram/minute or 60 g/hour while fructose, galactose and others can only be absorbed at a rate of 0.6 g/minute or 36 grams/hour. Since they have different transporters in the gut, combining different sugars (i.e. glucose/maltodextrin with fructose) can achieve absorption rates of 75-90 g/hour and this represents an absolute maximum intake level. At least in men, this level of intake during a cycling time trial improves power outputs by an enormous 15% (8). Since gender differences in fuel use disappear at higher intensities of exercise, I would expect women to show a similar response. While 75-90 g/h represents an absolute maximum intake level, this will not be required for all or even most types of workouts. Rather, the optimal amount and type of carbohydrate that should be consumed will depend on the duration and intensity of the exercise.

For low-intensity (aerobic, technical, light weight training) or short workouts that are less than 30 minutes, there is no benefit of carbohydrate intake unless the person has been on a low-carbohydrate diet. Once workouts reach 30-60 minutes at moderate intensities, only small amounts of carbohydrates are required. Here there is an odd strategy to consider. Swishing small amounts of carbohydrate, approximately 2 grams in 1oz/25 ml of fluid, for 5 seconds every 10 minutes and then spitting it out improves performance to the same degree as actually consuming carbohydrates (9). More fluid will still be needed but this can be useful for dieting athletes who need to control their total calorie/carbohydrate intake while maintaining exercise performance. There is an exception to this which are time trial events (maximal effort competitions lasting 40-60 minutes) performed during the luteal phase. Despite their duration, performance will be impaired unless ~40 grams/hour of carbohydrate are consumed during the event (10). This will also help to protect immune system function which can be impaired by high-intensity exercise (10a). Glucose, fructose or maltodextrin are would all be appropriate here.

Once endurance workouts reach the 1-2 hour mark, a carbohydrate intake of 15-30 grams per hour is recommended (in some cases, more than this may be required). This can come from any source of carbohydrate and would be an appropriate level of intake for strength/power, physique, high-intensity performance or mixed sports athletes so long as sufficient fluid is also consumed. While recommending carbohydrates to strength/power or physique athletes may seem odd based on their training, my experience is that even small amounts of carbohydrates improves training quality, especially for lengthy workouts.

Endurance workouts lasting from 2-3 hours should have a carbohydrate intake of 30-60 grams per hour with a mixture of fast acting carbohydrates being used. Maltodextrin/glucose with fructose in a roughly 2:1 ratio would be optimal here. If 30 grams per hour were consumed, that would be 20 grams glucose/maltodextrin and 10 grams of fructose or up to 40 grams glucose/maltodextrin and 20 grams fructose if the maximum amount is consumed. For very long-duration endurance events of 2.5-3+ hours, carbohydrate intakes of 60-90 grams per hour from a mixture of carbohydrate sources would be optimal. At 90 g/h, a mixture of 60 grams glucose/maltodextrin and 30 grams of fructose would be appropriate.

While carbohydrate is by far and away the most important nutrient to consume during exercise, adding small amounts of protein may also be beneficial (11). Some studies find that protein can directly improve endurance performance although this tends to only be the case if inadequate amounts of carbohydrates are consumed in the first place. This provides another strategy for dieting athletes to maintain their performance when their total carbohydrates/calorie intake is reduced. Of as much importance, consuming protein during exercise reduces the (admittedly small) amount of protein that may be broken down during training which could benefit long-term adaptation. A mere 4-8 grams of protein/hour is more than sufficient and this should come from a rapidly digesting protein such as whey.

Fluid Intake

While the need for carbohydrate and/or protein during exercise can vary significantly depending on the workout, at least some fluid intake will be required or at least beneficial (if only to avoid dry mouth) for all but the shortest or lowest-intensity workouts. Any workout lasting longer than 45-60 minutes will require some fluid intake and this is doubly true for exercise done on hot/humid environments or for women in the luteal phase or using any birth control that raises their body temperature. Women's bodies actually regulate body temperature and fluid balance differently than men's which impacts on their fluid requirements. Overall, women have lower sweat rates than men and this occurs for a few reasons (12). The first is that women generate less heat due to having less LBM, slower running speeds and lower power outputs (when women and men are matched for fitness, the differences disappear). Since they have a larger surface area than men, women also dissipate heat more effectively. Changes in estrogen and progesterone along with certain types of birth control can alter this due to water retention.

The net result of these differences is that, at least during the follicular phase, women actually have an advantage over men during exercise in the heat as they begin sweating later, sweat less (losing less fluids) and don't overheat as quickly. As is generally the case, this reverses itself during the luteal phase where the increase in basal body temperature and changes in other aspects of a woman's physiology may put her at greater risk for overheating, especially under hot and humid conditions (13). The fluid/sodium loading I described above can help with this but ensuring sufficient total fluid intake during exercise in the heat and humidity in the luteal phase is critically important (13a). While not nutritional per se, heat acclimation (living or training under hot/humid conditions) can help as well and here too there is a gender difference with women taking longer (10 vs. 5 days) to fully acclimate than men (13b). Pre-cooling strategies such as cooling vests or consuming ice slush (crushed ice that helps to keep core temperature down) may be necessary for long-duration endurance performance under certain conditions. I'd note that the above is mainly seen in untrained women and, with regular training, women's bodies start to sweat sooner (as do men's) and at least some of the differences disappear. Women just starting an exercise program may find that their fluid requirements actually increase as their fitness levels go up for this reason.

Given that most of the differences in fluid requirements are related to differences in body size and body composition, simply scaling down the guidelines developed for men is generally sufficient. For readers wanting specific numbers, an hourly fluid intake of 0.08-0.16 oz/pound (~5.7-11.4 ml/kg) would be appropriate. A 132 lb (60 kg) female athlete would need between 10-21 oz (340-680 ml) while 165 lb (75 kg) female would require from 13-26 oz (384-768 ml) per hour. For workouts lasting less than 2 hours, drinking to thirst is generally sufficient. For workouts longer than 2 hours, thirst can "fall behind" actual hydration causing an athlete to become dehydrated if they are not attentive to their fluid intake early in the workout or competition.

I'd mention again that sweat rates can vary significantly between any two women and the above values should be taken only as a starting point. Some athletes will need more fluid than the above and others will need less. One approach to determining individual fluid requirements during exercise is to weigh before and after with a goal of losing no more than 2-3% of starting body weight. This represents 2.5-4 lbs (1.1-1.8 kg) for a female athlete weighing 132 lbs (60kg). If more than 3% of body weight is being lost, fluid intake during exercise must be increased. If weight loss is in this range, fluid intake is appropriate. At no time should weight be gained during exercise (see below).

The above numbers represent recommendations for endurance type of activities and other types of training will generally have much lower requirements although this depends on the type of training and where it is being done. A strength/power or physique athlete training indoors in a cool gym will not have nearly the fluid requirements of a sprinter or soccer player training outdoors in the heat. Using the lower values of 0.08 oz/lb (5.7 ml/kg) fluid per hour or simply drinking to thirst would be appropriate in these conditions. I'd note that the common practice for physique athletes to carry a 1 gallon (128 oz/3700 ml) bottle of water during their workouts is absolute overkill. For the 150 lb sample dieter, this represents 0.85 oz/lb of fluid, enough for 4 hours of continuous aerobic activity in the heat and excessive for any realistic gym workout. While avoiding dehydration is critical, overhydration can be equally detrimental.

Exercise Associated Hyponatremia

While dehydration is far and away more common, there is a rare condition that can develop during exercise called exercise associated hyponatremia or EAH that I want to address. Under normal conditions during exercise, sweating causes a greater loss of water than sodium, causing the body's sodium concentrations to increase. However, some athletes lose extremely large amounts of sodium in their sweat and, if this is combined with an excessive intake of low sodium fluids or pure water, the concentration of sodium in the body will decrease. If that athlete was already consuming a low-sodium diet along with large amounts of pure water, they are likely to be at an even greater risk. If this occurs and the concentration of sodium in the body falls too low or is maintained at a lowered level for extended periods, EAH may occur causing confusion, mental alterations cerebral swelling, brain damage and even death.

EAH is almost exclusively seen during long-duration endurance activities that are 2-3 hours or more in length although it seems conceivable that it could occur in any athletes training for extended periods under hot and humid conditions. Perhaps surprisingly it is the slower/poorer performing competitors who are at the greatest risk. They are on the course longer and their slower speeds make it easier for them to consume more fluids (i.e. its difficult to drink as much when running faster). If they try to force drink as much as possible, and this is always indicated by weight gain during exercise, EAH may develop. If they collapse and are rehydrated with nothing but water, sodium concentrations fall further and death may occur.

While rare in general, women are at a greater relative risk than men for developing EAH and suffer more physical symptoms than men if it does occur (14). One reason for the higher risk is the generally slower speeds seen in women compared to men which might allow them to more easily drink too much fluid. Women frequently start with more body water to begin with due to menstrual cycle or birth control related water retention, potentially lowering sodium concentrations. Female athletes frequently reduce sodium levels to very low levels which can exacerbate the problem. If they happen to lose more sodium than sweat during exercise or consume too much pure water, they will be at risk for developing EAH.

As rare as EAH is, the consequences are extremely serious and potentially fatal. I am primarily bringing it up in this section to make the point that excessive fluid intake (especially pure water in the absence of sufficient sodium and potassium) can be just as detrimental as too little fluid. With a few short-term exceptions such as dealing with water retention or making a weight class, athletes and active individuals should liberally salt their foods (again I recommend the combined sodium/potassium salts such as Lo- or Lite-Salt). I provided a number of reasons for that recommendation in Chapter 20 and to that list, the admittedly small risk of EAH can be added.

Practical Aspects of During Workout Nutrition

In contrast to the previous two phases of around workout nutrition, during workout nutrition has an enormous practical issue having to do with the relative ease with which food or fluids may be carried during training or competition. This problem tends to vary by sport with running generally having the largest problems. Runners have been found to consume less fluid during training and competition than other endurance athletes and this is primarily due to the practical issues of drinking while running. Traditionally shaped water bottles are impossible to hold although newer designs have handles and even devices like a Camelbak (a fluid containing backpack) add weight that must be carried by the runner. During competitions, runners are usually limited to drink stations in the first place and it's difficult to drink much fluid when running quickly. The same holds true for training runs. Unless an athlete is willing to run shorter loops or drop off water bottles at points along their run course ahead of time, they will either consume too little fluid or add to their body weight by having to carry it. This also limits the ability to consume carbohydrates and/or protein. Carbohydrate gels exist but do nothing to help with hydration.

Other sports don't share these issues by and large. Cyclists can carry water bottles on their bike or put whole foods in their jerseys, swimmers can put water bottles with fluids and/or nutrients on the pool deck, rowers can carry fluids/nutrients in the boat for long training sessions, etc. Even sports that involve running such as soccer, field hockey, basketball or track and field don't have the same issues.   Not only are fluid requirements not as high but the training is all done in the same area, allowing fluids to be left on the sidelines or with training bags. The start and stop nature of the sports also makes it far easier to drink. Here there is a potential practical issue that breaks during training or competition tend to be less standardized and more set by the coach and the practice or competition structure. Athletes may not be able to consume fluids or nutrients when they want to but when they are given a break and allowed to do so. During competition, there may be breaks between plays, quarters or a half-time that gives at least some freedom to nutrient and fluid consumption.

Other Issues

While the above represents ideal during workout nutrition recommendations, there are a handful of other issues I want to address. In addition to providing fluids, carbohydrate and protein during workout nutrition should provide at least some electrolytes, especially sodium, to help offset exercise related losses (this should all but eliminate the small risk of EAH). An intake of 460-920 mg of sodium per 32 oz (960 ml) or 115-230 mg per 8 oz (236 ml) with 1/4 as much potassium would be appropriate.

Looking at the form of during workout nutrition, traditionally fluids have been used as this provides both fluid and carbohydrate intake (solids may also cause stomach upset). Commercial sports drinks such as Gatorade or Powerade in the US or Lucozade in the UK are available and generally contain roughly 14 grams of carbohydrate per 8 oz (236 ml) of fluid. This would provide 45 grams of carbohydrate for an athlete consuming 24 oz (708 ml) of fluid per hour. They also invariably contain sodium and potassium in appropriate amounts. Some newer products also contain protein, generally in a 4:1 ratio of carbohydrate to protein. Whey protein can be added to commercial sports carbohydrate drinks easily enough. Athletes can readily mix their own sports drinks by using the appropriate amount of fluid and carbohydrate (some prefer diluted fruit juice), adding a small amount of rapidly digested protein powder and an additional 1/4 tsp of Lo-Salt per 32 oz (~1000 ml) of fluid for sodium and potassium.

As I mentioned above, carbohydrate gels, small packets of rapidly digesting carbohydrates are available for use by athletes. As they provide no fluid to the body and water will still be necessary, I don't see much point to them over a nutrient containing drink to begin with. Certainly they are convenient (and lighter) and may be the only option for runners or other athletes who can't carry water bottles or fluid with them. In general, it is rare for athletes to eat solid foods during competitions although there are exceptions. The most common tend to be long-distance cyclists riding 4 or more hours or ultra-endurance athletes, who may eat some amount of solid, easily digestible food during their longer workouts or competitions. Jelly sandwiches, fruit and various types of low-fiber, low-fat carbohydrates are typically chosen and commercially available food bars (or their homemade versions) could be used. Water will still have to be consumed to ensure that fluid requirements are met. Technically, strength/power, physique and other athletes could consume solid foods during their workouts but this tends to be somewhat rare.

Putting it All Together

I've summarized all of the above information in the chart below. The lower values can be used for lower intensity workouts and all non-endurance athletes will usually find them to be more appropriate as well. Team/mixed sports may need proportionally more carbohydrates for some training sessions that are particularly long or contain a large amount of high-intensity work. For any workout or competition longer than 2 hours, both sodium and potassium must be present to ensure that there is no risk of EAH.

Duration	Fluid Intake	Amount Carbs	Type of Carb	Protein
<30 minutes	None/To thirst	None	None	None
30-60 minutes	To thirst	Mouth Rinse	Most forms	None
Time Trial (Luteal)	To thirst	30-45 g/h	Most forms	4-8 g/hour whey
1-2 Hours*	To thirst	15-30 (60) g/h	Most forms	4-8 g/hour whey
2-3Hours	0.08-0.16 fluid oz/pound (5.7-11.4 ml/kg)	30-60 g/h	Glucose or glucose+fructose	4-8 g/hour whey
>2.5 Hours	0.08-0.16 fluid oz/pound (5.7-11.4 ml/kg)	75-90 g/h	Glucose+fructose, solids possible	4-8 g/hour whey

*Includes other training sessions such as strength/power/physique, HIIT or team practices

I'd finish by noting that cool, but not cold fluids, improve absorption of fluid from the stomach and help to keep body temperature down somewhat. Additionally, while it may be convenient to spread fluid and nutrient intake out during exercise (i.e. drinking 4-6 oz/120-180 ml of fluid every 15 minutes), it actually turns out that larger amounts consumed less frequently work just as effectively. The fluid and carbohydrate simply sits in the stomach waiting to be digested and this may provide a strategy for runners and other athletes who have limited opportunities to consume fluid or carbohydrates during training. This has to be weighed against the potential for stomach upset some experimentation may be necessary.

Post-Workout Nutrition and Recovery

Post-workout nutrition refers to anything consumed from immediately after the workout to roughly 2-4 hours afterwards at which time normal eating resumes. This phase has three primary goals which are to repair and rebuild muscle tissue, refill muscle glycogen and replace lost fluids/rehydrate. Replacing lost electrolytes (sodium and potassium) is equally important and, as a female specific issue, sufficient calcium intake after a workout is critical to ensure optimal improvements in bone mineral density (BMD). Although not related to nutrition per se, women recover from heat stress differently than men and it should come as no surprise that women's requirements for post-workout recovery differ from that of men's (15).

For decades, it was felt that consuming nutrients immediately following a workout was critical for optimal recovery and adaptation due to improvements in blood low and nutrient uptake into muscles. Glycogen storage is fastest immediately after training and delaying carbohydrate intake by 3 hours reduced glycogen synthesis by 50%. Similarly, delaying protein intake following a resistance training workout reduced the overall anabolic response to training. This led to the concept of the anabolic window, a relatively short time period following training where nutrients had to be consumed or optimal results would not be had. In more recent years, this idea has been challenged. First and foremost, any anabolic window appears to be much longer than previously thought (16). As importantly, hitting daily nutrient targets is of far more importance overall than ensuring immediate post-workout nutrient intake (17).

There are a number of reasons for this change. Looking at glycogen replenishment, even the slowest rates of glycogen synthesis are able to refill muscle glycogen stores within 24 hours so long as total carbohydrate intake is sufficient and the only time that rapid rapid initial glycogen replenishment matters is when time periods less than 8 hours are examined. In the most general sense this means that anyone training only once per day will always have sufficient time to refill muscle glycogen between two workouts. The types of exhaustive workouts that are either limited by or which significantly deplete muscle glycogen are are generally done infrequently which makes rapid glycogen resynthesis that much less important. Exhaustive aerobic, HIIT or sprint sessions are rarely done more than 2-3 times per week meaning that 48 hours will usually pass between those sessions. High-volume physique training is done frequently during the week (often 5-6 times per week) but body parts are generally rotated or varied across days of the week which means that several days will pass between workouts for the same muscle. In all of these situations, there is more than enough time to refill muscle glycogen regardless of speed. Only those athletes who will be performing high-volume and/or high-intensity workouts or competitions involving the same muscle groups within 4-8 hours of one another need to be concerned with rapid rates of muscle glycogen synthesis. In all other situations, only the total carbohydrate intake between workouts matters.

In a more general sense, the fact is that unless someone has not eaten for 4-5+ hours before a workout, they will still have at least some nutrients available for use at the end of the workout. In fact, as I pointed out when I discussed the pre-workout snack, eating before training is potentially more effective as those nutrients are available immediately following the workout. Anything eaten following the workout must first be digested and it may be 30 minutes or more until nutrients are available. But there are situations where someone may not have eaten within 4 hours of a workout. This might be due to their schedule although it is most common for morning workouts where there simply isn't time (or someone chooses not) to eat. In this case, post-workout nutrition becomes critical as it is the first source of nutrients that will be available to the body after the workout has ended. Whether they have eaten prior to the workout or not, the Category 1 dieter must consume at least some protein (preferably from a fast digesting source such as whey) following weight training workouts as this will help to prevent LBM loss (17). As mentioned earlier in this chapter, the postmenopausal woman should do the same.

The point of the above section is not to argue against post-workout nutrition. It is never detrimental in any sense and, whether truly required or not, is a convenient time to consume nutrients to facilitate the recovery and adaptation process sooner rather than later. However, outside of a handful of situations, the idea of an anabolic window that closes shortly after the workout is over is incorrect and ensuring post-workout nutrition may not be as mandatory a dietary requirement as previously thought. That said, let me look at what might represent ideal post-workout intakes of nutrients for various situations and goals.

Repairing and Rebuilding Muscle Tissue

While glycogen resynthesis has been the typical focus of post-workout nutrition, it's becoming clear that repairing and rebuilding muscle tissue is a key aspect of long-term recovery and adaptation to training so I will look at it first. Both dietary protein and carbohydrates are important to this process, having independent but overlapping goals. The primary role of dietary protein is to aid in the repair of damaged tissue along with the synthesis of new proteins and this a fundamental way that training improves fitness, by signaling the body to make more proteins involved in endurance, strength, muscle size, etc. Only dietary protein can support these changes (carbohydrate cannot) and an intake of 0.13-0.22 g/lb LBM (0.3-0.5 g/kg LBM) would be appropriate. The lower intake ius appropriate for endurance/HIIT training and the higher value should be used for strength/power/physique or sprint training. This yields a protein intake of 15-25 grams for our sample female with 117 lbs LBM. Due to their amino acid profile (high in the Branched Chain Amino Acids, especially leucine), animal source proteins are superior to vegetable source proteins and dairy proteins are superior to soy (19,20). Isolated pea protein is also high in leucine (21).

While dietary protein is by far and away the most important nutrient to support this goal, there are potential additional benefits of both dietary fat and carbohydrate. Certain types of dietary fats, primarily the essential fatty acids (EFA's) that I discussed in the last chapter appear to sensitize skeletal muscle to the effects of protein and this is yet another reason to consume them regularly. The impact of carbohydrates on the repair process is actually somewhat debatable. At most it has a small impact on the process, probably by decreasing protein breakdown, but the effect is small or non-existent if sufficient protein is being consumed. Carbohydrate is still important to refill muscle glycogen but, as above, not as critically important as once thought. Just as with the pre-workout snack, some strength/power/physique athletes prefer to consume only protein after training as refilling muscle glycogen is not critical.

Refilling Muscle Glycogen

The second primary goal of post-workout recovery is to refill muscle glycogen following training and I will address two specific situations. The first is for those athletes who want to start the recovery processes immediately but have no need for rapid glycogen resynthesis. Here, a carbohydrate intake of roughly 0.31-0.45 g/lb (0.7-1.0 g/kg) consumed within an hour of training and again two hours later is more than sufficient and this might represent 45-70 grams of carbohydrate in each meal. The highest values will only be required after the most exhaustive workouts (i.e. 2 hours at a fairly high intensity) and most will probably find that the lower values are more than sufficient. For sprint or lower volume resistance types of workouts (i.e. low repetition weight training), this value can be cut further and 25-35 grams of carbohydrate with an equal amount of protein will be enought. In this situation, the type of carbohydrate is more or less irrelevant. Studies have used sugars, maltodextrins, starches, liquids (which also provide fluid), solids and for the most part it simply fails to matter what is consumed so long as the correct amounts are eaten. Solid meals containing carbohydrate, protein, fat and fiber will also work..

The second, and more complex situation, is one where an athlete must rapidly refill muscle glycogen. This will be maximized with a carbohydrate intake of 0.45-0.54 g/lb (1-1.2 g/kg) per hour for the first four hours after training will maximize glycogen storage. For our 150 lb female athlete this would be an intake of 65-81 grams of carbohydrates every hour for four hours for a total of 260-320 grams of carbohydrates over this four hour span (22). Eating smaller snacks every 15-30 minutes has an even greater impact but may not be realistic. At the four hour mark, normal eating would resume although, realistically the athlete has now re-entered the pre-workout meal phase of around workout nutrition. Ideally, carbohydrate intake should begin as soon as realistically possible after the end of training since glycogen synthesis rates will be at their absolute maximum. While there appears to be little difference overall between solid and liquid carbohydrates or even different types of carbohydrates, liquids (which also provide fluid) and other concentrated, rapidly digesting carbohydrate sources may be preferred to avoid the stomach upset that may accompany eating such a large amount of solid food in a short period of time.

While the above represents an ideal approach to rapid glycogen resynthesis, it has the often seen problem of potentially exceeding some women's daily calorie or carbohydrate intake levels, especially under dieting conditions. Certainly the only time that the above will be remotely necessary is for those athletes with extremely high energy expenditures (typically endurance athletes) and a higher calorie intake but women may still run into problems. A solution to this is to add protein (which should be done anyway) to a relatively lower amount of carbohydrate as this will increase glycogen storage despite the lowered amount of carbohydrates (23). Combining 0.13-0.0.18 g/lb (0.3-0.4 g/kg) LBM protein with 0.36 g/lb (0.8 g/kg) carbohydrate can stimulate the same amount of glycogen storage as larger amounts of carbohydrate and will allow lower calorie/carb intakes to be effective. So instead of consuming 81 grams of carbohydrate post-workout, our sample athlete could consume 15-20 grams of protein and 54 grams of carbohydrate. This has the overall effect of enhancing overall recovery and stimulating glycogen storage post-workout while reducing total calorie and carbohydrate intake.

Rehydration, Electrolytes and Calcium

The third primary goal of post-workout nutrition is rehydration. Here the recommendations will be far less specific as the amount of fluid required for rehydration depends entirely on how much was lost during training in the first place. Generally speaking, longer and more intense workouts cause more fluid loss but environmental conditions and individual differences play a huge role (as I've noted, sweating rates varying enormously between any two individuals). The most accurate way to estimate fluid requirements following training is to weigh before and after with the goal of re-achieving starting bodyweight prior to the next training session For every pound (0.45 kg) of weight lost, a total of 24 oz or 750 ml of fluid will be required for replacement (this represents the amount of fluid lost from the body along with a 50% increase to cover normal hydration needs). An athlete who lost 6 lbs (2.7 kg) would need to consume 144 fluid oz (4.5 l) in total to rehydrate in the hours following the workout. This isn't to say it should be consumed all at once, this just represents the amount required before the next workout occurs.

Independent of fluid intake per se is the need to replace lost electrolytes. As with fluid intake, determining how much needs to be restored or making specific recommendations is difficult as sodium losses can vary 7 fold between any two individual (athletes losing a tremendous amount of sodium often find that their clothes are slicked white). The best solution to this is to simply ensure sufficient fluid intake while, as I have mentioned before, salting foods liberally to ensure optimal absorption. Pure water is actually quite poor for rehydration as large intakes simply result in greater urinary losses. In contrast, fluids with sodium or potassium present (or drinking water with a meal containing both) enhances fluid retention significantly. For those athletes who prefer to drink pure water by itself, Lite- or Lo-Salt can be added with 1 tsp per 32 oz (960 ml) being an appropriate amount. Commercial electrolyte waters such as coconut water are also available but tend to be more expensive.

One aspect of post-workout recovery that is overlooked is that of calcium intake. This is more of an issue for woman then men given women's relatively limited time to build peak bone density and the long-term risks that not achieving peak bone density can have. At least certain types of training (those involving high impact or peak forces such as resistance training, jumping or sprinting) tends to stimulate both bone synthesis and breakdown. Just as dietary protein is required to support protein synthesis following training, calcium intake is required to support optimal improvement in bone density. And while most of the impact of calcium on bone health will come from sufficient intakes on a day-to-day basis, at least some of that calcium should come after the workout with the post-workout meal being a convenient time to ensure that some is consumed. No specific guidelines exist but 200-300 mg of calcium would seem appropriate.

Is Milk the Optimal Post-Workout Food?

Combining all of the different components I've described above, an optimal post-workout meal or food for maximizing recovery would contain a high-quality source of protein, some carbohydrates, possibly dietary fat while also providing fluids, sodium, potassium and calcium. There actually is a single food that meets all of those criteria and that food is milk, which some feel may be an optimal sports drink (24). In one simple package, milk provides high quality dairy protein (a mixture of fast digesting whey and slow digesting casein), a mixture of carbohydrates, fluids, sodium, potassium and the most well absorbed form of calcium that can be consumed. Milk has been found to be superior to water in terms of rehydration while chocolate milk has been found to improve recovery and adaptation to training (25-27). Consuming milk following training improves changes in body composition along with having a positive effect on bone health (28, 28a). While not providing fluid, ice cream would provide all of the above while also helping to cool the body after exercise. This could be useful after exercise under hot or humid conditions.

Despite it's near perfect combination of nutrients along with being convenient and readily available, milk does have some potential disadvantages. As I mentioned already in Chapter 20, not everyone can digest milk or consume it without stomach upset. Those with lactose intolerance either have to use relatively more expensive lactose removed milk or keep a supply of the milk digesting pills I mentioned in the previous chapter handy. Perhaps the largest drawback of milk is that, used alone, it can take a fairly large amount to meet all but the lowest nutrient recommendations above.

Eight fluid ounces (~240 ml) of regular milk contains 8 grams of protein, 12 grams of carbohydrate and variable amounts of fat (of some interest, high-fat milk may be more effective for muscle building than low-fat milk but nobody is quite sure why). To fulfill her nutrient requirements, the 150 lb sample dieter would have to consume nearly 24 fluid oz (720 ml) of milk to reach her goals of 25 grams of protein and this would provide 36 grams of carbohydrate which is a tremendous amount of fluid to drink at once. For endurance athletes, the opposite situation tends to hold and consuming enough carbohydrate from milk would tend to provide excessive amounts of protein (which is not a problem in and of itself) along with requiring tremendous amounts of fluid. Here, chocolate milk may be a better choice here as it has roughly 24 grams carbohydrate per 8 fluid oz (240 ml). Sixteen fluid oz of chocolate milk would provide 16 grams of protein with 48 grams of carbohydrate which is right in line with the post-training recommendations above. Chocolate milk is often better tolerated by people with lactose intolerance as well for some reason.

While milk alone may be near a near perfect post-workout food, there is no reason that it would have to be the sole source of nutrients Following a strength training type of workout, protein powder could be added to milk to bump up the protein or the milk could be consumed in addition to another protein containing food. The endurance athlete could consume milk in addition to whole foods providing carbohydrate and (as needed) additional protein to reach their post-workout nutrient goals.

Putting It All Together

I've summarized the information discussed above on post workout nutrition in the chart below. I've indicated the suggested amounts of protein, carbohydrate, fluids, electrolytes and calcium and provided recommendations for different kinds of sports/activities. Physique should be taken to include any weight training performed to increase muscle size. In the very few situations that it may be relevant, I've provided recommendations for rapid glycogen replenishment.

	Physique	Strength/Power	High-Intensity	Team/Mixed	Endurance
Protein	0.18-0.22 g/lb LBM	0.22 g/lb LBM	0.22 g/lb LBM	0.13-0.18 g/lb LBM	0.13 g/lb LBM
Carbs: Normal	1-2X protein Optional	1-2Xprotein Optional	1-2X protein Optional	0.3-0.45 g/lb	0.3-0.45 g/lb
Carbs: Speedy w/o Protein	0.45-0.54 g/lb/h hourly for 4 hours*	Unnecessary	Unnecessary	0.45-0.54 g/lb/h hourly for 4 hours*	0.45-0.54 g/lb/h hourly for 4 hours
Carbs: Speedy w/ Protein	0.36 g/lb + 0.13 g/lb LBM protein hourly for 4 hours*	Unnecessary	Unnecessary	0.36 g/lb+0.13 g/lb LBM protein hourly for 4 hours*	0.36 g/lb +0.13 g/lb LBM protein hourly for 4 hours
Fluids	To Thirst	To Thirst	To Thirst	Variable*	24 oz/lb lost
Na+/K++	Yes	Yes	Yes	Yes	Yes
Calcium	Yes	Yes	Yes	Yes	Yes

*Na+/K+ are sodium and potassium. Physique athletes occasionally need speed glycogen recovery, usually when they are carb-loading for a competition or using very specific types of diets. Some team/mixed sports may be performing two exhaustive workouts per day although this is probably less common overall. For fluid intake, many team sports train outdoors in the heat and fluid and electrolyte losses can be large.

To put the values above into more concrete terms, let me look at two sample athletes in different situations. The first is the 150 lb, 22% body fat female with 117 lbs of LBM I have been using throughout this book. She has just performed a 90 minute weight training workout and will be consuming 0.22 g/lb LBM protein with an equal amount of carbohydrate immediately post workout. This means that she will need to eat 25 grams of protein with 25 grams of carbohydrate (200 calories). The second athlete is a 130 lb female endurance athlete with 16% body fat so she has 110 lbs (50 kg) of LBM. She has just finished an exhausting aerobic workout and has to perform a second workout roughly 8 hours later. She is trying to reduce her body fat so immediately after training she will be consuming 0.13 g/lb LBM of protein with 0.3.6 g/lb of carbohydrate hourly for the first four hours following training. So she will be eating 15 grams protein and 46 grams of carbohydrate every hour for the first four hours following training before moving to normal eating and preparing for the second workout. Depending on the nature of that workout she might need a pre-workout snack, during workout nutrition and additional post-workout nutrition.

Both athletes would should choose a high quality protein with a mixture of carbohydrates while providing fluid, sodium, potassium and calcium as this will meet all of the requirements for optimal post-workout recovery. While solids appear to be as effective as fluids, not all athletes are hungry for solid food following an intense workout. Liquids often provide convenience on top of providing at least some fluid intake. To avoid stomach upset and provide rapid digestion, the second athlete is probably best served by including at least some amount of fluid in the first meals after training before transitioning to solid foods in the later hours following her first workout. A mixture of solid and liquid foods is often optimal.

Post-Workout Recovery

While not related to nutrition per se, there are two female specific issues related to post-workout recovery that I do want to address. Training, in the most general sense, stresses the body and causes a disruption of homeostasis. It is that disruption that ultimately, stimulates changes in fitness in response to training. This means that recovery from training cannot optimally occur until the body has returned to normal. Post-workout nutrition is aimed at that in the first place but there are other issues that are not only important but where women may differ from men and need to adopt different recovery practices.

Blood flow to muscles is one aspect of this. During training, blood flow to working muscles is increased which both increases nutrient delivery along with waste product removal. After training (or during training in-between individual bouts of exercise), blood flow and blood pressure decrease. This decrease occurs to a greater degree in woman than in men and blood pressure sometimes drops below resting values. This compromises blood flow into and out of the muscles, potentially hampering recovery. Performing light aerobic activity prevents this decrease and women may benefit from doing this after workouts (referred to as cooling down) to a greater degree than men. Compression socks, which increase blood return from the lower have also been shown to slightly improve recovery in women (29).

Related to this are issues related to heat generation and heat stress with exercise. As I mentioned above, women's bodies thermoregulate differently and and women are less likely to overheat than men during exercise, at least during the follicular phase of the menstrual cycle (this changes during the luteal phase or with some types of birth control). But this reverses itself following exercise with women's bodies actually storing heat to a greater degree than men, and cooling off more slowly. This delays the return of the body to homeostasis and might potentially impair recovery. This also suggests that women may benefit more than men from some currently used post-workout cooling strategies than men. Ice baths have long been used although this can impair the adaptations that occur to training and cooling vests may be a better choice. Drinking cold fluids after training should reduce core temperature slightly (recall my mention of ice cream post workout) and even draping a cool towel over the back of the neck helps to dissipate heat. These strategies are likely to be most beneficial for those women who have done long workouts in hot or humid conditions and even moreso during the luteal phase. While outside of the scope of this book, the use of cold following a muscular injury appears to be more beneficial for women as well.

Summarizing Around Workout Nutrition

Before finishing the chapter with an examination of fasted training, I want to summarize the information I've presented on all four phases of around workout nutrition for different general training situations and sporting categories. For each I'll show each phase of around workout nutrition and how it might optimally be set up. This isn't meant to indicate that every phase will be needed or necessarily should be used and they interact with one another as I discussed above.

Individual variation in scheduling, needs, and responses will all play a role in what combination is or is not optimal or preferred and some amount of experimentation will be necessary over time for any given person to find their own preferred or ideal eating schedule around training sessions. Trainees performing different types of training across a week may find that different combinations are needed around those different training sessions. So a team sport athlete might be performing team practices, various types of endurance/HIIT workouts and strength training, each of which will have its own specific requirements.

Strength/Power, Physique and High-Intensity Performance Workouts

Strength/power, muscle growth and high-intensity performance workouts are all more alike than they are different in terms of their fuel use and goals and I will give similar recommendations for them. With the possible exception of physique type workouts, this type of training doesn't generally use a tremendous amount of muscle glycogen and have as their goal improving muscle size, strength or power output. The values below would be appropriate, assuming 60-90 minutes or more of intense training per workout.

	Pre-Workout	Pre-Workout Snack	During	Post-Workout
Protein	Normal	0.22 g/lb LBM	4-8 g/hour	0.22 g/lb LBM
Carbs	Normal	1-2X protein intake (optional)	15-30 g/h	1-2X protein intake (optional)
Form	Solid	Easily digestible	Liquid	Preferred
Fluid	To thirst	To thirst	To thirst	To thirst
Electrolytes	Normal	Normal	Normal	Normal
Calcium	Normal	N/A	N/A	200-300 mg

So the sample 150 lb female dieter with 22% body fat and 117 lbs of LBM would eat a normal meal 3-4 hours before the workout, 25 grams of protein with up to 25-50 grams of carbohydrates 1-2 hours before the workout, 15-30 grams of carbohydrate and 4-6 grams of protein per hour during the workout and another 25 grams of protein with up to 25-50 grams of carbohydrate post-workout. For strength/power and physique athlete, carbohydrates before and after training are optional though high-intensity sports training will tend to benefit from their intake. Normal eating would resume 2-4 hours after the workout.

Team/Mixed Sports Training

Team and mixed sports training may be one of the most difficult categories of sports to give concrete nutritional recommendations for due to the structure of the workouts. If there is any constant in team training it is that it is generally done in a vary start and stop fashion but beyond that training can vary from purely technical or tactical training to scrimmages and this will alter the calorie expenditure, fuel use and nutritional requirements from almost negligible to fairly high. I've shown some general values below.

	Pre-Workout	Pre-Workout Snack	During	Post-Workout
Protein	Normal	0.13-0.18 g/lb LBM	4-8 g/hour	0.13-0.18 g/lb LBM
Carbs	Normal	1-2X protein intake	15-30 (60) g/h*	1-2X protein intake
Form	Solid	Easily digestible	Liquid	Preferred
Fluid	To thirst	To thirst	To thirst	To thirst
Electrolytes	Normal	Normal	Normal	Normal
Calcium	Normal	N/A	N/A	300 mg

*60 g/hour of carbohydrate will only be necessary for the most intense types of
training and most workouts will require only 15-30 g/hour.

So the sample 150 lb female dieter with 22% body fat and 117 lbs of LBM would eat a normal meal 3-4 hours before the workout, 15-20 grams of protein with up to 40 grams of carbohydrate 1-2 hours before the workout, 15-30 grams of carbohydrate (up to 60 grams/hour for extremely intensive training) and 4-6 grams of protein per hour during the workout and another 15-20 grams of protein and up to 40 grams of carbohydrate post-workout with normal eating resuming 2-4 hours later. In rare occasions such as training camps or certain types of competitions with multiple games on the same day, the rapid glycogen resynthesis schedule from earlier in the chapter would be used in the first 4 hours following training.

HIIT and Endurance Training

While individual endurance sports each have their own specific nuances of training, they tend to be more similar than not in terms of the types of workouts that are done during training. At the same time, compared to many others sports, endurance training shows some of the largest variance in training that may be done with each having potentially different nutritional requirements. An easy 30-60 minute aerobic session might require nothing more than normal eating and fluids while an exhaustive 2-4 hour aerobic workout including intervals might require all four phases of around workout nutrition for optimal results. The huge variations in what might be optimal precludes me from making any type of meaningful chart and I'd refer endurance athletes to the previous sections instead to determine what their needs might be.

Fasted Training

While it has been generally accepted that at least some amount of around workout nutrition should be used for optimal performance, there are also situations where fasted training (done without eating) may be done or be beneficial. Frequently this occurs for practical reasons, situations where someone trains early in the morning and is unable to eat anything beforehand for one reason or another (i.e. stomach upset). There is also a dietary strategy called Intermittent Fasting (IF'ing, discussed in the next chapter) where people deliberately wait until later in the day to eat and often choose to train without eating beforehand.

Perhaps the most commonly recommended type of fasted training is easy aerobic training done for the goal of optimal fat loss or during a diet. This approach developed in the physique community decades ago and came out of the fact that more fat is used during exercise under those conditions. Logically it seemed that this should result in greater fat loss but I mentioned in a previous chapter that it's debatable if this is actually true or not (30). Recall that the total amount of fat burned during most types of exercise is small to begin with and women's bodies simply switch back to using glucose for fuel the rest of the day making any impact small, if it exists at all. That said, the Category 1 female who is struggling with lower body fat issues may still benefit from fasted aerobic work and the some of Stubborn Fat Protocols discussed in Appendix 1 are meant to be done fasted. For the most part, other trainees seeking fat loss should perform their aerobic work whenever it is convenient or they are most likely to do it consistently.

Moving to athletic and performance training, it has been taken as a matter of faith that all but the lowest intensity and duration aerobic sessions should include some amount of carbohydrate intake but there may be situations where this is untrue. As with the above, there is at least some indication that training fasted may improve muscle's ability to use fatty acids for fuel and this would potentially increase endurance by sparing muscle glycogen. At a greater extreme, it's been suggested that deliberately performing endurance training with lowered muscle glycogen levels may improve the adaptations seen to training (31). This requires more than training fasted as only liver glycogen is depleted after an overnight fast while muscle glycogen is unaffected. Accomplishing the goal of training under low glycogen conditions requires performing two hard workouts with no carbohydrates in-between or following a low-carbohydrate diet.

While these strategies have been shown to cause various biochemical changes to occur in muscle, performance improvements are rarely seen (in some cases it is actually harmed). As I discussed previously, athletes find it impossible to complete high-intensity training sessions when muscle glycogen is depleted and some work finds that the body's ability to use carbs for fuel (i.e. during sprinting) is impaired. Some researchers are actually calling the changes "carbohydrate impairing" rather than "carbohydrate sparing" for this reason. Most sports scientists point out that endurance athletes, due to the sheer amount of training they perform are probably doing at least some amount of it with lowered glycogen without deliberately trying to do so. It's also being suggested that, while low-intensity training might benefit from fasted training, high-intensity workouts should still be supported with adequate carbohydrate intake. This potentially gives the best of both worlds, generating greater adaptations to the lower intensity endurance training while still supporting high-intensity training.

However, as usual most of the work on this topic has been done on men and I question whether or not it will have the same effect in women. As I've discussed, women's bodies already spare glycogen during low- and moderate-intensity aerobic exercise compared to men and this likely leaves less (or no) room for further improvement. Supporting this, a recent study found that women showed better training adaptations when they ate beforehand whereas men benefitted more from training fasted (31a). Women show superior endurance to men in certain activities and, in a very real sense, men attempting to fat adapt themselves with this type of dietary strategy are trying to make their physiology more like that of a woman's.

Moving to resistance training (very little work has been done on other sports), limited work suggests that there might be a superior training response when training is done fasted and proper post-workout nutrition is implemented (32). In that study, actual muscle growth was not measured and it's unclear if there will be actual long-term benefits to training after having eaten. From a purely anecdotal standpoint, many in the IF'ing community train fasted (often consuming isolated amino acids which I think is somewhat pointless) and seem to make at least similar gains from their training as those who eat beforehand. There is at least some tendency in that community to perform relatively shorter, lower-volume (but higher intensity) weight training sessions and this tends to have an impact on whether or not fasted training can be done. For longer workouts, many get superior performance by eating before the workout. Trainees will have to experiment to see what is best for them within the guidelines I have provided.

Like many dietary strategies, training fasted has both its pros and cons. In some situations it may be appropriate or at least neutral in its effects while in others its effects are more questionable or event detrimental. Perhaps the ultimate decision, outside of practical ones is whether or not performance during the workout suffers from training fasted rather than fed. As I mentioned above, trainees can vary enormously in their relative ability to eat or not eat before workouts (and this depends on the type of workout being done). Some can't eat anything within hours of training without stomach upset and may find fasted training superior while others must have eaten or their training suffers. Even if muscle glycogen is not depleted, many find that lowered blood glucose harms performance. Women already rely more heavily on blood glucose than men and recall that it may become more unstable during the luteal phase. So their ability to train fasted or not might vary across the menstrual cycle. Birth control might also impact on this.

Chapter 23: Meal Frequency and Patterning

Whether involved in training or not, the next aspect of setting up a daily diet revolves around meal frequency, the number of meals eaten per day, and meal patterning, how those meals are distributed throughout the day. There is an additional issue of how calories are distributed across the week. While it has been most common for people to use identical distributions every day, fundamentally there is not only no reason that calorie intake should be the same every day but also good reasons to vary them. For each topic I'll look at some of the commonly held myths or misconceptions along with different approaches to each and where they might be relatively more or less appropriate. I'll also present some relatively "new" approaches that some readers may not be familiar with. Outside of the occasional practical issue there are no gender differences that really exist for this topic. There are also only a handful of situations where hormonal modifiers are relevant and I will only address them as needed.

Meal Frequency: Myths and Misconceptions

Meal frequency refers to the number of times someone eats in a day and this can include meals or snacks. As is so often the case with nutrition, there is a tremendous amount of commonly accepted knowledge about meal frequency in terms of fat loss, muscle gain and health but much of it is incorrect. Perhaps the most general and commonly repeated idea is that a high meal frequency (i.e. eating 6 small meals per day or roughly every three hours) has a number of enormous metabolic and other benefits and that any eating plan that does not include this frequency of eating is sub-optimal. Entire books and lifestyles have been based around this concept and it's not uncommon to hear of obsessed dieters sneaking away from their work station or skipping social events to maintain this type of rigid eating schedule.

One commonly made claim is that is that eating more often will increase or "stoke" metabolic rate but this is based on a misunderstanding of the thermic effect of food (TEF), the increase in calorie burn that occurs after eating. As I described earlier in the book, TEF is estimated at about 10% of total calorie intake so someone eating 1800 calories per day will burn roughly 180 via TEF. For all practical purposes this means that the TEF to eating one larger versus multiple smaller meals is insignificant approaching zero and research has found this to be true in both women and men (1,1a). Six 300 calorie meals will create a 30 calorie TEF six times (180 calories total) while three 600 calorie meals will create a 60 cal TEF 3 times (still 180 calories). One large meal per day may actually create a slightly larger TEF but the differences is only a few calories. Meal frequency simply has no meaningful impact on energy expenditure.

It's similarly claimed that skipping a single meal or going more than three hours without eating will put the body into "starvation" mode, slowing fat loss and causing the body to store fat. This is often coupled with the above idea such that skipping breakfast slows metabolism eating breakfast stokes the metabolism for the rest of the day. In small animals with short lifespans, it is true but here a single meal represents a large proportion of their life span (at least one animal will die if it misses a single meal). In humans, a single meal is meaningless and fasting for 4 days actually increases metabolic rate (2).

Additional claims for a high meal frequency include increased fat loss or LBM sparing while dieting but this only holds true at the extremes of meal frequency (i.e. 2 vs. 6 meals per day) and even there only when protein intake is too low. When protein intake is high enough the differences disappear and any meal frequency between 3-4 meals per day shows no difference in either fat loss or LBM maintenance while dieting (2a). Given that an average meal takes 4-5 hours to digest, this would be expected. Other commonly made claims are that a high meal frequency will keep blood sugar stable or control hunger better. The first is sort of true but the studies invariably compare unrealistic meal frequencies (i.e. 3 meals to 17 small snacks) that have no relevance to normal eating patterns. Even the claim that eating more frequently controls hunger is questionable. A recent study found that eating more frequently made people hungrier in addition to having no impact on overall fat burning (3). PCOS women may benefit from a higher meal frequency and 6 meals per day was found to improve insulin sensitivity more than 3 meals (4). As both weight loss and exercise improve insulin sensitivity, I doubt this has any real relevance overall.

Finally, it's often claimed that a high frequency of eating is needed to maximize muscle growth or adaptations to training but shockingly little research has examined this. Given the relatively long time that mixed solid meals to digest, eating every 3-5 hours at a minimum would seem to be a reasonable approach. Across the roughly 16 non-sleeping hours of the day, this yields a meal frequency of roughly 3-5 times per day. Similar to the meal frequency data above, 4 meals per day containing protein is superior in terms of maintaining protein synthesis to only 2 meals but 8 meals has no additional benefit (5).

Is There an Optimal Meal Frequency?

Hopefully the above will convince my readers that more of the claims that a high meal frequency is either beneficial or required are false and that, within a moderate range of 3-4 meals per day, there is little to no difference in almost any measured parameter. In a general sense, this means that the optimal meal frequency will depend on the needs and preferences of the individual. Someone's work, school or life situation all play a role and many women have family or children's schedules to take into account. If training is being performed, the amount and type impacts not only on her total daily food intake but at least some of those calories will come around her workouts. All of these factors and more will go into the determination of what might be the optimal meal frequency in any given situation.

One issue that is often forgotten is total calorie intake and there are situations where a lower meal frequency (and potentially altered meal patterning) may be superior. This situation primarily occurs in smaller Category 1 women dieting to the extremes of low body fat percentage (BF%) who are on relatively fewer calories. Very small meals appear to not send an effective fullness signal and the practical implications of this is that fewer, larger meals may keep dieters fuller than more but smaller meals when total calorie intake is low. The same can hold for Category 2/3 dieters using aggressive deficits.

Consider this book's sample dieter on a calorie intake of 2000 calories/day. If she tries to eat 6 meals per day, each meal is just slightly over 300 calories which is small but still reasonable. If she were to reduce her meal frequency to four meals per day each will be 500 calories per day. While both of these might be realistic in terms of maintaining fullness, the situation becomes significantly worse as her calorie intake drops further. If later in the diet her calorie intake has dropped to 1400-1600 calories per day, a 6 meal per day frequency puts each meal at 230-260 calories per day while 4 meals would keep each meal at 350-400 calories. At 1200 calories per day, each of 6 meals is only 200 calories, barely a snack. At three meals per day and a post-workout snack of 200 calories, each meal would be just over 300 calories. It's not a large amount of food at each meal either way but the latter is better by degrees.

Clearly women (or proportionally larger men) with a higher caloric intake needn't worry about this as much since they have more daily calories to work with. Larger female dieters or highly trained athletes performing enormous amounts of exercise are frequently in this situation. When the daily diet allows for 2000+ calories per day to be eaten, it's much easier to maintain a high meal frequency with each meal being larger overall. In some cases, generally female athletes expending an enormous number of calories per day, a higher meal frequency may be more or less required. A 150 pound athlete eating 3000 calories per day may find that fewer larger meals causes stomach upset or discomfort due to their large size and eating more frequently is beneficial. This has to be weighed against real world work and school schedules in terms of whether it is realistic or not.

Meal Patterning: Introduction

Meal patterning refers to how the day's meals, calories or nutrients are distributed or spaced throughout the day. Since any one or even all three can vary, the number of possibilities becomes enormous and about any pattern that can be conceived has probably been tried and/or found to be effective by someone. And while it's common to see specific patterns being argued as optimal for all situations, it's better to look at meal patterning within the context of the specific situations to which it is being applied.

A number of factors go into determining what type of meal pattern might be more or less appropriate for a given situation. The first is meal frequency itself. If meal frequency is higher, those meals have to be more spaced out since people are only awake for a certain number of hours per day. The actual macronutrient intake of the diet has an effect here although it mainly impacts on when those nutrients are eaten during the day. Work, school and life schedules play a role as there may be times when eating a meal is not realistic. This is a common problem for collegiate athletes. Actual training times during the day also impact when meals must fall. Athletes or serious trainees should also get in the habit of having a slow digesting protein at bedtime as this will help support recovery and adaptation to training (6).

As I look at some of the common meal patterns, I will be making a few basic assumptions about people's schedules. The first is that people sleep 8 hours per day, wake up at 7 am and going to bed at 11pm with 16 hours per day in which they might conceivably eat. The second is that if around workout nutrition is being used, anything being eaten before during or after a workout it will be considered as a single meal. This will be true even if all three phases of around workout nutrition are not implemented. For athletes, one meal containing at least protein will always come at bedtime as well and this will all impact on the patterning (and frequency) of the other meals. As I look at each pattern, I'll address it in general along with it's potential pros and cons and what situations it might be more or less appropriate for.

Even Meal and Nutrient Distribution

Perhaps the most common meal pattern is an even distribution where the day's calories and macronutrients are spread fairly evenly across the day. They needn't be exactly identical, just within a fairly close range in terms of their overall composition. The interval between meals needn't be exact and is often determined by a person's life, work or school schedule. As I mentioned above, for women who are exercising, at least one meal is likely to be around the workout itself with the others spaced relatively evenly throughout the day. For high-level athletes training twice daily, two of the day's meals will likely be coming around training with the others spaced fairly evenly between and around them. I've shown some representative patterns for different meal frequencies below.

Time	7-9am	9-11am	11am-1pm	1-3pm	3-5pm	5-8pm	8-11pm
3 Meals	Meal			Meal		Meal	
4 Meals	Meal		Meal		Meal		Meal
5 Meals	Meal		Meal	Meal		Meal	Meal
6 Meals	Meal	Meal		Meal	Meal	Meal	Meal

For the sample dieter on 2000 calories, a three meal distribution would be three ~660 calorie meals eaten roughly 6 hours apart, a four meal distribution would be 500 calories every 4 hours or so, a five meal distribution 400 calories every 3 hours and a 6 meal schedule 330 calories every 2.5 hours or so with each meal being more or less identical. You can see how the 6 meal per day schedule is nearly impossible to follow unless someone is a full-time athlete or perhaps works at home. The above examples aren't meant to be absolute suggestions and even a 6 meal pattern would be distributed a little more evenly than shown. While simple and convenient to set up, the even distribution isn't automatically the best approach as there are many good reasons where an uneven distribution of calories will be a better overall approach.

Uneven Meal and Nutrient Distribution: Introduction

An uneven meal distribution can refer to a number of different approaches but the most general concepts are that either the size, nutrient composition or both of the meals are varied throughout the day. Looking first at uneven calorie distribution, the simplest approach would be to divide the day's calorie into relatively smaller or larger meals. It's probably better to think of these as snacks and meals and I'll arbitrarily define a snack as containing 200 calories or less and a meal as containing 200 calories or more.

The general public tends to follow an uneven distribution of their food, eating three larger meals (breakfast, lunch and dinner) with one or more snacks eaten between those meals. If the sample dieter eating 2000 calories ate three 200 calorie snacks, that would leave 1400 calories divided evenly across the other three meals and each would contain 460 calories. Someone might eat breakfast before work, have a mid-morning snack, lunch, an early afternoon snack, dinner and then a snack before bedtime. Athletes or serious trainees often end up with at least a similar structure in that they may have a pre-workout snack, post-workout meal and then a pre-bedtime snack containing at least some protein (20-25 grams of a slowly digesting protein only contains 80-100 calories) or protein and carbohydrate in addition to their three main meals. In this situation, each meal or snack may be reasonably similar in terms of the relative amounts of protein, carbohydrates, fat and fiber they contain although the absolute amounts will vary with a 500 calorie meal containing more total grams of each compared to a 200 calories snack.

To variations in the size of each meal, there may can also be variations in the distribution of the day's protein, carbohydrates, fat and fiber. Strictly speaking any combination of single or multiple nutrients could be included in any given meal or snack but certain combinations tend to be better than others. The most important "rule" here is that any meal or snack should always include ~0.15 g/lb or 0.3 g/kg of protein (~20 grams for a 132 lb/60 kg female) regardless of whether any other nutrients are eaten. To this may be added fiber, fat, fat and fiber or all three other nutrients depending on the circumstances. With the possible exception of during a workout, carbohydrates should not be consumed by themselves. Even there protein is still beneficial but it may not always be practical to consume. As I mentioned in an earlier chapter, a common tendency for non-athlete women, especially when their diets contain too many carbohydrates and too little protein to begin with, is to have snacks or even meals that are either nothing but carbohydrate (fruit, some types of candy) or, worse yet, carbohydrates and fat with too little protein (many types of candy and even many meals that contain little to no protein). This invariably leaves them far hungrier than they would be if they ate sufficient protein with those foods at every meal.

While the above can technically generate an enormous number of possible combinations (and there have long been some very silly ideas about food combining out there), I only consider a handful of them to be worth considering in practical terms. These tend to revolve around how carbohydrates are distributed at any given meal with meals being relatively lower or higher in carbohydrates with relatively constant protein, fat and fiber. Low-carbohydrate meals will contain protein, protein/fat, or protein/fat/fiber combinations and higher carbohydrate meals will either focus on protein and carbohydrates (before and during workouts) or contain all nutrients (all other meals).

Uneven Meal and Nutrient Distribution

Perhaps the oldest idea about calorie distribution is to make breakfast the largest meal, lunch the second largest and dinner the smallest (i.e. "Eat dinner like a king, lunch like a prince and dinner like a pauper."). This probably stems from the idea that we are most active during the day and least at night or that eating a large amount before going to bed will result in fat gain (since the calories aren't being used), this latter idea being untrue for a number of reasons. That said, a larger breakfast meal has been shown to improve insulin sensitivity, lower androgen levels and improve fertility in women with PCOS (7). But as with meal frequency, these will occur with fat loss and regular activity to begin with. Female athletes with PCOS might want to explicitly avoid this meal pattern as elevated testosterone levels are part of what makes them successful as athletes. Research is mixed on whether eating relatively more earlier in the day or later at night is superior for weight and fat loss (studies have found both) and I suspect that any effect is due to alterations in dieter's total calorie intake. So long as calories are being controlled or restricted, I doubt there is any major effect. I would note that eating large amounts of calories may be detrimental to health although this might simply be due to people eating more calories total and gaining fat (8).

In the Western world, it is far more common for people to eat a relatively small breakfast, larger lunch and dinner the largest meal of the day. This tends to be related to social and lifestyle factors (i.e. morning is busy, lunch is eaten at work and dinner is eaten at home) but there are many good reasons to structure the day's eating this way when dieting. One is that it allows proportionally more calories to be eaten in the evening when most social or family situations (often involving food) occur. For women who are training intensely and train in the evening, putting proportionally more calories at this time tends to improve recovery and performance. Perhaps the most valuable reason to put more calories in the evening (moreso for smaller Category 1 dieters) is related to hunger and most people's work schedules. Many, if not most, work during the day and find that their hunger is reasonably well controlled due to being busy or at least distracted from eating. Similarly, most people are at home in the evenings when they are inactive, bored and surrounded by food which can make adherence to a fat loss diet more difficult. This pattern will not hold for women who work at night or perform shift work (which is its own complication). In this situation, moving even a few hundred calories from earlier to later in the day can help enormously with hunger and appetite control. For women with families, it may also help them to avoid having to cook multiple dinners since they are able to eat more total food. This can be combined with flexible eating strategies and allow for social events to be included on a limited basis while still adhering to the diet.

While the reduction in calories can technically come from any nutrient, it would be most common to move carbohydrates to later in the day leaving protein, fat and fiber for earlier meals. The extra carbohydrates eaten at night often help with sleep (by raising serotonin levels) which is often disturbed while dieting. If training is being done in the evening, this allows those carbohydrates to fuel the training. This strategy generates an overall dietary pattern where the earlier meals of the day tend to be based around protein, fat and fiber while the evening meals contain all four macronutrients. At the extremes, some dieters will save nearly all of their starchy carbohydrates until bedtime eating only protein, dietary fat and fibrous carbohydrates earlier in the day. Given their tendency to have some problems with blood sugar (especially during the luteal phase), women may benefit from consuming perhaps a half piece of fruit (12.5 grams of carbohydrates) with each of their earlier meals. This will stabilize blood sugar levels while leaving plenty of dietary carbohydrates for later in the day.

Women who train in the mornings or at lunch-time will have more difficulty applying this type of strategy since at least some dietary carbohydrates would need to be placed around the workout, limiting how many can be moved to the evening hours. Athletes training twice a day may also have problems unless their morning or lunch workout is of relatively lower intensity. It's more than possible to do an easy aerobic workout in the morning without needing to consume carbohydrates afterwards and this will allow the day's carbs to be targeted around the important training sessions. Since athletes are typically eating more calories and carbohydrates to begin with, the above is less of an issue to begin with.

For the postmenopausal woman, eating relatively more calories, and more specifically protein, later in the evening may have an added benefit of helping to stave off age-related muscle loss. Aging causes muscle to become insensitive to the tissue building effects of dietary protein and putting up to 70% of the day's total protein in the evening meal has been shown to overcome this resistance (9). If resistance training is performed in the evening, the effect should be even better. This does not benefit younger women for whom a more even distribution of protein is superior.

Skipping Breakfast

Taking the above approach to an even further extreme is the idea of skipping breakfast completely. This idea will probably come as a surprise given some of the ideas that exist regarding the importance of breakfast so let me address those briefly. I discussed above how the idea that breakfast stokes the metabolism or that skipping a meal slows metabolism is incorrect. Skipping breakfast does appear to be a common behavior in overweight individuals which has led many to conclude that doing so causes weight gain but it's more likely that people start skipping breakfast after they have gained weight (just as many start using diet products after they gain weight) rather than it causing the weight gain in the first place.

Skipping breakfast often causes people to eat more later in the day but this still tends to reduce their total daily food intake (10). If someone skips a 500 calorie breakfast and that causes them to eat 200 more calories later in the day, they have still eaten 300 less total calories overall. Even the claim that skipping breakfast hurts mental performance is questionable. It certainly appears to be true in children in terms of school work but for adults, it's more a matter of people's normal eating habits. When people who normally eat breakfast skip it, their mental performance suffers but the opposite is also true: people who typically skip breakfast have their mental performance suffer if they do eat (11).

Just as reducing the size of meals earlier in the day allows for more calories to be eaten later in the day, eliminating breakfast entirely does the same on a larger scale as the several hundred or more calories that might have been eaten then can be moved to later in the day or the evening times/around workouts. This doesn't really work for women who train first thing in the morning but even lunchtime workouts can be preceded by a small snack if needed and this will still save calories for later in the evening to help deal with hunger and the other issues I addressed above. I'd note that it can take a few days to adapt to skipping breakfast and many find that gradually decreasing the size of breakfast over several days works better.

Intermittent Fasting (IF)

The above can be taken even further by skipping breakfast as well as lunch and waiting until later in the day to start eating at all. This type of approach, currently popular in at least some subcultures, is usually called Intermittent Fasting or IF'ing. The basic idea is that fasting for more extended periods or only allowing food to be consumed during certain periods of the day or week (also called time restricted feeding or TRF) may have a number of health and other benefits (12). IF'ing can actually describe to a number of different eating patterns but here I'm focusing on individual days of eating.

Early studies on IF'ing compared one large meal per day to multiple smaller meals and the single meal approach was at least as good if not superior to the multiple meal approach. At least one study found a small fat loss in the single meal group which should demonstrate how wrong the ideas of skipping meals and starvation mode are. While a single meal IF approach may be appropriate for women who are not training or not training intensely, it requires modification for female athletes or the serious trainee.

For athletic purposes IF'ing is typically modified to include 3-4 meals clustered around training with a fasting period of 14-16 hours and an "eating window" of 8-10 hours. If someone ate their final meal at 8-10pm, this would mean waiting to break the fast until roughly 12-2pm. For an evening workout, a small snack might be eaten at this time with around workout nutrition potentially being included. A larger post-workout meal is eaten with one or two more meals eaten before bedtime. Probably the most well known approach to this type of athletic IF'ing is Martin Berkhan's Leangains approach which combines IF'ing with resistance training. Unfortunately, very little direct research on IF'ing for athletes has been done. Most of what does exist is on athletes who observe Ramadan, a religious fast where food and water are only allowed before sunrise and after sunset. Here, outside of some issues related to dehydration, performance has not been found to be compromised (13). Two recent studies, both in men, have also examined this approach with the second suggesting that the IF'ing pattern might be superior for fat loss (14,15).

Athletic IF patterns tend to work best with evening workouts for people training only once per day. It is less effective for morning or lunch workouts since food intake is ideally clustered around training, eliminating the potential benefits of eating more food in the evening. Performance athletes training twice daily can have problems with IF'ing unless their morning workouts are fairly low intensity and can be performed without needing carbohydrates before, during or after. An easy aerobic, technical or even low volume weight training workout could be done in the morning fasted with the higher intensity workout done in the evening when eating has resumed to support it nutritionally.

While I will address the issue of IF'ing for women below, I'd mention here that Martin has found that some women experience low blood sugar with the full 16 hour fast and are better off starting with a 14 hour fast instead. If the previous day's final meal is at 8-10pm, this means that regular eating should resume between 10 am and 12 pm (only breakfast is skipped). Fruit at the first meal helps with blood sugar levels and this is likely to be even more important during the luteal phase. The meal needn't be large and a small meal/snack at 5pm would be eaten for an evening workout followed by a post-workout and dinner meal. A bedtime snack containing at least protein (but which can include other nutrients as well) can help to stave off middle of the night hunger. True fasting does cause problems for some people and a small protein meal early in the day can help to maintain energy and blood glucose.

Summarizing Daily Meal Patterning

I want to finish this section by looking at the major patterns I've described side by side including an even distribution (with no workout), even distribution with post-workout and bedtime snack, skewed evening distribution and athletic IF'ing approach. I'll use the sample diet of 2000 calories with the follicular phase diet of 140 grams of protein, 235 grams of carbohydrate and 56 grams of fat per day and assume meals at 7-8am, 12-1pm, 4-5pm, a 6pm workout, post-workout meal, 8pm meal and pre-bed snack.

	7-8am	12pm-1pm	2pm	4-5pm	6pm WO	7pm Post WO	8:30pm	10:30pm
Even	500 35/58/14	500 35/58/14		500 35/58/14		None	500 35/58/14	
Post WO	400 22/46/14	400 22/46/14		400 22/46/14		200 25/25/0	400 22/46/14	200 25/25/0
Evening		230 20/20/8	240 20/20/9	240 20/20/9		350 25/50/5	600 30/75/20	350 25/50/5
IF'ing		240 20/20/9		240 20/20/9		350 25/50/5	840 50/95/28	350 25/50/5

The meal notation is calories and then grams of protein, carbohydrates and fats.

At 2000 calories per day, the differences in patterning aren't very large since each of the day's meals can be be reasonably sized. As calories decrease, uneven distributions become far more beneficial.

Weekly Calorie Patterning

In addition to daily meal patterning, there is the issue of weekly calorie distribution. As with daily calorie distribution, an enormous number of patterns are possible or have been used successfully but there is no singularly appropriate pattern for all situations with training, goals, etc. determining what is best.

Even Calorie Distribution

An even weekly calorie distribution is exactly what it sounds like which is that every day has roughly the same number of calories and nutrient intake levels. It is unlikely to be exact from day to day outside of some of the more obsessive/detail athletic populations but, at least within a general range, calorie and nutrient intakes are not being systematically varied. While calories can technically be set at, above or below maintenance, an even distribution tends to only be appropriate when the day's daily activities are very similar. Depending on the training being done, this may or may not be the case.

Uneven Calorie Distributions

As with daily meal patterns uneven calorie distributions can include alternations in calories or nutrient intake levels although these tend to go hand in hand. If one of the macronutrients is increased or decreased, caloric intake will change accordingly, unless another is changed as well. With no exception I can think of, protein intake should never change unless it is being increased slightly and this means that any changes will occur through carbohydrate and/or fat intake. In the real world, most people end up having an uneven calorie distribution naturally, usually eating more on the weekends than during the work-week. Here I am going to focus on more structured/deliberate approaches to uneven weekly calorie distributions. The research here has invariably been done on dieting in overweight or obese individuals and I will focus on that first to define some terms before addressing some of the modifications that can or should be made for athletes/serious trainees or when goals other than fat loss are desired.

Intermittent Caloric Restriction, Alternate Day Fasting and Cyclical Dieting

Intermittent Caloric Restriction (ICR) is a catch-all term that exists somewhat under the heading of IF'ing. In the most general sense ICR refers to any approach that alternates ~1-4 diet (sometimes more) or "fasting" days with 1-2 days of relatively normal eating days. The word fasting is a bit misleading as the studies typically provide 25% of maintenance calories (i.e. a 75% deficit) in a single meal on the fasting days. The normal eating days are done without restriction, often called ad-libitum (or ad-lib) eating with most eating anywhere from maintenance or slightly more to 5-20% below maintenance (15a). ICR patterns can be contrasted to typical caloric restriction (CR) where calories are reduced every day of the week.

While the data on is only now starting to accumulate, ICR is at least as good and may be superior to straight calorie restriction in terms of sparing lean body mass (LBM) , improving dietary adherence and limiting the hormonal and metabolic adaptations to dieting (16). Intriguingly, ICR also generates the same or even superior fat losses compared to traditional CR due to the enormous deficit created by the fasting days. And ICR does this while potentially being less stressful psychologically and physiologically.

Although ICR is more of a general term, there are specific patterns that have been studied and which may be worth considering for non-athlete Category 2/3 dieters. One is called Alternate Day Fasting (ADF) which alternates fasting with ad-lib eating on a day-to-day basis and which generates 4 fasting and 3 ad-lib eating days across a 7 day week. This could be switched to 4 straight fasting days followed by 3 ad-lib days which will generate the same enormous deficit while allowing the weekends (when most people eat more and have social obligations) to be higher in calories. This is sometimes called cyclical dieting.

Longer fasting periods are possible and one study compared 11 days of fasting followed by 3 days of ad-lib eating with 14 days of straight CR (17). The ICR subjects actually lost more fat (while reporting less hunger) and their resting metabolic rate decreased less than the CR group. Another used only 2 days of fasting per week followed by 5 days of normal eating and both weight and fat loss still occurred (18). This approach would allow the general dieter to gradually lose fat while still eating normally most of the week.

Fundamentally, ICR looks very much like the refeed/moving to maintenance concept I described in Chapter 21 and readers may recall that my comment that refeeds per se might not be appropriate in the early stages of dieting. This is actually contradicted by the ICR studies and I think the difference is that the dieters in the ICR studies aren't deliberately trying to raise calories but simply eating normally on the ad-lib days. I've compared straight CR at a 40% daily deficit to various ICR patterns below.

	Mon	Tue	Wed	Thu	Fri	Sat	Sun	Avg. Deficit
CR	40%	40%	40%	40%	40%	40%	40%	40%
ICR	Fast	Fast	Maint.	Fast	Fast	Maint.	Maint.	38-43%
ADF	Fast	Maint.	Fast	Maint.	Fast	Maint.	Fast	38-43%
Cyclical (2/5)	Fast	Fast	Maint.	Maint.	Maint.	Maint.	Maint.	15-21%
Cyclical (4/3)	Fast	Fast	Fast	Fast	Maint.	Maint.	Maint.	38-43%
Cyclical (5/2)	Fast	Fast	Fast	Fast	Fast	Maint.	Maint.	46-53%

*Fast is fasting at 25% of maintenance calories. Maint is maintenance or 10% above.

I've shown a range of deficits for the ICR pattern and the actual number depends on whether or not the ad-lib day is at maintenance (larger number) or 10% above (lower number). With the exception of the 2/5 pattern, which still generates a weekly deficit that will cause slower fat loss over time, all of the ICR patterns generate the same or larger deficits than straight CR. The cyclical 5/2 pattern generates a much larger total deficit and an 11/3 pattern (not shown) would generate a deficit of 56-60% below maintenance for that time period, generating significant fat loss. As importantly, the ICR patterns achieve this with fewer total (albeit harder) dieting days which can mean less stress, better adherence and all of the benefits I discussed in the chapter on Flexible Eating Strategies. To be honest, and I say this as someone who has written about this type of approach for many years, I see ICR approaches as the future of dieting for fat loss in general public. Even for long-term weight maintenance ICR may have benefits in that the occasional "fasting" day can be inserted if the individual is starting to backslide and regain the lost weight/fat.

ICR/Calorie Cycling for the Athlete and Serious Trainee

While the idea of ICR, ADF and cyclical dieting are relatively new to the realm of general weight loss, similar approaches have been used by athletes in one form or another for years. In the physique community, they are generally referred to as as Calorie or Carbohydrate Cycling, the latter term referring to the fact that it is most often carbohydrates that are being varied on a day-to-day basis. Since dietary protein and fat intake typically doesn't change, this has the effect of varying calories as well. A variety of patterns have been used and I will use the terminology of Calorie Cycling as the equivalent of ICR, Every Other Day (EOD) refeeds as the equivalent of ADF and Cyclical Dieting will still be called Cyclical Dieting.

With the exception of the IF'ing and Ramadan studies I mentioned above, almost no research has been done on ICR or calorie cycling patterns in athletes. Despite this, there is interest in the ability of these types of approaches for athletes as they might help them to maintain a lowered body weight (especially important for weight class athletes) or body fat percentage (BF%), to lose fat while maintaining performance or avoid fat gain while improving performance or increasing muscle mass (19). Women derive the added benefits of reducing hormonal and menstrual cycle disruption while dieting.

To be useable by athletes, ICR patterns must be modified in several ways. The first is related to the actual calorie intakes and there are several issues here. While ICR patterns for general weight loss uses only two calorie levels athletes will be setting at least three different calorie levels which are below, at and above maintenance (I say at least as there may be situations where more than one below maintenance level is set or used). Added to this is the fact that many athletes may have a daily maintenance level that changes significantly throughout the week. As I described in Chapter 16 and 17, this can vary by sport. Physique and other strength/power athletes have training days that are more alike than different (with non-training days simply being off days) while other types of sports can have much more variability from day to day. A cyclist spinning easily for an hour may burn a few hundred calories during training while a 4 hour hard ride with HIIT may burn 1500 or more calories easily.

Related to this is the actual structure of the ICR pattern which is used and there are two issues here. The first is the number of below, at or above maintenance days that are used per week and this depends on whether fat loss or muscle/fitness gain is the primary goal (I will look at each separately below). The second is how the days are distributed throughout the week. For the general dieter, how many fasting or normal eating days are used per week or where they fall during the week is mostly an issue of preference and convenience. In contrast, athletes must set the number of days at any given calorie level along with their distribution throughout the week to support their training, recovery and adaptation while still allowing them to reach their body composition goals. For optimal results, variations in calorie and carbohydrate intake should be synchronized with the athlete's training structure and goals for optimal results. The primary factor here is the number of high-intensity workouts per week and this varies from sport to sport. For that reason, none of the three patterns listed above will be appropriate in all situations.

Calorie Cycling for Muscle, Strength/Power and Fitness Gains

Since it is relative simpler (primarily in terms of the different calorie levels), I want to first address how ICR might be used to gain muscle mass, increase strength/power or improve other aspects of fitness while limiting fat gains. The overarching goal here is to create a calorie surplus where it is needed (i.e. around primary workouts) while keeping the overall calorie level of the week close to maintenance (or even very slightly below) to avoid excessive fat gain. In general, only three distinct calorie levels will need to be set when ICR is being used for this goal. The first is maintenance which should be equal to the day's Total Daily EnergyExpenditure (TDEE). The second is above maintenance which should never be more than 10% (15% for women with PCOS/subclinical hyperandrogenism) above maintenance or ~ 200-300 calories in most situations. The final intake level is below maintenance which will generally be no more than 10-20% below maintenance with one exception.

It's important to realize that adaptation to training is a continuous process and that, regardless of any benefits on body composition, reducing calories too much in the days after an important workout can impair the athlete's progress. Not only should the calorie reduction never too be too large but, ideally, should not come on the day after a high intensity or important training day. For the sample dieter, her maintenance level will be 2370 calories (matching her TDEE). On below maintenance days, a 10-20% deficit would be 230-460 calories giving her a goal range of 1900-2100 cal/day with the calorie reductions coming from meals not around the workout. On the above maintenance days, 10-15% would be 230-360 calories per day giving her a target range of 2600-2700 cal/day. Calories on the above maintenance days should be added around the workout itself, either pre-, during- or post-workout.

How many days at each calorie level will depend on the specifics of the athlete's training and the primary factor is the number of primary or key workouts (defined here as those workouts meant to improve the target fitness goal). First let me look at the situation where only two key workouts per week are done and an ICR pattern would be appropriate. This is common for endurance sports where one long workout and one quality interval workout might be done per week. These are typically spread out (i.e. Wednesday and Saturday) across the week although they might be done on two consecutive days (i.e. on weekends when more time is available). Some high-intensity performance sports or team/mixed sports might also follow this pattern as well. In all of these situations, the high calorie days would be placed on the training days with 2 below maintenance days and the rest of the days of the week at maintenance.

	Mon	Tue	Wed	Thu	Fri	Sat	Sun
Pattern 1	O -10%	L+Ma	H+10%	M+Ma	L-10%	H+10%	L+Ma
Pattern 2	L+M	L-10%	M-10%	O+Ma	L-10%	H+10%	H+10%

O = Off, L = Low Intensity Training, M = Moderate Intensity Training,
H= High Intensity Training, Ma = Maintenance calories

Both cycles are set up around two high intensity training days, spread apart in Pattern 1 and back-to-back in Pattern 2 with a mixture of low- and medium-intensity workouts and one off day per week. The primary training days are matched with above maintenance calorie intakes while both below maintenance days come two days after primary workouts so as not to interfere with recovery and adaptation.

In many situations, typically high-intensity performance athletes and some strength/power athletes it's more common to have three high-intensity training sessions per week, almost universally on alternating days per week. It's not unheard of for serious recreational trainees or physique athletes to only train three times per week but it seems fairly uncommon for most. In most cases, at least four days per week of training would be done with each workout being at a fairly high-intensity. The same holds true for many strength/power athletes, especially powerlifters and strongmen although some Olympic lifters train almost daily. In all of these cases, an EOD approach to calorie cycling tends to be most appropriate and I've shown some potential schedules below. Only high-intensity training days are shown.

	Mon	Tue	Wed	Thu	Fri	Sat	Sun
3-Day EOD	H+10%	-10%	H+10%	-10%	H+10%	-10%	M to -20%
4-Day EOD	H+10%	-10%	H+10%	-10%	H+10%	H+10%	M to -20%

H = High-Intensity Training

Both examples should be fairly self-explanatory with higher calorie intakes being used on the training days, below maintenance calorie intakes being used on the non-training or recovery days and Sunday being anywhere from maintenance to 20% below. As there is no way to avoid having a lowered calorie day following a training day the deficit must be moderate on those days. This type of approach, while conceptually interesting, can limit gains for some athletes and they may be better off simply alternating longer gaining phases (accepting some fat gain) alternated with short dieting periods. Another potential approach is presented below.

	Mon	Tue	Wed	Thu	Fri	Sat	Sun
3-Day EOD	H+10%	M	H+10%	M	H+10%	M	-30-50%
4-Day EOD	H+10%	H+10%	M	H+10%	H+10%	M	-30-50%
5-Day Cycle	H+10%	H+10%	H+10%	H+10%	H+10%	M	-30-50%

H = High-Intensity Training, M= Maintenance Calories to +10%

In all three cycles, calories are set above maintenance on the primary training days and at maintenance or at a slight surplus (to further facilitate recovery) on the non-training days with one exception. That exception is on Sunday where a fairly aggressive deficit could be used after a day off from training to offset the previous week's surplus. In this case anywhere from a 30-50% deficit could be used which would be 700-1175 calories below maintenance for the sample dieter. This would leave the dieter eating mostly protein, vegetables with perhaps a bit of fruit but this will offset fat gain without harming recovery.

Conceptually at least, cyclical dieting could be used for muscle, strength/power or fitness gains with limited fat gains. Generally one of two approaches have been used although I can't say that either were really used to any significant degree. The first was to keep calories slightly below maintenance during the week with higher calories on the weekends in conjunction with serious training. While workable, this limits the amount of quality training which can be done every week. The second alternated 5 days of above maintenance calories with two days below maintenance and was generally called reverse cyclical dieting. The problem here is that reducing calories on the day after a primary training day will impair adaptation and progress to that training which is sub-optimal. For this reason, I would recommend using either the ICR or EOD/ADF types of approaches discussed above for this goal.

Calorie Cycling for Fat Loss

As has been the case throughout this book, fat loss tends to be a more common goal, has more issues to address and I will spend proportionally more time discussing it. The goal here is to effectively lose fat for either performance or appearance reasons while preventing LBM or performance loss. This is in addition to the potentially more important issues of avoiding or at least limiting the negative hormonal effects along with the potential menstrual cycle dysfunction that can occur. The basic strategy, as I've described in various chapters of this book, is to create a sufficient weekly deficit to generate fat loss while increasing calories to maintenance or slightly higher (in the case of refeeds) with some frequency based on factors such as the weekly training structure, diet Category and goal BF%.

The primary difference between Calorie Cycling for fitness gains and fat loss is in how the calorie levels will be set up. Maintenance will always be that day's maintenance (in some cases this can vary significantly from day to day) while above maintenance days, if used, will be no more than 10% above. It's when the below maintenance calorie days are set that the differences show up. Recall from Chapter 17 that fat loss calorie levels can be set by percentage (i.e. small, medium, large deficits) or by goal weekly weight loss although both more or less create the same deficit. So assume that the sample dieter at 150 lbs is targeting a 1% weekly weight loss at the start of her diet. This is 1.5 pounds per week and at an estimated 3,500 calories per pound, she needs a total weekly deficit of 5250 calories per week or 750 calories per day. If she were using an even calorie distribution she would create the deficit every day of the week.

With an ICR/Calorie Cycling approach, she will instead divide that weekly deficit across the number of active dieting days. In the chart below I've shown how this works based on a maintenance calorie level of 2350, the weekly deficit and anywhere from 6 dieting days and 1 maintenance day to 4 diet days and 3 maintenance days. The daily deficit is calculated by dividing the weekly deficit by the number of diet days and I've shown the percentage deficit that will occur on the diet days. For reasons I will explain below, I've also shown the same for a goal of 0.5% per week and 140 pounds (0.7 lbs and a weekly deficit of 2450 calories). The numbers in the chart are unrelated to how those days are scheduled within the week.

	1% Weekly Weight Loss					0.5% Weekly Weight Loss				
Maint	Weekly	Diet	Maint	Daily	%	Weekly	Diet	Maint	Daily	%
2350	5250	6	1	875	37%	2450	6	1	400	17%
2350	5250	5	2	1050	45%	2450	5	2	490	21%
2350	5250	4	4	1300	55%	2450	3	4	800	35%

Maint is daily maintenance, Weekly is the weekly deficit, Daily is the daily deficit, Maint and Diet are the number of each per week and % is the percentage reduction from maintenance

You can see that as the number of total dieting days decreases, the size of the daily deficit in both absolute and percentage terms goes up fairly significantly. For a 1% weekly weight loss goal, the required daily deficit goes up from 875 calories and a 35% reduction with 6 dieting days up to 1300 calories and a 55% reduction when there are only 4 diet days. Attempting to have less than 4 diet days per week leads to unrealistic or impossible approaches which is why I have not shown them. If four days at maintenance were attempted, a 75% daily deficit would be required and just to make the point, if only 2 days of active dieting were used, the required daily deficit would be 2600 calories, exceeding the dieter's daily maintenance (this would entail eating almost nothing and doing hours per day of exercise). For slower fat loss rates (i.e. 0.5% per week), four days at maintenance might be workable since the required deficit is smaller but I will only consider weeks with a maximum of 3 days at maintenance going forwards.

As shown above, even three days per week at maintenance can result in fairly large daily deficits but this is offset by at least two factors. The first is that fewer maintenance days are generally needed earlier in the diet when the weekly deficit tends to be largest, lessening the daily deficit on the diet days. This isn't universal and I will present weekly patterns containing 1,2 and 3 maintenance days per week below. Related to this is the fact that dieters are usually targeting a slower rate of weekly weight loss by the time they are using a larger number of maintenance days and this is shown in the right half of the chart. If our sample dieter is only targeting 0.5% weekly weight loss late in the diet, her total weekly deficit has dropped to only 2450 calories and her daily deficits in both absolute and relative terms has dropped enormously as well. Even with three days at maintenance, the required daily deficits are not insurmountably large.

The number of maintenance days used per week (1-3 as described above) will depend on a number of factors. The number of high-intensity workouts per week is a primary one with more workouts requiring more days at maintenance to support them. The dieter's category plays a major role and the number of days at maintenance will increase as a dieter moves from Category 3 to 2 to 1. Goal BF% is a critical player and the more extreme a level of low BF% is being sought, the more days at maintenance will be required to offset the negative hormonal changes. This is especially true as the diet length increases and the number of days at maintenance will actually be increasing later in the diet. As I mentioned in Chapter 21, this runs counter to the prevailing idea that a diet must become more extreme as the diet progresses but it is late in the diet when the body's adaptations are at their greatest, meaning more days at maintenance are required.

I'm going to look at Calorie Cycling for fat loss a little bit differently than I did for muscular and other fitness gains. Primarily I want to make a distinction between dieting performance athletes and those involved in the physique sports since their needs are somewhat different. Primarily this revolves around the need for the performance athlete to maintain performance in their sport which, strictly speaking, isn't the goal of the physique competitor (maintaining performance is, at most, important for avoiding LBM loss). Along with this are differences in the nature of training being done. Performance athletes are, as often as not training the same muscle groups in their key workouts while physique competitors most commonly train different muscles groups on different days. The physique competitor is usually trying to reach the lower limits of BF% while the performance athlete may or may not be. First let me look at the issue of calorie cycling for performance athletes and how 1,2 and 3 days at maintenance might be used.

1 Day at Maintenance Per Week
Let me look first at diet cycles with only one day per week at maintenance. Since this diet structure allows for the most dieting days, the deficit on any of those days will be smaller as per the chart above which means that even athletes with more than one high-intensity training day per week should be able to use it. As well, performing the other high-intensity days with lowered daily carbohydrate intake will lower muscle glycogen which, recall from Chapter 14 enhances fat loss in women. As well, with only one day per week at maintenance, that day can technically fall on any day of the week although it would be most common to place it either on or the day before the most important workout of the week. There are pros and cons to both approaches.

Recovery and adaptation tends to be optimized by slightly having higher calories on the training day but performance may not be optimal. The athlete will typically be performing the workout with at least somewhat lowered carbohydrates stores which, depending on the workout being done, could cause problems (i.e. decreased performance or early fatigue). Having 1-2 normal carbohydrate meals prior to the workout can offset this and would be recommended for most athletes as fasted training on a background of lowered glycogen tends to invariably harm performance unless exercise intensity is low (i.e. if only a low intensity aerobic workout is being done, doing it fasted may burn additional fat for energy). If the workout is longer than an hour, and this should only be the case for endurance athletes, carbohydrate consumption would begin after the first hour and would continue or the rest of the day.

This may not work for all athletes, some report getting somewhat sleepy when they raise carbohydrates while dieting and eating at maintenance the day before a primary workout may be ideal to ensure adequate glycogen stored might be the most appropriate choice. The increase in calories should come after a light workout to enhance muscle glycogen storage and this tends to support performance during the next workout to the greatest degree. Since maintenance of performance tends to be the primary goal during dieting, this is an option worth considering. I've shown the two different 1-day cycles below. I've arbitrarily placed the primary training day on Saturday but it may fall anywhere in the week. Only that workout is indicated and other days may include training or be days-off depending on the week's structure.

	Mon	Tue	Wed	Thu	Fri	Sat	Sun
Option 1	Diet	Diet	Diet	Diet	Diet	T+M	Diet
Option 2	Diet	Diet	Diet	Diet	L+M	T+D	Diet

T= Primary Workout, L = Light workout, M = maintenance, D = diet day

There's not much more to be said about the above cycle except that, while it can be effective in many situations, it may be unable to support the training of athletes with multiple high-intensity workouts per week. Later in an extreme diet, 1 day at maintenance will also not be sufficient to reverse any hormonal or menstrual cycle disruptions. In both cases, the next approaches will be required.

2 Days at Maintenance Per Week

In the situation where 1 day per week at maintenance is not sufficient to maintain performance or limit hormonal adaptations, a second day of maintenance per week will be required . This does reduce the number of dieting days to 5 which increases the necessary daily deficit on each of those days which may or may not be a problem depending on the target weight/fat loss. This will depend on the individual dieter and whether or not their training or exercise performance suffers.

With this cycle, there are two options for how the days can be distributed. The first would be to put them on sequential days and this is nothing more than a cyclical diet where 5 days of dieting are alternated with 2 days at maintenance. This can be a good approach for the athlete who occasionally performs two primary workouts back-to-back and there are two ways to integrate the maintenance days with training. The first would be to put both maintenance days on the training days to support recovery for both. This may compromise performance during the first training session and the first maintenance day could also be on the day before with the second day falling on the first workout day (fueling the second).

Probably the more common way to apply this cycle would be to have the two days at maintenance spread throughout the week as it's more common for most athletes to have their primary workouts spread out in this fashion. This tends to work best when there are two primary workouts per week and a strength/power athlete (i.e. powerlifter with two heavier and two lighter days per week) or sprint type athlete (who might do speed work on Monday/Friday) could use this pattern successfully. Here again, the maintenance days could be placed on or before the primary training day depending on whether the goal is optimal performance or optimal recovery and adaptation. I've shown the some sample patterns below, again focusing only on the primary training days and days at maintenance. Other training days are low-intensity/off and all non-maintenance days are indicated only as diet.

	Mon	Tue	Wed	Thu	Fri	Sat	Sun
Back to Back Option 1	Diet	Diet	Diet	Diet	Diet	T+M	T+M
Back to Back Option 2	Diet	Diet	Diet	Diet	L+M	T+M	Diet
Back to Back Option 3	Diet	Diet	Diet	Diet	L+M	T+M	T+Diet
Spread Pattern Option 1	Diet	Diet	T+M	Diet	Diet	T+M	Diet
Spread Pattern Option 3	Diet	L+M	T+Diet	Diet	L+M	T+Diet	Diet

T= Primary Workout, L = Light workout, M = maintenance, D = diet day

Weekly structures with two maintenance days per week can cover a fairly large number of training situations but there may still be some where the amount of high-intensity training being done cannot be supported or hormonal/menstrual cycle problems are occurring and a third maintenance day is needed.

3 Days at Maintenance Per Week

In the situation where two days at maintenance per week are insufficient, a third day at maintenance may be necessary to support training or avoid hormonal problems. As I showed above, potentially the largest drawback here is that the daily deficit will go up further as there are only 4 dieting days per week. If a 1% weekly weight loss rate or higher is being targeted, this may make those days little more than lean protein, vegetables, essential fats and a small amount of fruit due to the significantly lowered calorie intake. This is certainly possible for some athletes, especially since it is only done four days per week. If a slower weekly rate of weight loss is targeted (or acceptable), much of this problem will be avoided.

There are three primary weekly patterns that can be used when 3 days of maintenance eating are being included. The first would be to have a single maintenance day during the week along with two maintenance days back-to-back (I'll call this a 1+2 pattern). This has the same potential benefits as above in terms of the back-to-back days and the third day can support another high intensity workout earlier in the week. An endurance athlete doing one HIIT workout and one or two longer workouts on the weekend might use an approach like this. A second pattern would be to have the higher calorie days alternate with diet days throughout the week. This generates an EOD approach identical to the one described when I talked about fitness gains although the daily calories levels are different. This tends to be most appropriate for athletes who have three high-intensity training days spread throughout the week alternated with lower intensity training days. All three days could technically be placed consecutively although this would be somewhat uncommon. Athletes performing two hard workouts back to back might use this and could eat at maintenance the day before and on both two workout days supporting both performance and recovery.

	Mon	Tue	Wed	Thu	Fri	Sat	Sun
1+2 Pattern Option 1	Diet	Diet	T+M	Diet	Diet	T+M	T+M
1+2 Pattern Option 2	Diet	L+M	T+Diet	Diet	L+M	T+M	Diet
EOD Option 1	T+M	Diet	T+M	Diet	T+M	Diet	Diet
EOD Option 2	L+M	T+Diet	L+M	T+Diet	L+M	T+Diet	Diet
3 Days in a Row Option 1	Diet	Diet	Diet	Diet	L+M	T+M	T+M

T= Primary Workout, L = Light workout, M = Maintenance, D = Diet day

In a dieting situation, it would be nearly unheard of to either use or need more than three maintenance days per week and the above patterns should be able to meet the need of any potential athletic situation that might occur. Outside of the occasional sport, few athletes perform more than three high intensity workouts per week and this would almost never be done while dieting in the first place.

Calorie Cycling for Physique Athletes

Finally let me look at Calorie Cycling for physique athletes (much of this also applies to any Category 1 athlete dieting down to the extremes). As I mentioned above, the primary goal of the physique athlete is not performance per se but reaching the goal appearance in terms of BF% while maintaining LBM. I'd note that maintaining performance during weight training workouts is important from the standpoint of LBM maintenance but it's only secondary in that sense. Additionally, as I've mentioned throughout this book, the training of the physique competitor tends to be distinct from that of other sports in that different muscle groups in the body are trained in different workouts (this is in contrast to the fact that most sports train the same muscle groups at all workouts). The structure of the week may vary enormously between any two competitors depending on how they group the body parts and sequence them throughout the week as well. This makes the glycogen depletion that occurs with training much less of an issue. Only the highest volumes of training would cause this to occur but any workout that extensive wouldn't be repeated frequently to begin with. Finally, since they are usually attempting to reach the lower, if not lowest limits, of female BF%, the physique athlete faces far more negative adaptations in terms of hormonal changes, menstrual cycle dysfunction, energy expenditure, hunger and others than other athletes.

The practical implications of this is that how many days at maintenance are needed per week will primarily depend on where in the diet the competitor is with the number of days at maintenance increasing later in the diet when she is leaner. As I noted above, while this runs contrary to how most conceptualize dieting, it simply works better for all the reasons I've discussed throughout the book. In this situation, I recommend increasing the number of days at maintenance after every Diet Break and this will roughly correlate with the reductions in her BF% and the cutoff points I have provided below

	Initial BF%	Ending BF%	Min Days	Max Days
First block of dieting	24	18	1	3
Second block of dieting	18	14	2	3
Third block of dieting	14	10	3	3

Min Days = minimum days at maintenance, Max Days = maximum days at maintenance

You can see how the required frequency of maintenance days increases as the diet progresses and the athlete's BF% is decreasing (dieters who are not going below 14% body fat will not use the third block of dieting numbers). In the first block, following the recommendations in this book, the dieter should not cross the critical energy availability (EA) threshold to begin with and the inclusion of the day at maintenance is to refill muscle glycogen and offset the generally small negative hormonal responses. By the time she is at 18% and going lower, she will be approaching and might just cross the EA threshold at which point a full 2 days at maintenance will be needed. Realistically, by the time she is 14% or below, she will be below the critical EA threshold and three days at maintenance will be required.

In the chart, I've indicated both minimum and maximum days of maintenance in each block with the minimum number of days increasing with each active dieting block. But you will also see that it is possible to start with up to 3 days at maintenance from the outset of the diet and I want to look at the pros and cons of that approach. The primary con to using more days at maintenance from the outset of the diet is that individual dieting days will be harder in terms of the required calorie deficit to make the weekly goals. As I discussed above, this is offset by the fact that there are fewer diet days to begin with (i.e. 4 hard diet days might be tolerable in a way that 7 would not) and the increased number of days at maintenance. A slower rate of fat loss could also be targeted to keep the size of the deficits more reasonable but this will further increase dieting time. The primary pro to using a larger number of maintenance days per week from the outset is that such approaches potentially allow physique competitors with a weak muscle group to improve it while they are dieting. In general gaining muscle while losing fat is difficult (approaching impossible in well trained and lean individuals) but combining certain training structures with this cyclical calorie alternations makes it at least possible to gain small amounts of muscle.

This leads into a similar discussion of how the days at maintenance would be placed into the week. With a single day at maintenance, the maintenance day can fall anywhere in the week as needed. Friday or Saturday as common as this allows at least some potential for social interaction since the athlete can eat normally but it would be common to put it on or on the day before a particularly important workout. For example, if a physique athlete knows that they tend to lose size in a specific muscle group or two, the could place the maintenance day around that workout. The same comments hold for 2 days at maintenance and the days could be spread throughout the week (i.e. Tuesday/Friday or some similar spacing) as desired. Here a cyclical approach where the maintenance days are back to back might be considered to try to improve a weak muscle group. Here, the first maintenance day would be placed before the workout and the second on the day of as this would support both intensity and recovery for that training.

For the three days per week at maintenance, any of the three patterns described above would be potentially usable although putting at least two of the days back to back would give the most potential to bring up a weak point. In some cases, three days of above maintenance eating could be used with weak point muscle groups placed during the days at maintenance. My own Ultimate Diet 2.0 is structured very similarly to this with roughly 4 days of hard dieting alternated with 3 days above or near maintenance and a specific training structure that integrate with that pattern. While not a large number of women have used it, those that have often reach very low levels of BF% often without menstrual cycle disruption and while gaining small amounts of muscle. Although I did not plan it this way, UD2 it is probably more optimized to the needs of Category 1 women than it is to men (although it works for both). An EOD approach can also work well to maintain intensity during more workouts of the week along with never allowing more than 1-2 days of active dieting before potentially improving hormonal levels. As I discussed in Chapter 14, this this may help to avoid the normal hormonal adaptations (and anecdotally does just that).

To avoid needless repetition, I won't show all of the possible combinations of 1,2 and 3 days at maintenance diet structures and will only focus on those aimed at bringing up weak points. I would only recommend placing two muscle groups on these days, perhaps one larger and one smaller muscle group (i.e. glutes, biceps) as bringing up more muscle groups than this at once will be almost impossible.

	Mon	Tue	Wed	Thu	Fri	Sat	Sun
2 Days Option 1	Diet	Diet	Diet	Diet	M	WP+M	Diet
2 Days Option 2	Diet	Diet	Diet	Diet	Diet	WP+M	M
3 Days Option 1	Diet	Diet	T+M	Diet	M	WP+M	Diet
3 Days Option 2	Diet	Diet	T+M	Diet	Diet	WP+M	M
3 Days Option 3	Diet	Diet	Diet	Diet	M	WP+M	M

WP = Weak Point Muscle Group(s), M = Maintenance

While the above doesn't exhaust every possibility, you can see how calories can be increased to maintenance around those days to support both the training itself along with recovery and growth from that workout. Make no mistake that growth in these muscle groups will not be large and most of it is likely to occur earlier in the diet when BF% is relatively higher but for physique competitors. However, even small improvements in those weak points can make a difference on competition day.

Criticisms of IF'ing/ICR for Women

To wrap up this chapter, I want to examine a variety of criticisms regarding women and IF'ing (and here I am using the term to refer to both daily IF'ing along with the various types of intermittent caloric variations I discussed above). At least one popular article online has argued that IF'ing is somehow damaging to a woman's physiology with claims of increased anxiety, hair loss menstrual cycle dysfunction and other problems occurring (20). This seems to be based on anecdotal reports along with some misinterpretation of the admittedly limited research on humans. I'd refer interested readers to a well written analysis of some of those criticisms (21). Certainly there is limited research on women and IF'ing and, as with most obesity research, most of that is on overweight women Only a handful of studies have included normal weight women and I discussed earlier in the book that lean/Category 1 women are at a greater likelihood of menstrual cycle disruption than other women. But this is true of any lowered EA state and I'm see little reason why IF'ing would be specifically worse in this regard.

Given that most IF approaches use an alternation of calories with calorie increases to maintenance or above at some frequency, I might expect less of a problem overall due to the benefits of raised calories and carbohydrates on restoring hormonal status and function (and recall Eric Helm's anecdotal experience with ICR discussed above). There is extremely limited data in this regard with some of it coming from Ramadan fasting where a small percentage of women (20-30%) showed some form of menstrual cycle dysfunction (22). So it's possible that there is a percentage of women who are more at risk with this type of eating pattern. I do find it telling that the apparent anecdotal reports on the negative effects of IF'ing come from a paleo forum. Readers may recall that very low-carbohydrate intakes per se have the potential to cause menstrual cycle dysfunction in women and this is common with many paleo approaches.

I'd note that, in many cases, therapeutic fasting has been shown to have benefits for women. It may improve reproductive function (probably through weight loss) in PCOS women and can decrease symptoms of anxiety and depression while having positive effects on self-esteem and improving mood generally (23). As with so many issues specific to women, the potential positives or negatives of fasting/IF'ing is likely to be very situation specific (i.e. Cat 3 vs. Cat 1, active vs. inactive). That said, clearly any women who do show early negative responses with IF'ing types of approaches should move away from them but this comment could be made for any dietary approach or strategy and overall I find the above criticisms of IF'ing far from compelling.

That said, I do think there are some potential issues associated with IF'ing that often go unaddressed although these really apply to both women and men. One is that, for some people at least, IF'ing approaches cause more problems than they solve. Some dieters do find that fasting even most of the day causes them to lose control of their food intake when they do start eating and this causes them to exceed their daily calorie goals. IF'ing for fat loss only works if calories are controlled or monitored and many failures can be tracked to nothing more than people eating too much during their eating window. Starting the first meal with protein and fiber can help with this but it can still cause problems for some people. This seems more true for people who are attempting to limit themselves to a single meal and the day often turns into alternations between complete fasting and binge level eating. The same holds for weekly calorie variations especially the more extreme alterations where extremely low calories on one or more days are often more than offset by a loss of food control on the normal eating or carb loading days. Once again, if any given individual has problems in this regard, IF'ing is not the right approach for them.

This brings up the next potential problem with IF'ing patterns I want to address which is that, superficially at least, they often look like the starve/binge patterns seen in some types of Eating Disorders (ED's). It's been suggested that IF'ing might have not only adverse physiological effects but also the potential to increase the number (or severity) of ED's or body satisfaction although very little research has been done on this topic. In one study (using an ADF pattern) in overweight individuals, the reverse was found to be true; the subjects had no increase in symptoms of an ED and had no or a positive increase in body image (24). In contrast, an older study using an extreme ICR (4 days at 600 or less calories followed by 3 uncontrolled days) found increases in hunger with increasingly higher calorie intakes on the uncontrolled eating days along with psychological changes not dissimilar to what is seen in bulimia (25).

Of some interest, these were not restrained eaters/chronic dieters in the first place as you might expect and the extreme ICR approach still caused some fairly concerning changes. This is admittedly an extreme ICR approach in that the low-calorie days were very low and, anecdotally at least, women who use more moderate ICR approaches seem to avoid this. All of that said, I would generally not suggest ICR approaches for women with a pre-existing ED or who are in recovery. But even women who have not had previous problems should be aware of this potential issue. If ICR approaches start to become alternations of extreme calorie restriction and binge eating, a more standard dieting approach may be superior.

Some Final Comments about Meal Frequency and Patterning

While I have discussed different daily and weekly calorie patterning separately which may make it sound as if they are mutually exclusive, this is not the case. Not only can they be combined but there are often good reasons to do so. The major issue here, as discussed earlier in the chapter, is the interaction of meal frequency (and thus patterning) with calorie intake. When fewer calories are being eaten in a given day, a lower meal frequency is often beneficial to help maintain fulness. As well, using a skewed type of pattern where more calories are moved towards the evening (or a full-blown IF approach is used) can be beneficial. This also allows what carbohydrates are allowed on that day to be targeted around training if it is being done/being done in the evening.

In contrast, on higher calorie and carbohydrate days, a higher frequency and more spread meal pattern may be superior simply to keep the size of the meals smaller and more manageable without stomach upset. This is especially true when carb-loading protocols, which may involve intakes of 4.5-5-5.5 g/lb (10-12 g/kg) or higher of carbohydrate intake per 24 hours are being used and where consuming this in a few enormous meals is impractical. In any case where ICR approaches of any sort are being used, fewer/larger meals and/or an IF'ing approach might be used on the lower calorie days while more meals and a more spread pattern might be best on the higher calorie days. I've shown this below for ICR (2 split maintenance days), EOD and cyclical dieting patterns.

	ICR			EOD			Cyclical		
	Calories	# Meals	Pattern	Calories	# Meals	Pattern	Calories	# Meals	Pattern
Monday	Low	4	IF'ing	Low	4	If'ing	Low	4	IF'ing
Tuesday	Low	4	IF'ing	High	6	Even	Low	4	IF'ing
Wednesday	High	6	Even	Low	4	If'ing	Low	4	IF'ing
Thursday	Low	4	IF'ing	High	6	Even	Low	4	IF'ing
Friday	Low	4	IF'ing	Low	4	If'ing	Very High	8	Even
Saturday	High	6	Even	High	6	Even	Very High	8	Even
Sunday	Low	4	IF'ing	Low	4	If'ing	Maintenance	5	Even

There' is also absolutely no reason that the choice of meal frequency, patterning or weekly calorie patterning won't or can't change throughout the year when a trainee's goals change. Physique athletes tend to focus on muscle gain (while limiting fat gain) most of the year but will insert either short diets or full-blown competition diets as they prepare for competition. Calories will be higher during the gaining phase which may mean that a higher daily meal frequency and more spread pattern will be preferred. If some type of calorie cycling to limit fat gain is being used, lower calorie days may still benefit from lowered meal frequencies or different meal patterns or distributions. The same holds for other athletes and what is done in the general preparation phase when training is geared towards developing fitness will be different than what is done during the competition period when the focus is on competition performance. The athlete may have to introduce a specific phase to optimize body composition as well and I will address when this is best done in a later chapter.

264

Chapter 24: Supplements

Having examined the details of setting up an optimal diet in detail, I want to move into a discussion of dietary supplements. Some of what I will discuss will be of a fairly general nature and relatively gender non-specific but the majority of this chapter will be aimed at supplements that are specifically relevant to women or that may have differential effects in women. I'll first discuss general use supplements (applicable to most readers) with a detailed discussion of soy protein/phytoestrogens before looking at supplements specific to the luteal phase, amenorrhea, PCOS and menopause. I'll finish by looking at fat loss and performance related supplements. There will be some overlap in the sections as many products that are beneficial in one situation are also be relevant to another. To avoid repetition, I will generally discuss the supplement in detail the first time it is mentioned and then only refer to it briefly.

Introductory Comments about Supplements

The topic of dietary supplements is one often marked by extreme differences of opinion. On the one hand are those who feel that dietary supplements are required and the multi-billion dollar supplement industry markets endless products to different populations. Supplements aimed at the general public promise improved health or energy or the prevention of disease while those aimed at athletes are claimed to improve performance, strength, endurance or muscle size. New products promising fat loss arrive constantly with few delivering the promised results. At the opposite extreme is the occasionally voiced idea that all supplements are useless so long as a balanced diet is eaten or that supplements may harm health. Certainly in some cases the latter can be true: some supplements are problematic consumed in excess and dieters are notorious for taking double or triple the recommended dose which causes problems.

Claims are occasionally made that relatively innocuous supplements such as multi-vitamins are not only useless but may harm health. Correlational studies sometimes find this to be the case where supplement intake results in people having worse health or increased body weight. But just as the relationship with diet products and weight gain is reversed, I think this is too. A very common pattern is that when people take dietary supplements, they feel as "having covered their bases" they can eat whatever they want and do whatever they want lifestyle wise. The act of taking the pill causes them to give themselves free reign to not care about any other aspect of their diet and engage in poor eating and lifestyle habits (1). And it is the poor eating and lifestyle habits rather than the supplement that are the real problem. This has been seen with diet supplements, where people justify eating more food than they otherwise would when they take such supplements (2). The product either has no effect or the person actually gains weight due to their food intake overwhelming any (small) impact of the supplement.

While supplements have their place, the simple fact is that they can never make up for poor eating or activity patterns. No legal fat loss supplement will cause meaningful fat loss without a change in diet or activity patterns and no sports supplement can improve an athlete's performance without proper training and nutrition. At best supplements can add to the results of proper diet and exercise or help to address specific problems or issues but that's all. As their name suggests, they should supplement proper diet and activity patterns and nothing more. I'll finish by noting that supplements generally only have a benefit on health or performance when they are correcting a deficiency in the first place but this does not mean that taking more will have an additional effect. Excessive nutrient intake can cause problems and my recommendations are aimed at ensuring optimal/required levels but no more. There are also supplements that, while not correcting deficiencies, address issues that women (but not men) face.

Do Active Individuals Need Dietary Supplements?

A long running debate is whether or not athletes and serious trainees have increased vitmain and mineral (the micronutrients) requirements that may require dietary supplementation. As I discussed in Chapter 20, it's clear that exercise can cause the loss of some nutrients such as iron, zinc, magnesium and others and this will raise daily requirements for athletes. As I discussed, it's often argued that the increased food intake of athletes will easily cover this. This assumes that the athlete is eating enough and making food choices which provide the necessary nutrients in both sufficient amounts and from well-absorbed forms. As often as not neither of these is true. Females often chronically undereat (and this is exacerbated when dieting) and many make foods choices such as removing red (or all) meat or dairy products that limit the intake and absorption of iron, zinc and other critical nutrients. Even bodybuilders, often thought to represent the pinnacle of health and optimal nutrition, often show micronutrient deficiencies (2a,2b).

Regardless of any argument or theory, the reality is that people both in the general along with athletes and active individuals often show nutrient deficiencies with women being at a potentially greater risk for certain deficiencies due to their food choices and calorie intake. Zinc, iron, calcium, Vitamin D and magnesium are often far below optimum. This can cause issues with overall health, bone density and athletic performance as I discussed previously. Ideally, all of these nutrients would be obtained from a perfectly set up diet in the first place and this is the world that many mainstream nutritionists seem to live in. In the real world, this type of nutrient intake is rarely the case. Certainly the recommendations I made in Chapter 20 go a long way towards achieving this but there will be readers of this book who will not eat those foods on a regular basis. They may have no taste for certain food, can't afford those foods (red meat can be especially problematic) or are following as specific dietary approach such as a vegetarian/vegan diet that precludes eating those foods. In this case supplementation will be necessary as, without them, it will be nearly impossible for a woman to meet her nutritional requirements, especially when they are dieting.

While I feel that dietary supplements may be useful or in some cases required to correct a deficiency or meet daily requirements, it's critical to realize that the nutrients from food are absorbed more effectively than from isolated supplements. Invariably there are other nutrient or co-nutrients found in food that improve absorption and/or have additional health benefits. Recall that both red meat and chicken have a factor that improves iron absorption and dairy foods contain optimal amounts carbohydrates, protein, sodium and other nutrients that improve calcium absorption.

While this certainly points to an ideal situation being one where all nutrients are obtained from whole foods, this is still not always possible. And it also points to a compromise approach for those situations, such as when calories are restricted, when certain foods cannot be eaten in the necessary quantities. That approach is to combine the dietary supplement with a reduced amount of the whole food that would otherwise provide them. This allows calories to be controlled and reduced while providing the nutrients and co-factors that improve the absorption and utilization of the supplement (i.e. the food will improve absorption of the supplement). Rather than consuming 8-oz of dairy (providing 200-300 mg of calcium), a calcium supplement could be taken with 4-oz of dairy. An iron supplement could be taken with a reduced amount of red meat or chicken for the same reason.

General Use Supplements

All of the supplements I want to describe in this first section are simply for general use and/or health. They are meant to act as a nutritional insurance or to address known deficiencies that occur in women.

Multi-Vitamin/Mineral

Irrespective of whether they truly help or not, I consider a basic multi-vitamin/mineral to be worthwhile for both the general public or active individuals, simply to cover nutritional bases. As above, nobody eats a perfect diet all the time and for Category 3 dieters, there is some indication that there are nutrient deficiencies that occur with obesity (3). While these aren't a likely cause of fat gain directly, the number of processes that they may be involved in related to body weight regulation is profound (4). While unlikely to have a major impact, correcting these deficiencies can only help when at loss or improved health is the goal. As well, taking a multivitamin/mineral while dieting may prevent the normal weight-loss induced increase in hunger that occurs (4a).

While many will likely disagree, I generally don't see the need to spend massive amounts of money on higher end multi-vitamins. Certainly many basic multi-vitamins don't use the highest quality ingredients and the absorption may not be fantastic but this can be made up by taking more than one pill per day, split morning and evening with meals. As any supplement should be adding to the day's intake to begin with, I do not see the issue of absorption as being particularly relevant in most cases. I'd note that it's quite common to find multivitamin/mineral products with both a female and male version. Typically women's versions contain iron (generally absent in men's products) or other nutrients important to support women's health or pregnancy such as folic acid.

Since a pill can only be so large before it cannot be safely swallowed, there are many nutrients that women are often deficient in that cannot be put in a typical daily multi-vitamin/mineral product. Calcium is a prime example with many pills containing 200 mg or 1/5th or less of a woman's requirements. Vitamin D levels are often fairly low and well-below current recommendations to correct deficiencies. Others I will discuss next often have to be supplemented separately as well. A multi-vitamin should be taken with a meal as there are likely to be nutrients or other factors found in the food being eaten that will improve absorption. Some vitamins (A,D and K) are fat-soluble and are best absorbed with a fat containing meal.

Probiotics

In the last few years there has been real interest in what is called the gut microbiota, which refers to the bacteria found in the stomach. There are multiple types of bacteria some of which have beneficial and some of which have negative effects with the ratio of the good and bad bacteria playing an enormous role in almost all aspects of human health including obesity, diabetes, and many others (5). There is even recent interest in what is being called the gut-brain axis with the types of gut bacteria impacting on mental function and mental illness. I should state up front that this is a rapidly developing area of research and the full picture of what the optimal proportion or ratio of different types of bacteria is still being determined.

There is at least some indication that a certain "bad" ratio of bacteria (an increased ratio of firmicutes to bacteriotides) may increase the risk of obesity but it's hard to tell cause from effect here. It does appear that part of the ratio of good to bad bacteria is genetically determined but even 3 days of overeating can significantly worsen the ratio while even small amounts of weight loss improve this ratio. That said, an increased ratio of bad to good bacteria may be associated with obesity and metabolic diseases (5a). It's also been found that women have a different ratio than men with more of the bad bacteria and this may actually predispose women towards Irritable Bowel Syndrome (5b).

Outside of weight loss, there are ways to improve the overall ratio of good to bad bacteria. One is to ensure adequate amounts of what are called prebiotics, foods such as yogurt, higher fiber carbohydrates or even fermented foods such as kimchi or sauerkraut which are metabolized in such a way as to improve the microbiota. The dietary recommendations in this book should ensure their intake. Also recall from Chapter 21 that the intake of small amounts of dark chocolate may also have an effect. There are also preformed prboiotic supplements available. There are endless types (including one that is aimed specifically at the bacteria in a woman's vagina which may help with yeast infections) and little indication of what type may be best at this point. Anecdotally, women with IBS or Crohn's often report a subjective different between different brands of probiotic supplements but unless symptoms are present, this is a supplement that most don't tend to "feel" any effect from. Until more research is available, taking a basic probiotic supplement daily should be sufficient.

Iron

I discussed iron in some detail in Chapter 20 in terms of its involvement in thyroid metabolism, exercise performance and mental function along with the two different types and where they are found in the food supply. I also looked at some of the reasons that women frequently end up having insufficient iron intakes which, over time, can lead to various levels of iron deficiency, ultimately culminating in anemia. The different levels of iron deficiency require blood work to assess and are beyond the scope of this book but symptoms of fatigue, depression, diminished appetite, pale skin and others may indicate that iron status is below normal. In those situations where a woman's diet is unable to provide sufficient iron or she is already deficient, iron supplementation may be required to ensure adequate intake and/or rebuild iron stores. For endurance athletes, iron supplementation (most likely correcting a deficiency) has been found to improve aerobic performance and lower heart rate during exercise (6).

Iron supplements are typically taken orally although iron injections or infusions are sometimes used to raise levels rapidly (this carries with it a small risk of toxic shock). For most of the time that they have been available, only non-heme iron (i.e. ferrous fumarate) have been available and doses of 100-300 mg/day have been used to restore iron levels. This often causes nausea, stomach upset or tarry poop and current recommendations are to take 50-60 mg of non-heme iron twice daily to restore levels. Depending on the degree of iron deficiency, this can significantly improve levels within 2-3 months. I'd mention again that the consumption of red meat has been shown to improve the body's iron stores significantly more than non-heme iron supplementation, pointing out the potential superiority of whole foods to supplements (7).

In recent years, a heme iron supplement has been developed. These are absorbed with the same efficiency as the iron from animal foods and can be taken at far lower doses than non-heme iron, avoiding side effects while improving the body's iron status as if not more effectively. I still feel that animal source foods such as red and other meats should be included in the diet as they contain other important nutrients and high-quality protein but women who have been diagnosed as being iron deficient could readily combine a heme iron supplement with an increase in animal foods containing iron to rebuild iron stores. In the US, the product is called Proferrin and other products such as Ironsmart are available.

http://www.proferrin.com
http://healthyimmunity.com/products/ironsmart.asp

I want to emphasize that iron supplementation should not be undertaken casually, especially at higher doses. Excessive iron intake is as bad as too little as iron can build up in the body and do damage (a genetic disease called hemochromatosis causes this to occur). The normally cycling woman is relatively more protected against this due to monthly blood losses but only women who have been diagnosed as being iron deficient or who's diet is inadequate should consider taking an iron supplement.

Calcium/Vitamin D

Since the combination of calcium and Vitamin D, along with several other nutrients, are so critical for bone health, I will discuss them together. As I discussed previously, calcium intake is often low due to the removal of dairy foods from the diet while Vitamin D deficiency is primarily due to a lack of direct sun exposure by many people in the modern world. This is important as Vitamin D is being found to play a role in nearly aspect of human health with low levels being associated with many diseases. Low intakes of both calcium and Vitamin D are associated with fat gain and a recent study found that women who supplemented Vitamin D at 2000 IU/day lost more weight than those who did not (8,8a). As I discussed in Chapter 20, dairy foods improve body composition while dieting and in response to training and the dairy calcium is at least partly responsible. I'd mention that obese (Category 3) individuals store Vitamin D within their fat cells with supplementation often failing to raise the levels in their bloodstream. In this population, losing fat raises Vitamin D levels as it is released from the fat cells themselves.

Due to their role in bone health, calcium and Vitamin D intake arguably play a more important role for women than men. Recall that women have a fairly limited time to develop peak bone density and a lack of sufficient calcium/Vitamin D and other nutrients may prevent this from occurring and cause problems much later in life. Combined with resistance and other high force activities, the combination of the two can improve bone density. Surprisingly this can even occur in postmenopausal women who are not on hormone replacement. Low Vitamin D levels have also been shown to be directly related to some of the health problems that occur after menopause, including muscular weakness (9, 9a). There is also a link between low Vitamin D levels and the development of diseases such as endometriosis, uterine fibroids and PCOS (10). For athletes, vitamin D is turning out to have a number of effects that impact on performance and low Vitamin D status can decrease the overall response to intense training (10a). Athletes who live in countries with extended winters are especially at risk here.

As I discussed in Chapter 20, calcium intakes range from 1000-1200 mg/day (with some recommending 1500 mg/day) for pre-menopausal women and I'd mention again that an intake of 1200 mg of calcium may reduce symptoms of PMS (10b). postmenopausal women on HRT only need 1000 mg/day of calcium while those not on HRT require 1500 mg/day. That same 1500 mg/day would be appropriate for the amenorrheic female although it's unclear if this has any protective effect on bone loss. Due to increased absorption, at least some of the day's calcium intake should come from dairy foods with supplements being added as required. The actual amount of calcium supplementation required will depend on the level of calcium intake already in the diet and their requirements This will have to be determined by reading labels but an average serving of dairy typically has 200-300 mg of calcium and at least some calcium will come from other foods in the diet. If someone is obtaining 800 mg of calcium from the diet, they might need anywhere from 200 mg to 700 mg to make up the remainder of their daily requirement.

Looking at supplements, calcium carbonate is one of the most well absorbed forms of calcium although others such as calcium citrate are also absorbed well with most commercial supplements containing other nutrients that are important to bone health as well. The impact on bone health is improved if the daily dose is taken in smaller doses with meals throughout the day; at the very least I would recommend splitting any supplementation morning and night.

Moving to Vitamin D, there is no real consensus as to what an optimal level of Vitamin D in the blood actually is. Blood concentrations of 30 ng/mL or lower indicate deficiency with a level of ~50 ng/mL possibly being optimal. From the standpoint of optimizing bone health, levels above 50 ng/mL are required for women. Similarly, it's unclear what represents an ideal or optimal dose of Vitamin D to correct a deficiency. Ideally blood work would be bone but the reality is that, unless someone lives in a perpetually sunny place and gets sufficient sun exposure, their Vitamin D levels are almost assuredly low. It takes 100 IU (2.5 mcg) of Vitamin D per day to raise levels by 1 ng/mL and someone with a level of 30 ng/mL would need 2000 IU's (50 mcg) per day to raise their levels to 50 ng/mL with higher doses being necessary if levels are lower than this. Practically speaking, for all but the lowest levels of Vitamin D, an intake of 4000-5000IU (100-125 mcg) per day should achieve levels of 50 ng/mL over time without having any risk for excessive intake (which may occur with much higher doses for extended periods of time).

Fairly recently, a maximum Vitamin D intake of 2000 IU per day has been suggested (there is much debate over this) and many may question why I am giving higher recommendations than this. A primary reason is that, realistically, it's better to have Vitamin D levels be higher than lower than the 50 ng/mL cutoff. As importantly is the fact that sufficient amounts of direct sun exposure stimulate the body to produce between 10,000 and 20,000 IU of Vitamin D and I question how a lower level of supplementation could possibly cause problems except in someone who already had high levels (which is generally rare).

If even small amounts of direct sun exposure can be achieved, it only takes 5-10 minutes for lighter skinned individuals and up to 30 minutes for darker skinned individuals to generate maximum Vitamin D production in the skin. Vitamin D supplements can be found in either the D2 or D3 form but the latter is absorbed with much better efficiency. Vitamin D is unique in that the entire weekly dose can be taken all at once (all other supplements need to be taken daily). For readers who don't like swallowing pills and who wanted to dose 4000-5000 IU (100-125 mcg) Vitamin D per day, a single weekly dose of 28,000-35,000 IU could be taken all at once. Since a majority of readers will be taking some supplements at least one daily, I don't particularly see why adding a Vitamin D capsule (they are small) to the mix will be a problem. Since it is a fat soluble vitamin, Vitamin D should be taken with a fat containing meal.

Fish Oils

When I discussed optimal nutrient and food choices in Chapter 20, I talked about different types of fats and specifically the fish oils. The two fish oils are referred to as EPA and DHA and are often called essential fatty acids or EFA's. Recapping that information briefly, fish oils are a type of poly-unsaturated fat (PUFA) which have a tremendous number of effects in the body including the modulation of inflammation, improving immune system function, potentially increasing fat mobilization and burning along with limiting fat storage. Fish oils have been shown to improve fat loss on a diet although the impact is not enormous. Specifically relevant to women, fish oils may have other benefits including a reduced risk of breast and colon cancer (and potentially uterine and skin cancer). They may reduce the risk of manic depression, certain types of dementias, high blood pressure, diabetes and others. I mentioned that DHA is critical for the development of a baby's brain and, in a somewhat related vein, sufficient fish oil intake may reduce the risk of postpartum depression after childbirth, improve the health of the newborn (10b).

With long-term use, fish oil supplementation may improve leptin sensitivity in the brain (which could decrease the impact of dieting on many aspects of physiology) and low levels of EPA/DHA in the brain are associated with a number of mood disorders and even depression and other mental illnesses. Fish oil supplementation has also been shown to reduce symptoms of PMS (11). Except for those cultures that eat fatty fish regularly, the intake of EPA/DHA is generally low or at least sub-optimal. And while this chapter is about supplements, I'd reiterate that fish oils are absorbed more effectively from fatty fish. However, outside of those countries and cultures where fatty fish is consumed, my experience is that many if not most don't have a taste for those types of fish making a supplement necessary.

While the minimum requirements for fish oils are quite small, I recommend a total combined daily intake of 1.8-3.0 total grams of EPA/DHA with women under 160 lbs using the lower dose and women heavier than that using the higher dose. As I mentioned in Chapter 20, similar doses have been found to improve symptoms of Rheumatoid Arthritis (RA) and a recent study found that women who were given 2.4 g/day of preformed fish oils lost nearly 3 pounds of fat while gaining over a pound of LBM in 6 weeks (11a). A fairly average fish oil capsule will contain roughly 300 mg of combined EPA/DHA meaning that 6-10 pills per day would be required to achieve my recommended dose. This isn't universal and different brands of fish oils may contain different amounts of EPA/DHA and readers will have to determine how many are required to reach the above amounts. For those who don't like swallowing pills, there are also liquid fish oils such as Carlson's which are lightly flavored and can be used as salad dressing. I do not recommend that flax seed be used, however. While it contains the parent fatty acids (ALA and LA) which are converted to EPA/DHA, the conversion is very inefficient except in vegetarians.

Finally I should mention krill oil which is often touted as a more concentrated/superior form of fish oil. In one study, 2 grams of krill oil was superior to 2 grams of fish oils in reducing PMS symptoms (12). No research I am aware of has compared krill oil, which is significantly more expensive, to the higher intakes of fish oil I am recommending but women with severe PMS may wish to consider it.

Since they are very reactive to heat and light, fish oil supplements should be kept in a dark bottle in a cool place such as the refrigerator. Some people experience fish burps when they take fish oil supplements but this can usually be eliminated with the use of enteric coated capsules and by keeping them cool.

Zinc/Magnesium

While zinc and magnesium aren't related in the same way that calcium and Vitamin D are, they do have a handful of interactions which are relevant to women and I will discuss them together for convenience. As mentioned in Chapter 20, both nutrients are often deficient although for effectively opposite reasons. The most absorbable form of zinc is found in animal foods and removal of those foods contribute to zinc deficiencies while magnesium is found in many vegetable foods with inadequate intake of those foods contributing to magnesium deficiencies.

Magnesium plays a tremendous number of roles in body but one of critical importance is that sufficient magnesium intake is important (along with calcium, Vitamin D and others I discussed in Chapter 17) for optimal bone health (13). Zinc is also involved in a number of biological processes but one of importance to dieters is that a low zinc status lowers thyroid hormone levels and potentially metabolic rate. In a case study of two zinc deficient female athletes, zinc supplementation at only 26 mg/day for several months improved zinc status and improved thyroid hormone levels. In one of the subjects resting metabolic rate (RMR) increased by 200 calories per day while the second saw an unbelievable 500 calorie per day increase (14). Zinc depletion has been shown to lower levels of active thyroid hormones as well.

I talked about the importance of sleep earlier in this book and how insufficient sleep can contribute to increased appetite and weight gain along with being disrupted while dieting. The combination of zinc and magnesium helps many to sleep more effectively (I'll discuss more sleep supplements later in the chapter as well). In the luteal phase, the combination may have even more potential benefits. As I discussed in Chapter 2, the changes in estrogen and progesterone during the second half of the normal menstrual cycle cause changes in serotonin and dopamine that can cause cravings, increased appetite and mood changes. Zinc and magnesium have been shown to improve serotonin signaling which helps with at least part of this issue (15). I also mentioned that chocolate is thought to be especially craved due to it's high magnesium content and some women report decreased cravings with magnesium supplementation. Magnesium supplementation may also reduce symptoms of PMS, cramping and menstrual migraine (15a).

A daily intake of 25 mg of zinc and 400 mg of magnesium would be effective and these can be taken an hour before bedtime to help with sleep or at other times of the day so long as they do not cause sleepiness. Different forms of zinc are absorbed more or less identically and the form chosen here is of no relevance. Most pills seem to be 50mg and they can be bitten in half or taken every other day. Cheaper forms of magnesium such as magnesium oxide are very poorly absorbed and this is a place where paying more for a higher quality magnesium citrate will be worthwhile.

Protein Powders/MRPs/Protein Bars

In several chapters of this book, I have commented that women often under consume or actively avoid protein unless they are involved in physique or strength/power sports. This may be due to fear of various health risks associated with certain foods, the fat content or simply not having a taste for protein foods. While whole foods are generally better choices to raise protein intake, there are also concentrated protein powders that can offer an easier and/or more convenient way to increase their protein intake to my recommended levels. Protein powders are also convenient for women with busy schedules along with being useful for many aspects of around workout nutrition. On a fat loss diet, the combination of resistance training with post-workout protein helps to reverse the normally negative effects of dieting on muscle metabolism \, helping to spare LBM loss (16).

There are a vast number of different protein powders available but the ones I want to focus on first are the dairy proteins. Perhaps the most well known of these is whey protein, a rapidly digesting protein that provides amino acids to the body quickly. It mixes well in most liquids or foods and tends to be most beneficial around workouts when rapid digestion is preferred. Whey is especially valuable around or after menopause as its fact digesting nature helps to offset the normal age-related muscle loss. There is also casein protein, a slowly digesting protein that provides amino acids to the body over much longer periods. Casein doesn't mix as well as whey, usually requiring a blender or mixing bottle, and can have a slightly chalky texture. This can help with fullness on a diet, especially if mixed with some fat and fiber.

Finally is Milk Protein Isolate (MPI) which is a mixture of 20% whey and 80% casein which has both the benefits of drawbacks of the other two proteins. The whey digests rapidly while the casein is slower but it has the same chalky texture and mixing difficulties. Dairy protein powders can contain some calcium but the amounts can vary widely from as little as 100mg in some forms of whey up to nearly 700 mg in some brands of MPI so this is potentially a good source of dairy calcium. Most diary protein powders have also had the lactose removed so that lactose intolerant individuals can use them without problems.

There are also a number of vegetarian protein powders although these vary enormously in quality and taste. Hemp protein is available and I mentioned previously that pea protein may be as effective as whey following resistance training. Soy protein is probably the most commonly used vegetarian protein powder and I will discuss it separately in the next section.

Nutritionally, a typical scoop of protein powder will contain 25-30 grams of protein although this can vary. Commercial products can contain variable amounts of carbohydrates and fats as well but these will be listed on the label. They can be mixed into water or used to make blender drinks. For a more meal-like type of drink, mixing protein powder into yogurt or milk, adding some type of fat (peanut butter is a favorite), a small piece of fruit and one of the commercial fiber powders can make a thick smoothie with a controlled amount of calories and a lot of nutrition. A packet of Sugar-Free jello can be used to thicken it for even better texture. Endless recipes incorporating protein powders can be found online.

Related to protein powders are meal replacement products (MRPS), which I discussed in Chapter 20. Typically a liquid or mixable powder, MRP's contain a mixture of protein, carbohydrate, fat, fiber and micronutrients and are meant to replace a whole food meal. While these products should never make up the totality of a daily diet they can provide convenience and a quick meal to help busy women meet their daily nutrient needs. They should be used for less than two total meals per day. Similar to MRP's are protein bars, nutrient dense food bars generally containing all the macronutrients, possibly some fiber, along with vitamins and minerals. Newer products taste almost like candy bars (helping to quell cravings for sweet foods) and they can provide convenient nutrition for busy women. Busy athletes often have trouble meeting their calorie and nutrient requirements and protein bars provide a quick, convenient source of calories and nutrients. Protein bars are not always as filling as whole food meals and I would caution against their overuse while dieting as they can leave someone hungrier than eating a meal would.

Soy Protein/Phytoestrogens

While I focused on dairy protein powders in the above section, I want to talk about soy protein separately. Here I will actually be including soy based foods such as tofu and tempeh, soy milk, soy oil, and many others (soy protein has been used in many processed foods due to its low cost although this seems to be shifting in recent years). Soy protein powders also fall into this category and the primary compounds I will be discussing, called phytoestrogens, are available as isolated supplements. Strictly speaking, soy foods and isolated supplements are not interchangeable as there may be compounds in soy foods that are having an independent effect on the body but I will treat them as effectively identical. When I am making a distinction between soy protein and phytoestrogens I will make it clear which I am discussing.

I am discussing soy protein separately from other proteins and foods for a number of reasons. The first is that, while soy certainly has effects on male physiology, it has arguably been recommended more to women overall. More importantly, soy proteins have been surrounded by a fair amount of controversy in recent years. Early indication of potential health benefits (first observed in cultures that ate soy regularly) drove a huge interest in soy protein but later studies also identified potential negatives. Along with that came individuals who had personally run into problems with soy. Entire books completely decrying it's consumption exist. Even in research, the pros and cons of soy are heavily debated and, as is so often the case, the truth of the matter lies somewhere in the middle (17). In short, low or moderate doses of soy often have distinctly different effects than high doses and the specific population being examined is a huge determinant of whether or not soy is beneficial, neutral or potentially harmful.

How Does Soy Work?

While whole soy foods contain many different biological compounds, it is the phytoestrogen content that I will be primarily focusing on here. Let me mention in passing that there is currently concern over man-made estrogens (called xenoestrogens or environmental estrogens) which may be having a number of negative effects on human and animal physiology but this is beyond the scope of this book. So far as the phytoestrogens, the primary two are genistein and diadzein. Phytoestrogens are plant based compounds that are structurally similar to estrogen. As such they can exert a tremendous number of effects in the body, many of which may vary between women and men (18). I won't detail all of the mechanisms by which phytoestrogens act in the body but the end result is that phytoestrogens alter a woman's normal estrogen metabolism in a number of ways. Of primary importance here is that phytoestrogens bind to the estrogen receptor and appears to do so more strongly than estrogen itself. This blocks her naturally produced estrogen from binding to the receptor although estrogen levels are unchanged. At the same time, phytoestrogens send a weaker signal than a woman's own estrogen and this is where things grow complex.

The overall effect of the above is that the effects of phytoestrogens in a woman's body depend enormously on her current estrogen levels. In a woman who's estrogen levels are relatively normal (i.e. the normally cycling female), phytoestrogens will have the effect of decreasing total estrogenic signaling due to phytoestrogens binding to the receptor and blocking estrogen while sending a weaker overall signal. In contrast, when estrogen levels are low and there is little to no signal to begin with (i.e. amenorrhea or menopause without hormone replacement), phytoestrogens will increase estrogen signaling since there is little to none to begin with. While confusing, this distinction is important as it impacts directly on whether or not phytoestrogens have the potential to be overall beneficial or negative in terms of their effects.

Potential Benefits of Soy Protein/Phytoestrogens

There are a number of potential pros and cons associated with the intake of phytoestrogens although studies invariably find fairly mixed results. As mentioned, at least some of this is due to the population being studied and whether they are starting with higher or lower estrogen levels. People also vary in how well or poorly they metabolize phytoestrogens with both high and low metabolizers and high metabolizers potentially experiencing effects not seen in the low metabolizers. A final issue is whether soy protein/foods (which contain other compounds) or isolated supplements are being studied.

Perhaps the most well-known potential benefit of phytoestrogens in women is the potential to reduce breast cancer risk later in life. While breast cancer is extremely multifactorial, with a large genetic component, at least one major factor is a woman's lifetime estrogen exposure. Due to their effects (i.e. binding to the estrogen receptor but sending a weaker signal), phytoestrogens have the effect of lowering this, reducing overall breast cancer risk. At least some research suggests that soy intake must be started at an early age for there to be an effect, which would be occurring in cultures where soy is a staple of the diet making it questionable if similar results would occur in women consuming soy later in life. Soy does reduce levels of LH and FSH (19). While this doesn't lower estrogen or progesterone levels it increases the length of the menstrual cycle by 1-2 days. This could mean up to 24 fewer menstrual cycles over a lifetime, reducing the risk of some types of cancer. Soy also reduces symptoms of PMS (20).

There are other potential benefits of soy, primarily for postmenopausal women. Readers may recall that many of the negative effects that occur around or after menopause are due to the reduction in estrogen levels. This includes shifting body fat patterns, increased cardiovascular risk, menopausal symptoms (i.e. hot flashes and others), osteoporosis and both breast and endometrial cancer. For those women who are not using HRT, phytoestrogens would maintain at least some estrogenic signaling to offset this (21). While it will be far lower than what would be seen with HRT, some should be better than none in this situation. While unstudied to my knowledge, the same could very well apply in the case of women with functional hypothalamic amenorrhea in that soy/phytoestrogen intake could replace at least some of the missing estrogenic signal.

Potential Negatives of Soy Protein/Phytoestrogens

While soy clearly has a number of potential benefits, these are often inconsistently seen and have to be weighed against several potential negatives. Even the impact of phytoestrogens on breast cancer are inconsistent with some studies showing that they can increase the overall risk. This could be related to several factors including some interaction with genetics but is most likely related to the doses being used. Overall, so long as soy protein/phytoestrogens are consumed in relatively moderate amounts, any impact on breast cancer risk is at most neutral.

One very real negative of soy protein is that it has the potential to negatively impact thyroid metabolism (many of the negative reports online are related to this) although this too depends on the specific situation (22). In animals, soy protein has actually been found to increase levels of T4 (inactive thyroid hormone) but this doesn't appear to occur in humans. Rather, most studies (including 8 studies on women) have found no measurable impact on thyroid hormone in people with normal thyroid function. In contrast, soy has potential negative effects on women who are hypothyroidal and have low thyroid hormone levels to begin with. In this case, appears to impair the absorption of thyroid medication although this effect disappears if the medication is taken 12 hours away from the soy protein. There is also some theoretical concern that soy protein could impair an enzyme important to thyroid hormone metabolism. However, this is only seen when iodine intake is too low to begin with. Since iodized salt is a primary contributor of iodine in the diet, the general restriction of sodium in the diets of health-conscious women is likely part of any problems that may have occurred. So long as sodium/iodine intake is sufficient, the intake of soy has no negative impact on thyroid hormone production or metabolism.

A somewhat theoretical concern regarding soy is its potential to act as what is called an endocrine disruptor (I mentioned xenoestrogens above). This simply means that they have the potential to disrupt the body's normal hormone (endocrine) system with their increasing presence in the modern world being linked to a number problems. In some animals, for example, normal sexual development is being impaired due to the presence of these compounds in the water supply. This exposes the adult animals and their offspring to high levels of xenoestrogens for their entire life. In terms of soy protein, this raises potential concerns for two groups of women. The first is for pregnant women for whom soy intake could expose the developing fetus to high levels of phytoestrogen, negatively impacting on the baby's overall physiology. Similar concerns have been raised regarding the use of soy protein in infant formulas (22a). It's also conceivable that excessive soy could pose a problem for girls both before and during puberty. Here soy proteins could have a similar impact on overall development (I'd note that the presence of xenoestrogens in the environment is thought to be one cause of girls hitting puberty earlier).

Let me be clear that there is little to no direct research on most of these issues. It would be unethical to study the impact of soy on fetal development in humans but animal research does suggest a potential risk. While informative, there can be vast differences in animal and human physiology. What little human research exists for soy formula in babies finds no meaningful difference in development between soy and breastfeeding although breastfeeding is still considered the first choice (22b). I am unaware of any research systematically examining the impact of soy protein on pre- or post-pubertal girls but, once again, my feeling is that anything with the potential to negatively impact development is best avoided. Certainly the intake of soy products in Asian cultures indirectly suggests no impact of soy protein but there are other considerations here. There are often ethnically based adaptations to the local food supply that alters metabolism. More importantly is the fact that the actual soy intake in Asian cultures is relatively low in the first place. As I'll discuss below, higher intakes of phytoestrogens often have distinct effects than lower intake levels. Overall my general feeling is that it's better to err on the side of conservatism and avoid anything with the remotest potential to negatively impact on a developing fetus, baby or pubertal female.

The Optimal Dose of Soy and Phytoestrogens

As with so many aspects of human physiology, whether something has positive or negative effects depends heavily on the dose and whether or not soy/phytoestrogens show positive, negative or no effects depends on this as well. Almost without exception the research that has found a negative effect from phytoestrogen intake has used very high doses. In contrast, small and moderate doses have at worst a neutral effect on physiology if not having a benefit overall. This distinction is critical to make due to a fairly normal part of human psychology where people assume that if some is good, more must be better. When any nutrient is claimed to be healthy, at least some people will start megadosing and this is when they get into problems.

Soy protein is no different. Having heard it was healthy (and potentially protective against breast cancer), women started consuming it in large amounts. Since soy protein was fairly cheap compared to higher quality proteins, food companies started using it as much to save money as to put it on the label and market it based on its soy content. The end results of this is that soy intakes in Western countries went from very low to extremely high almost overnight. But what was lost in all of the soy mania is that the daily intake of soy based foods in Asian cultures is actually quite small. The daily intake of soy protein in Asian cultures is in the realm of 10 grams per day providing roughly 10-30 mg of phytoestrogens per day. Which is interesting when you consider that most of the studies showing beneficial (or neutral) effects of soy were providing phytoestrogen intakes of roughly 50-100 mg/day with negative effects occurring above that. Most soy proteins have 1-3 mg phytoestrogen per gram of protein so a 100 mg/day intake would allow no more than 30 grams of soy protein per day.

But many people went far above that either deliberately or eating large amounts of soy-fortified foods. As an example of just how ludicrous this can get, there is a case study of a woman with fertility and hormonal issues who was found to be consuming 40 grams of phytoestrogens per day. Not 40 grams of soy protein but 40 grams of phytoestrogens or roughly 13,000 times the recommended intake. This would be akin to someone taking 13,000 baby aspirins because they heard it helped prevent heart attacks. I am not saying that this is typical or common but I strongly suspect that most of the people who experienced major problems with soy were simply consuming far more than is beneficial. Invariably when people write about their personal horror stories with soy, those problems can be tracked to their consuming too much to begin with and then blaming the soy for their own excessive intake.

Soy Recommendations

Having looked at the issue of soy and phytoestrogens in a general sense, I want to look at where it might or might not have relevance within the context of this book. I want to say up front that some of what I will write is somewhat speculative due to their being no direct research on the topic. It seems fairly clear that the largest potential impact of soy will be in postmenopausal women who are not using HRT. Here the potential to reduce the risk of some cancers, neurodegeneration along with many of the symptoms of menopause would seem to make them a worthwhile consideration (I will discuss other useful supplements for menopause below). The same might hold for peri-menopausal women although I'm unaware of any research on this specifically. Postmenopausal women using HRT as well as women who have undergone partial hysterectomy and are on estrogen only HRT, would be unlikely to benefit from soy and it might actually reduce the effects of the HRT to begin with by blocking the estrogen receptor.

For the adult pre-menopausal woman, the situation is far more complex. In at least a general sense, phytoestrogens would seem to be potentially beneficial in terms of reducing the risk of breast and other cancers later in life. This effect is somewhat questionable based on what I discussed above but, at moderate intakes, any effect will only be neutral. Women with severe PMS symptoms would want to consider soy (along with other supplements discussed in this chapter) since it can reduce those symptoms. For female athletes, estrogen has an important effect on muscular remodeling and adaptation (this will be discussed in more detail in Volume 2) and I would question the use of soy as this would reduce these potential effects of estrogen. Additionally, as discussed in Chapter 20, soy protein is inferior to other proteins for recovery and supporting increases in muscle mass. This wouldn't be relevant to the female seeking general fitness and health but more serious trainees would probably benefit from avoiding soy proteins and consuming other high-quality proteins instead. Women on thyroid medication or who have been diagnosed as hypothyroidal must either avoid soy protein or, if they choose to use it, must ensure adequate iodine and this is best accomplished by ensuring sufficient sodium intake.

That said, in the normally cycling Category 1 female who is dieting to the extremes, the decrease in LH due to soy protein could conceivably contribute to menstrual cycle dysfunction and loss of cycle due to a low Energy Availability (EA). There is at least some indication that soy might reduce the release of cortisol from the adrenal gland and this might be useful for the psychogenically stressed dieter (23). Avoiding excessive diet and exercise and other types of stress relief would be a superior approach. The potential negative of soy in the normally cycling Category 1 female is likely to reverse itself when and if amenorrhea occurs and estrogen levels drop. In this case, the consumption of soy protein would maintain at least some estrogenic signaling (identical to what occurs in the postmenopausal woman). While speculative, this could maintain the effect on fat mobilization, hunger suppression, leptin sensitivity and all of the other effects of estrogen that are lost when amenorrhea occurs. This might have the additional benefit of preventing the often extreme breast shrinkage (caused by a loss of estrogen signaling) that can occur while dieting to this level.

For women using combined hormonal BC, it would seem pointless to use soy specifically. The BC is already replacing estrogen in the body and soy would seem to reduce the overall effect of the BC in this regard. At most the effect may simple be neutral. There is at least some suggestion that soy protein is useful for the treatment of obesity although it's hard to tell if this is due to soy itself or just a higher protein intake (24). In several studies of post menopausal women, soy protein was shown to either increase LBM or decrease visceral fat (24a). Finally, in women with PCOS, phytoestrogens have been found to improve hormonal markers and insulin resistance and this would be beneficial for those women trying to improve their fertility and health (25). I would expect this to apply to women with subclinical hyperandrogenism as well. PCOS/subclinically hyperandrogenic athletes would be better off avoiding soy as reducing androgen levels would tend to reduce the benefits that the elevated levels confer.

The issue of soy protein is complex and controversial and that controversy is unlikely to be settled any time soon. It's clear that in some situations, soy can be of benefit and others it may be detrimental. Outside of postmenopausal women not on HRT, there are arguably more questions than there are answers at this point and women must make their own choice about whether or not to use soy. Women who do choose to consume soy protein or to use isolated phytoestrogens should aim for a total daily intake of 50-100 mg at the maximum or 25-30 grams of total soy protein per day. Given the prevalence of soy in the food supply, it might be better to target the lower level on the assumption that there will be some intake to begin with before any more is added. Isolated supplements containing genistein and diadzein are also available although they frequently contain other compounds of fairly questionable benefit.

Sleep Supplements

Earlier in the book I discussed sleep and how insufficient amounts of sleep is turning out to be a risk factor for overeating and weight gain. Women are already more likely to have disrupted sleep during the luteal (and especially late luteal) phase and dieting and fat loss per se can make this worse. Finding ways to improve and/or ensure sufficient sleep is therefore critical and I want to look at non-supplement approaches briefly first. One easy strategy to improve sleep it to consume carbohydrates at bedtime as this raises serotonin levels which promotes sleep. As discussed in Chapter 23, this is a good reason to shift more calories to the evening while dieting.

The next step is proper sleep hygiene. This refers to a cluster of behaviors such as avoiding caffeine or high-intensity exercise in the evenings, going to sleep and waking up at the same time of night, sleeping in a cool dark room and others (full lists or proper sleep hygiene can be found online). Once sleep hygiene has been addressed and corrected, a variety of supplements may help if sleep is still disrupted. I'd note that the neurochemistry of sleep is complicated and there is a great deal of individual response to different sleep supplements. Some experimentation may be required to find the compound or combination of compounds that is ideal for any given reader of this book.

Perhaps the most well known sleep supplement is melatonin. This is a compound produced in the pineal gland as darkness falls which stimulates sleep. The normal night-time increase in melatonin is inhibited by direct light entering the eye and a very common cause of poor sleep in the modern world is working at the computer, on a tablet, on a phone late at night as light entering the eyes prevents melatonin from increasing. As discussed in Chapter 2, women in the luteal phase are more sensitive to this effect. While it's ideal to simply avoid these devices at night, this is not always possible. There is a free computer program called f.lux which adjusts the light quality of electronic screens based on the current time of day.

If this is still not sufficient, melatonin may be supplemented as well. Supplements range enormously in dose from 300-500 micrograms (mcg) up to 5mg or more. Many find that the smallest doses work just fine and that higher doses cause strange dreams or leave them feeling almost hung-over the next morning. Both short-acting and time-released melatonin is available and the combination of the two may be worth considering. The short-acting form helps people to fall asleep while the time-released keeps them asleep.

There are other supplements that may also be beneficial. Theanine (found in tea) helps to quite the mind and has shown benefit for general anxiety as well with 100-200 mg taken before sleep as a typical dose. Valerian root can also be beneficial with a dose of 450 mg taken an hour before bed. Gaba Amino Butyric Acid (GABA) is another relaxation/anti-anxiety supplement that helps some to sleep and the dose is 500 mg an hour before sleep. Both the zinc/magnesium combination I discussed above and 5-HTP discussed below can also help.

Luteal Phase/PMS Supplements

Having looked at supplement which apply to all women, I want to begin looking at supplements aimed at specific female situations, starting with the luteal phase of the normally cycling woman. As I described in Chapter 2, this is when a large amount of a woman's physiology changes, often for the worse with negative changes to mood and energy levels along with increased hunger and food cravings occurring. This is most extreme during the late luteal phase and some of these products may have their greatest benefit in the last week of the cycle. For the most part, these supplements would only apply to the normally cycling woman although some women with PCOS/hyperandrogenism still experience similar changes at points in their extended cycle. For the most part, women using hormonal birth control (BC) don't have the same types of issues although high-dose/high-potency progestins occasionally cause problems with hunger and cravings. I will discuss amenorrheic and postmenopausal women separately in the chapter.

For decades, endless products have been recommended to help reduce some of the negative of PMS. As I've discussed, some of the general use supplements seem to have benefits in improving the symptoms of PMS. The fish oils, calcium, magnesium and phytoestrogens have all shown at least some benefit in this regard and recommended amounts have been given previously. Increasing potassium while lowering sodium intake may also help with water retention during the late luteal phase (as well as the late follicular phase). Beyond that, many other compounds such as Evening Primrose Oil (EPO) and St. John's Wort are often claimed to have benefits but, by and large, research has not found them to have any real benefit. Only one, Vitex Cagnus, discussed next, has been shown to have any real benefit (26).

Vitex Cagnus

The herb Vitex Cagnus, also knows as chasteberry, has been used in traditional medicine for various purposes and has many potential benefits for women during the luteal phase. While Vitex may work through multiple mechanisms, the primary one of interest here is that it binds to the dopamine (DA) receptor in the brain. DA is involved in pleasure, hunger and cravings and the increase in the latter two are at least partially related to falling DA levels during the luteal phase (this drop in DA occurs with dieting in general). Although not actually studied for hunger or craving control, Vitex should help to control both. Additionally, decreasing DA levels causes the hormone prolactin, which is involved heavily in breast milk production following pregnancy, to increase and this is at least partially responsible for the breast tenderness that often occurs. In this regard, Vitex has been studied extensively and improves symptoms of PMS including breast tenderness (27). Vitex is a herbal product, available in herb, drop and other forms and this can make dosing recommendations difficult. Many herbal products are either not standardized for the active ingredient or do not list how much of the active ingredient is present. For example, a herb that contains 200mg standardized for 10% of the active ingredient would contain 20mg of the active ingredient (200 mg * 0.10 = 20 mg). Various products exist including some standardized products but a typical herbal containing the dry vitex cagnus extract would be dosed at 400-500 mg/day taken in the morning.

5-HTP (5-HydroxyTryptophan)

A derivative of the amino acid tryptophan, 5-HTP is an amino acid which is converted to the chemical serotonin in the brain. During the luteal phase, serotonin levels in the brain decrease (this also occurs during dieting in general) and this contributes to the changes in mood and increase in carbohydrate cravings and hunger. While zinc and magnesium can help with this by increasing serotonin signaling, 5-HTP is a more direct approach. A dose of 50-100 mg taken up to three times per day, including an hour before sleep, can help with mood and carbohydrate cravings while also improving sleep.

Aspirin/NSAID

While drugs rather than supplements, a final consideration is the addition of aspirin or other Non-Steroidal Anti-Inflammatory Drugs (NSAIDs) to reduce the pain or discomfort of cramping. As I discussed in Chapter 2, this can occur during the late-luteal phase and into menstruation and is due to the release of prostaglandins which stimulate uterine contractions to shed the endometrium. Both aspirin and NSAIDs block the production of these compounds and in at least some women (50%) these drugs can help to alleviate menstrual cramps (28). There is no indication of which NSAID might be best and, as I mentioned in Chapter 2, a small percentage of women (18%) appear to be resistant to the effects of the drugs. Women who experience severe cramps are encouraged to experiment with either aspirin or an NSAIDs during the late-luteal and into the early follicular phase (if cramping continues) to see if it helps.

Amenorrhea

In addition to the general use supplements, women who have developed functional hypothalamic amenorrhea (FHA) will need to raise their calcium intake to 1500 mg/day. To this I would add the speculative potential of soy protein or phytoestrogens to maintain at least some estrogenic signaling. For the most part, the luteal phase supplements are not necessary although Vitex or 5-HTP might play a role in helping to control hunger for those dieters attempting to reach the low extremes of BF%. I mentioned in Chapter 12 that an underappreciated effect of amenorrhea is a disruption of normal melatonin rhythms with a phase-shift occurring whereby melatonin stays up during the day (causing lethargy and depression) but decreases later at night (causing sleeplessness). This may be reversible with the use of small doses of melatonin taken earlier in the evening (28a). Amenorrheic women may wish to try 300 mcg of melatonin 4 hours and again 2 hours before bedtime. This could be combined with a light box providing ~10,000 lux for 30-60 minutes obliquely into the eyes in the morning as this will reduce melatonin levels.

A second possible supplement is called actyl-l-carnitine or ALCAR. A derivate of the amino acid l-carnitine (which is involved in fat metabolism), ALCAR has a number of effects in the brain one of which is to increase LH pulsatility when it has decreased (29). One study found that 6 out of 10 subjects had spontaneous menstruation with 2 g/day of ALCAR for 6 months and this might have potential to reverse FHA when it has occurred (30). A combination of 250 mg ALCAR + 500 mg carnitine per day was also shown to improve LH levels while decreasing cortisol levels (30a). Correcting the low EA state is still of critical importance but ALCAR (with or without carnitine) may be worth considering for those women with FHA who are trying to resume normal menstrual cycle function.

PCOS/Subclinical Hyperandrogenism Supplements

So far as supplements for women with PCOS or subclinical hyperandrogenism, all of the general use supplements are still indicated here and many have specific benefits in PCOS. For example, fish oils improve metabolic profile and lower androgen levels in women with PCOS (31). Zinc at 50-300 mg/day has both general health an insulin sensitizing effects while the combination of magnesium (220 mg/day) and zinc (50 mg/day) reduces inflammation (32,32a). Women with PCOS are often found to have low Vitamin D levels although this may be due to more being stored in fat cells (33). Supplementing 4000 IU o Vitamin D/day has been found to improve metabolic health (33a). Combined with a low-calorie diet, 50,000 IU/week of Vitamin D improves menstrual cyclicity (33b). As mentioned, phytoestrogens improve insulin sensitivity, hormonal status and other issues associated with PCOS and 50 mg/day is the dose. Two mg of melatonin improves hormonal status while partially normalizing the menstrual cycle (34).

As mentioned above, the luteal phase supplements might potentially be beneficial for some women with PCOS. Even with a lengthened cycle, a luteal phase will eventually occur although there will be no way to predict when this will happen but those supplements may be useful at this time. Women with subclinical hyperandrogenism may have slightly more consistent menstrual cycles and find that those supplements are useful if the typical issues of cravings, hunger and/or PMS are present.

In addition to the above, there are a number of supplements that have been specifically examined in PCOS, primarily aimed at improving overall metabolic health, insulin sensitivity or the infertility that is so common. While insulin sensitizing drugs such as Metformin have been used to treat PCOS, a number of supplements have been shown to have broadly similar (or in one case, equivalent) results. Alpha-lipoic acid (ALA, not be confused with a fatty acid found in flaxseed and other oils) is an insulin sensitizer. Six-hundred milligrams twice per day of a special slow release form been found to improve insulin sensitivity in lean women with PCOS (35). N-Acetyl Cysteine (NAC) does the same at doses of 1.8-3.0 grams/day and was actually found to be more effective than the drug Metformin (36,37). Cinnamon at 1.5 grams per day for 3-6 months also improved insulin sensitivity (38). Chromium picolinate, a compound that was popular with athletes many years ago improves insulin sensitivity at dose of 200 micograms per day (39). A new compound called monacolin-k at 3 g/day has also recently been shown to have benefits although it does not appear to be commercially available yet (40). Finally, CoQ10 at 100 mg/day has been shown to improve insulin sensitivity and glucose metabolism (40a).

While the above have only been studied in limited fashion, perhaps the most studied supplements are folic acid (a B-vitamin), myo-inositol and chiro-inositol with the latter two having the most work done on them (41). In a number of studies, either by themselves or in combination, they have been shown to improve insulin sensitivity, health markers and/or ovarian function/fertility (42-44). Additionally, myo-inositol and chiro-inositol have been found to have differing effects with myo-inositol improving metabolic health and chiro-inositol improving menstrual cycle function. The typical doses used in the studies are 400 micrograms (mcg) of folic acid, 4 grams of myo-inositol and 1 gram of chiro-inositol. There is some indication that this combination works better with the addition of N-acetyl Cysteine.

Product	Effect	Dose
Vitamin D	Improved metabolic health	4000 IU/day
Phytoestrogens	Improved insulin sensitivity and metabolic health	50 mg/day genistein/diadzein
Melatonin	Improved hormonal status and partially normalized menstrual cycle	2 mg at night
Alpha-lipoic Acid	Improve insulin sensitivity	600 mg twice/day
N-Acetyl Cysteine	Improved insulin sensitivity	1.8-3.0 grams/day
Cinnamon	Improved insulin sensitivity	1.5 grams/day
Chromium Picolinate	Improved insulin sensitivity	200 mcg/day
Monacolin-K	Improved insulin sensitivity	3 g/day
CoEnzyme Q10	Improved insulin sensitivity and glucose metabolism	100 mg/day
Folic Acid	Improved insulin sensitivity, metabolic health, fertility	400 mcg/day
Myo-Inositol	Improved metabolic health	4 grams/day
Chiro-Inositol	Improved menstrual cycle function and fertility	1 g/day

Peri- and Postmenopausal Supplements

For the most part, the peri- or postmenopausal woman should be using the general use supplements I described above. As described in Chapter 20, calcium intake should be 1000 mg/day for women not on HRT while 1500 mg (with sufficient Vitamin D) is critical for the postmenopausal woman not on HRT to support bone health. Iron intake can be reduced to 8 mg/day since there is no longer monthly iron loss occurring from menstruation. Clearly the luteal phase supplements would be unnecessary although some of them will be mentioned again for treatment of some of the symptoms that occur at menopause.

Hot flashes, mood swings, trouble sleeping, vaginal dryness and many others may occur in response to the change in hormonal status (45). As mentioned earlier in the book, the use of HRT will impact on how prevalent these symptoms are but not all women can or will choose to use HRT after menopause. Those women may wish to consider soy protein (20-30 g/day) or phytoestrogen supplementation (50-100 mg/day) as discussed above. A product called <u>Amberen</u> (found at amberen.com) containing succinates has recently been shown to improve the symptoms of menopause by raising estrogen levels (45a,45b).

Many other supplements have also bee found to reduce some menopausal symptoms (46). Black cohosh has long been used for treatment of various female specific issues and a fairly large amount of research suggests that it can reduce both hot flashes and mood swings. The mechanism of black cohosh does not appear to be through estrogen signaling and may be caused by an increase in brain serotonin (which decreases as estrogen drops) which I've mentioned is involved in mood, appetite and many other processes. Zinc, magnesium and 5-HTP, discussed previously, have similar effects and may be worth considering. The dose of black cohosh is 40mg/day and it may have the potential to interact with other drugs. Readers will have to look up specific medications online. St. Johns Wort (a herbal compound that has been trialed for depression) has additive effects with black cohosh in helping to improve mood and/or depression. The dose is 900 mg/day.

Vitex Cagnus, discussed above in relations to the luteal phase supplements, appears to have mood benefits for postmenopausal women and this may actually be through a slight mimicking of progesterone in the body (increasing dopamine signaling would also improve mood). The dose is the same as above, 500 mg of chasteberry taken in the mornings. Ginkgo is a herb that is popular among users of nootropics (compounds that are supposed to improve brain function) and improves blood flow to the brain. A dose of 120 mg/day appears to improve memory and overall cognition, both of which can be affected during peri- and post-menopause due to the drop in estrogen. There are a host of other supplements that are claimed to improve postmenopausal symptoms including dong quai (a Chinese herb), ginseng, wild yam, and evening primrose oil but these are either inadequately studied or have no effect. Many products aimed at menopausal women will contain a grab-bag of these products but at wholly ineffective levels and I'd recommend that women wanting to try the above supplements should obtain them separately at appropriate doses. While it would be ideal to trial each supplement individually to determine their individual effects, postmenopausal women looking for relief may simply not care to go through this process so long as they are getting some relief to begin with.

Melatonin

While I discussed melatonin supplementation as a general sleep supplement, it may have an even more pronounced benefit for the peri- or postmenopausal woman. With increasing age, and especially at menopause, melatonin levels start to fall and this is associated with many of the negative effects such as changes in mood, sleep, hot flashes, sexual interest and function (47). Various studies looking at supplementation of melatonin in peri- and postmenopausal women have found a reduction in these effects, an improvement in sleep, a potential benefit on bone health and even a loss of body fat and small gain in LBM over the course of a year (48-52). Doses range from 1-5 mg per night with no indication of what might be optimal. I would mention again that some people find that higher doses either leave them feeling almost hung over in the morning or give them extremely strange dreams. I recommend starting at a lower dose and increasing it gradually based on individual response.

Myo-Inositol

I described the enormous potential benefits of myo-inositol in PCOS above but it may have some benefit for women going through menopause. Specifically, 2 grams of myo-inositol taken twice daily had benefits on both thyroid metabolism and insulin sensitivity while 3 mg of melatonin and 2 grams of myo-inositol at bedtime only improves insulin sensitivity (52a).

DHEA

Early in the book, I mentioned that DHEA (produced in the adrenal glands) is one of the primary androgens in women and this becomes even more true after menopause has occurred. When the ovaries stop producing hormones, adrenal hormone production because a primary source of hormones in a woman's body (as I discussed briefly in Chapter 3, there is currently great interest in androgen replacement for postmenopausal women). In addition to it's other effects, DHEA can be converted to other hormones such as testosterone and estrogen which will provide at least some estrogen signaling. For this reason, it has been suggested that supplemental DHEA might have a particularly benefit for the postmenopausal women by providing DHEA to be converted to other hormones without the potential risks that can accompany HRT.

A tremendous amount of work has been done on DHEA and supplementation has been shown to improve bone density, decrease many of the side effects related to menopause such as vaginal dryness, potentially increase muscle mass or decrease muscle loss, improve insulin sensitivity, decrease body fat levels, possibly decrease the risk of breast cancer, could decrease the risk of heart disease, help women to maintain cognitive function, increase libido, improve the skin, decrease cancer risk and reduce overall mortality (53). Amazingly, nearly every negative symptom associated with menopause without HRT seems to be improved with nothing more than DHEA supplementation.

Overall, DHEA has been shown to be incredibly safe with few negatives. The primary side effect is increased facial hair and acne but this is not surprising given that DHEA is an androgen and will have androgenic (masculinizing) effects. So far as dosing of DHEA, the majority of studies have used either a DHEA cream or as little as 50 mg day in capsule form. Given that DHEA is a hormonal precursor, women may wish to discuss it's use with their primary health care provider. Female master's athletes should be aware that DHEA is banned by many sporting federations.

I have summarized the menopausal supplements with their effects and doses below.

Product	Effect	Dose
Soy Protein	General estrogen signaling	25-30 g/day
Phytoestrogens	General estrogen signaling	50-100 mg genistein/diadzein per day
Amberen	General estrogen signaling	
Black cohosh	Reduced hot flashes	40 mg/day
St. John's Wort	Improved mood/depression	900 mg/day
Vitex Cagnus	Improved mood	500 mg chasteberry
Ginkgo bilboa	Improved memory and cognition	120 mg/day
Melatonin	Improved sleep, bone health, body composition and menopausal symptoms	1-5 mg at night*
Myo-Inositol	Improved thyroid metabolism and insulin sensitivity	2 g twice per day
DHEA	Benefits too numerous to list (see text)	DHEA cream or 50 mg/day capsule*

*High doses of melatonin cause next-day drowsiness or strange dreams in some people.
DHEA is a hormonal product and should be discussed with a primary health care provider.

Fat Loss Supplements

If there is a single category of popular, heavily marketed and enormously lucrative dietary supplements it is those aimed at fat loss. The entire industry is filled with hundreds of products, with new ones appearing annually, most of which do absolutely nothing for the consumer except to lighten their wallet. Many if not most of these products are based on animal research on mice and rats and, with almost no exceptions, do these products ever translate into a meaningful effect in humans. The general uselessness of such products has led to an oft-held belief that there are no compounds that can accelerate or facilitate fat loss but this is also untrue. There are a variety of compounds, tested in humans that have been shown to impact on some aspect of the fat loss process. They may increase energy expenditure, blunt appetite, increase fat mobilization or have other effects. The overall effect of these products is typically small and only work within the context of a proper diet/exercise program. None are required but some may be useful.

With one exception, all of the compounds I am going to talk about in this section are generally termed thermogenics (24). This is a class of compounds that frequently has multiple effects in the body but primarily leads to the burning of calories and the generation of heat ("thermo" = heat, "genesis" = making). The overall impact of these compounds is not enormous, typically causing an increase in resting metabolic rate (RMR) of ~5+% which might amount to an extra 100-150 calories burned per day. Over a month's time this might increase fat loss by roughly one pound (0.45 kg). While the thermogenic effect is not profound, these compounds often have other beneficial effects such as blunting appetite or mobilizing fat from fat cells. They frequently help to offset the normal diet related drop in metabolic rate and some have been studied in terms of long-term weight maintenance. Since most of the thermogenic compounds in use are stimulants, part of their effect may be due to an increase (NEAT).

While beneficial, the largest potential drawback to thermogenics is that they are stimulants with all that implies. While almost always well-tolerated under research conditions, there can be minor side effects including increases in heart rate and blood pressure. Taken too late at night, they can impair sleep and some people feel anxious or jittery when they use them. While these effects are typically fairly short-lived and disappear rapidly, people with pre-existing high blood pressure may need to avoid these products at least until they have lost fat and things have normalized. People prone to anxiety may be unable to use all but the mildest of these compounds and one (yohimbine) should be avoided completely.

As importantly, given the potential side effects, is the too-often seen tendency among dieters to think that more is better and to double or triple the dose in the hopes that fat loss will double or triple. A number of very publicized deaths associated with one of the compounds (ephedrine) I will discuss below is primary related to people taking too much (ephedrine was also popular in rave culture and was being used with many other drugs). When I discuss these compounds, I will generally give recommendations on how to avoid side effects and avoid any risk and I strongly suggest that readers follow them. If any negative effects are seen, the product must be discontinued as any small benefit will not be worth it.

Readers can safely assume that any product not listed is ineffective or doesn't have good human research to support it's use. Products such as Conjugated Linoleic Acid (CLA), garcinia cambogia, rasberry ketones and many more exist but do little to nothing There will be endless new products every year and it's usually safe to assume that they will be equally ineffective. This is actually true of most products where, historically, perhaps 1 in 100 products (if that) end up having any effect. Let me reiterate that none of these compounds is required for fat loss although they may be potentially useful and helpful in certain circumstances. The diet and exercise program should always be the primary focus.

Caffeine

Caffeine is arguably the single most universally used compound in the world and has slight metabolic effects in the body in terms of fat loss (I will discuss it's effects on exercise performance later in the chapter). Most people probably obtain caffeine in beverages such as coffee, tea, soda, energy drinks, etc. with the actual caffeine content of different drinks varying fairly enormously. There are also pills available, typically providing 200 mg of pure caffeine and various herbal forms such as guarana, kola nut or yerba maté are also used. Pure caffeine and coffee are not identical and coffee specifically has been found to play a role in diabetes prevention and weight control due to other compounds that are present (55).

Caffeine has a small impact on energy expenditure with 600 mg/day causing ~100 extra calories per day to be burned. As above, while small, this might increase fat loss by ~1 lb/month. It's important to note that the addition of even small amounts of cream or sugar to coffee can easily offset this increase. Speciality coffees with whip cream, flavoring, sprinkles and other additions easily contain hundreds of calories, overwhelming the small increase in energy expenditure. While research has also shown that caffeine can decrease food intake in men, this effect is not seen in women (55a). Caffeine, at an intake of 5 mg/kg/day (300 mg/day for a 132 lb/60 kg woman) was also found to prevent weight regain following an ICR type of diet (55b). Caffeine typically generates few side effects except in those who do not habitually consume it (or who stop for several days). Even these go away with regular use.

There are gender differences in caffeine metabolism. During the follicular phase, women and men metabolize caffeine identically but in the luteal phase, women show higher peak levels after ingestion with the caffeine being metabolized more slowly (it stays in her system longer). The same change in metabolism of caffeine occurs with the use of hormonal BC (56). Practically, this means that women who are using BC or in the luteal phase and who are sensitive to caffeine in terms of sleep interruption may need to reduce the amount of caffeine they are taking or consume it earlier in the day. Women sensitive to the stimulant effects may find that their tolerance changes during different phases of their cycle as well.

As I mentioned in Chapter 13, caffeine has the potential to increase the cortisol response to certain kinds of stress in women and overuse of caffeine can be a problem. Category 1 dieters often find themselves increasing their caffeine intake to enormous levels simply to maintain their energy levels and this could be potentially problematic. If cortisol is already elevated for psychological, diet and training reasons, driving it even higher with caffeine abuse could potentially contribute to the ultimate development of adaptive hypocortisolism. Some have suggested that excessive caffeine may increase PMS symptoms and women with more severe symptoms may wish to try reducing their dose until menstruation begins.

It is somewhat difficult to give an actual recommendation for daily caffeine intake. Given what I'll discuss regarding some of the other thermogenics, most of which work better with caffeine, I'd tentatively suggest 400-600 mg as an upper daily limit with this being potentially decreased during the late luteal phase. The caffeine content of drinks varies enormously. A typical cup of coffee is about 60 mg, a diet soda is about 30mg of caffeine, a typical caffeine pill contains 200 mg and some energy drinks can contain up to 400 mg of caffeine. A 400-600 mg upper limit of caffeine would allow 2-3 pure caffeine pills, up to 10 cups of coffee, 1 energy drink or, while excessive, nearly 20 cans of diet soda per day.

Capsicum/Cayenne/Hot Pepper

Capsicum is the active ingredient found in cayenne pepper and has at most mild effects on energy expenditure, fat mobilization and fat burning. Taken before exercise, it can increase the use of fat for fuel and may even activate the beige/brown fat I mentioned earlier in the book. Unlike the other compounds in this chapter, capsicum is not a stimulant. The effects of capsicum only lasts a few hours which means that multiple doses per day would be taken for maximum effect. Since cayenne pepper is used for cooking, it is not uncommon for capsicum to be eaten although the amounts used tend to be culturally based. In India, the intake of capsicum may be as high as 25-100 mg/day while it may be as low as 1.5 mg/day in other parts of the world. There are also ethnic differences in how much capsicum people can tolerate at once. People raised on hot pepper can eat them more easily than those who weren't.

The potency of capsicum is measured in what are called Scoville Heat Units (SHU) which can range from 0 (for a bell pepper) up to 1,600,000 (for a pepper called the Carolina Reaper). Cayenne pepper is generally between 30,000-40,000 SHU and commercial supplements are typically in this range (there are more concentrated forms). Research has typically used 2.5-10 mg/day which is roughly 3-10 grams of whole peppers. For those not culturally acclimated to eating hot peppers, capsicum supplements would be a better choice since there will be no spicy taste in the mouth. They should be taken with food as they can cause some degree of stomach discomfort. People who have trouble swallowing pills may wish to avoid capsicum as it's not unheard of for a gelcap to get stuck and dissolve in the throat causing severe pain.

Green Tea (ECGC) with Caffeine

Green tea, or rather it's active ingredient EGCG (epigallocatechin-3-gallate), is another compound that has been studied as a thermogenic. Like cayenne and caffeine, the effects are fairly mild, raising energy expenditure by perhaps 5% over normal. Combined with caffeine, the effect is even more potent. ECGC also seems to lack the stimulant based side-effects inherent to other compounds. While it's theoretically possible to consume ECGC in brewed tea, the amounts required tend to be enormous and isolated supplements will likely be superior. The recommended dose is 130-160 mg of EGCG with 100 mg of caffeine taken up to three times per day for a total of 390-480 mg ECGC and 300 mg of caffeine. Herbal supplements all tend to be dosed differently but should indicate either how much of the active ingredient is present or the percentage standardization so that it can be calculated.

Nicotine with Caffeine

Given it's association with smoking (and it's related health risks), I debated whether or not to include nicotine as a potential thermogenic dieting aid in this book. However, isolated nicotine, in patch or gum form, is not the same as smoking due to the presence of thousands of other chemicals in commercially produced forms of tobacco. Like the previous compounds, nicotine has mild metabolic effects, increasing energy expenditure by about 5% and this effect is enhanced if it is used with caffeine. As importantly, nicotine has a profound appetite suppressing effect and this alone could make it useful. The effects of nicotine are short lived, around 2 hours which means that any stimulant effects will dissipate rapidly. For maximum effect it would need to be taken frequently but this might give nicotine its greater potential for occasional use as needed. For example, it could be used to control night time hunger without interrupting sleep. The effective dose is 1 mg of nicotine with 100mg of caffeine.

Ephedrine with Caffeine

The final thermogenic compound I want to discuss is ephedrine, a compound I suspect many readers will be familiar with. A stimulant often found in asthma medications, ephedrine came to light as a potential fat loss compound decades ago. Almost without exception it is combined with caffeine (and occasionally other compounds) and most refer to it as the ephedrine/caffeine or EC stack. There was brief interest in the potential of aspirin to have additional benefits but it is generally unnecessary. In the 90's, the EC stack (or it's herbal equivalents ma huang and kola nut) were enormously popular. Due to misuse, there were a number of deaths associated with its use but this was invariably related to taking excessive amounts or combining it with other drugs. While the above may seem alarming, EC has been studied extensively for decades and no problems were found except for small increases in heart rate and blood pressure, both of which go away fairly rapidly. Some experience stomach upset and EC can cause some degree of anxiety or jitters in some people as well. But these effects are typically minor and well tolerated and the real problems with EC only show up with extreme mis-use. Used correctly and intelligently, EC has a stunning number of potential benefits for both weight/fat loss as well as long-term maintenance.

Of all the compounds I've discussed, EC has the most potent thermogenic effect and overall, it can increase fat loss by roughly 2 lbs (0.9kg) per month over placebo (57). This isn't an enormous amount compared to what can be achieved with diet and exercise, of course, but EC has other potential benefits. There is typically a large blunting of appetite that occurs (though this may wear off) along with increased fat mobilization and burning in muscle. The effect of ephedrine on metabolic rate can not only accelerate fat loss but help to offset the drop in metabolic rate that occurs during dieting. Of some interest, EC is almost completely unique among fat loss compounds in that its thermogenic effects actually increase over time even as the side effects lessen (58). Nobody is quite sure why but it may be related to activation of the brite/beige fat I discussed earlier in the book. EC may also help with long-term weight maintenance by offsetting the seemingly permanent decrease in adaptive thermogenesis that occurs.

As I mentioned above, the largest potential negative effect of EC are its general stimulant effects. Someone with pre-existing high blood pressure, for example, might be better off avoiding EC until some amount of fat loss has occurred (I'd note that most of the research was done on obese individuals including women and there were few problems). Even in that situation, following the recommendations I will provide momentarily should avoid negative effects in all but the most sensitive individuals. If problems still occur, the combination should be discontinued. Given that many athletes are dieting and seek fat loss, ephedrine has potential benefits here as well. I will discuss the potential benefit and drawbacks of ephedrine on exercise below.

In the earliest studies, the typical dose of EC was 20 mg of ephedrine with 200 mg of caffeine and this was usually given three times per day (i.e. 8am, 12pm, 4pm). Since it is a stimulant, taking a dose much later than 4pm can interrupt sleep although there is huge variability here. Remember that women's metabolism of caffeine is slower during the luteal phase and in response to certain types of BC and, while not studied to my knowledge, this could contribute to sleep problems.

While the above might represent an optimal dosing schedule, I recommend that anyone who has never used EC before (and this is especially true if they are in Category 3 and/or have pre-existing issues with high blood pressure or anxiety) start much more gradually. I would first recommend a half dose (10 mg ephedrine, 100 mg caffeine) taken once per day in the morning. This will ensure that sleep is not interrupted and give the person a chance to assess their tolerance to the compound. Mild side effects are very common but typically dissipate within a few days. If this dose is tolerated, either a second half-dose can be added at lunch or the morning dose can be increased to the 20 mg/200 mg level. A few days later, a second half-dose at lunch can be added. This gradual increase can continue, only so long as the compound is well tolerated up to the maximum of 20 mg ephedrine/200 mg caffeine taken three times daily.

For the most part, herbal ephedra is no longer widely available (in the US it is banned outright) and even if it were I recommend ephedrine as it has less side effects. Ephedrine is usually found in asthma medications such as Bronkaid and Primatene in the US and Chesteez in the UK although it is not available in all countries. Ephedrine is often combined with guaifenesin; this is an expectorant (it makes people cough) and is there to prevent the production of methamphetamine. Pills typically contain 20-25 mg ephedrine although some may be limited to 8 mg/pill such that 2-3 pills (16-24 mg) will be needed to get a 20 mg dose. The caffeine can be obtained from any source so long as roughly 200 mg is consumed. In the US ephedrine is highly regulated with daily and monthly purchase limits in place but even the lowest levels allow for 3 doses per day for a month. I cannot speak to other countries. Pseduoephdrine, also found in many cold medications, does not have the same metabolic and fat loss effects as ephedrine.

A question that comes up is when EC should best be added when dieting. Some prefer to start using it immediately to enhance fat loss although others prefer to save it until later in the diet when metabolic rate is starting to adapt and hunger is increasing. Given that the hunger blunting effects often disappear with chronic use, the second approach may make slightly more sense. I'd note that adding 1-3 grams of the amino acid L-tyrosine to the EC stack can increase it's appetite suppression effects. For short, more aggressive diets, starting EC at the beginning makes the most sense to accelerate fat loss. When dieting is more prolonged, it may be more beneficial to save it until perhaps the half-way point of the diet or even later. When hunger is starting to increase drastically and fat loss is starting to slow, EC can be a life-saver.

Yohimbine

The final compound I want to discuss in this section is yohimbine (the herbal form is called yohimbe). Yohimbine is not truly a thermogenic in the sense of increasing energy expenditure or generating heat. Rather it's potential fat loss effects are fairly indirect and related only to the loss of stubborn lower body fat. For this reason, only the Category 1 dieter looking to achieve the lower limits of body fat will potentially benefit from yohimbine or should even consider using it. Even there I would suggest waiting until the upper body is fairly lean (roughly 15-17% body fat by older measurement methods and 18-20% by DEXA) before considering yohimbine. Category 2 and 3 dieters will see no benefit from yohimbine and should consider the other compounds described above instead.

Yohimbine works by inhibiting alpha-2 receptors in the body which readers may recall are found in large amounts on women's lower body fat cells and which inhibit fat breakdown and mobilization. By inhibiting the inhibitor, yohimbine has the ultimate effect of increasing fat breakdown and release. Yohimbine has a secondary effect of increasing blood flow into stubborn fat which facilitates fat loss as well. While often cold to the touch, many find that lower body fat is warmer when yohimbine is used due to the increased blood flow. This gives yohimbine potential for improving lower body fat loss (59). As with the other compounds discussed, caffeine can further improve these effects. With regular use, yohimbine actually builds up in the body and often has a greater effect over time. However, yohimbine can also cause water retention to occur, potentially masking any fat loss that is happening. What generally happens in this situation is that fat in the hips and thighs start to become dimply and squishy, in contrast to its normal solid and smooth texture. Water loss usually occurs within a few days with the visual appearance of the area improving. Eliminating yohimbine for a few days will allow this to occur and I do recommend that physique competitors using yohimbine cease it's use at least a week out from the show. Like ephedrine, yohimbine is a banned substance in many sporting federations.

Yohimbine can be found in one of two forms: yohimbine HCL (the synthetic form) and yohimbe bark (the herbal form). I cannot strongly enough recommend against using the herbal form of this compound. Not only are herbal products often dosed poorly but other compounds in yohimbe bark can cause enormous side effects. People find that they both sweat and have chills and the overall response can be very negative. A pure yohmibine HCL should be found or the product should not be used at all.

Since insulin blocks the effects of yohimbine, the ideal way to take it is after an overnight fast prior to aerobic activity. This would typically be the morning although women following one of the IF'ing types of meal distributions might be performing aerobic activity in the early afternoon. In many cases, women may not be able to do fasted cardio. In this case, yohimbine can be taken 3-4 hours after a meal when insulin levels have decreased. In the situation where women are lifting weights and doing aerobic work afterwards, the best way to take yohimbine would be right as the weight workout starts so that it is reaching peak levels in an hour when the aerobic work is done. For an hour workout, this would mean taking the yohimbine at the very beginning, for a 90 minute workout it would be taken 30 minutes into training.

The recommended dose of yohimbine is 0.09 mg/lb (0.2 mg/kg) so the sample 150 lb female would use 150 lbs*0.09 mg/lb or 13.5 mg and this would be taken with 100-200 mg of caffeine. Yohimbine HCL (the synthetic form) is limited to 2.5 mg per pill so this would mean 5-6 pills (12.5-15mg) would be needed. As with the EC stack, I recommend everyone start with a half dose to assess their tolerance for the compound. The dose can be gradually increased to the maximum over a few days if it is well tolerated. To ensure that the mobilized fatty acids are burned for energy, yohimbine should be taken roughly an hour prior to low- or moderate-intensity aerobic activity. While far from universal, many who use yohimbine notice a slight tingle or itch in their hip and thigh area, probably due to increased blood flow. I will present a protocol using High-Intensity Interval Training (HIIT) in Appendix 1 but yohimbine and weight training tends to make people feel awful. Either they are generally overstimulated or get nauseous.

It is common to see bottles of yohimbine state that women should not use the product but this is based on an old misconception about how yohimbine works. Yohimbine HCL was originally used for erectile dysfunction in men and is often still prescribed for such. At that time, it was assumed that yohimbine was working hormonally, probably by raising testosterone, and this would certainly make it a poor product for women. But this is not the mechanism of action and yohimbine simply increases blood flow to the genitals. This effect is also seen in women meaning that a woman's hip and thigh fat may not be the only place that tingles during exercise.

The biggest potential risk with yohimbine is that it can increase anxiety in some people. Certainly all stimulants can do this to some degree but large doses of yohimbine are used specifically in research studies to trigger anxiety attacks. Anyone prone to anxiety of any sort must not use the compound as the potential negatives far outweigh any benefits. As well, yohimbine should never be combined with EC as the side effects tend to multiply. If both compounds are being used in a day, yohimbine should be taken at least 4 hours away from a dose of EC. Usually this would mean yohimbine in the morning and ephedrine at lunch and possibly in the afternoon but other schedules are possible.

While yohimbine is a potentially useful compound for Category 1 women dealing with stubborn lower body fat, it is not for everyone. Whether the side effects are too severe or it is banned in their sport, not everyone will be able to use it (in some countries, it can't be obtained in the first place). There are non-yohimbine based approaches to women's stubborn fat in Appendix 1.

Performance Supplements

The final category of supplements I want to look at are those that may have some benefit for sports performance. As with fat loss supplements, hundreds if not thousands of products have come and gone over the years and this will never cease to be the case. Athletes are always looking for that extra edge or magic pill to take them to the next level and supplement companies exploit that desire endlessly. My list here will actually be fairly short and I'll only note that the cutting edge of sport nutrition supplementation is finding products that may have specific benefits. Since this isn't a book on that particular topic, I will be focusing on a handful of supplements that have such enormous benefits or relatively global applications to most females. As with around workout nutrition, performance supplements are generally only relevant to the serious trainee or athlete. Performance supplements are also only relevant once a trainee's training and nutrition program (including around workout nutrition) is already in place. Like fat loss supplements, they may add a few percent of improvement to a proper program but cannot ever replace it.

Caffeine and Ephedrine

While I discussed caffeine and ephedrine above in terms of their potential metabolic and fat loss effects, I want to briefly look at them again, both separately and together, in terms of sports performance. Caffeine alone has been studied extensively and an overall picture of its effects on performance has been found. Almost without exception, caffeine improves endurance performance in events ranging from 60 seconds in duration up to 2 hours or more and this seems to be the case for all sports that have been studied (60,61). There is often enormous variability in the performance increase with caffeine with some people being clear caffeine responders and others being non-responders.

In terms of weight room performance, the impact of caffeine tends to be somewhat variable. Most find an increase in muscular endurance, the number of repetitions that can be done with a given weight, without much impact on maximal strength unless absolutely enormous doses are used (62). As usual, most of the work on this topic has been done on men and there are few studies on either endurance or strength performance in women. What little exists suggest that women get at least the same benefit (and possibly more) in endurance performance and one study did find a small (but enormously variable) increase in the maximum amount a woman could bench press with caffeine (63).

The recommended dose of caffeine to improve performance is 1.35-2.6 g/lb (3-6 mg/kg) roughly an hour before exercise and this would represent 200-400 mg of caffeine for the 150 lb sample lifter. Smaller women would use less than this and the lower doses would be within the realm of the recommended doses of caffeine I described above. For extremely high quality workouts or competition, higher doses could be beneficial but they should always be tested in training first as they may overstimulate the athlete and cause technique to suffer. High doses of caffeine on an empty stomach can cause stomach upset and in some sports requiring very fine coordination, the stimulant effects of caffeine can impair performance. I'd note again that women in the luteal phase of their menstrual cycle or who are using BC metabolize caffeine differently and this could potentially alter the response to caffeine that is seen.

For the most part, ephedrine by itself has never shown any real performance benefits and I won't discuss it further. However, in the same way that the combination of EC is more potent than either compound in terms of metabolic and fat loss effects, the combination may improve performance more than either compound alone (64). One very real effect of EC on performance is that exercise at any given intensity feels easier. This allows for a higher intensity of effort to be used which means that running or cycling speeds or the amount of weight lifted would be increased. Being able to train at a higher intensity should increase performance gains although it might just as likely cause an athlete to overtrain.

The doses of ephedrine and caffeine in the research studies have been fairly enormous. Typical amounts are 2.2 mg/lb (5 mg/kg) of caffeine and 0.25-0.45 g/lb (0.8-1 g/kg) of ephedrine. This amounts to 330 mg of caffeine and 47-65 mg of ephedrine taken all at once for the 150 lb sample lifter which is far more than the 20 mg ephedrine/200 mg caffeine combination used for fat loss. Anecdotal evidence suggests that the same 20/200 dosing will improve performance (many lifters find that they are stronger in the weight room for example). I not aware of any research that has included women or compared their response to men to see if it differs although overall metabolism of EC seems to be more or less identical.

As with caffeine, higher doses of EC might be beneficial for particularly intense workouts or competition but they must be tested during training due to their potential for side effects. Since EC can raise body temperature, there is at least hypothetical concern that using it during the luteal phase while training or competing in the heat could add to the potential for overheating. Finally, ephedrine is a banned substance in some federations although it may be allowed below a certain concentration. Before using ephedrine in training or competition, athletes must determine if it will cause them to fail a drug test.

Creatine Monohydrate

Creatine monohydrate is perhaps one of the single most well studied performance supplement in the history of supplements with hundreds of studies done over several decades. Within skeletal muscle is a compound called creatine phosphate (CP) which provides short-term energy for high intensity activities lasting around 10 seconds or so (i.e. sprinting and some types of weight training). Creatine is also found in other tissues within the body. Creatine is found primarily in red meat and can also be synthesized in the body from certain amino acids. Relevant to this chapter, supplementation of creatine monohydrate has been found to increase levels of CP within the muscle which has the result of increasing potential energy production. It also causes some degree of water retention within the muscles.

Unsurprisingly, there are gender differences in creatine metabolism and how women respond to supplementation compared to men (65). Women store less total creatine in their body than men but this is primarily due to having less total muscle mass (women's generally lower intake of red meat may also contribute). At the same time, women show either the same or slightly higher concentrations of creatine within their muscles. When supplemented with creatine, women's levels do not increase to the same degree as men and their body weight goes up less. In one study, supplementation caused an average weight gain of 1 lb (0.45 kg) in women compared to 2+ lbs (1+ kg) in men (66).

Despite those differences, creatine has been shown to improve performance in almost all sports and this improvement occurs across all ages and genders with women showing similar improvements to men (67). Strength, power and muscular endurance improve as does high intensity exercise performance. One possible exception to this are sports where the body has to be moved against gravity and where the small weight gain may be problematic. This includes running and cycling (especially on hilly routes) along with sports such as gymnastics, ballet, and others. The slight weight gain could also cause a weight-class athlete to have difficulty making their weight class. Even here, athletes can use creatine to improve the quality of their high-intensity training sessions before being removed prior to competition to drop the excess weight.

While creatine has traditionally been thought of as a performance oriented supplement, it has other potential benefits (with more being found every day) some of which may be even more important to women than to men (68). It has several potential benefits for pregnancy which are beyond the scope of this book but, more importantly may have other therapeutic benefits. In conjunction with exercise, creatine helps to offset the loss of muscle mass and bone density in older women (69). Creatine supplementation has also been shown to help with some types of depression (70). Women have a higher incidence of depression than men and might derive more benefit from creatine due to differences in brain metabolism.

Early studies on creatine generally used a dosing pattern of 20 grams of creatine per day (in 4 doses) for 5 days with a daily maintenance dose of 3-5 grams per day. Later it was found that taking smaller amounts of creatine for longer periods of time are just as effective. An athlete could take 10 grams per day for 10 days before moving to maintenance and even 3-5 grams per day for a month will eventually saturate muscle creatine stores with a maintenance dose of 3-5 grams per day maintaining them for as long as it is taken. Unless there is some extreme need to rapidly load creatine, I recommend using the lower doses for longer durations as they are more convenient and have less risk of causing stomach upset or diarrhea. Vegetarians typically have lower muscular creatine levels, probably due to their lowered meat intake, and creatine supplementation might be of even more benefit to them.

While creatine monohydrate has been the most common form used, there are others that were brought to market, usually with claims of better absorption. None of those claims were true and creatine monohydrate is as effective as any of the other forms. About the only other form of creatine that might be worth considering are the micronized forms as this tends to cause less stomach upset in sensitive individuals. Consuming creatine with some type of carbohydrate tends to improve absorption due to the insulin response and athletes can simply put their daily 3-5 g dose in the meal before or after training (some physique and strength/power athletes prefer to use creatine both before and after training sessions). I'd reiterate that there can be a small weight increase with creatine and those women who are prone to mental stress from this may wish to avoid it. Any athlete for whom increased water retention or bodyweight might cause problems during competition should discontinue creatine supplementation 1-2 weeks before competition to allow the increased water weight to dissipate.

Beta-Alanine

A relatively newer supplement, beta-alanine is a compound with solid research backing that may be able to improve longer duration maximal-intensity activities lasting from 30 seconds up to roughly 10 minutes. This would include moderate repetition weight training, most forms of HIIT, running events from the 400m to the 1600m (or any sport with events lasting in that time range) and there may even be a benefit for sports that have a sprint or HIIT component such as soccer (71). During these types of activities, acid is produced within the muscle (this causes the burning sensation) which is one cause of muscular fatigue. Among other substances, this acid is buffered within muscle by a compound called carnosine, the levels of which are raised by beta-alanine supplementation.

Beta-alanine should be dosed at 3.2-4.6 g/day in divided doses of 2 grams or less for at least 2 weeks with greater benefits seen after 4 weeks. Beta-alanine may be even more effective when used with creatine, especially for athletes who want to increase strength, power or muscle mass. In one study, the combination of 10g/day of creatine and 3.2 g/day of beta-alanine allowed a larger training volume to be done and this generated greater gains in strength and muscle mass in the long-term. To my knowledge there is no research on gender differences in beta-alanine and performance. However, women (and vegetarians) have lower levels of muscle carnosine so, just as with creatine, supplementation might benefit them even more than men.

DHEA

While I discussed DHEA in reference to adaptive hypocortisolism in Chapter 13 and again for postmenopausal women above, I want to address it briefly relative to training and performance. In Chapter 3, when I discussed BC, I mentioned that effectively all forms have the potential to decrease a woman's testosterone levels by roughly 50% through several different mechanisms. For female athletes or even the serious trainee trying to maximize her gains, this is significant with BC potentially impairing their gains in strength or muscle mass. DHEA provides a potential solution to this problem as it has been shown to restore free testosterone levels in women taking BC (72).

Specifically, 50mg of DHEA per day was sufficient to completely reverse the effect of a combined BC containing the second generation progestin levonogestrel. It was not, however, able to completely reverse the impact of a combined BC containing the fourth generation progestin drospirenone (which is known to be more anti-androgenic than other progestins). Regardless, DHEA supplementation offers a potential solution for the female athlete or serious trainee who must or simply choose to use BC. Let me state again that DHEA is a hormonal compound with potentially androgenic (masculinizing effects) and there can be side effects from its use such as acne, hair growth and others. I would recommend that any women choosing to use DHEA start with 25 mg/day (ideally blood work for DHEA and DHEA-s would be obtained to set an optimal dose) to assess their response to it. Athletes must be aware that DHEA is banned by many if not most sporting federations and could cause them to fail a drug test.

Chapter 25: Estimating Dieting Times

The next topic I want to examine is how to estimate dieting times: that is, how long it might take to realistically lose a given amount of weight or fat. This is generally important as dieters tend to have extremely unrealistic ideas about how rapidly they will be able to reach their goals. As I've mentioned rates of fat loss are always slower than the mathematical predictions based on energy balance due to metabolic slowdown, the composition of what is being lost, etc. That alone tends to increase the active dieting time by 25-50% and that is increased further by the Pre-Diet phase, Full Diet Breaks, etc. with a good rule of thumb being that it will take 50-100% longer to reach a goal than predicted (or desired). A diet calculated to reach a goal in only 12 weeks might realistically take 18-24 weeks.

For the general dieter, that rough value may be sufficient although it can still be useful to have a rough idea of how long it might take to reach a goal (or what a realistic goal in a given time frame is). Where estimating dieting times becomes truly critical is for those dieters, usually athletes, who are on a time schedule. A physique competitor or weight class athlete who must reach a specific goal by a specific date needs to know when they should begin dieting and this chapter will show how that can be determined in different situations. Let me first look at the general method of estimating dieting time.

Calculating Active Dieting Time

The first step in determining the total dieting time is to estimate the active dieting time. This represents the number of weeks of actual dieting that will be required to reach the goal (total dieting time will be longer). Three factors go into determining the active dieting time. The first is the total amount of fat/weight that needs to be lost to reach the dieter's goal. The second is the goal weekly weight loss (0.5, 1.0 or 1.5%) that the dieter will be targeting and which was used to set up the diet itself. Finally is the dieter's goal BF%. I showed the calculations for determining total fat and weight loss in Chapter 18 and readers will need to calculate that value if they haven't already. I also gave recommendations for different weekly weight loss goals in Chapter 18 which I have repeated below in a slightly different format.

	0.5%	1.0%	1.5%
General Category 3	Probably too slow	Yes	Yes (esp. initially)
General Category 2	Possible	Yes	Yes
General Category 1	Yes	Yes	2-4 Weeks Maximum
Athlete ending above 15%*	Yes	Yes	Mini-Cut
Athlete ending below 15%*	Once below 15%	Until reaching 15%	Mini-Cut OR When behind on diet

*This category includes the serious recreational trainee

As I described in Chapter 18, the choice of weekly weight loss for the general female dieter depends on their Category. For the general Category 3 dieter the 0.5% rate will be assuredly too slow and the higher rates of weight loss will usually be superior. Starting with the faster rate for the first 4-8 weeks to generate significant fat loss before moving into a more moderate 1% deficit long-term can be very effective here. In Category 2, while the 0.5% deficit is possible, the rate of weekly weight and fat loss may be disappointingly slow and the higher rates can be used. While the general Cat 1 dieter can use the 1.5% per week (assuming the diet is properly set up), it should be for short periods only and the slower rates of weekly weight loss will be more appropriate for extended diets.

Looking at both athletes and the serious recreational trainee, the choice of weekly weight loss rate will vary depending on the ending BF% goal. If the athlete will be ending their diet above 15% body fat (and realistically 18% is a more likely goal), either the 0.5% or 1.0% rate will be appropriate. As I discussed earlier in the book, the slower rate gives a greater potential to make fitness gains but the faster rate will end the diet sooner so that the athlete get back to fully fueled training. The 1.5% rate may be workable for short "mini-cuts" to keep BF% in check in the off-season but training must be reduced during that time period to avoid overtraining. It can also be used if a dieter's fat loss has fallen behind in an attempt to catch up. For the athlete who will be finishing below a body fat of 15% and this includes many types of physique competitors along with some performance athletes, the best approach will be to use a 1.0% weekly goal until 15% is reached. At this point, the 0.5% rate should be used to complete the diet.

Before looking at other issues, I want to show the basic calculation involved in estimating dieting times based on the dieter's initial weight, total weight/fat loss required and goal weekly weight loss. Say we have a serious recreational trainee who is 150 lbs at 24% body fat (115 lbs LBM) who wants to reach 18% body fat. She needs to lose ~12 pounds of total weight/fat and will target a 1% weekly weight loss. The calculation of her active dieting time appears in the box below.

> **Step 1: Convert Weekly %Weight Loss to a Decimal**
> Divide the weekly weight loss percent by 100
> 0.5% = 0.005, 1.0% = 0.01, 1.5% = 0.015
> **Step 2: Determine Weekly Weight Loss**
> Multiply body weight by the value from Step 1
> 150 pounds * 0.01 = 1.5 lbs/week
> **Step 3: Determine Total Weeks of Active Dieting**
> Divide Total Weight Loss by Average Weekly Weight Loss
> 12 lbs required weight loss / 1.5 lb/week = 8 weeks

So the theoretical amount of active dieting time that would be required for her to reach her goal would be 8 weeks. But her total estimated dieting time will be longer than this. This is where the goal BF% comes into play as more extreme diets will require greater increases in dieting time. I will be using a cutoff point of 15% body fat here although, practically, 18% body fat is the lowest that all but the most extreme dieters will typically target. When a dieter's goal body fat is above 18%, they should use the adjusted percentages shown in the table below to calculate their active dieting time. I've shown some intermediate weight loss goals of 0.75% and 1.25% as these may be appropriate under some conditions.

Weekly Weight Loss Target	0.5%	0.75%	1.0%	1.25%	1.5%
Adjusted Value for Calculation	0.375%	0.56%	0.75%	0.94%	1.13%

The top value is what should be used to set up the actual diet as described in Chapter 17 but it is the second value that should be used to estimate dieting time. That is, if a dieter is targeting 0.5% weekly weight loss, they should use 0.375% to calculate their dieting time. I've shown the adjusted calculation in the box below for the same 150 lb female dieter who needs to lose 12 pounds. While she uses 1.0% weekly weight loss to set up her diet, she will use the 0.75% value for the actual calculation.

> **Step 1: Convert Weekly %age Weight Loss to a Decimal**
> Divide the adjusted percentage weight loss by 100
> 0.375% = 0.00375, 0.75% = 0.0075, 1.13% = 0.0113
> **Step 2: Determine Weekly Weight Loss**
> Multiply body weight by the value from Step 1
> 150 pounds * 0.0075 = 1.1 lbs/week
> **Step 3: Determine Total Weeks of Active Dieting**
> Divide Total Weight Loss by Average Weekly Weight Loss
> 12 lbs required weight loss / 1.1 lb/week = 11 weeks

So while her theoretical dieting time was 8 weeks total, her actual active dieting time may be as long as 11 weeks, nearly a 40% increase. This value isn't absolute as there can be large scale variations in the metabolic adaptations, changes in NEAT, etc. with some women reaching their goals relatively faster or slower than predicted. Primarily it is to give a more realistic dieting time and act as a safety buffer for those dieters on a time schedule as it is better to start too early rather than too late.

In contrast to the situation above, the dieter who's goal body fat is below 15% should use 0.5% across the board to calculate their dieting time. This is true even if she is starting her diet with a 1% weekly goal and only switches to 0.5% as she crosses 15% body fat. While possible overestimating dieting time slightly, using this value ensures that the dieter has enough time to reach their goal without problems such as significant LBM losses, early menstrual cycle or hormonal dysfunction, etc. It's always easier to slow down the rate of fat loss when someone is ahead of their goals than it is to catch up when they are behind and using 0.5% ensures that there is sufficient dieting time. So consider the sample dieter I've used throughout this book at 150 lbs/22% body fat who needs to lose 22 lbs to reach 10% body fat.

> **Step 1: Determine Weekly Weight Loss Using 0.5%Current Bodyweight**
> 150 pounds * 0.005% = 0.75 lbs/week
> **Step 2: Determine Total Weeks of Active Dieting**
> Divide Total Weight Loss by Average Weekly Weight Loss
> 22 lbs / 0.75 lbs/week = 29.3 weeks rounded up to 30 weeks

Since it's impractical to diet for a portion of a week, her estimated dieting time is rounded up to the next higher whole number. While I won't show the calculation, if she were to estimate her dieting time based on 1% per week until 15% body fat and 0.5% after that, it would yield 21 weeks of active dieting, almost exactly 50% less than the calculated 30 weeks. If the number of weeks of active dieting were the only factor involved in determining dieting time, calculating the start date of a diet would be trivial: a 16 week diet would be started 4 months before the goal date. But there are other factors to consider.

Adding the Other Factors

While the above calculation provides the active dieting time, there are other factors that must be added to that value to determine the total dieting time. The first is the Pre-Diet phase which may not be needed at all or last up to 8 weeks depends on the specific situation. Whether or not it technically adds to the dieting time also depends on the situation. For the beginning dieter, it does factor into dieting time while for many athletes it is really the last month of their previous training phase. The second addition is the Full Diet Break which will need to be added at appropriate interval depending on the duration of the diet and the dieter's Category. Recommended frequencies for Full Diet Breaks appear below.

Category	1	2	3
Frequency of Break	6-10 weeks	10-14 weeks	14-18 weeks

Depending on the situation, anywhere from zero up to 3 full diet breaks (for very extended diets) will be necessary. How much time this adds to the diet depends on how long of a diet break is used. One week is the absolute minimum duration but two-week diet breaks can be appropriate in certain situations. For longer diets, it's generally best to use 1-week diet breaks and this means that up to 3 total weeks may be added to the diet. For athletes or the serious recreational trainee (but not the general dieter), an additional week will be required for any final dietary manipulations (i.e. peak week, making weight, etc.)

A final factor, relevant only to the normally cycling female, is the additional 1-2 weeks that may be required to ensure that the diet starts in the follicular phase. This may not necessarily mean that time has to be added to the diet so much as that it's start should be shifted. In some cases, the Pre-Diet Phase, if it is being used, can be set so that it ends in the late luteal phase which means that active dieting will begin in the follicular phase. Women with any hormonal modifier need not worry about this.

Depending on the specific situation, all of the above might be added to the total dieting time. So consider the serious recreational trainee from above at 150 lbs who needs 11 weeks to lose 12 pounds prior to a vacation She will not need to perform a Pre-Diet phase and since she is in Category 1 and technically only needs a single one-week diet break around the 6-10 week mark of her diet. Since her diet is only 11 weeks long to begin with she can probably ignore the break as her diet will end right about the time any problems might start (her vacation will act as a diet break). Assuming she doesn't use the diet break and is going on vacation on July 1st, her diet would start in the second week of April. If she needed to adjust the diet so that it started in the first week of her menstrual cycle, she would conceivably need to add 1-2 weeks and start her diet in the last week of March. Her diet schedule appears below.

Week	April				May				June				July
Week	1	2	3	4	1	2	3	4	1	2	3	4	1
Eating	N	D	D	D	D	D	D	B	D	D	D	D	Holiday

*N = Normal eating, D = Dieting, B = Diet break (if used)

With the above general method explained, I want to look at population specific issues for the general dieter, serious recreational trainee and different types of athletes. For the final group, I will divide dieter by whether or not they are targeting a BF% above or below 18% rather than by sports category.

The General Dieter

Other than understanding that the actual time to reach their weight and fat loss goals are likely to be longer than predicted or hoped for, I don't generally think that the general dieter should worry too much about predicting their dieting times. Certainly, having a rough idea of the expected dieting times to reach a short- or long-term (or even dream) goal can act as a reality check on how long reaching those goals are likely to take and knowing this beforehand can have two potential outcomes. For some dieters, knowing the actual duration that might be required to reach a long-term goal can be discouraging and this is why I recommend focusing on shorter term goals instead. Alternately, having realistic expectations that can actually be met within the goal time frame can be encouraging.

In the general dieting population, I feel that dieting should be looked at a long-term process (and a learning experience). Poor dietary and lifestyle habits don't develop overnight and they certainly don't reverse themselves overnight. Focusing only on the end goal can be frustrating while focusing on the process (and realizing that mistakes will be made and can act as a time to make changes aimed at future success) is often superior. This is especially true when looking at the issue of long-term weight maintenance. Here it is the habits developed during the diet that tend to be associated with success and this is a problem with diets (or dieters) that only focus on short-term changes. While often achieving large-scale weight losses, these approaches have almost no chance of succeeding in the long-term as no true behavior changes have occurred. This isn't to say that keeping the long-term goal in mind is bad but that focusing on what hasn't yet been achieved instead of what has been accomplished can be detrimental.

For those general dieters who still want to estimate their dieting time, the above method will be used. First they should determine the total weight loss needed and I'd reiterate that the Category 2 and 3 dieter should really be using their short-term goal weight loss rather than their long-term or dream goal targets. They should then determine what weekly weight loss target they will be using to set up their diet. Since no dieter in this population will be dieting below 18% body fat, they will use the adjusted values from above. To that calculation, the following will be added.

	Pre-Diet Phase	Full Diet Break	Final Week
Category 1	4-8 Weeks	2 Weeks Every 6-10 Weeks	No
Category 2	4-8 Weeks (optional)	2 Weeks Every 10-14 Weeks	No
Category 3	4-8 Weeks (optional)	2 Weeks Every 14-18 Weeks	No

As indicated in the chart, not all general dieters will require the Pre-Diet Phase although it may be beneficial. The general Category 2 or 3 dieter can technically move directly into dieting since they are not at risk for impairing menstrual cycle function, etc. However, the normally cycling general Category 1 dieter faces both the risk of menstrual cycle dysfunction along with excessive LBM loss if they aren't involved in an exercise program. At least a 4 week Pre-Diet phase should be used to start a proper training program prior to beginning all but the most moderate diets (and the Pre-Diet phase will be part of total dieting time). Unless dieting times for very large weight losses are being estimated, diet breaks are best used between blocks of active dieting. There will never be any need to add an additional week after the diet ends and the normally cycling dieter may adjust the start of their diet to begin in the follicular phase.

Example 1

A Category 3 female who weighs 250 pounds is targeting a 10% (25 lb) weight loss. She is targeting a 1% weekly weight loss and will use 0.75% to calculate her active dieting time.

> **Step 1: Convert Weekly %age Weight Loss to a Decimal**
> Divide the adjusted percentage weight loss by 100
> 0.75% = 0.0075
> **Step 2: Determine Weekly Weight Loss**
> Multiply body weight by the value from Step 1
> 250 pounds * 0.0075 = 1.9 lbs/week
> **Step 3: Determine Total Weeks of Active Dieting**
> Divide Total Weight Loss by Average Weekly Weight Loss
> 25 lbs required weight loss / 1.9 lb/week = 13 weeks

Since she is in Category 3, she will not need to use a Pre-Diet phase and can move immediately into dieting (exercise can and should be introduced gradually if at all possible). As Category 3 dieters only need a diet break every 14-18 weeks which is more than her actual dieting time that too can be eliminated. She will not need an additional week at the end of the diet and the only possible adjustment would be to begin the diet during the follicular phase to take advantage of better controlled hunger. This doesn't actually change the duration of the diet but only when it might ideally start. So her actual dieting time will be 13 weeks with no modifications. At the end of that 13 weeks, she would take at least a 2 week Full Diet Break which will give her an opportunity to practice eating at maintenance. The break can be longer as needed or desired and eventually she is likely to move back into active dieting, targeting her next short-term goal. Assuming she starts her diet on January 1st, the block of dieting will look like this.

	Jan				Feb				Mar				April			
Week	1	2	3	4	1	2	3	4	1	2	3	4	1	2	3	4
Eating	D	D	D	D	D	D	D	D	D	D	D	D	D	B	B	D

*N = Normal eating, D = Dieting, B = Diet break

For comparison, I want to look at how the duration above will change if she is targeting a full 50 pounds of weight loss. Rather than do a single calculation for the full 50 lbs, I'll start with the 13 weeks for her to get to 225 pounds and then determine the dieting time for an additional 25 pounds of weight loss. The difference is that I will adjust the weekly weight loss (still at 1%) for her new body weight in Step 2

> **Step 1: Convert Weekly %age Weight Loss to a Decimal**
> Divide the adjusted percentage weight loss by 100
> 0.75% = 0.0075
> **Step 2: Determine Weekly Weight Loss**
> Multiply body weight by the value from Step 1
> 225 pounds * 0.0075 = 1.9 lbs/week
> **Step 3: Determine Total Weeks of Active Dieting**
> Divide Total Weight Loss by Average Weekly Weight Loss
> 25 lbs required weight loss / 1.6 lb/week = 15.6 (16) weeks

So while it should only have taken her 13 weeks to lose the first 25 pounds, you can see that the next 25 is predicted to take 16 weeks due to the reduced total weight loss she will be experiencing. Adding this 16 weeks to her original 13 weeks gives 29 weeks of active dieting time. The Pre-Diet phase and final week are still not needed but she will need to take a diet break at roughly the halfway point and this will add 2 weeks to her total diet for a total of 31 weeks (nearly 8 months). Even this assumes everything goes perfectly and it may still take longer for her to lose 50 pounds (I described a study in Chapter 18 where nearly half of female dieters lost less than 37 pounds in 48 weeks). Once again, this is a big reason that I think setting long-term/dream goals and then focusing primarily on short-term goals is superior for this group. Dieting durations become overwhelmingly long as the total amount of fat loss desired goes up.

Example 2

A non-exercising 145 pound Category 1 female wants to lose 10 pounds. She will target a 1% weekly weight loss and use 0.75% to calculate her active dieting time.

> **Step 1: Convert Weekly %age Weight Loss to a Decimal**
> Divide the adjusted percentage weight loss by 100
> 0.75% = 0.0075
> **Step 2: Determine Weekly Weight Loss**
> Multiply body weight by the value from Step 1
> 145 pounds * 0.0075 = 1.1 lbs/week
> **Step 3: Determine Total Weeks of Active Dieting**
> Divide Total Weight Loss by Average Weekly Weight Loss
> 10 lbs required weight loss / 1.1 lb/week = 9 weeks

\

Since her total weight loss is fairly small, the diet's duration is also relatively short (though most women would hope for this to happen twice as quickly). However, due to being in Category 1 and not exercising, she must perform a minimum 4 week Pre-Diet Phase where she introduces proper exercise (primarily resistance training) to avoid LBM loss and the potential for weight rebound when the diet is over. Since her active dieting time is only 9 weeks she will not need a diet break and there is no need to have an additional week at the end of the diet. Her total diet will last roughly 13 weeks at which point she will move into maintenance. Assuming a January 1st start, her overall dieting plan would look like this:

	Jan				Feb				Mar				April			
Week	1	2	3	4	1	2	3	4	1	2	3	4	1	2	3	4
Eating	P	P	P	P	D	D	D	D	D	D	D	D	D	Maintenance		

*P = Pre-Diet Phase, D = Dieting, B = Diet break

Another Approach for the General Dieter

In addition to using the above, I want to present the general dieter with another potential tool that they can use which is an online weight-loss calculator developed from numerous studies on fat loss (1). The calculator can be found at:

http://goo.gl/QorxO2

And will let users enter their weight, activity levels, goal weight/fat loss, calorie deficit and other variables which are then used to predict a theoretical weight loss curve over time. The calculator does only estimate weight loss (rather than fat loss) and there are a huge number of estimations and assumptions built into it. One is the rate of metabolic adaptation that might occur which can vary enormously between any two women. Some may lose less and others more quickly than predicted. Of more importance, the calculator is making some assumptions about the proportions of fat and LBM that are being loss that may not be correct. A recent study in Category 2 women found that the calculator drastically underestimated the total weight loss in response to both moderate (500 cal/day) and severe (1000 cal/day) deficits (2). There are a number of reasons for the discrepancy not the least of which is that the calculator predicted a large loss of LBM. However, due to engaging in resistance exercise, the women actually lost no LBM and this decreased the total amount of weight loss (but not fat loss) that actually occurred. I would expect the calculator to be nearly useless for the general Category 1 dieter or active individuals.

Strictly speaking, the calculator is not calculating the time to reach a specific goal but rather the expected losses over a given amount of time. This can still be informative as it will indicate the amount of real-world weight loss that might occur over a given time frame for a specific calorie deficit.

The Serious Recreational Trainee

The serious recreational dieter falls in-between the general dieter and competitive athlete in terms of their overall need to estimate their dieting time. Certainly there can be time constraints in this population that is either self-imposed or for a special event (i.e. holiday) or physique transformation contest. But, as often as not the goals are simply more about improving appearance without any specific time pressure. Even here, having an idea of how long it might take to reach a certain goal is useful, if for no other reason than to provide an oft-needed reality check on what time frames are required to reach a goal.

While it's not impossible that a serious recreational trainee would be in Category 3, it's far more likely for them to be in Category 2 or the higher range of Category 1. Looking at realistic time frames, a Category 2 recreational trainee would likely be targeting Category 1 (24% or below) while a Category 1 trainee might be targeting 18-20%. Generally, weekly targets of 0.5-1% are appropriate in this population although the 1.5% rate can be used for short (2-4 week) diets. Since a goal BF% below 18% should not generally be targeted, the adjusted percentages from above should be used for the calculation of active dieting time. To that the following will be added.

	Pre-Diet Phase	Full Diet Break	Final Week
Category 1	2 Weeks*	1-2 Weeks Every 6-10 Weeks	Possibly
Category 2	2 Weeks*	1-2 Weeks Every 10-14 Weeks	Possibly

*If used at all

By definition, the serious trainee is already engaged in intense exercise and this means that the Pre-Diet Phase may not be required. If it is used at all, 2 weeks at maintenance calories prior to starting the diet should be more than sufficient. Since the serious recreational trainee is already training, the Pre-Diet phase isn't necessarily considered part of the actual dieting time but really just a maintenance phase at the end of the previous training phase. Whether or not the Full Diet Breaks will even be needed will depend on the dieter's initial and goal BF% and generally only one (and an absolute maximum of two) will be required. In general, a final week probably won't be required but it's not uncommon for recreational trainees to schedule a photo shoot (or be involved in some sort of transformation competition) where they use some of the manipulations that physique competitors use in the final week. If desired, the start of the diet might be adjusted to begin in the follicular phase as needed.

Example 1

A Category 1 female at 135 lbs and 22% body fat wants to reach 18% body fat and this will require a fat loss of 7 lbs. Since she only has a small amount of fat to lose, she will set up her diet based on a 0.75% weekly weight loss meaning that she will use 0.56% to estimate he dieting time.

Step 1: Convert Weekly %age Weight Loss to a Decimal
Divide the adjusted percentage weight loss by 100
0.56% = 0.0056
Step 2: Determine Weekly Weight Loss
Multiply body weight by the value from Step 1
135 pounds * 0.0056 = 0.75 lbs/week
Step 3: Determine Total Weeks of Active Dieting
Divide Total Weight Loss by Average Weekly Weight Loss
7 lbs required weight loss / 0.75 lb/week = 9.3 (10) weeks

So her active dieting time will be 10 weeks and to this she will first add a 2 week Pre-Diet Phase. Although a Full Diet Break is indicated between 6-10 weeks of dieting, with a diet only last 10 weeks she can probably skip it. She will schedule a photo shoot after the diet is over and add a final peak week (acting as a break) such as a physique athlete would use for a total dieting time of 11 weeks. For a photo shoot in the first week of May, she should start dieting in the first week of February. If a Pre-Diet phase were included, this would begin in the second week of January. I've shown the latter case below.

	January				February				March				April				May			
Week	1	2	3	4	1	2	3	4	1	2	3	4	1	2	3	4	1	2	3	4
Eating	N	N	P	P	D	D	D	D	D	D	D	D	D	D	D	Peak	Photos	N		

*N = Normal eating, P = Pre-Diet Phase, D = Dieting, B = Diet break

For the normally cycling serious trainee, the above might need to be adjusted forwards or backwards by 1-2 weeks to begin the diet in the follicular phase.

Example 2

A Category 2 female at 155 lbs and 35% body fat wants to reach 22% body fat and this will require a fat loss of 26 lbs. She will target a 1% weekly weight loss and will use 0.75% to estimate her active dieting time.

Step 1: Convert Weekly %age Weight Loss to a Decimal
Divide the adjusted percentage weight loss by 100
0.75% = 0.0075
Step 2: Determine Weekly Weight Loss
Multiply body weight by the value from Step 1
155 pounds * 0.0075 = 1.15 lbs/week
Step 3: Determine Total Weeks of Active Dieting
Divide Total Weight Loss by Average Weekly Weight Loss
26 lbs required weight loss / 1.15 lbs/week = 22.6 (23) weeks

---

Due to the significant loss of body fat that she is targeting, her active dieting time is nearly 6 months and this is a reality for this type of goal. By the time a 2 week Pre-Diet Phase (if used) and at least 2 1-week Diet Breaks are added, her total dieting time would be 28 weeks or 7 months. While this duration of continuous dieting might be possible (and in certain situations may be required), it is unrealistic for most dieters. Here, the calculation acts less as an estimate of the dieting time and more as a reality check on the goal, indicating that it is not realistic to reach that BF% in a single uninterrupted diet. While the above might represent a long-term or dream goal but (as I discussed in Chapter 18), it would be superior in this situation to diet down in more realistic length blocks alternated with periods at maintenance.

Attempting to first go from 155 lbs/35% to 144/30%% body fat only requires a total loss of 11-12 pounds which could be accomplished in ~11 weeks of active dieting and 13 weeks of total dieting after a 2-week Pre-Diet phase is performed. Having reached that sub-goal, that level could be maintained for 1-2 months (possibly focusing on gaining small amounts of muscle) before dieting further to 133 lbs/25% body fat. This would require an additional 11-12 pounds of fat loss and ~11 more weeks of active dieting. Since no Pre-Diet phase would be required, this will represent the total dieting time. She would enter maintenance again and could diet down further as desired. While this approach takes longer, it is more likely to succeed by breaking unrealistically long dieting times into more realistic and achievable blocks.

Athletes Ending Above 18% Body fat

Rather than look at each type of dieting athlete separately, I will subdivide them based on their goal BF% since that is what determines what specific method they will use to estimate their dieting time. The first group I will look at are those athletes who will not be dieting below ~18% body fat. This will include the majority of strength/power athletes, most weight-class athletes (excepting possibly lightweight rowers who may need to reduce BF% to lower levels) and at least some types of performance athletes (i.e. volleyball, basketball, some swimmers and cyclists). The only physique athlete that might be in this group is the bikini competitor as they may only need to reach 18-20% body fat for competition.

A majority of these athletes will have either a specific date by which they need to reach their goal or at least a general range of dates by which they need to reach top shape. Knowing how long the diet is likely to take is important here to know how early it needs to start and this is in contrast to the general dieter and serious recreational trainee for whom this is not usually the case.

While it's not impossible for athletes in any of these groups to be in Category 3, the reality is that those athletes are typically in the super heavy weight classes of strength/power sports (where BF% is more or less irrelevant) or in sports where higher BF% are allowed or preferred. Most commonly, athletes will either be in the higher range of Category 1 or Category 2. Since they will not be going below 18% body fat, athletes in this group will use the adjusted values from above to perform the dieting time calculations and to that they will add the following.

	Pre-Diet Phase	Full Diet Break	Final Week
Bikini	Optional*	1 Week Every 6-10 Weeks	Yes
Strength/Power	2-4 Weeks	1 Week Every 6-10 Weeks (Cat 1) 1 Week Every 10-14 Weeks (Cat 2)	Yes
Weight-Class	Possibly*	1 Week Every 6-10 Weeks (Cat 1) 1 Week Every 10-14 Weeks (Cat 2)	Yes
Performance	Generally No	1 Week Every 6-10 Weeks (Cat 1) 1 Week Every 10-14 Weeks (Cat 2)	Yes

*Depending on whether or not they are performing regular aerobic exercise already

Whether or not a Pre-Diet phase is required in this group depends on the specifics of the sport. If regular aerobic work is already being done, as is usually the case for bikini competitors, some weight class (i.e. mixed martial arts) and performance athletes, a Pre-Diet phase will not be required. If aerobic work is not being done, a minimum 2 week Pre-Diet phase should be performed and this is really just part of the previous training phase more than part of the actual diet. Depending on their category, a one week Full Diet Break will be required every 6-10 or 10-14 weeks. Since the total fat loss required isn't enormous and the diets shouldn't be excessively long, 1-2 total diet breaks are all that will usually be required. Finally, all athletes will be need a final week at the end of their diet. Bikini athletes have a peak week while strength/power and weight class athletes may be manipulating water. Performance athletes need to refill muscle glycogen and recover before their competition, often performing peaking workouts as well.

Example 1

A bikini athlete at 125 lbs/22% body fat (97.5 lbs LBM) wants to reach 18% for a competition. This requires 6 lbs of fat loss which will be adjusted upwards to 7 lbs to account for potential LBM loss. She will use an intermediate weekly weight loss target of 0.75% which means that she will calculate her dieting time with a multiplier of 0.56%.

Step 1: Convert Weekly %age Weight Loss to a Decimal Divide the adjusted percentage weight loss by 100 0.56% / 100 = 0.0056 **Step 2: Determine Weekly Weight Loss** Multiply body weight by the value from Step 1 125 pounds * 0.0056 = 0.7 lbs/week **Step 3: Determine Total Weeks of Active Dieting** Divide Total Weight Loss by Average Weekly Weight Loss 7 lbs required weight loss / 0.7 lbs/week = 10 weeks

So she will need 10 weeks of active dieting to reach her fat loss goals. Assuming she needs no Pre-Diet Phase she would need at most a 1-week Full Diet Break about halfway through her diet along with a final peak week prior to her competition for a total of 12 weeks of dieting time. Knowing this she would count back from her competition date to start exactly 3 months prior. If her competition was on July 1st, she would need to start her diet on April 1st and her schedule would look like this.

	April				May				June				July	
Week	1	2	3	4	1	2	3	4	1	2	3	4	1	
Eating	D	D	D	D	D	D	B	D	D	D	D	P	Competition	

*D = Dieting, B = Diet break, P = Peak Week

If she were normally cycling and the start of her diet occurred during her luteal phase, she would need to move the start of her diet back two weeks for a total of 14 weeks and could use a slightly lower weekly weight loss target initially to avoid reaching peak condition too early (although this is far less of a problem than reaching it too late). What she does after her competition can vary. In some cases, athletes only target a single competition in which case she can go back to normal eating and training. In others, they will plan to compete multiple times once they are already in shape. T How this is approached depends on the specifics of the situation but the details are beyond the scope of this book.

Example 2

A female swimmer is 145 lbs/28% body fat (105 lbs LBM) and wants to reach 20% body fat for her competition phase. This requires a 14 lb fat loss which is adjusted upwards to 15 lbs for LBM loss. She will target a 1% weekly weight loss rate meaning she will use a 0.75% value to calculate her dieting time.

Step 1: Convert Weekly %age Weight Loss to a Decimal Divide the adjusted percentage weight loss by 100 0.75% / 100 = 0.0075 **Step 2: Determine Weekly Weight Loss** Multiply body weight by the value from Step 1 145 pounds * 0.0075 = 1.1 lbs/week **Step 3: Determine Total Weeks of Active Dieting** Divide Total Weight Loss by Average Weekly Weight Loss 15 lbs required weight loss / 1.1 lbs/week = 13.6 (14) weeks

Unless she is coming out of a complete training break, she will not need a Pre-Diet Phase and the only additions will be 1 and possibly 2 1-week Diet Breaks during her diet along with 1 week at the end of the diet for recovery and this will mean a total dieting time of 16-17 weeks. While this is not excessively long, this is 4 months during which her training may be somewhat limited by her reduced calorie intake. In future seasons, it would probably be better for her to maintain a lower BF% in future seasons to limit the amount of dieting required to reach her goal. If she limits her BF% to no more than 24% in future seasons, her overall dieting time to reach 20% will be cut in half. Since she is not targeting a specific date (unless her first competition is particularly important) but rather her overall competition period, she doesn't have the same need to start on an exact date as other athletes. The swimming season begins in September and she should aim to reach top condition fairly early in the season so her diet should start roughly in May.

	May				June				July				August				September
Week	1	2	3	4	1	2	3	4	1	2	3	4	1	2	3	4	
Eating	D	D	D	D	D	D	D	B	D	D	D	D	D	D	D	R	Competition

*D = Dieting, B = Diet break, R= Recovery

This could be varied. If August were planned as a particularly intensive month of training, she would probably be better off starting her diet in April and dieting through May, June and July so that she can support the August training with sufficient calorie intake as she enters the competition period.

	April				May				June				July				August	September
Week	1	2	3	4	1	2	3	4	1	2	3	4	1	2	3	4	Intensive Training	
Eating	D	D	D	D	D	D	D	B	D	D	D	D	D	D	D	R	Maintenance	Competition

*D = Dieting, B = Diet break, R = Recovery

Due to the fact that her diet is relatively prolonged, which may impair her ability to train effectively, it may be better to divide the full diet into two shorter diets with a month-long break between them to maintain, rebuild fitness, etc. The break could be scheduled to coincide with a particularly heavy training block. Assuming it occurs in June, she would diet in April and May, maintain through June and then finish her diet in July and August into her September competition season.

	April				May				June				July				August				September
Week	1	2	3	4	1	2	3	4	1	2	3	4	1	2	3	4	1	2	3	4	
Eating	D	D	D	D	D	D	D	R	N	N	N	N	D	D	D	D	D	D	D	R	Competition

*D = Dieting, B = Diet break, R = Recovery

Athletes Ending Below 18% Body fat

Finally are those athletes who will be targeting a final body fat of 18% or lower. This primarily includes all non-bikini physique athletes (bodybuilding, physique, fitness, and figure) along with most endurance athletes such as runners, cyclists, swimmers and triathletes. Other athletes such as sprinters and some soccer players may compete at low BF% levels such as this as well. Dieters in this category face a number of issues that women in the other groups do not. The first is that they are frequently targeting the lowest limits of human BF% that a woman might achieve. That alone brings with it all of the possible problems I described earlier in the book in terms of menstrual cycle disruption/dysfunction (including amenorrhea), negative hormonal changes, bone density loss, immune system dysfunction and others. More practically, the realities of dieting to that level of body fat means that extremely prolonged dieting times are not only required but more or less unavoidable and I want to look at why this is the case.

A primary factor is that athletes in this category generally have a limit to how lean they can be when starting their diet. Ideally, an athlete trying to reach the lower limits of BF% would start out fairly close to their goal (as I've recommended for athletes trying to reach 18% or above) but trying to maintain a ver low BF% year around causes enormous problems. Physique and strength/power (but to a lesser degree endurance and other high-performance athletes) often find that making gains in muscle or performance is difficult at even 18% body fat which ultimately limits them reaching their potential or making meaningful gains between competition. Additionally, there may be constant hunger, food focus and higher stress levels since the person is essentially dieting all the time. They end up restricting calories year round and this causes some to remain near or even below the critical energy availability (EA) threshold with all of the consequences on menstrual cycle function, bone density loss and others that I described in Chapter 12.

Even if they aren't below the critical EA threshold at this point, they will typically drop below it very quickly when they begin their diet and induce hormonal dysfunction. A case study that I will discuss in detail in Chapter 34 found exactly that in a female physique competitor who started her diet at too low a

BF5, with an already low EA, crossing the critical threshold immediately upon starting her diet and losing her menstrual cycle just as rapidly. At the same time, starting at too high of a BF% makes it nearly impossible to reach the lower limits of BF% in any reasonable time frame. Any woman starting much higher than 22-24% body fat will find that her predicted dieting time may approach the better part of a year which is physically and mentally exhausting. Realistically, and I'll show this at the end of the chapter, a woman in the high 20% body fat range cannot reach the lower limits of female BF% (though she might get to the middle teens) in any reasonable time frame.

Ultimately a balance must be struck between starting off lean enough to reach the ultimate goal while not being so lean that other problems occur. Practically, 18-22% is about the right range and even 18% will be too low for some with most women attempting to reach the lower limits of BF% ideally starting in the 22-24% range. Even more ideally they would have maintained this level of body fat for several months prior to starting their diet. This will allow them to entire their dieting phase with the highest calorie intake (and Energy Availability) while still being at an appropriate body fat level. Other athletes, who may have to start their diet fairly soon after their off-season may not have this option but physique athletes typically train year round with few long breaks and can aim to do this.

All of these factors can add up very long diets often in excess of 6 months to drop from 22-24% to 10% body fat. For athletes, physique or otherwise, used to shorter but more extreme diets, this can cause a bit of mental shock since they may be used to doing it in half that time (or have heard top competitors claim to get into shape in 12 weeks or less). But dieting in this fashion has enormous benefits. For the physique athlete, it allows for more dietary flexibility, less restrictive diets and less total cardio. This adds up to less psychological and physiological stress overall. For all types of athletes dieting to the low extreme of BF%, performance (and LBM) is often better maintained due to the lessened requirement for severe restriction and menstrual cycle dysfunction tends to be delayed as the critical EA threshold is not crossed as quickly. Full-blown amenorrhea may be avoided completely by dieting in this fashion. At the very least it will be vastly delayed. Ultimately, the benefits of a longer diet far outweigh the negatives.

While performance athletes may be targeting a longer competition phase, in which case they may not need to reach peak body composition at a specific date, the physique athlete will always have a specific date by which they must reach peak condition. They may be dieting for a single competition or for a series of competitions but, unless the first competition is being used to test out various peak week strategies, they will need to start their diet with sufficient time to reach their goal by that specific date.

As I described earlier in the chapter, typically the dieter in this category can start with a 1.0% weekly weight loss target earlier in the diet and move to 0.5% once they reach about 15% body fat/roughly the middle of the diet (for short mini-cuts they might use 1.5% per week but this is a short-term approach only). However, they should always use 0.5% weekly weight loss to calculate their total active dieting time. To that active dieting time, the following will be added (I'm assuming that all athletes attempting to diet to sub 18% are starting in Category 1).

	Pre-Diet Phase	Full Diet Break	Final Week
Physique	Depends*	1 Week every 6-10 weeks	Yes
Performance	Generally No	1 Week Every 6-10 Weeks	Yes

*Depending on whether or not they are performing regular aerobic exercise already

The physique athlete may or may not need a 2-4 week Pre-Diet phase depending on the amount of aerobic work they have been doing in the off-season. If they have been doing none or little (less than three sessions per week), and this isn't uncommon when gains in muscle mass are the goal, the Pre-Diet phase should be inserted and 4 weeks will probably be required to gradually increase the amount of aerobic work being done. Performance athletes, unless they are coming straight out of their off-season will not need the Pre-Diet phase under most circumstances. If the Pre-Diet phase is required, it doesn't exactly add to the total diet duration but represents the final phase of their training prior to starting active dieting.

To this a 1-week Full Diet Break should be inserted every 6-10 weeks with the breaks becoming more frequent as the dieter gets leaner. If there is time a 2-week diet break would be ideal but the diet is already long enough and 1 week is generally a better choice. Due to the extended nature of the diet, there will be 2 or 3 diet breaks, adding 2-3 total weeks to the diet. Both groups of athletes will need to add a final week, the physique athlete for any peak week manipulations and the performance athlete for general recovery and to refill muscle glycogen prior to their first major competition.

Example 1

A female runner is 125 lbs at 19% body fat (101 lbs LBM) and wants to get to 12% for her competition season. This will require a total fat loss of roughly 10 pounds which will be adjusted up to 11 pounds to account for LBM loss (she may lose more if she is not resistance training). She will likely start her diet aiming for a 0.75% weekly weight loss and move to 0.5% once she crosses 15% but she will use 0.5% weekly weight loss to estimate her active dieting time.

> **Step 1: Convert Weekly %age Weight Loss to a Decimal**
> Divide the adjusted percentage weight loss by 100
> 0.5% / 100 = 0.005
> **Step 2: Determine Weekly Weight Loss**
> Multiply body weight by the value from Step 1
> 125 pounds * 0.005 = 0.6 lbs/week
> **Step 3: Determine Total Weeks of Active Dieting**
> Divide Total Weight Loss by Average Weekly Weight Loss
> 11 lbs required weight loss / 0.63 lbs/week = 17.5 (18) weeks

Her active dieting time is 18 weeks and she will not need to perform a Pre-Diet phase under most circumstances. She will also need to plan a single week of recovery for recovery after her diet before her main competitions start. Since her diet is only 18 weeks, she can technically get away with one full diet break and use the recovery week as the second one. Alternately she could plan for two full diet breaks and have them a bit more frequently. The typical running season starts around May or June but unless she has an important competition early in her season, she can technically finish her dieting in the early part of her competition phase. At the latest she should plan on starting her diet in the first of January (conveniently after the holidays are over). I've shown her schedule with both one and two diet breaks and her diet continuing through the beginning of the competition season below.

	January				February				March				April				May				June
Week	1	2	3	4	1	2	3	4	1	2	3	4	1	2	3	4	1	2	3	4	
1 Break	D	D	D	D	D	D	D	D	D	P	D	D	D	D	D	D	D	D	D	R	N
2 Breaks	D	D	D	D	D	D	P	D	D	D	D	D	D	D	P	D	D	D	D	R	N

*D = Dieting, P = Diet break, R = Recovery, N = Normal

Example 2

The final example is the book's sample female at 150 lbs/22% body fat (117 lbs) LBM. She will be dieting to 10% for a physique contest and this will require 20 lbs of fat loss and this will be adjusted to 22 lbs of total weight loss to account for potential LBM loss. She will start with a 1.0% weekly weight loss although this will be adjusted as the diet continues to 0.75% and finally to 0.5% at the end of the diet although she will use 0.5% weekly loss to estimate her active dieting time.

> **Step 1: Convert Weekly %age Weight Loss to a Decimal**
> Divide the adjusted percentage weight loss by 100
> 0.5% / 100 = 0.005
> **Step 2: Determine Weekly Weight Loss**
> Multiply body weight by the value from Step 1
> 150 pounds * 0.005 = 0.75 lbs/week
> **Step 3: Determine Total Weeks of Active Dieting**
> Divide Total Weight Loss by Average Weekly Weight Loss
> 22 lbs required weight loss / 0.75 lbs/week = 29.3 (30) weeks

You can see that her active dieting time is already extremely prolonged but, once again, this is necessary to optimize the diet/avoid the problems associated with shorter diet durations and more extreme approaches. Ideally this competitor would be coming out of 2-3 months of maintenance/consolidation training from her last muscular gaining phase and the final month of that training would act as her Pre-Diet Phase where she would be at maintenance calories and start to bring in aerobic work gradually. With an active dieting time of 30 weeks and a requirement to take a Full Diet Break every 6-10 weeks, she will need three breaks and add 3 weeks to her total. Finally are her peak week manipulations which add a single week. Ignoring the Pre-Diet phase, which really represents the end of her previous training rather than the start of her diet, her estimated total dieting time will be 34 weeks or 8.5 months.

Although it's not uncommon for physique competitors to enter multiple contests in the modern era since they are already near peak condition (some physique sports also have qualifiers for championships), her first competition will still be occurring at a specific date. Unless she intends to use it as a test-run for her peak week manipulations, this means that she should be in peak condition at least a week prior to the contest. Assuming she is targeting a May 1st competition, she would count back 8.5 months and plan to start her actual diet in the middle of August with the Pre-Diet phase beginning in the middle of July. Since this represents the extremes of dieting, I've provide some more information in the charts below including how she would adjust her percentage goal bodyweight loss each week along with how many days per week she would need to move calories to maintenance has her diet progresses.

	July	Aug	Sep	Oct	Nov	Dec
Weight Loss			1.0% 1.0%	1.0%	0.75%	0.75%
Days Maintenance			1 d/wk 1 d/wk	1 d/wk	2 d/wk	2 d/wk
Weeks	3 4	1 2 3 4	1 2 3 4	1 2 3 4	1 2 3 4	1 2 3 4
Phase	P P	P P D D	D D D D	D D D B	D D D D	D D D B

	Jan	Feb	Mar	Apr	May
Weight Loss	0.5%	0.5%	0.5%	0.5%	
Days Maintenance	3 d/wk	3 d/wk	3 d/wk	3 d/wk	
Weeks	1 2 3 4	1 2 3 4	1 2 3 4	1 2 3 4	1
Phase	D D D D	D D D B	D D D D	D D D Pk	Comp

*P = Pre-Diet D = Dieting, B = Diet break, Pk = Peak Week, Comp = Competition

As the chart shows, the Pre-Diet phase starts in the middle of July, at this point she will be eating at maintenance and gradually increasing her aerobic work as needed. Her first block of dieting begins in the third week of August with a 1% weekly weight loss goal with the inclusion of 1 day of maintenance eating per week. The first diet break occurs after 10 weeks at which point she targets a 0.75% weekly weight loss goal and adds a second day at maintenance eating. After 8 weeks, she takes her second diet break before finishing the diet with a 0.5% weekly weight loss goal and three days per week at maintenance. Ideally she should reach peak condition in the third week of April with the final week being her peak week.

Final Comments on Dieting to Low BF%

As I've mentioned several times, there are often much needed checks in terms of what is realistically achievable in terms of reducing BF%. This is especially true when targeting the lower levels of BF% where dieting times can become enormously long in the best circumstances. Related to this is the fact that even small differences in initial BF% can have enormous effects on the estimated dieting time. To examine both issues, I've provided estimated active dieting times for a range of weight/BF% levels and goals.

Wt	Initial BF%								
175	35	22	25	28	31	50	54	58	61
170	30	12	15	19	22	37	41	45	59
160	26	4	8	11	15	26	31	35	40
155	24	N/A	4	8	11	21	26	30	34
150	22	N/A	N/A	4	8	16	21	25	30
145	21	N/A	N/A	2	6	13	18	23	27
140	20	N/A	N/A	N/A	4	11	16	20	25
135	19	N/A	N/A	N/A	2	8	13	18	22
130	18	N/A	N/A	N/A	N/A	6	11	15	20

Please note that the above only includes active dieting time. For women at a higher initial BF%, the numbers are actually on the high side as I calculated dieting times based on a 0.5% weekly weight loss goal while, realistically, faster rates would be used until 18% was reached. The numbers jump significantly from 18 to 16% due to the need to use the slower rates of weight loss. Regardless of the exact numbers, the above chart is meant to illustrate the point about dieting times relative to both initial and ending BF% goals. To those values would have to be added the Pre-Diet Phase (if needed), any Full Diet Breaks and a final peak week as needed. This could potentially add 4-7 weeks or more to the numbers above.

Even without those additions, it's clear how initial BF% can drastically change the dieting time needed to reach a specific goal. For example, our 150 lb female will require 30 weeks of active dieting (34 weeks total) to reach 10% if she starts at 150 lbs with 22% body fat but this drops to 25 weeks of active dieting time (28 weeks total dieting time) if she starts at 140 lbs and 20% body fat. While starting even leaner would reduce this even further, as I noted above, Category 1 females have a lower limit in terms of how lean they can realistically be at the start of their diet. A woman at 35 % body fat would require 31 weeks to get to 18% in one straight diet while attempting to get to the 10-12% required for a physique competition would take over a year of active dieting (and far more total dieting time). This is simply unrealistic and targeting a competition two years away and dieting down in stages would be the better approach in this situation. Until she is in Category 1 to start, she has little no realistic chance of reaching the lower limits of BF% without dieting for too long without a break and/or attempting to use an extreme approach that may cause significant problems for her.

The chart also illustrates how much less total dieting is needed for those women targeting higher levels of BF%. To get from 22% body fat to 18% body fat required 8 week of active dieting and perhaps 10 weeks of total dieting time while a woman at 26% would require the same 8 weeks to get to 20% body fat. Clearly when more moderate fat loss goals are in place, they can be achieved proportionally much more quickly.

Chapter 26: Identifying and Breaking Plateaus

In an ideal world, once a proper fat loss diet and exercise program were set up, even taking into account the slower rate loss than is expected or predicted, fat loss would occur in a continuous fashion until the goal was met. In the real world, this is never the case. Fat loss is rarely continuous and linear on a week-to-week basis (and certainly not on a day-to-day basis) but tends to occur in starts and stops (muscle gain occurs in the same fashion by and large). Fat may be lost continuously for some time period prior to appearing to stop for some time before a much larger than expected loss is seen seemingly overnight. While frustrating, this is a normal part of the fat loss process that people have to accept will occur.

Overlapping with the above is the fact that weight and fat loss will eventually plateau in a real (rather than apparent) sense. Fat loss may be much lower than predicted (or expected/desired), slow to a rate that is more or less meaningless or stop completely at some point in the diet. This type of plateau is not only immensely frustrating to the dieter, who feels as if they are putting in a lot of effort for no results, but dieters on a schedule may be unable to reach their goals in time if their fat loss slows or stops completely.

The normally cycling woman has the additional variable of the menstrual cycle and its associated changes in water weight which can also impact on both appearance and body composition measurements. It's important not to confuse these normal shifts in body weight with true plateaus in fat loss. I mentioned in a previous chapter, and will reiterate below, that the normally cycling woman must compare like weeks of the cycle (i.e. early follicular to early follicular in the next month) to gauge her progress in any meaningful way. Women with hormonal modifiers, with the possible exception of some types of birth control (BC) that may impact on water weight, don't have to worry about this as much.

There are fundamentally, four causes of plateaus, although I will only look at three of them in this chapter in terms of what they represent, how to identify them and how to address them. The first is simply non-adherence to the diet which is fairly self-explanatory but quite common. Related to this is the mis-estimation or mis-tracking of calorie intake which is less well recognized but extremely important. The third, and one I have mentioned earlier in the book is water retention due to stress and excess cortisol levels. The fourth, and the one that I will discuss in the next chapter has to do with the actual metabolic adaptations that occur in response to fat loss and that require the diet and exercise program to be adjusted over time. I will end the chapter by briefly addressing plateaus in muscle growth.

What is a Plateau?

Since the nature of fat loss is that it rarely occurs nonstop or in a straight line in the first place, it's important to decide if a true plateau has occurred before trying to determine if there is a problem that needs to be addressed. Far too many dieters (over)react to what are nothing more than short-term stalls in weight or fat loss by drastically altering calorie intake, activity levels or both when all they really need is patience. At the same time, ignoring a true plateau for too long can be just as detrimental, especially for those dieters who have to reach a specific goal in a certain time frame. So what defines a plateau?

In the most general sense, a plateau refers to an extended time period when there is no meaningful or measurable change in weight, body fat or body composition. Either they have stopped changing completely or slowed to the point that they aren't moving the person towards their goal at a reasonable rate. One problem here is that even the best body fat/body composition methods show some degree of error and variation. A woman using calipers, with a 2-3% potential error, who loses 1% body fat may not be able to actually measure it, especially if fat is being lost from areas not being tracked. Alternately, if the calipers do show a 1% change, the dieter can't know if it was a true change or not. DEXA, often considered one of the most accurate methods has similar error inherent to the method. All of these methods can only really pick up changes in BF% over longer time periods. But this is no help to the dieter in the short term.

In this sense, scale weight may be slightly more accurate as modern digital scales can measure fairly small changes in bodyweight accurately. So while calipers may have an error of 2-3%, a scale might pick up a 0.5 lb (0.22kg) or less change in body weight easily. A rolling weekly average has to be used (as described in Chapter 6) as day-to-day fluctuations can easily overwhelm true changes but weight can sometimes give a better indication of what is actually going on. For athletes, this is problematic as fat rather than weight loss is the typical goal. Here, so long as performance is staying relative stable (i.e. poundages in the gym, performance in other training) and weight is being lost, the majority of what is being lost should be fat (women's lower propensity to lose LBM makes this even more likely). Certainly the scale has its own set of problems, discussed in detail in Chapter 6 but there are solutions (i.e. combing the scale with other tracking methods) that can easily overcome them.

First, let me examine what a plateau is not. It's not a lack of day-to-day changes in scale weight or measurement and I'd reiterate that scale weight can go up while someone is dieting due to changes in water, sodium intake, and food in the GI tract. Unless a dieter is on an extreme diet and achieving large-scale changes in body weight, even a single week without change may be common as the errors inherent in the measurement are larger than the actual changes (i.e. a 3 lb day-to-day change in weight exceeds a predicted weekly 1 lb weight loss). Again, a weekly rolling average can help to smooth this out but a lack of weight loss from one week to another doesn't necessarily mean anything and dieters must understand this.

In general, I'd define a true plateau as a lack of meaningful or measurable changes in weight or body fat/body composition for more than 2-3 weeks. For all but the slowest amounts of fat loss, most methods of measurement should be able to pick up real changes over that time frame. The light Category 1 dieter can have the most problems as the weekly rates of predicted weight loss may become very slow indeed. A 130 lb female targeting 0.5% weekly weight loss is only looking at 0.65 lbs per week which is easily overwhelmed by small changes in water weight, etc. Over 2-3 weeks, the total losses should be 1.3-1.9 lbs which should be detectable by most methods. In this case, visual changes can be more informative as they often start to occur on a near daily basis in lean dieters. This is due to the fact that even a 0.5 lb loss of fat is a fairly large proportion of her total remaining fat so small losses can have profound visual effects.

Even defining a plateau as a 2-3 week span with no measurable change is a problem for the normally cycling woman due to the impact of the menstrual cycle on water retention. I've repeated a chart from earlier in the book to show how the dynamics of the menstrual cycle might impact on body weight for a 150 lb female targeting a 1% weekly weight loss of 1.5 lbs/week along with the changes that might occur across several months of dieting (Month 3 and 3a will be explained below)

Phase	Month 1	Month 2	Month 3	Month 3a
Early Follicular	150 lbs	148.5 lbs	148.5 lbs	148 lbs
Late Follicular	152 lbs	150.5 lbs	150.5 lbs	150 lbs
Early Luteal	148 lbs	146.5 lbs	146.5 lbs	146 lbs
Late Luteal	155 lbs	153.5 lbs	153.5 lbs	153 lbs

Once again, the numbers are for illustration only and any individual woman might show greater or lesser changes across the cycle. For this reason I recommend that women track their personal changes over at least one month prior to starting to their diet so they know what they personal pattern will be. When I originally presented the chart it was to show that weight loss progress cannot be tracked on a week-to-week basis due to the menstrual cycle related changes. Comparing the early- to late-follicular phase of Month 1 to one another makes it appear that the dieter is backsliding while comparing the late luteal phase of Month 1 to the early follicular of Month 2 makes it appear that a tremendous amount of progress is being made. Only like weeks of the cycle can be meaningfully compared in this regard.

But this same dynamic in terms of tracking makes the determination of a true plateau more difficult as well as my suggested 2-3 weeks will mean comparing unlike weeks. Rather, the only way to determine if a plateau has occurred is to compare like weeks of the cycle. From Month 1 to Month 2, it's clear that progress is being made as the 1.5 lb goal weight loss was achieved during each week of the cycle. Let me note again that the identical change might not occur in each week of the cycle with the late luteal being the most likely to diverge from the rest (it might best to ignore that week entirely in many cases). Moving from Month 2 let me explain the chart. Month 3 represents, as shown, zero weight loss across all weeks and I would suggest the dieter conclude they had reached a plateau after the early luteal phase rather than waiting a full month. Month 3a represent a small weight loss (0.5 lbs) that is below the target goal and again the dieter should conclude that a true plateau has occurred.

All of the above is much less of an issue for women with hormonal modifiers. Women who are oligomenorrheic may show some changes in water retention and body weight but they occur fairly unpredictably depending on her cycle length (I will only say that if weight spikes suddenly it is assuredly water weight from hormonal changes). Hormonal birth control that uses a 3 week on/1 week off pattern could conceivably show changes in water weight during the withdrawal week but this can be determined prior to the diet as well. So long as the woman on this type of BC is tracking weekly, she can decide if she's hit a plateau after 2-3 weeks of no change. Peri- and postmenopausal women have no real cycle of note and the amenorrheic woman will have lost any cyclical changes in water weight that normally occur. Once a plateau has been identified, the next step is to determine what is causing it to fix the issue.

Not Adhering to the Diet

One of the most common causes of fat loss plateau, arguably more common in the general public (but not unheard of in the serious trainee or dieter), is simply not adhering to the diet. The reality is that most dieters will deviate from their diet to one degree or another and this fact alone, rather than metabolic adaptations per se, can often explain the less than expected weight loss that occurs (1). We live in an environment where highly palatable food is always available and most social events revolve around eating. This, along with increasing hunger on a diet, leads people to eat more than planned or desired, offsetting or eliminating their goal deficit and slowing weight/fat loss below the goal rate.

For the general dieter, this isn't necessarily a huge issue and I'd re-emphasize that dieting in this group should be seen as a long-term process and learning experience. Mistakes will occur and can be corrected over time. Going back to the idea of rigid and flexible restraint, thinking that a diet is either perfect or failed does more harm than good. A weight loss stall of a few weeks isn't of any real importance in the context of a very long-term diet that may last months or longer. In contrast, the dieting athlete on a time schedule can't afford to lose much dieting time to non-adherence and this occurs more commonly than may be realized. While many imagine the dedicated lean athlete ignoring their body's hunger for extended periods until they reach their goal, this is not always the case. The most dedicated athlete is still human and hunger (along with a general feeling of deprivation) can cause them to overeat and slow or stop fat loss. As I discussed in Chapter 15, this is often due to the disinhibition that so often occurs in rigid dieters. Regardless of the reason, dieters on a time frame must be able to stick to their diet consistently.

There are various strategies to combat this problem. The general dieter who finds themselves repeatedly breaking their diet should consider taking a Full Diet Break and move to maintenance until they are ready to actively diet again. In this case, trying to adhere to a diet and continuously failing does far more harm than good. Not only is weight and fat not being effectively lost, but the constant sense of failure causes mental stress and harm people's sense of self-efficacy (the belief that they can achieve a goal). In this situation, it is far better to succeed at maintenance than to constantly fail at dieting.

For all dieters, the Flexible Eating strategies/attitudes I discussed previously can have an enormous impact as it can be psychologically easier to adhere to a diet earlier in the week when someone knows that they can have a free meal or raise calories to maintenance in no less than 5-6 days. The Intermittent Caloric Restrictions (ICR) approaches I discussed in Chapter 23 can be equally powerful here as there are never more than a few days of active dieting before a normal eating can resume. Not only do such approaches break the normal feeling of endless deprivation, they have the potential to offset diet induced hunger along with allowing dieters to schedule higher calorie days to better fit their lifestyle. In situations where a dieter knows that they have a social event to attend where they may not be able to resist eating more, an Intermittent Fasting (IF) day can be performed to "save" calories for the evening.

Irrespective of the above, if a dieter's fat loss plateau can be traced to not adhering to the diet, then there is no need to look for any other cause. The causes of the non-adherence should be addressed and that will be all. Assuming that the dieter is adhering to their diet, there must be another cause.

Mistracking and/or Underestimating Food Intake

Related but subtly different to the not adhering to the diet is the second cause of fat loss plateaus which is mistracking or underestimating actual food intake. Non-adherence is an issue of the dieter, generally knowingly not sticking to their diet while mistracking is an issue of thinking that they are eating a different amount of food than they actually are. Mistracking and underestimating food intake is an enormously common issue and studies repeatedly show that true food intake may be under-estimated by as much as 30-80% depending on the population being studied (2). Someone who thinks or reports that they are eating 1800 calories might actually be eating 2400-3200 calories per day, preventing any meaningful fat loss. The existence of food underreporting has led to some very poor conclusions and ideas over the years. For example, it's often claimed that the lean and obese eat the same number of calories per day (therefore obesity must be caused by something else) but this incorrect. Obese individuals simply report eating the same amount as lean individuals while the obese are, in actuality, eating much more.

Under-reporting of food has been found in almost all people to one degree or another although obese individuals tend to show the greatest amount of it (also underreporting dietary fat). Even registered dietitians, who you would think would be good at this, are found to under-report/mis-estimate their actual food intake. I want to make it very clear that I am not saying that people are deliberately "lying" about their food intake although this accusation is often made. More commonly, food underreporting is due to most people having a poor idea about portion sizes and the calorie count of foods. Much of this is due to changes in the modern environment where gradually increasing serving sizes have given people a skewed idea about what a real-world portion might represent (food companies add to the problem by playing games with the serving sizes on foo labels). As an example, I'd ask readers to ask themselves how large a 4oz (113g) chicken breast is and try to visualize it before reading the next sentence. The answer is that it is roughly the size of a deck of cards and I'd further ask readers how close their estimate was. Unless someone has spent considerable time previously measuring their food intake, the answer will be not very. Any assumptions about calorie or macronutrient content are also likely to be inaccurate.

Many also fall into the trap of thinking that certain foods don't really count or can't possibly add up to that many calories. Sauces, various types of toppings, even cream in coffee can add up over the course of a day (gourmet coffees with chocolate, whip cream and more can readily add hundreds of calories to the diet). Dieters of all kinds will pick and snack at small bits of food (especially if they are cooking) and assume that it doesn't amount to much in the big scheme but these calories add up rapidly. People also tend to mis-estimate the calorie content of foods which are deemed or promoted as being healthy, thinking they have few calories or can be consumed without limit. Fruit juices are a good example of this where a single large class can have 100-200 calories of mostly simple sugars. Salads can have their own set of problems: while vegetables are extremely low in calories, the full-fat cheese and salad dressings and other additions to a salad can increase the calories to above that of a hamburger.

In some cases the issue is less one of mistracking/mis-estimating as not tracking at all. In Chapter 15 I discussed the potential pros and cons of popular un-calculated rules based diets that generally tell people that they can eat as much as they want before tricking them into eating less. As I mentioned, these approaches often work stunningly well in the early stages but progress grinds to a halt over time. Dieters assume that so long as they eat only diet appropriate foods, portions or calories don't matter. Over time, hunger increases, energy expenditure decreases, adherence starts to suffer and the dieter ends up eating more food even if they aren't conscious of it. When food companies release high calorie versions of foods that are appropriate for those diets, calorie intake goes up even further. Eventually the person is no longer creating a deficit and both weight and fat loss cease.

While the above phenomenon tend to be more prevalent in the general public, there can also be problems in athletes. In general, this group is far more aware of the calorie values and portion sizes of foods due to having spent time tracking and measuring to begin with but that doesn't prevent them from making mistakes. As I mentioned above, they are often found to "forget" to report their high-calorie or high-fat food intake (or binges), usually to appear healthier than they are. Frankly, if any group is often deliberately lying about their food intake it is this one. Which is somewhat ironic when it is usually the overweight dieter who is accused of this. Even when food is not be deliberately "forgotten" it's not uncommon for food intake to gradually increase during a diet due to increasing hunger. A previously tightly measured cup of starch or vegetables gradually becomes slightly overfilled, increasing calorie intake and mis-measurement of peanut butter is endemic in the physique community.

A carefully measured tablespoon containing an exacting number of calories slowly becomes an overfilled spoon where the sides and bottoms are licked clean. What was a single serving has become a serving and a half and done 4 times per day, the individual is now eating several hundred more calories than they think. For a smaller female on a small deficit, this all but eliminate fat loss. It's also not unheard of for athletes to fall into the trap of thinking that calorie intake doesn't matter so long as they stick to a specific dietary approach (i.e. clean eating, 6 meals/day, paleo). But it always does.

Regardless of the specific cause of mistracking/underestimating true food intake, the end result is the same: the number of calories that the person says or thinks that they are eating is below what they are actually eating, often significantly so. Lean women will report no fat loss on 1200 calories per day (and hours of aerobics per day) when they are actually eating double that amount (in the case where their calorie intake is accurate, water retention is often masking any changes as I will discuss below). Overweight women often report equally low calorie intakes with no weight loss but invariably they are simply mis-estimating their true calorie intake and eating far more than they think.

While arguably more rare, problems with food intake and mistracking can sometimes go in the opposite direction with some overestimating how much they are eating. Recall that, in some women, exercise blunts hunger to the point that athletes end up unconsciously undereating or dropping below the critical Energy Availability (EA) threshold. Athletes trying to gain muscle often think they are eating more than they think as well. In all situations where mis-tracking or mis-estimating food intake may be a problem, the only way to solve the problem is to go through the process of measuring and tracking food intake to determine how much is actually being eaten.

Benefits of Tracking Food Intake

While the process is somewhat tedious, I'm not sure that there is a more beneficial task that dieters, especially in the general public can go through the process of measuring and tracking their food intake as there are multiple short- and long-term benefits to be had from this. The primary short-term benefit is allowing the dieter to determine if mistakes in their actual food intake are the cause of a plateau. This is far more important for the lean dieter on a time schedule but even frustrated general dieters are often able to get their weight and fat loss moving again once they realize that they are eating more than they think they are and to adjust their food intake accordingly. When and if the general dieter is ready to move to a more calculated diet as described in this book, they will need to have some idea about food portions as well and the process of measuring and tracking will give them an advantage in this regard.

Since active people and athletes have typically gone through the process of tracking their actual food intake previously, the long-term benefits of tracking food intake are really of the most benefit to the general dieter. And these benefits are truly enormous. Given how bad most people are at estimating food intake, going through the process of tracking is incredibly informative in that it helps dieters to learn what real-world food portions and their caloric contents actually are. In the modern world, this is invaluable.

Tracking food intake also help people to become more mindful and aware of what they are actually eating since they now have to pay explicit attention to it (the simple act of writing down the day's food intake often causes people to eat less and lose weight with no other changes). Unlike animals who generally eat only when they are hungry, humans often eat mindlessly or for reasons other than hunger and this can add hundreds of calories to the diet. I mentioned in Chapter 21 that the part of the brain involved in this turns on automatically in lean people in response to food intake but not in overweight individuals. With practice the function of this part of the brain improves with dieters becoming more aware of their overall eating habits. By tracking other information, other contributors to overeating can be identified.

How to Track Food Intake

While it can be somewhat of a hassle, the actual method of tracking food intake is not terribly difficult. All that needs to be done is that everything that is consumed (whether solid or liquid) must be tracked, measured and recorded. Here I do mean everything (except perhaps plain water): if a dieter puts it in their mouth it must be rtracked. If nothing else, this will point out just how much small amounts of seemingly unimportant foods can add up over the day, increasing calorie intake significantly.

In tracking what is being consumed, the food must be measured precisely. This requires a food scale along with measuring spoons and cups as this will allow both solid and liquid foods to be measured. Even here it is possible to mis-measure foods. Food scales are not a problem but it's common to overpack a tablespoon with peanut or other nut butters (liquid oils spill over the side) or to overfill a 1 cup measure. The solution to this potential problem is to put the measuring cup or spoon on the food scale to see if it was over or underfilled. To do this, the cup or spoon should first be weighed (and many scales can be set to zero with the cup/spoon on it) before measuring out the portion of food. Reweighing will indicate only the weight of the food and that can be compared to the proper weight for that serving. For example, a tablespoon of peanut butter should weigh exactly 16 grams and, if measured correctly, this should fall just under the lip of the spoon. If, upon weighing, the actual amount if less or, more commonly, more than 16 grams, it has been mis-measured and this will further help the dieter to better understand proper servings sizes. It is more difficult to measure liquids in this fashion although they are relatively more difficult to under-estimate as an excessive amount will spill out of the measuring device.

Once the amount of food or drink being consumed has been measured, the calorie and macronutrient content of the food can be obtained by reading the label. If a label isn't available, there are numerous websites online that have this information available. This information, the food eaten, the amount eaten and, optionally, the macronutrient (protein, carbohydrate, fat grams) content should be recorded for every meal. In years gone past, this would be done with pen and paper but there are both websites and apps that will allow this information to be entered, totaled and saved . Most have food databases built-in or are linked to online resources and will keep track of calories, protein, carbohydrate and fat when the food and amount is entered.

Other information can be recorded as necessary and often knowing when and why someone is eating can be as valuable as knowing what and how much. Emotional state and environment all impact on food intake and keeping a record of this can help people to identify their own personal food triggers. Whether due to stress, sadness or happiness, people overeat for different reasons and identifying those is a first step to identifying solutions or alternate activities to address the problem.

How Long to Track Food Intake

For the general dieter who has never tracked food intake before, I would generally recommend tracking every day's food intake for a minimum of two weeks and this must include weekends. Food intake commonly changes and goes up during this time and only tracking the weekdays can give an inaccurate indication of how much and what is actually being eaten on a regular basis (3). Eating out during this time can be problematic since only the most obsessive dieter is going to get out their food scale at a restaurant. Many restaurants do provide calorie and nutrient information for meals but this is far from universal and there is always the question of accuracy. Ideally it might be best to avoid eating out during these two weeks but this may not be realistic. In the big scheme, one or two meals that go untracked over a two week span will not have an enormous impact in terms of the information collected.

By the end of this two week span, dieters will not only have a much better understanding of their true daily calorie intake but also of what real-world food portions actually are. As another long-term effect, they will now have a much better ability to estimate their calorie intake and gauge portion sizes, both for meals eaten at home or at a restaurant, without having to measure as constantly or regularly. Going forwards, most dieters will not need to measure and track their food all the time although the occasional two to three day spot check (including one weekend day) can always be useful to both refresh and further improve their ability to accurately estimate their food intake. This type of short spot check is also all that is usually required for the dieting athlete who already has experience tracking and measuring their food. If a plateau has occurred, these few days of measuring all of their food can identify any problems that exist.

If the cause of a fat loss plateau can be traced to underestimating or mis-tracking food intake, and the dieter is still pursuing fat loss, the solution is to ensure that calorie intake is returned to the appropriate and/or goal level going forwards and this should cause fat loss to resume. If, instead, calorie intake is actually at the proper level, the cause of the plateau still lies elsewhere.

Water Retention

Even if a dieter is perfectly adherent and their calorie intake is accurate, a plateau in weight and fat loss may still occur for one of two primary reasons. The first of these, and the one that I will end this chapter with is water retention. This is not really a true fat loss plateau in that fat loss has not truly stopped or even slowed (as is the case with the two situations above). Rather, it is more of an apparent plateau where any losses that are occurring are not showing up on the scale or body composition measurements due to water retention. Bioelectrical Impedance (BIA) is enormously sensitive to changes in water weight and other methods of body composition measurement can be impacted as well with water retention effectively "masking" any actual fat losses that may be occurring. While I am primarily focusing on stress and cortisol related water retention here, this can be additive to the effects of the menstrual cycle. Some types of hormonal birth control also cause water retention which might add to this effect.

Briefly, as I discussed in some detail in Chapter 13, the combination of large calorie deficits and excessive amounts of exercise raise cortisol levels chronically to begin with. If that type of dieting and exercise is initiated with no build up, the effect is magnified further. Even when a progressive build-up does occur, this combination can still cause problems and it's usually best if only one or the other is present. There are exceptions to this, usually in smaller Category 1 females at the end of an extreme diet. Here, calories will be relatively low with an often large amount of aerobic activity and this is simply required to maintain fat loss and reach the extreme goals being targeted. When this is added to a certain psychological profile that is common in dieters (along with the fact that dieting itself is an additional psychological stress) the effect is magnified. Any life stresses add to this further. The reduction in both thyroid hormone and leptin allow cortisol levels to increase further all of which can add up to water retention.

While water retention is common while dieting, determining if it is present is not always easy. Typically there are at least some visual changes and women may experience water retention in the calves and ankles or simply in general. There is often a general feeling of puffiness, often in the face (individuals with Cushing's disease, a condition of massive cortisol overproduction, develop an almost moon faced appearance) although it can occur everywhere. This not only looks different than body fat but feels different to the touch. Although very subjective lean physique athletes find that their muscular definition is blurred and this is a sign that water is being retained. Just as they may have experienced throughout their life during the menstrual cycle, when women are retaining water due to excess cortisol production, they feel bloated and "fat" with appearance worsening and clothes fitting more tightly. In many ways, given their past experience with the effects of water retention during the menstrual cycle, I would expect women to be more aware of what this feels like than men.

Some have tried to dismiss the effect of water retention on apparent plateaus, preferring to focus on metabolic adaptation. However, the effect I'm describing has been known since the 1950's if not earlier, being referred to as starvation edema. In The Minnesota study I described in Chapter 9, the men stopped losing weight at the predicted rate at one point while also showing severe signs of water retention. The exact mechanism was unknown at the time but, given the extremeness of that situation, cortisol was assuredly involved. Adding to this, it's common for dieters who have been apparently stalled for 2-3 weeks to experience a rapid loss of weight (sometimes called a whoosh) overnight with an improvement in appearance and body composition. Since it is biologically impossible to have lost that much fat in one day, it can only be the body losing water (this is no different than what occurs from the late-luteal phase into the beginning of menstruation). Whooshes tend to occur under several conditions. One is when fed up dieters take a few days off of exercise and raise their calories. Another is when they follow my advice to raise calories to maintenance (though this can just as easily cause a small weight gain due to the increased carbohydrate storage). Regardless, the commonality of these situations is that the increase in calories/carbohydrates along with a reduction in training is causing cortisol to drop.

There are other potential mechanisms at work here. It appears that, when fat loss has occurred, fat cells frequently refill with water (5). Essentially, the fat loss has occurred but has not yet become apparent (for lack of a better way of putting it). What often happens in this situation is that a woman's body fat becomes subjectively different to the touch. It may become squishy or dimpled and this is especially apparent in leaner dieters. Almost without exception, the whoosh occurs fairly soon thereafter with weight dropping and appearance improving rapidly. Finally, while I don't think much of BIA scales, they measure body water. Anecdotally, many dieters have noticed a major change in those readings right before a whoosh occurs. This would require consistent use but many bathroom scales have BIA built in.

While there are absolutely other factors such as metabolic adaptation, discussed in the next chapter, I think it's clear that water retention due to stress and cortisol is at part of the plateau phenomenon. So now let me look at some of the ways to address water retention.

Be Patient

While there are more proactive approaches to either avoiding or addressing water retention, discussed next, sometimes the best approach is to simply be patient when a plateau occurs (I am assuming here that the dieter is adherent and eating the amount that they think they are eating). Even when dieters are under fairly chronic stress due to exercise, diet, psychological or life factors, it's still uncommon for water retention to last more than 2-3 weeks before a whoosh occurs of its own accord. Water balance is fairly well controlled in the body and eventually the system will normalize itself. For the normally cycling woman this is most likely to occur in the early follicular or luteal phase but may happen at any time in the cycle. Specific stress reduction techniques during this time can be useful, especially for the psychogenically stressed dieter. Stretching, meditation, Yoga or even the occasional glass of wine (a natural relaxant and diuretic) can all be helpful. I am still not joking about the benefits of good sex.

I want to really drive home the point that the absolute worst thing a dieter can do when they hit an apparent short-term plateau is to drastically alter their calorie intake or activity levels as this will simply exacerbate any cortisol related problems. As I discussed in Chapter 13, this is the cycle that many dieters create or find themselves in where stress related cortisol increases cause plateaus which causes them to increase their activity or calorie restriction, worsening the problem.

Avoid Combinations of Excessive Calorie Restriction and Exercise

While I discussed this in detail in Chapter 13 and mentioned above, I want to reiterate the general need to avoid the combination of excessive calorie restriction with excessive amounts of exercise. One or the other may be present, but not both. If a dieter wants to cut calories extremely, they must reduce the amount of exercise they are doing. If they are doing a large amount of exercise, their deficit must be smaller. This is even more true for those dieters who are already psychogenically stressed or who have a great degree of pre-existing life stress. If such approaches are used they must be built up to gradually to avoid further overactivation of the stress system. As I mentioned above, there are often situations where small Category 1 dieters must combine these two but it should always be occurring gradually over the duration of their (often) long diets. Adding 10 minutes of aerobics to each workout per week over months is very different than immediately performing 2 hours/day. Ideally one day should be taken off from training per week as this alone will allow cortisol to fall although this may not be possible at the end of extreme diets due to the need to maintain a high enough energy expenditure to maintain fat loss.

Bring Calories to Maintenance at Sufficient Frequencies

Along with the above is that bringing calories to maintenance/performing refeeds with a sufficient frequency. This too will lower cortisol levels and often causes a whoosh. For the general public dieter, this is probably best accomplished with one of the Intermittent Caloric Restriction (ICR) approaches I described in Chapter 23. For athletic dieters, a more systematic approach to raising calories to maintenance in terms of synchronizing the days with training will be preferred although the end result is effectively the same. Anecdotally, women who do this tend to report less water retention and fat loss "stalls" than those women who maintain the same deficit chronically. Apparent plateaus may still occur and, if they do, there is a more active approach that can be taken.

The Dry Refeed/Return to Maintenance

While increasing calories to maintenance goes an incredible way towards avoiding cortisol mediated water retention to begin with, it can be modified in such a way to try to force a whoosh to occur. Called a dry refeed, this is a day with calories and carbohydrates raised to maintenance coupled with a deliberately low fluid intake. To understand how this might work, recall that carbohydrates store water in the body with every gram of carbohydrate storing between 2-3 grams of water. Using a value of 3 grams of water, this means that eating an additional 150 grams of carbohydrate would store 450 grams of water (about one pound). When muscle glycogen is depleted from dieting and training, that carbohydrate goes into the muscle (and liver) pulling water into both. Physique athletes take advantage of this fact when they engage in carbohydrate loading with sufficient water intake to make their muscles look fuller and slightly larger.

But consider what happens if those carbohydrates were consumed with an insufficient water intake. The carbohydrates will still be stored within the muscle and will still try to pull water in with them. Without water intake, that fluid should come from the bloodstream, with the additional benefit of pulling water from underneath the skin into the bloodstream. Muscles become fuller while appearance and muscular definition improves even if body weight doesn't actually change. Essentially the water is being distributed to at least some degree (consuming sodium can have a similar temporary effect, pulling water into the bloodstream and out of the skin, a strategy often used on contest day by physique athletes). I'd note that this effect will only be particularly noticeable in lean dieters and it may not be enormous. However, the dry refeed will still have the same benefits in terms of reducing cortisol levels. Even if body water is not redistributed as described above it may still be lost by the body via urination. Since fluids are being restricted during this time, more water should be lost than is being consumed. Bodyweight will fall, appearance will improve, body composition measurements should show positive change and the apparent plateau will be broken.

When I originally conceptualized the dry refeed, it was based around a 5-hour increase in carbohydrate intake which, as I discussed in Chapter 21, I no longer recommend or utilize. This means that it would be combined with either a 1-day or 2-day refeed/return to maintenance calories. For various reasons, primarily comfort, I would only recommend any degree of fluid restriction for 1-day at most. This could be on the first or second day of back-to-back maintenance days as desired. Even here, restricting fluids for the entirety of the day isn't necessary and only 5 hours of fluid restriction in the evening should be sufficient with normal, but not excessive fluid intake earlier in the day. If someone's last carbohydrate meal was at 9pm, they would begin fluid restriction at 4pm. During those 5 hours, only small sips of water would be consumed. This can make people very thirsty and chewing gum or sucking on ice cubes can go a long way towards making it more tolerable. A glass of wine at bedtime can facilitate the whoosh process due to it's diuretic effect and this can be combined with other stress reduction methods if desired.

If the dry refeed goes properly, weight should drop in all dieters although only the Category 1 dieter is likely to see a significant improvement in appearance. They should feel as if their muscles are full and women who lift weights in the day or two after will get an incredible pump. If a 2-day refeed is being used, physique athletes can use it to practice their carb-load protocol. Not everyone improves their appearance immediately afterwards (some take a day or two to look completely dry and full) and this is a good way to determine this prior to the competition. I want to emphasize that the dry refeed is not a strategy to use frequently (i.e. every time weight fails to drop at the expected rate). Since it should take 2-3 weeks to decide if a plateau has occurred, the dry refeed should not be done any more frequently than that. So far as timing, it's probably best for the normally cycling woman to use it during the early or late follicular phase when water retention is at its least. Women on a 3 week on/1 week off type of birth control would use it during the withdrawal week although the differences aren't as large here. Women with any other hormonal modifier can use the dry refeed as needed (again, only once every 2-3 weeks maximum).

Plateaus in Training Gains

While fat loss is far away a more common goal for women, many readers of this book will be interested in increasing their muscle mass, strength/power or some other aspect of fitness and I want to finish the chapter by looking at the issue of plateaus for those situations. For the most part in this section, I will be focusing on the goal of muscle and weight gain for the physique athlete or serious trainee and to a lesser degree strength and power performance. Certainly some strength/power athletes are seeking increases in muscle mass (or total body weight) but this isn't universal as many are trying to optimize their performance at their current body weight. Endurance athletes rarely seek muscle gains per se and mixed sports and high-intensity performance sports can vary significantly (usually any desire to gain muscle is relatively small). In all cases where muscle gain is the goal, this information will apply.

Like fat loss, the goal of muscle and weight gain is simple in the sense that both are either being gained or not being gained (fat gain is basically the same but few pursue it explicitly except for after the end of an extreme fat loss diet when the goal is to return to physiological normalcy). Unlike fat loss, which can technically occur in the absence of exercise, gains from training are related to the combination of the training program itself along with proper nutrition (generally including a slight surplus in calories although this depends on the specific sport) to ensure recovery and long-term adaptation. For this reason, a plateau could technically be occurring due to an improperly set up training program, inadequate/improper nutrition or a combination of poor training and poor nutritional support. Since I won't address training in detail until Volume 2, I will assume going forwards that the training program is set up appropriately and focus only on nutritional or other aspects that might be causing a plateau. To a great degree, everything I wrote in this chapter regarding fat loss applies to muscle/weight gain to one degree or another although usually in the opposite direction (there are other differences between the two goals that I will discuss as well). Weight and muscle should be gained over time, eventually it will slow or stop for one or more reasons and below I will discuss what defines a plateau along with the impact of water retention, non-adherence and mistracking of calories (as with fat loss, metabolic rate adaptations are discussed in the next chapter) .

Determining If a Plateau has Occurred

One of the major differences is the relative ability to even determine if a true plateau has occurred in the first place. In that muscle gain requires a calorie surplus, body weight should be going up to one degree or another (losing fat while gaining muscle can occur in some situations but is relatively more difficult to achieve) and some proportion of that total weight gain being made up of muscle (an unfortunate reality being that at least some amount of fat gain is common when athlete are aiming to gain muscle). Here there is a major difference between fat loss and muscle gain which is the rate of each. Rates of fat loss may be relatively quick, depending on the deficit and the amount of body fat, but gain in muscle are always extremely slowly.

While it depends on her initial body weight, as I showed in Chapter 17, a monthly rate of weight gain of 0.5-2 lbs per month (the latter only for the heaviest female athletes) is about the maximum that might occur. Contrast that to the 4.5-6 pounds of fat that could conceivably be lost. Even women with PCOS only gain muscle at a relatively faster rate and muscle gain is simply never fast. Gains in other types of fitness are often even slower. An endurance athlete might train for 4-6 or more weeks before seeing any real improvement and high-intensity performance athletes like sprinter may train for even longer before they improve their speed. Even strength/power athletes often only attempt to set new personal bests in a meet every 12-16 weeks although there is generally some indication of progress during the training cycle.

Adding to this is that muscle growth often seems to occur in starts and stops. Trainees will show little to no growth for some period of time before a major change occurs. I don't know the mechanism behind this and some of it probably just represents the slow rate of muscle growth in the first place. Even a monthly weight gain of 2 pounds can be easily overwhelmed by error in measurement and our ability to measure increases in muscle size are fairly limited. Any woman gaining weight rapidly enough to be able to track it effectively on the scale is gaining weight far too quickly to be doing anything but adding body fat at an accelerated rate. BF% measurements should be able to track changes in LBM but water, glycogen, etc. can all throw those values off. That's on top of the inherent 2-3% error in the method. Even a tape measure is only so accurate and someone gaining 1/4" on their biceps may not be able to measure it. It's not until fairly significant amounts of muscle have been gained that they are particularly visible or measurable.

Practically this all means that a time period of 2-3 weeks is far too short to decide if a plateau in growth (or any other component of fitness) has occurred and it may take 2-3 months before that decision can be made under the best of circumstances. In this case, a plateau would be determined in a number of ways. One would be if the actual weight (or hopefully measurable muscle) gain was slowing, stopping or simply below the goal level. If an athlete were targeting a 0.85% monthly weight gain and their actual weight gain was only 0.5% per month after 3 months, there would be a problem that needed addressing. Strictly speaking, the normally cycling woman (and women on some types of BC) have the same monthly dynamics to contend with as they do with fat loss plateaus but again there is a difference. Muscle gain can be at best tracked on a month to month basis in the first place which makes the presence of monthly variations in body weight and water kind of a non-issue. So long as weight and body composition is tracked at a consistent time each month, and I'd generally recommend a few days into the early follicular phase or the first week of BC, there is no real issue here.

One somewhat indirect approach to determining if a plateau in muscular gains has occurred is to look at strength gains in the weight room. While the detail of training will be discussed in Volume 2, the most general tenet of gaining muscle is that the muscle must be overloaded. There are myriad ways to do this but the simplest is that strength gains in a moderate repetition range tend to correlate with muscle gain over time. If a female physique athlete is adding weight to a set of 8-12 repetitions of an exercise over time, muscle growth should be stimulated. This means that a lack of strength gains over a reasonable time frame would at least somewhat suggest a plateau in muscle growth. This approach has it's own set of issues not the least of which is that rates of strength gain for women is also fairly slow. A lack of strength gains over a month's time for a non-beginner might be common although a lack of any progress over 2-3 months would tend to indicate a plateau had occurred (in many cases this will be due to poor training).

Regardless, at some point, just as with fat loss, the trainee will have to decide if they have reached a true plateau in weight or muscle gain. At which point they need to determine what is the cause. And just as with fat loss, there are multiple potential causes.

Water Retention

While water retention can be a large-scale issue for fat loss, it's relationship with muscle gain is a little bit odd. In this case, water retention can make it looks as if a plateau has not occurred when it may have. The issue here is that water retention will increase body weight, will show up as LBM by some methods of body composition measurement and may increase tape measure measurements slightly. Many find that holding extra water in the body makes them stronger in the weight room. Large amounts of carbohydrates (or carb-loading) and supplements such as creatine both increase body water, which shows up as LBM, and makes athletes stronger. This can make it look as if the athlete is making better progress than they actually are although the effect is never continuous. A small weight gain will occur relatively rapidly and then stabilize and this can simply be used as the new baseline from which changes are tracked.

Non-Adherence and Calorie Mistracking

Since they are so related I'll address non-adherence to the gaining diet and mistracking of calories at the same time as both can and do occur in athletes trying to gain weight. It's probably less common for true non-adherence to the diet to be an issue when gaining weight simply due the dynamics that occur when someone is not dieting. While some have poor appetites, most athletes enjoy eating and aren't fighting deprivation and hunger as when dieting (if anything the problem is keeping them from eating too much and gaining excess fat). Certainly athletes may be inconsistent with their food intake which usually manifests in simply not eating enough. If an athlete is not gaining muscle mass at the rate expected, it is worth looking at their nutritional consistency.

Similarly is the issue of calorie mistracking although, once again it works in the opposite direction to dieting. Here it's not uncommon for athletes to think that they are eating more than they actually are. While far from universal, some people (both women and men) have physiologies that turn off their hunger when they try to overeat. These are the people who swear that they eat a ton and can't gain weight. And while you may occasionally see them eat a huge meal, what you don't typically see is how little they eat the rest of the time. I'd remind readers that high-intensity training can make some athletes lose their appetite which can lead to a non-deliberate type of undereating. This is probably most common for endurance athletes due to the nature of the training but it can occur for all athletes. So in the case where an athlete may be eating too little, the same food tracking suggestions from the last chapter hold. In this case, they should ensure that they are eating as much as they think or are supposed to be to maximize their gains.

Chapter 27: Adjusting for Metabolic Adaptation

While the issues I addressed in the previous chapter can cause a false (water retention) or real (non-adherence, mistracking) fat loss plateau, they are technically avoidable. What is not avoidable is the metabolic slowdown and adaptation that is known to occur during a diet and which is a large part of why real-world weight and fat loss is lower than what is predicted or expected (1). Whether as a cause of a true plateau or simply slowing fat loss beyond the level needed to reach a goal by a specific time, all dieters will eventually experience metabolic slowdown and have to address it.. In this chapter, I want to briefly review those adaptations prior to examining concretely how they work to slow fat loss/eventually cause a true plateau. I will also look at various methods that can help to maintain fat loss at the desired rate or restart it after a plateau. Many of the issues I discuss in this chapter will also apply to the Full Diet Break or when a diet is finally ended in terms of how Total Daily Energy Expenditure (TDEE) will need to be adjusted. At the end of the chapter, I will briefly address this topic in terms of muscle and weight gain.

A Brief Review of Metabolic Slowdown

I looked at the metabolic adaptations that occur to dieting in detail in Chapter 9 but want to briefly review them again here. In short, all components of energy expenditure can and usually do decrease to one degree or another. With the exception of TEF (which is only really responsive to food intake), they decrease for two basic reasons. The first is due to the weight loss itself as a smaller body burns less calories at rest and during activity, both formal exercise and Non-Exercise Activity Thermogenesis (NEAT). But there is also an adaptive component, a decrease in energy expenditure beyond what would be predicted based on the fat loss alone. RMR drops more than predicted, there are adaptations to skeletal muscle so that fewer calories are burned during most types of activity than the weight loss alone would predict and the total amount of NEAT often drops.

Of the total drop, the largest contributor is the decrease in body weight while the adaptive component is typically much smaller, perhaps 5% in overweight individuals and reaching a maximum of 15-20% in the very lean. The change in TEF is negligible with the drop in exercise calorie expenditure being perhaps 10%. The largest part of the drop in TDEE is actually in non-exercise components of TDEE, especially reductions in NEAT which may be considerable. In general, women's bodies adapt somewhat more quickly and to a greater degree than men although there is enormous individuality between any two dieters.

Unfortunately there is little that can be done to offset this at the current time. Leptin injections can reverse some of the adaptations but never made it out of the research realm except for the treatment of amenorrhea. Athletes have long used various drugs to offset the metabolic drops that occur and some of the thermogenic supplements such as ephedrine/caffeine at least help to somewhat by increasing RMR slightly and/or increasing NEAT due to their stimulant nature. The recommendations in this book, avoiding pathological dieting practices, raising calories to maintenance at appropriate intervals and taking diet breaks help but nothing can completely prevent these metabolic adaptations from occurring.

A Concrete Example of Metabolic Slowdown

The consequences of the above adaptations are that, over time, fat loss will slow and eventually potentially stop as the body comes back into energy balance. Since I only looked at the physiology of this in Chapter 9, I want to give a more concrete example of this using the sample dieter at 150 lbs with a maintenance calorie intake of 2370 calories. She is targeting a 1% weekly weight loss or 1.5 lbs. This requires a weekly deficit of 750 calories per day which is created by performing 375 calories of aerobic exercise and reducing calorie intake by 375. Both of these will remain constant during the diet.

If she is losing 100% fat, her predicted fat loss should be 1.5 lbs/week and I'll assume exactly that. Over the next 3 weeks she should lose roughly 4.5 lbs (1.5 lbs/week * 3 weeks) and weigh 145.5 lbs. Her energy expenditure will have decreased and let's say it goes down by 100 calories per day. With no change to her diet or activity, her effective deficit will have been reduced to 650 calories per day which will lower her weekly fat loss to 1.3 lbs per week. At week 6, she will have lost 3.9 lbs (1.3 lbs * 3 weeks) and weigh 141.6 lbs and let's say her energy expenditure has dropped by another 100 calories per day. Her effective deficit will drop to 550 calories per day and weekly weight loss will drop to 1.1 lbs. At week 9, she has lost 3.3 lbs (1.1 lbs/wk * 3 weeks) to reach 138.3 lbs. Her energy expenditure has dropped by another 150 calories which reduces her effective deficit to only 400 calories per day and a predicted weekly fat loss of 0.8 lbs, only half of her goal. By week 12 she will only have lost 2.4 more pounds. If her her energy expenditure drops by another 100 calories, her effective deficit to 300 calories per day and her actual fat loss to only 0.6 lbs/week. If this pattern continued and her energy expenditure dropped by 100 calories every 3 weeks, her fat loss would drop to 0.4 lbs/week in week 15, 0.2 lbs/week in week 18 and fat loss would stop completely in week 21. In the chart below, I've shown her predicted and actual weight changes, the changes in her TDEE, the effective deficit and the predicted compared to actual fat losses.

	Start	Week 3	Week 6	Week 9	Week 12
Predicted Weight	150	145.5	141.0	136.5	132.0
Actual Weight	150	145.5	141.6	138.3	135.9
TDEE	2350	2250	2150	2000	1900
Calorie Reduction (cal/day)	375	375	375	375	375
Exercise Expenditure (cal/day)	375	375	375	375	375
Effective Deficit (cal/day)	750	650	550	400	300
Predicted Fat Loss (lbs/wk)	1.5	1.5	1.5	1.5	1.5
Actual Fat Loss (lbs/wk)	1.5	1.3	1.1	0.8	0.6

The numbers above are only meant to be illustrative and the adaptations that might be seen in any given dieter could be relatively larger or smaller which will impact on how quickly or slowly (and to what degree) the above occurs. Primarily it is meant to demonstrate what is happening to TDEE and how that changes the effective daily deficit as weight and fat loss occur. With no adjustment in diet or activity, weight and fat loss slow and will eventually stop as the deficit is either eliminated or becomes too small to matter. Weight and fat loss may start near the predicted rate but will slow and slow until a new stable body weight and BF% is reached. I'd note that while the metabolic adaptations in response to dieting eventually bring fat loss to a halt, they can never occur to such a degree that fat gain starts to occur as is occasionally claimed. At most fat loss will simply stop and be maintained at the new level.

There are two practical implications of the above. The first is that, if a dieter needs to maintain their fat loss at a consistent rate, they will have to progressively adjust their calorie intake, activity levels or both as the diet progresses. In the example above, if the dieter reduced her food intake by 50 calories and added 10 minutes per day of low intensity aerobic activity to burn 50 extra calories in week 4 of her diet, she would maintain her predicted deficit for the next several weeks at which point she would have to make another adjustment, further reducing food intake/increasing activity. Experienced dieters, especially in the physique community, tend to do this fairly automatically, making small adjustments to their diet or activity patterns weekly or every 2 weeks in order to stay on schedule.

The second implication is that when a dieter hits a true fat loss plateau, when TDEE has decreased to eliminate any deficit, diet or activity will have to be modified to achieve further fat loss. To this I'd add that the persistence of the metabolic adaptations after a diet is over means that TDEE will always be reduced relative to the pre-diet level. Food intake must always be reduced (relative to before the diet) or activity increased to maintain the new weight.

This leaves the question of how to actually estimate or adjust the diet in either case. This is problematic as the adaptive component can vary 5-fold between any two dieters. Only dieters with a great deal of previous experience are able to make the necessary adjustments more or less automatically although I want to provide at least some general guidelines for everyone else. All of the methods that I will provide are only estimates and that real-world fat loss will always be the final determinant of whether or not the adjustment was correct or not. If fat loss resumes at the goal weight, it was. If not, it wasn't.

Estimating the Drop in Metabolic Rate

In order to be able to adjust the diet to account for the drop in metabolic rate, it's necessary to have a rough idea of how much of a drop might realistically be seen for a given amount of weight and fat loss. While not perfect, this will give at least a rough estimate of how much the diet might need to be adjusted for a given loss. Our Category 1 dieting female has a TDEE of approximately 15.6 cal/lb (2350 calories at 150 lbs). If weight loss were the only factor that means that her TDEE should only drop by 15.6 calories for every pound lost which is more or less insignificant. For a 5 lb drop, the value would be just under 80 calories. Since their RMR and TDEE (as a multiplier of bodyweight) are already lower, Category 2 and 3 women will see an even smaller drop in terms of the total number of calories.

But there are the additional adaptive components of the metabolic drop itself that I discussed in such detail in Chapter 9 which have to be taken into account. This too will scale with Category, at least to some degree. As mentioned above, the adaptive drop in RMR might be as little as 5% for a Category 3 woman and up to 15-20% for a Category 1 dieter at the extremes of leanness or who develop amenorrhea. TEF will be reduced due to the decreased food intake although this tends to be a fairly small effect; a 250 calorie reduction in food only lowers TEF by 25 calories and this usually isn't worth worrying about too much. Changes in muscular efficiency will reduce the number of calories burned by 10-25% with higher values seen for lower intensity activity and vice versa. This will lower the calorie burn of any fixed amount of exercise and intensity or duration will have to increase to offset this. Finally there is the issue of NEAT where the change in body weight and muscular efficiency have an impact along with the total amount done in a day going down. Unfortunately, estimating the drop in the amount of NEAT is almost impossible although I will suggest one approach below.

Adjusting the Fat Loss Diet

While it would be technically possible to try to estimate all of the changes in each component above to come up with an average drop in TDEE, I've taken a slightly simpler approach. To do this I analyzed a number of different studies that have actually measured changes in TDEE in dieters of varying BF% and used those values to come up with a rough estimate for the drop in TDEE per pound lost (2-6). Those values appear in the chart below and I've included a 20% variance in either direction to account for the variation that may be seen. The Category 1 column has no range as there is simply not enough data in lean individuals to get more than a rough average. Both female bodybuilder case studies and the original Minnesota semi-starvation study found a value of 42 cal/lb and I've shown a 20% variance under range.

Category	TDEE decrease	Average	Range	3 lb loss	5 lb loss	10 lb loss
3	6-15 cal/lb	10 cal/lb	8-12 cal/lb	24-36 cal	40-60 cal	80-120 cal
2	14-34 cal/lb	24 cal/lb	20-28 cal/lb	60-84 cal	100-140 cal	200-280 cal
1	~42 cal/lb	N/A	34-50 cal/lb	105-150 cal	170-250 cal	340-500 cal

You can see there can be a fairly wide variety of responses, with the total decrease in TDEE increasing with larger amounts of weight loss. Unfortunately, there's no way to know ahead of time whether someone will show a larger or smaller adaptive response to dieting and fat loss. As mentioned above, real-world changes in fat loss will ultimately have to be used to fine-tune the changes that are being made to diet and I will discuss this below.

To use the above values, simply multiply the current total amount of actual weight loss (i.e. ignoring the rapid first week changes) times the value above to get a range of calorie values. That is the amount that the current diet would need to be adjusted by. So let's say that our 150 lb dieter has lost 3 pounds of fat over 2 weeks of active dieting. This would predict a drop in TDEE of 105-150 calories per day (34-50 cal/lb * 3 lbs) and she would have to adjust her diet by this much to maintain her goal rate of fat loss with further adjustments occurring in an additional 2 weeks. A Category 3 dieter who had lost 20 pounds might see a 160-240 calorie drop in TDEE (though some women may see much more) and she would have to make the same adjustments to her diet if her goal was to maintain the same rate of fat loss. I will discuss the specific changes that should be made to the diet or exercise program later in the chapter. First I want to look at another potential way of estimating the changes in TDEE to determine what changes to make to either the diet or exercise (or both) program.

Activity Trackers

Recent years have seen the development of activity trackers, devices worn on the body (frequently the wrist) that use a variety of technologies to keep track of daily activities and get a rough idea of TDEE. Even a basic step counter can give some idea of activity. Worn throughout the day, they interact with smartphones, apps or online software that gives a readout of activity, energy expenditure and other measurements. While none of the currently available trackers are perfect in terms of their accuracy (many are very poor for certain types of exercise), they can provide a fairly clear indicator of whether or not daily activity is changing on a diet and that alone often causes people to ensure that, at the very least, their non-exercise activity does not go down. A related benefit is that seeing their activity levels often causes people to want to beat them, effectively gamifying exercise.

While the technologies used by activity trackers varies (many use heart rate which can be quite inaccurate), the most accurate overall at the time of this book's writing in late 2017 are the Fitbit, Garmin Vivofit and MisFit Shine with all three being accurate at low-intensities but only the Vivofit being accurate during running (7,8). In coming years, improvements in the technology should allow accuracy to improve. While these devices can do a decent job of tracking overall activity, they will be unable to pick up adaptive changes in energy expenditure for RMR, TEA or NEAT. While useful, they are still, at best, an estimate.

In addition to their ability to give a general idea about TDEE and changes in activity, many activity trackers also act as sleep monitors, providing information about sleep quality. This is important not only for overall health but also for fat loss. This type of functioning can be used to determine if late in the day stimulant use or high-intensity exercise is negatively impacting on someone's sleep. It also becomes easier to more objectively determine if any of the sleep supplements I discussed in Chapter 24 are having any real effect. Various sleep hygiene strategies can be tested as well to see which improve sleep quality.

Perhaps the best way to use an activity tracker is to establish a baseline activity level prior to the beginning of active dieting (i.e. during the Pre-Diet phase if it is being used). Not only can this help to estimate maintenance calories for diet set up, it can indicate if activity is changing throughout the day or over time. Users may find that an intense workout earlier in the day causes NEAT to go down later in the day and that scaling that workout back actually leads to a higher TDEE overall. Changes in activity over the duration of the diet can also be monitored. Even if the device isn't necessarily accurate, a comparison between the baseline value and current value can be made which would give another rough indicator of how much TDEE has dropped. So if at baseline a dieter showed a TDEE of 2300 calories and a few weeks later, the device showed a TDEE of 2000 calories, that would necessitate an adjustment to the diet of 300 calories per day to maintain the current rate of fat loss.

How Often to Adjust the Diet

With an understanding of what adjustments should be made to avoid plateaus and keep fat loss moving at an appropriate rate, I want to look at how often the diet should be adjusted. It's important to remember that, for all but the largest deficits, the actual rate of fat and weight loss tend to be relatively slow and in many cases, adjusting the diet extremely frequently can be unproductive. As always, this changes with the dieter's Category as well as the presence of absence of a time frame to reach the goal. A Category 3 general dieter won't need to adjust their diet nearly as frequently as a Category 1 dieter for whom a slowing in fat loss may put them behind schedule or even make it impossible to reach their goals. Some general guidelines for how long to wait before adjusting the diet appear below.

Category	Frequency of Adjustment
1	2-4 weeks
2	4-8 weeks
3	8-12 weeks

You can see how the values change with decreasing category although only the Category 1 dieter on a strict time frame would need to adjust their diet every 2 weeks (keep in mind that) the normally cycling woman might have to wait 4 weeks to get an accurate measurement of whether or not they are losing less than the expected amount of body fat. Dieters who are not on a time frame and this includes both the general dieter or the serious recreational trainee can use the above guidelines. The general Category 2/3 is probably best off adjusting their diet after every Full Diet Break between blocks of active dieting since the changes occurring in that time frame should simply not be that large. The exception to this would the dieter who hits an enormous fat loss plateau (while being adherent/tracking food properly) during that time.

I want to make it clear that the metabolic adaptations to dieting are occurring gradually and it's not as if there is no change until the 4 or 8 week mark as the chart above might imply. Over 6 weeks of dieting, a 300 calorie total drop might be occurring as 50 calories per week, for example. There is simply a realistic limit to how often or how much a diet can or should be adjusted. The lean dieter on a tight schedule might be making small adjustments weekly or bi-weekly but other dieters will not need to do this. Dieters can become obsessive enough and it's far too easy to start adjusting the diet far too frequently in response to fairly small changes in fat loss. Until someone is being perfectly adherent and tracking their food to begin with, the reality is that the variation in the day's food intake will be greater than any changes that would need to be made over the short-term to begin with. Until a true plateau (i.e. 2-3 weeks of no loss) has occurred, no change to the diet should be made in the first place.

How to Adjust the Diet

Once the degree of metabolic adaptation has been determined or estimated, it will be time to adjust the diet and there are two issues that need to be considered. The first is whether a reduction in calories, increase in exercise or some combination should be used with the best choice depending heavily on the dieter's Category and the specific situation. I examined this briefly when I talked about setting the deficit originally but want to look at it at least briefly again here. As a secondary issue, if calories are being reduced, the question of which nutrient should be reduced becomes important.

Should Diet or Exercise be Altered?

In a general sense, metabolic adaptation can be compensated for by reducing food intake, increasing activity or using some combination of the two (technically thermogenic supplements could be added but here I will only focus on diet and exercise). I addressed this topic somewhat in a different context when I talked about creating the initial deficit, pointing out that dieters in different Categories and situations (i.e. serious recreational exerciser vs. physique athletes vs. high-intensity performance athlete) tend to have better and worse ways of creating their deficit in the first place. And while many of those comments hold for adjusting the diet for metabolic slowdown, I want to look at them briefly again.

Whether food intake should (or even can) be reduced or activity increased depends on where each is set currently. Someone who is already on lowered calories may not be able to reduce them further without having so little food to eat that they cannot adhere to the diet. In this situation, increasing amounts of activity, whether aerobic, HIIT or with conscious attempts to increase NEAT, may be the only practical way to maintain fat loss in the face of metabolic adaptations. Let me reiterate that too much high-intensity/HIIT exercise can readily overstress the body. One to two HIIT sessions per week is usually the limit and the intensity of aerobic work must be limited to some degree. Anything much higher than 140-150 heart rate (HIIT excepted) tends to be too much and increasing the duration of low- or moderate-intensity activities is usually a better choice. In this situation, depending on how low calories are, a combination of a slight calorie reduction with an increase in activity may be best. If metabolism has gone down by 150 calories, both a 150 calorie reduction or a 150 calorie increase in activity may be difficult while a 50 calorie reduction in food intake with a 100 calorie increase in activity (or 50% from each) may work and this level of change can probably be sustained when the next change is required.

The above situation is most commonly seen in the smaller Category 1 female which is why starting too aggressively, or not starting the diet early enough, can get these dieters into trouble. As I showed in Chapter 14, if they cut calories or add too much exercise too early, they are often left with nowhere to make further changes later in the diet. In contrast, a larger Category 2 or 3 female or highly active athlete who is eating more calories may be able to reduce their food intake by several hundred calories while still having a large amount of food to eat every day (the same holds true for larger men as well). A woman who is eating 1800-2000+ calories per day due to a high activity or body weight can remove 100-200 calories from her diet much more easily than a smaller woman on 1400 calories or less.

The same dynamic holds for exercise but in reverse. For those who are not performing much in the way of exercise, and this might typically be the Category 2/3 beginner who is just beginning an exercise program, increasing activity may be superior to reducing food intake. Some of this depends on how large of an adjustment needs to be made. Trying to increase activity by 200-300 calories per day takes a fairly significant increase in duration or intensity and this may be too much for someone relatively new to exercise. Increasing energy expenditure by only 100-150 calories might only take 15-20 minutes of moderate activity which could be achievable in some circumstances and fitness should have improved to allow another increase by the time the next adjustment is required.

In contrast, someone who is already performing a large amount of exercise, and this is most common with high-intensity performance, mixed and endurance athletes, adding more can be problematic. One advantage these athletes have is that their high training levels allow them to burn a considerable number of calories with even small increases in fairly low intensity activity. Just as with setting up the diet in the first place, small increases to warm-ups or cool-downs or even the main workouts can often burn the necessary 100-150 extra calories per day fairly easily but there will be a limit to this. Strength/power athletes are in a kind of odd place here. On the one hand they typically aren't performing a lot of aerobic work to begin with and this represents a place where they can conceivably increase the amounts they are doing. On the other hand, excessive aerobic activity at anything but fairly low intensities tends to harm performance. Brisk walking or non-impact aerobic work at low intensities can often burn quite a few calories. Adding aerobic work gradually over time also helps to avoid major drops in performance among these athletes.

A Note about Small Category 1 Dieters

Let me finish this section with a quick note. In recent years, due to the use of what can only be described as pathological dieting practices among extreme dieters (typically physique athletes) involving hours of aerobics and (at least reported) very low calorie intakes, the idea that anyone who is on low calories (1200 or less) and performing an hour or more of aerobic work per day is dieting incorrectly has become popular. As I've discussed, in a general sense this isn't incorrect in that this combination can cause problems for women physiologically (i.e. menstrual cycle dysfunction, excessive stress) especially if they jump into this approach from the time they start their diet.

However, there is a reality here that can't be ignored which is that lighter Category 1 females dieting to the extremes will almost invariably end up with fairly low calorie intakes near the end of an extreme diet. A fairly standard intake for dieting is 10 cal/lb and this means that a 120 lb female would be dieting on only 1200 calories per day to begin with unless her activity is very high. Further reduction in her calorie intake from that level will eventually become impossible which means that activity levels will have to increase, often to much higher levels than you would see in larger dieters (or males who often need no cardio to lose fat effectively). Daily aerobic activity levels of an hour or more may seem excessive and they are in one sense (though endurance athletes may do this as a matter of course but they build up to it gradually). But they may also be required in this situation to reach the dieter's goal.

But there are key differences between these two two situations. A woman who immediately starts doing two hours per day of aerobics and cuts calories too much is generating an incredible immediate stress to her body which can cause any number of problems that I've already discussed. She will cross the critical energy availability (EA) threshold immediately, raise cortisol and is dieting in a damaging way. In contrast, the small Category 1 dieter is likely starting with a fairly moderate calorie deficit along with moderate amounts of aerobic activity which are being gradually increased over the duration of a 6 month diet. That second dieter, reducing calories by 50-100 or adding 5-10 minutes of aerobic activity every few weeks is doing so gradually and progressively enough to avoid overstressing her body. So long as she is still raising calories to maintenance and performing diet breaks (something that the first dieter almost never does), she will be limiting the stress that is occurring. Any absolutist ideas about what should or should not be done are as mistaken as the idea that the critical EA threshold must never crossed.

Adjusting Macronutrient Intake

As I discussed above, whether or not calories will (or even can) be reduced or activity increased depends on the specific situation. If calories are already low, increasing activity may be the best option. If activity and food intake are high, calorie reductions may be better. In many cases, a mixture of the two will be best. Regardless, at some point realistically calories will have to be reduced to one degree or another and I want to look at which macronutrient (protein, carbs, fats) should be reduced. Let's assume a dieter needs to make a 100 calorie adjustment to her deficit and has decided to make it by reducing her food intake. Which macronutrient should she adjust? Unless intake is excessive for some reason, protein intake should never be reduced (it may actually need to be increased slightly under some situations). This leaves carbohydrates and fats and a 100 calorie change would require a 25 gram reduction in carbohydrates or a roughly 11 gram reduction in fat (a combination of the two could be used).

As it has the highest calorie density, reducing dietary fat would have the least impact on the total volume of food being eaten. This might help with fullness but there are other concerns. For the normally cycling Category 1 female, reductions in dietary fat beyond a certain point might increase her risk for menstrual cycle dysfunction although women with any hormonal modifier needn't worry about this. There is also the fact that moderate fat diets are often superior to lower fat diets in many ways. Dietary fat slows digestion which keeps people fuller between meals and gives food a better mouth feel so that it may be more enjoyable, improving adherence. All of which means that reductions in dietary fat beyond a certain point (and recall the minimum values I provided in Chapter 19) may cause more problems than they solve.

That would suggest that reducing dietary carbohydrates as the better approach and in many cases it will be. In most diets, achieving the necessary deficit will require some reduction in carbohydrates almost no matter what else is done. Certainly the lower energy density of carbohydrates means that more food will have to be taken out of the diet if 25 grams of carbohydrates, rather than 11 grams of fat, are removed. At the same time, it would be most common to remove more concentrated starchy carbohydrates when reductions are made, leaving the higher volume fibrous vegetables as the primary carbohydrate source. This minimizes the issue with food volume but raises another problem due to excessive reductions in carbohydrate intake leaving athletes underfuelled for their training.

The latter issue is far less of a problem so long as calories are being raised to maintenance with sufficient frequency as one effect of this is to refill muscle glycogen stores. As well, the athletes with the highest carbohydrate requirements in the first place have the highest overall calorie requirements so their carbohydrate intake is already higher. Removing 25 grams from a diet containing 150 g/day of carbohydrate is far different than removing it from a diet containing 350 g/day of carbohydrate. For less active or inactive individuals, the need for sufficient to carbohydrates to support exercise is not an issue and reducing carbohydrates is often the best approach.

Returning to dietary fat, an additional issue is that dietary carbohydrates may reach a point where further reductions takes the dieter into the realm of Very Low-Carbohydrate/Ketogenic Diet (again defined as a carb intake of 80-100 g/day or less). In situations where there is some degree of insulin resistance present (i.e. PCOS, Category 3) this is not a problem and may be superior to begin with. In contrast, in leaner athletes, ketogenic diets are often not well tolerated. Many find that their energy is down, their training and mood suffer, and they suffer mental fatigue (offset by sufficient mineral intake) or simply feel terrible. Relevant to the normally cycling Category 1 female, ketogenic diets may be associated with menstrual cycle dysfunction (though this might be avoided with sufficient days at maintenance). In this situation, reductions in dietary fat may be the only option to maintain carbohydrate intake.

While I've addressed this topic by considering only exclusive reductions in carbohydrate or fat, it is equally possible to cut both carbohydrates and fats by a small amount, in this case 100 calories would require a 12.5 g carbohydrate reduction (roughly 1/2 serving of starchy carbohydrate) and 5 grams fat reduction (about 1/3rd of a tablespoon of oil) which would be hardly noticeable. This approach be necessary near the end of the diet when the dieter just doesn't have the ability to reduce either carbohydrates or dietary fat by the required amount.

Finally I would mention that whether or not a woman is using a follicular or luteal phase diet may play a role in her choice of what nutrient to reduce. For a woman using a luteal phase diet, where carbohydrates are lower and fat is higher to begin with, reducing fat may be the easier and better choice since there is already a higher intake. For a follicular phase diet, the reverse would be true and reducing carbohydrates might be relatively easier since the total intake is higher. For women using both diets, carbs could be reduced from the follicular phase diet and fats from the luteal phase diet although this may introduce unnecessary complexity to an already complex approach.

I would note that most of the extreme situations will generally be seen in the normally cycling Category 1 dieter near the end of a prolonged/extreme diet. Calories simply end up so low and activity can't be increased too much more that there is no best option. There may be no way to keep dietary fat above the lower limit or in the optimal range to maintain menstrual cycle function or to keep carbohydrates from falling below a level where the diet will become ketogenic. In one sense, this is ameliorated by the fact that many dieters in this situation will either be close to developing amenorrhea or will have done so already. I will talk about this in detail in Chapter 32 but it tends to eliminate some of the problems I've discussed in terms of diet and menstrual cycle function. If the menstrual cycle has been lost, any issues with reductions in carbohydrate or fat content are no longer relevant from that standpoints.

Once the decision has been made to reduce either carbohydrate or dietary fat intake, a related question is which meal(s) of the day to remove them from. This is also context dependent, primarily being determined by whether or not the person is involved in intense training. For the recreational trainee or someone doing little to no exercise, it doesn't matter very much when either carbohydrates or fats are removed from the diet. Removing them from meals earlier in the day may be better as it leaves more of each for later in the day but there is no fundamental requirement for which meals should be adjusted and it can be done based on the dieter's preference.

For the dieter involved in intense training who is reducing carbohydrate intake, the reductions must come from any meal not eaten around the workout. This enables the athlete to create the necessary deficit while still supporting both performance during and recovery from training. I discussed a similar concept when I discussed meal patterning where dieters may already be setting up their diet to skew carbohydrate intake more around training. This just becomes more pronounced later in the diet. At the extremes, some dieters will end up in a situation where carbohydrates are only being eaten before and after training and perhaps at the next meal with the other daily meals consisting primarily of protein, fat and fiber. If a serious trainee or athlete is reducing their dietary fat, where that reduction comes from is less important. It would probably be best to remove it from meals earlier in the day rather than later simply due to the general problem with nighttime hunger (where dietary fat may help keep the dieter fuller longer). But as with the general dieter, this is more an issue of preference or convenience.

The Sample Dieter

To give a concrete example of how the above would be applied, I want to return to our sample dieter at 150 lbs/22% body fat who is dieting down to 10% body fat for a physique competition. When she set up her diet originally, her TDEE was 2350 calories and she created her initial deficit with 375 calories of food restriction to 2000 calories and 375 calories of aerobics. Neither are particularly excessive although the 375 calories of aerobic work might require 45 minutes at a moderate intensity. Several weeks into her diet, she needs to create an additional 105-150 calorie deficit to maintain fat loss at her desired rate and I'll split the middle and say that she is targeting a 125 calorie adjustment. Just to keep the math simpler, she will add ~5 minutes to each aerobic session which will easily burn 25 calories leaving her with the need to reduce food intake by 100 calories per day to 1900 calories. Since her carbohydrate intake is still decently high, she will reduce them by 25 grams in both phases of the diet and I've shown the new values below.

	Original Follicular	New Follicular	Original Luteal	New Luteal
Calories	2000 cal/day	1900 cal/day	2000 cal/day	1900 cal/day
Protein	140 g/day	140 g/day	140 g/day	140 g/day
Carbohydrates	235 g/day	215 g/day	156 g/day	131 g/day
Fat	56 g/day	56 g/day	90 g/day	90 g/day

In both cases, her dietary fat intake is above the lower limit cutoff which should decrease the potential for menstrual cycle dysfunction. Her carbohydrates are getting close to the cutoff for a ketogenic diet in the luteal phase diet but are still sufficiently high to avoid problems. This should also allow training performance to be maintained, especially if she brings calories and carbohydrates to maintenance with sufficient frequency (this early in the diet it will probably only be once per week).

At some point she will have to adjust her diet further and I do want to look at a situation where one of the problems I mentioned above may show up. After three more weeks of dieting, she has lost just over 3 pounds and needs to adjust the diet above again and needs to reduce her calorie intake by 150 calories. She'll burn the additional 50 calories with another 10 minutes of aerobic exercise, bringing her to an hour total which means she will need to reduce her calorie intake by 100, or another 25 grams of carbs or 10 grams of fat. I want to look at what happens if she decides to reduce her carbohydrate intake further.

	Original Follicular	New Follicular	Original Luteal	New Luteal	Adjusted Luteal
Calories	1900 cal/day	1800 cal/day	1900 cal/day	1800 cal/day	1800 cal/day
Protein	140 g/day	140 g/day	140 g/day	140 g/day	140 g/day
Carbohydrates	215 g/day	190 g/day	131 g/day	106 g/day*	130 g/day
Fat	56 g/day	56 g/day	90 g/day	90 g/day	79 g/day

Once again, her follicular phase diet is fine with both dietary carbohydrate and dietary fat at appropriate levels. But she runs into one of the problems I described in the luteal phase as a full 25 grams carbohydrate reduction takes her total carb intake to just over 100 grams, which is near the cusp of being a full-blown ketogenic diet. In this case, since her dietary fat is higher to begin with in the luteal phase, it makes more sense to reduce dietary by a mere 11 grams rather than to reduce carbohydrate further. This results in the diet shown in the Adjusted Luteal Phase column which is still problem free.

The above problem will tend to crop up more and more as she has to reduce calories further and at some point it may become impossible to keep carbohydrates above the threshold for being a ketogenic diet or dietary fat above the optimal level to avoid menstrual cycle dysfunction. If she hasn't lost her cycle by this point, she may have to accept a carbohydrate intake below 100 grams per day. Since there will be 2 or possibly 3 days at maintenance with higher carbohydrate intake by this point, it should be less of an issue compared to being on a full-blown low-carbohydrate diet. Alternately, she may have to keep gradually increasing her aerobic activity to keep her fat loss moving at the appropriate rate to avoid further reductions in calorie intake. As I mentioned in the note above, this is just the reality of dieting for smaller Category 1 dieters at the extremes and is not an issue so long as the increases occur gradually.

Metabolic Rate Adaptation to Weight gain

In the same way that metabolic adaptations can limit fat gain over time and be a cause of plateaus, it can have at least similar effects in terms of muscle and weight gain (as with the previous chapter, other fitness goals are more difficult to track in this regard and I will focus only on muscle/weight gain). And just as with the cause of plateaus in fat loss, once the issues of water retention, adherence and calorie mistracking have been addressed, it must be examined. Because just as any fixed calorie deficit will cause fat loss to eventually slow and stop, the same will hold true for any calorie surplus with any gains eventually stopping. Here the mechanisms are more or less identical and occur for the same reasons, although in the opposite direction. I'd also note that, in general, those adaptations do not appear to be as potent or effective in preventing weight gain as they are in preventing fat loss for most people.

Briefly summarizing those metabolic adaptations, a larger body will burn more calories at rest although the impact is not large here as gains in muscle mass have only small effects on RMR (i.e. one pound of muscle burns an extra 6 calories per day). It's somewhat debatable if RMR itself goes up in an adaptive sense, that is in excess of what would be predicted by body weight alone. At most, there seems to be a small and fairly short-lived effect that occurs early in the overfeeding period before dissipating. At least some of the increase in energy expenditure seems to come from increases in TEF but, as usual, the effect is quite small with a 200 calorie surplus per day only increasing TDEE by 20 calories per day.

Looking at exercise, a heavier body will burn more calories during activity of any sort. Of possibly more importance is the fact that most trainees will either do more training or be able to work more intensely in the training that they are doing when they are eating sufficient calories and that will further increase calorie expenditure (recall that the calories burned during most forms of exercise is still relatively small). The same dynamic will occur for NEAT with more calories being burned during those activities. There may also be changes in muscular efficiency with overeating which would also cause more calories to be burned. Of possibly the most importance, many find that the amounts of NEAT that they perform goes up when they are eating more calories. At least some of this is in the unconscious part of neat, fidgeting, changing posture and the rest. But simply having sufficient energy on a day-to-day basis may mean that NEAT can go up. Changes here are enormously variable but many who have trouble gaining weight or muscle often see their NEAT levels increase significantly. This tends to go hand in hand with having an appetite system that shuts down more easily and the combination is part of why these people are relatively protected against obesity in the modern world. But it can also make creating a constant surplus difficult when muscle/weight gain is the explicit goal.

Building Metabolic Capacity

Before addressing what changes can be made, I want to address a concept currently popular in the physique community called building metabolic capacity. The idea here is that, by using small increases in calorie intake, RMR can be increased significantly beyond what would be expected based on body weight. As I've discussed this is not supported by any research, most of which shows that overfeeding has at best a small effect on RMR or TDEE, causing nothing but excessive fat gain. Yet online there are numerous anecdotal reports of trainees maintaining their current body weight and body composition on much higher calories than might be predicted. I think there are a few factors that explain this disconnect.

One is that the trainees reporting this were usually doing excessive aerobic activity on low calories prior to undertaking this approach. As I mentioned in Chapter 14, by taking themselves above the critical EA threshold, a reversal of negative hormonal adaptations is likely to be occurring and it is completely plausible that there are actual improvements in RMR and other aspects of TDEE. However, this is really just allowing a relative normalization of RMR without truly increasing it over what would be expected and I think that a few other factors are at work here.

It's fairly clear that RMR per se does not increase significantly over what would be expected based on bodyweight. At the same time, these same athletes usually report being heavier (albeit more muscular) and that alone would increase RMR, just not due to any adaptive response. TEF will be up slightly but, once again, any effect is likely to be small. But the other factors will be playing a role here. Being heavier and doing more and/or more intense training will increase calorie expenditure in its own right and that will increase TDEE. Finally is NEAT and, between often reducing excessive aerobic volumes and increasing food intake, this is likely where the major changes are occurring. The athletes are no longer chronically exhausted from training on low calories and their NEAT either normalizes or even increases above normal, increasing their apparent TDEE beyond what might be expected. Simply, the idea that metabolic capacity is being built is not supported by any research and any effects on TDEE are due to the above mechanisms.

Adjusting Training and Diet

Just as with plateaus in fat loss, adjustments to either exercise or diet could technically be made when a trainee has reached a plateau in weight or muscle gain although here again there are differences, especially in terms of the exercise component. A major one is that, while fat can technically be lost without exercise, gaining meaningful amounts of muscle without excessive fat gain requires that at least resistance exercise be performed. In that sense, reducing the amount of exercise being done seems illogical. While this is at least partially true, there are places where excess activity might be preventing muscle gain. Perhaps the most common is when female trainees are determined to maintain a large volume of aerobic and/or HIIT work during their muscle gain phases. For performance athletes this is often required (i.e. a sprinter must perform sprint training) but for the physique or strength/power athlete it is not with both having the potential to either passively or actively harm gains in muscle, strength or power.

Passively aerobic and HIIT work burns calories which may eliminate or decrease the daily surplus. In premise this can be compensated for by eating more (this assumes that appetite is not excessively blunted). More actively, as I have mentioned and will discuss somewhat more in the next chapter, there is often an interference effect between aerobic/HIIT training and resistance training where the former impairs gains in the latter. That is, essentially aerobic and HIIT work send the muscle a signal to become smaller and more enduring and this can offset the signal that resistance training sends the muscle to become larger and stronger. It is a little more complex than this but, in general, excessive aerobic and/or HIIT work will tend to impair gains in muscle, strength and power and I recommend against it. A few easy aerobic sessions per week are often beneficial for recovery and to maintain appetite but I would recommend against more than perhaps 3 days per week of 20-30 minutes at a relatively low intensity and would not recommend that HIIT be done at all. If more than this is being done, it should be reduced or eliminated as that alone may be all that is required to overcome a plateau.

Given the necessity of resistance training for increasing muscle mass, it may seem strange that it could harm rather than help muscle gain but there are situations where this is absolutely the case and the training program is not set up optimally to make gains. There are two common but related situations here. The first is when an excessive amount of training is being done. It's not unheard of for those trainees seeking muscular gains to train 1.5-2 hours per day 6 or more days per week. With the possible exception of strength/power athletes, who often have very long workouts due to resting for extended periods between heavy sets, this is simply too much training to be effective under most circumstances. This approach often comes with trainees working at too low of an intensity to make meaningful gains. Many women will be in the gym for 2 hours doing set after set after set of relatively submaximal work while resting for very short periods of time and, simply, this is not the most effective way of stimulating gains in muscle, strength or power. In this case, reducing the total amount of training being done while increasing the intensity of that work is the superior approach and making this change may be all that is needed to break a plateau in or total lack of gains. I will provide some general guidelines for this in the next two chapters and training will be discussed in detail in Volume 2.

Once training has been addressed, the next change that can be made is in the diet. Assuming that water retention, adherence and calorie mistracking (discussed in the last chapter) have been addressed, a lack of gains in muscle mass or strength comes, in the simplest sense, to an insufficient calorie surplus. Here the fix is to increase calorie intake slightly until the goal weight and muscle gains begin to occur. Here, just as I would never recommend that women use more than a 10% total surplus (perhaps 15% in PCOS/hyperandrogenism), to begin with, I would not recommend that women make more than a 10% increase in their calorie intake at any given time. If the sample dieter with a TDEE of 2350 was already eating 2600 calories per day and was failing to make gains, she should increase her calorie intake by no more than 260 calories per day, for a total of ~2900 calories per day.

That level of intake would be maintained to see if it was sufficient to overcome the plateau (and as I mentioned in the last chapter, this might take 2-3 months before a decision was made) and, if not, would be increased by another 300 calories until her rate of muscle mass, weight or strength gains were appropriate. Unless protein intake is insufficient for some reason, any changes should come from carbohydrates or fats. In most cases, adding dietary fat will not be as beneficial as increasing dietary carbohydrates and this is where I would recommend any changes be made. A 300 calorie increase in carbohydrate intake would mean a 75 gram/day increase. At least some of this can be put in the pre- or post-workout meal but, if those are already at an appropriate level, the calories/carbohydrates can be spread across the other meals of the day as desired.

Chapter 28: Training Guidelines

While I will discuss the topic of training for women in great detail in Volume 2 of this book, I can't assume that all readers are familiar with exercise concepts in either a general or specific sense. For that reason I want to provide some guidelines on various types of exercise as it applies to the goal of dieting and fat loss. While specific sports may include such activities as plyometrics, scrimmages/practices and other forms of training in their weekly structure, the primary types of exercise I will be focusing on are weight training, aerobic exercise and High-Intensity Interval Training (HIIT). I will also briefly examine jumping exercise due to its potentially profound effects on bone density.

Since I have discussed each of those three previously in this book in terms of their impact on body composition or body fat, I will primarily focus here on general training principles for each and how they might be applied for different goals, especially fat loss. I want to reiterate that while all three types of training have their place in a proper fat loss program, if only one can be performed for some reason, it should ideally be resistance training. That along with a properly set up diet will cause fat loss while sparing the loss of lean body mass (LBM). Aerobic and HIIT exercise helps but is not required.

General Principles

Before looking at each specific type of exercise, I want to examine some general concepts that apply to all types of exercise. The first is the principle of Specificity (also called Specific Adaptations to Imposed Demands or SAID) which says that the type of adaptation or improvement in fitness is specific to the type of exercise done. Stretching improves flexibility, aerobic/HIIT exercise improve cardiovascular fitness, resistance/weight training improves muscular size and strength although there can be overlap. For beginners, aerobic exercise and HIIT may increase muscle size slightly and weight training may improve aerobic exercise performance. Weight training can also improve flexibility if it is done through a full range of motion. That said, if someone has a specific fitness goal, specific training will be the best approach.

The second general principle I want to look at is usually called the FITT equation. FITT stands for Frequency, Intensity, Time and Type which is best thought of as how often, how hard, how long and what type of exercise is being done. In many cases, specific types of exercise don't neatly fall into the categories described by FITT but, in general, it can be used to define the parameters of a given type of exercise along with minimum, maximum and/or optimum levels for specific goals. When I look at different types of exercise, I will look at each component although not always in that specific orer.

Let me mention that the components of FITT, especially the first three, interact in a number of important ways with many combinations being either mutually exclusive or simply a bad idea from an injury and burnout standpoint. For the most part, only one or occasionally two components can be high without the other two having to be lowered. I've shown some potential combinations below.

Frequency	Intensity	Time
Low	High	High
Low	Low	High
High	Low	High
High	High	Low

The first line indicates that a large amount of high intensity work must be done with a low frequency. A low frequency of low intensity work will allow a large amount (time) to be done. A high frequency of low intensity training allows a large amount to be done while a high frequency of high intensity activity means that only a small amount can be done at any one time. It is also possible to set one value at a moderate level and the other values will change. For example, moderate frequency, moderate intensity exercise can be done for moderate durations. In general, the type of exercise doesn't play a major role in the above although high-impact activities such as running or jumping that put a lot stress onto joints or bones can't usually be done with a high frequency or time unless that level is built up to over many years. In contrast, low-impact activities such as cycling, swimming, etc. can be done much more frequently.

The third and perhaps most important principle of training is that of Progression or Progressive Overload. In a very real sense, the fatigue and overload caused by exercise is what stimulates it to adapt and improve. Once that adaptation has occurred, training must progress further or the body will have no reason to adapt and fitness will no longer improve. Progression can occur in frequency, intensity or time and changes to each can be appropriate under different circumstances.

As an example of progressive overload, consider someone who decides to start running three times per week. At first they are only capable of running one mile per workout before becoming fatigued but, over the next several weeks the body will adapt and that one mile will no longer be challenging. If that person never runs more than a mile, their fitness won't improve further. To apply progression they might increase frequency, running one mile four times per week. Alternately they could increase intensity, attempting to run that mile faster. Finally, they might increase time and run 2 miles instead of 1. Eventually their body will adapt to this as well with another increase being required to improve fitness. At the point that they are happy with their current level, training can be maintained without progression.

Finally is the concept of Detraining, the loss of fitness that will occur if the exercise stimulus is reduced or taken away. If the person above had worked up to 3 miles per run done three times per week and cuts back to only 1 mile three times per week, their fitness will eventually decrease. If they stopped running entirely, their fitness would eventually return to where they started.   Detraining often takes a fairly long amount of time to occur in any meaningful amount and I mention that as beginners often fall into the trap of thinking that missing a single workout or two means that everything done to that point has been lost. This is akin to thinking that a single day off a diet reverses all the changes and neither are true. With one or two missed workouts, almost no fitness will be lost and even a full week with zero exercise will cause very little backsliding. As well, lost fitness always comes back faster than it was first developed. The sooner someone resumes their exercise program, the sooner they will return to their previous fitness level and be able to start making further improvements.

Aerobic/Cardiovascular and HIIT Exercise

Since aerobic/cardiovascular work and HIIT share a number of concepts, are often done with the the same types of exercises and are often used for broadly similar purposes, I will discuss them together. While similar in nature, there is one primary difference between the two types of exercise which is in how they are done. With few exceptions, aerobic exercise is performed continuously and for relatively extended periods of time (20-60 minutes or longer). The extended nature of aerobic exercise requires that it be done at a relatively lowered intensity (and it is the lowered intensity that allows it to be done for extended periods). Since the term will come up again, let me note that due to aerobic exercise often being done at a relatively steady or unchanging intensity, it is often called steady state exercise. In contrast, HIIT is done by first performing a short warm-up followed by some number of high-intensity intervals (usually ranging from 15-90 seconds) interspersed with lower-intensity recovery periods (who's duration may vary), followed by a cool-down. A typical HIT workout may take 15-25 minutes (although some workouts are longer). In this situation, the high-intensity nature of HIIT prevents large amounts from being done.

Intensity

As one of the main distinguishing factors between aerobic and HIIT exercise is the intensity, I will start by discussing that rather than frequency. The intensity of both aerobic and HIIT exercise has been set in a fairly large number of ways over the years but I will only focus on a few of them.   Perhaps the most common approach to setting exercise intensity for aerobic or HIIT work was to use heart rate.   While different methods exist, a typical approach would be to set the exercise intensity as some percentage of maximum heart rate (MHR). So aerobic work might be done at 60-75% of and HIIT might be done at 85-100% MHR. While relatively simple, this approach has a number of problems associated with it.

The first has to do with MHR itself which can be determined in one of two ways. Traditionally, MHR has been estimated with 220-age being the most commonly used equation. Thus a 20 year old has an estimated MHR of 200 and a 40 year old an estimate MHR of 180.   But this equation has problems. The first is that the equation was originally developed on men and is inaccurate for women who have a slightly lower MHR (1). While the difference is small, 220-age will overestimate a woman's true MHR. Of equal importance is that any given trainee may have a MHR that is drastically different than the predicted value. It's not unheard of to find 40 year old athletes with an MHR of 200 and the equation would give them a completely incorrect number. MHR can be tested directly, by performing 5 minutes of maximum intensity activity but this is both impractical and potentially dangerous for all but trained athletes.

Even if MHR can be determined accurately, another problem arises in that any recommended percentages for training are based on an average response. One person might find that exercising at 75% of MHR is an appropriate intensity while another may only be able to sustain 60%. Giving both the same recommendations may have one person doing too much and another doing too little. In recent years, performance athletes have tended to use individually determined thresholds to set exercise intensity. A common anchor point is to determine the highest intensity that can be maintained for an hour with aerobic work being done at or below this level and HIIT being done above it. In an ideal world this type of individual approach would be used for everyone to set proper exercise intensity (2). This is true for a number of reasons not the least of which is that exercising at the appropriate exercise intensity can impact on adherence (3). For beginners especially, exercise above a certain difficulty level causes a great deal of discomfort and a lack of enjoyment and this causes many to drop out. When exercise is done below that intensity, adherence is improved. Unfortunately, it is impractical to determine individual training thresholds for the general trainee or dieter at this time. Heart rate becomes even more problematic for HIIT workouts. During exercise, heart rate takes at least three minutes to reach a stable level but most intervals will be shorter than this and HR will not be a good indicator of the actual exercise intensity.

For all of the above reasons, I recommend that trainees use a method called Rating of Perceived Exertion (RPE) to gauge the intensity of aerobic/HIIT training. The RPE scale goes from 1-10 with 1 representing nothing and 10 representing maximal effort. I've presented the RPE chart below with the RPE values themselves, verbal descriptions and what might be a representative heart rate during exercise (let me reiterate that these may vary enormously between people). I've given some examples of what types of exercise fall into each category along with providing some names common to the online fitness industry. I've also indicated some rough calorie expenditures might be for a 130 pound female exercising for an hour.

RPE	Difficulty	HR	Type of Exercise	Common Name	Cal/Hour
0	Nothing at all		Sitting down	N/A	Very very low
0.5	Extremely Weak (Very easy)		Standing	N/A	Very low
1	Very Weak (Very Easy)	80	Brisk walking	LISS	Very low
2	Weak (Light)	120	Walking on incline, Slow cycling	LISS	200 (3 cal/min)
3	Moderate (Challenging)	130	Jogging Moderate cycling	MISS	300 (5 cal/min)
4	Moderate (Challenging)	150	Jogging Moderate cycling	MISS	400 (6 cal/min)
5	Strong/Heavy (Very challenging)	160	Hard running Fast cycling	HISS	500 (8 cal/min)
6	Strong/Heavy (Very challenging)	180	Hard running Fast cycling	HISS	650 (11 cal/min)
7	Very Difficult	180+	Interval Training	HIIT	See Below
8	Very Difficult	180+	Interval Training	HIIT	See Below
9	Very Difficult	180+	Interval Training	HIIT	See Below
10	Extremely Strong/Maximal	Max	Sprint Training	Sprinting	See Below

While an RPE from 1-6 is technically the range for aerobic work, exercising at an RPE below 3 is unlikely to do much for either fitness or health although it might be appropriate for a complete beginner in the earliest stages. Exercise at that intensity also burns very few calories per hour. As the RPE increases, so does the difficulty and calorie burn and an RPE of 6 can usually only be done for one hour maximum and only by very motivated trainees. The notations LISS, HISS and MISS are commonly used in the online fitness community and stand for Low-, Medium- and High-Intensity Steady State exercise. Above an RPE of 6, the duration that exercise can be maintained drops rapidly and exercise above that level is done in an interval/HIIT style. While some types of HIIT might eventually achieve a 10RPE by the end of the workout, exercise at that level is usually considered as sprint training.

Before moving on, let me explain the lack of calorie burn information for HIIT and sprint exercise. As I've described, both types of training are done by alternating relatively short bouts of very high intensity exercise with bouts of very low intensity exercise. While the high-intensity bouts burn a very high number of calories per minute, this tends to be cancelled out by low calorie per minute burn of the recovery periods between intervals. Combined with the generally shorter duration of the workout, this means that HIIT workouts usually burn far fewer calories during the workout than a traditional length aerobic workout. And while much has been made of the calories burned after HIIT, not only is the effect fairly small but, as discussed previously, it's even smaller for women. This isn't to say that HIIT is useless and I've mentioned that it has other benefits for women such as glycogen depletion. It's simply that in terms of the actual calorie expenditure, HIIT is frequently inferior to longer duration aerobic exercise.

Frequency

The frequency of aerobic work or HIIT refers to the number of total sessions which are done per week and this number can vary widely. Strength/power athletes may perform effectively zero sessions per week of either while endurance athletes may perform daily, or even multiple daily, aerobic sessions combined with some amount of HIIT as well. Most trainees will fall somewhere between those two extremes.

The primary factor (as per the FITT equation) that determines how often a given workout can be done is intensity. As exercise intensity goes up, the frequency of exercise must go down and vice versa. So LISS, given it's low intensity nature can usually be done daily. In some cases, MISS may be able to be done daily but this can become too much if other types of training such as HIIT or resistance training that stress the same muscle groups are also being done. In most cases, 3-4 sessions of MISS per week will likely be the upper limit. HISS can be done even less frequently and most would be hard pressed to do it more than perhaps twice per week if that often. An hour of properly done HISS is absolutely exhausting and it's worth noting that competitive endurance athletes do very little work at this intensity. For all other athletes, HISS should be used very sparingly if it used at all.

Finally there is HIIT which, due to it's very high-intensity nature should generally be limited to 0-2 workouts per week. As with MISS and HISS, this becomes more true is other high-intensity training such as weight training is being done that uses the same muscle groups (generally the legs). This is to avoid burnout and injury, both of which occurred when HIIT first became popular and dieters started doing it daily along with their weight training. Since HIIT is limited in its total frequency, any dieter or trainee who wants or needs to do other non-resistance training will have to perform LISS or possibly MISS (HISS and HIIT can not usually be combined in the same training week). In a dieting situation, if HIIT were being done twice weekly, LISS would be the best choice for the other days. The two can actually be combined to help with stubborn fat loss and I will detail these protocols in Appendix 1.

Time

Since aerobic/steady state exercise is more or less defined as exercise that can be done continuously for extended periods, time generally represents the duration of the workout itself. This isn't universal and for HISS type aerobic workouts, it would be common to perform a 10-15 minute low-intensity warmup to prepare the body prior to a 60' HISS session followed by a 10-15' cool down for recovery. So while the HISS segment is only 60', the total workout might take 80-90'. The typical MISS workout might need a brief (5 minutes) warm-up and cool-down if that and LISS workouts can be done without a warm-up or cool-down period. Since HISS should either be avoided or limited for most people, I will refer to time for aerobic workouts in terms of the time spent at the target intensity level only.

In terms of duration, 20 minutes of continuous activity is generally considered as the minimum duration to have any real effect although beginners can accumulate exercise of the course of the day (i.e. 5-10 minutes done multiple times in a day). As fitness improves, 20 minutes will no longer be sufficient and the duration can be increased with 60 minutes per session being the upper limit for general health or dieting situations. It would be better to add another day of exercise than to increase the duration if the trainee wants to do more. How much aerobic work would be done for performance athletes depends heavily on the sport with endurance athletes frequently doing 2-4 hours or more per session depending on the sport. In some dieting situations, usually smaller females dieting to the extremes, more than 60 minutes per session might be necessary. In this case, splitting it into two different workouts (i.e. 45' done twice daily) would be a better choice than performing one enormously long session.

Discussing HIIT in terms of time is a little bit more complex as there are 5 different components that will contribute to how long the workout takes. The two simplest to examine are the warm-up and cool-down periods which occur before and after the actual workout. As described previously, the warm-up is used to prepare the body for the high-intensity efforts and the cool-down is used to bring the body back down towards baseline for recovery. While athletes may do extended (20-30 minute) warm-ups before intense HIIT workouts, 5-10 minutes before and after will be sufficient for most trainees.

The third component is the duration of the high-intensity interval itself which I will call the work interval. This can range from less than 10 seconds (typically called sprint training) all the way up to 3-5 minutes or more. While sprint interval training (SIT) consisting of 6 seconds all out and 24 seconds rest has been used in some studies, I generally feel that, for non-athletic and fat loss applications, work intervals of 15-90 seconds will be the most appropriate with intervals of 45-60 seconds or longer being most beneficial in terms of depleting muscle glycogen for women (men can use slightly shorter intervals due to differences in fuel use and the amount of fatigue which occurs).

The fourth component is the duration of the low-intensity interval that occurs between work intervals, and I will refer to this as the rest interval (RI).   There are two common methods of setting the RI. The first is to wait until heart rate returns to 120-130 beats per minute regardless of how long it takes although few use this method anymore. More commonly used is to set the duration of the RI as a ratio relative to the work interval. A 1:1 ratio would mean that the RI is the same as the work interval (i.e. 45 seconds hard, 45 seconds easy) while a 2:1 ratio would mean that the RI is twice the length of the work interval (i.e. 30 seconds hard, 60 seconds easy).

In general, the shorter the work interval, the longer the relative rest interval. Ignoring the specific SIT protocols used in some research, it's not uncommon for a true all out sprint training to require a 15:1 rest interval with 150 seconds of rest being taken after only 10 seconds of effort.   At 30 seconds of all-out effort, anywhere from 2-4 minutes of rest (a 2:1 to 8:1 recovery interval) might be used. For a 60 second interval, only 60 seconds (1:1) might be necessary and a lower intensity 90 second interval might only need 45 seconds (0.5:1) rest. As I will discuss in much more detail in Volume 2, women generate less fatigue and recover more rapidly than men during HIIT. So in the same way that they will benefit from slightly longer work intervals, they can generally also use slightly shorter RIs than men.

The final component of time is the total number of intervals (including both the work and rest interval) that are being done. Someone performing 5 repeats of 45 seconds hard and 45 seconds easy (90 seconds total for the work and rest interval) will be be performing 7.5 minutes of HIIT (5X90 seconds) plus their warmup and cool down time. Someone performing 10 repeats of 30 seconds hard and 30 seconds easy (60 seconds total) will be performing 10 minutes of HIIT plus warm-up and cool down.

In the chart below, focusing on work intervals ranging from 30-90 seconds, I've shown what might be a typical number of total intervals along with an appropriate rest interval.   I've also shown an appropriate RPE for each duration of interval to be done at.

Interval Duration	Rest Interval	# Intervals	RPE
30 seconds	120-180 seconds	10-15*	9-10
60 seconds	60-120 seconds	5-10	8-9
90 seconds	60-90 seconds	5-6	8

*A commonly used HIIT workout in research is to perform 4X30 seconds all out with a 4.5 minute rest interval but this tends to be completely exhausting.

You can see that the same relationship of duration, intensity and time still hold even for individual HIIT workouts. As the duration of the interval goes up, the total number that can be done goes down as does the overall intensity of each interval.   So while a 30 second interval might allow the trainee to go nearly all out and perform a fairly large number of intervals, completing a 90 second interval will mean doing less total intervals and working at a slightly lower intensity. This shift in intensity explains why the relative rest interval duration decreases as the interval increases in duration. After an all out 30 second effort, several minutes will be required before it can be realistically done again. In contrast, the relatively lower intensity nature of the 90 second interval means that it can be repeated 1-1.5 minutes later.

While I will talk about programming more below, I will say here that beginners are best served by starting with a lower number of the shorter intervals first and they should not be done at maximum intensity to start. Over time, the intensity of the interval can be brought up to the highest that can be maintained for the entire time and the number of intervals can be increased gradually. And while women do recover more quickly from individual intervals than men, I would still recommend starting with the longer rest interval and decreasing it gradually if the workouts are being completed without excessive fatigue.

Type

The final consideration for both aerobic and HIIT exercise is type. Here there are both commonalities and differences between the two. Given that it originally developed to improve the performance of endurance athletes, traditionally HIIT was done using the same types of activities as the sport the athlete was involved in. Runners ran, cyclists rode their bike, rowers rowed, etc. And at a fundamental level, so long as it can be done at a high enough intensity, almost any activity that can be used for aerobic training can be used to perform HIIT. Running, cycling, rowing, the Elliptical machine, stair climbing machines and others can be used for both aerobic and HIIT type exercise. Walking is one exception in that it can't be done at a high enough intensity to be considered HIIT (in many cases, it is impossible to even reach MISS levels of intensity with walking).

Looking first at aerobic exercise, with the exception of athletes who will perform the majority of aerobic training in their actual sport, the type of activity chosen is far less important than the fact that the exercise is done. In that sense, the choice of aerobic activity should be based on preference, availability and/or safety. By preference I mean an activity that the person enjoys enough to do consistently. Availability means being able to perform the activity on a regular basis. Areas with unpredictable weather may make outdoor exercise problematic and activities that require very specific places to perform them may be difficult to perform regularly. Few will perform an inconvenient activity consistently.

Safety is another issue and this can reflect several issues. Outdoor cycling can be dangerous if someone lives in an area without bike paths or where traffic is high or drivers dislike cyclists (cycling is also not the cheapest activity to get involved in).   Due to having generally wider hips, running can often be problematic for women in terms of injury risk. This isn't universal and women built to run tend to have narrower hips and have a more linear body type. Even some gym equipment may not fit all women and over time this can cause overuse injuries. Overall, the best aerobic exercise should be enjoyable, available and safe enough to be done consistently and this trumps any claimed superiority for a specific activity.

Looking at some specific activities, walking is often found to be the activity people can do the most readily, most likely due to it being a basic human movement pattern. However, the intensity tends to be limited since 4.0 miles per hour is about the fastest most can walk.   Treadmills can be inclined but at some point walking will be insufficient or have to turn into jogging and running which many women are simply not built to perform safely. Cycling avoids this problem but beginners often find that their leg muscles give out before their cardiovascular system. The Elliptical (EFX) machines tend to be good choices in that they spread the stress out across the upper and lower bodies on top of decreasing joint impact but many have foot platforms that are too wide or narrow which can cause knee or hip problems. As two final comments let me first note that while outdoor activities (if available) can be more enjoyable than indoor activities, controlling intensity may be difficult. Someone attempting to cycle in a hilly area will find it nearly impossible to maintain a true steady state level of activity.

Let me finish by pointing out that there is no reason trainees can't perform different types of exercise. Having multiple options can not only avoid boredom but give more flexibility in training. When the weather is good, outdoor exercise can be chosen. When it's not, a different indoor activity can be done. Even for women who train solely inside in the gym, there's no reason different machines can't be done on different days or even within the same workout (i.e. 20 minutes on three different machines to total 60').

Moving to HIIT most of the above comments hold although safety becomes the dominant issue over even preference or availability.   Compared to steady state aerobic training, HIIT generates a large amount of fatigue and some activities become dangerous under this condition.   Running tends to be the most problematic as technique and form can deteriorate enormously, increasing the risk of injury significantly. Sprint running carries an enormous injury risk and many have pulled or torn hamstrings by going to the track and trying to run at full speed without proper training. Many other activities do not have this problem and the majority of HIIT studies have used cycling for this reason.   On a bike, when someone fatigues, they either slow down or stop pedaling but nothing beyond that happens (this is true of outdoor cycling as well). The same holds true for rowing machines, ellipticals, step machines and other non-running activities where increasing fatigue simply causes the exerciser to slow down or stop without injury. For non-athletes, I also generally recommend using indoor exercise types. About the only type of outdoor activity that might safely be done for a HIIT workout would be cycling and this creates practical problems with hills, traffic and controlling interval and rest durations accurately.

Let me finish by mentioning, in recent years, less traditional activities have been done in an HIIT style. This includes activities such as kettlebell work, sleds, some types of strongman activities, and various types of barbell complexes (a series of exercises done without a break one after another). These tend to be used by strength/power athletes as they are more specific to their sport although some types of exercise classes use free weights or other implements to perform HIIT workouts.   This can start to crossover with some types of weight training, discussed next, although the goals tend to be somewhat different for HIIT workouts.

A key aspect here is also safety and movements should be chosen where fatigue will not increase injury risk. For most that means picking relatively less technical exercises to perform the workout with. Some bodyweight exercises (effectively old school calisthenics), kettlebell swings, battle ropes, medicine ball exercises, sled pulling or pushing and others can generally be done safely in HIIT style. Movements such as Olympic lifts or even highly complex weight room movements tend to become dangerous done in this style as technique starts to deteriorate in the face of fatigue.

HIIT vs. Aerobic Exercise

Before moving onto the topic of weight training, I want to compare and contrast HIIT to aerobic exercise. First I'll look at some of the potential (or claimed) benefits of HIIT including its effects on general health, fat loss and being potentially more time efficient. Then I'll look at the potential negatives of HIIT (which are effectively the benefits of aerobic exercise) including the difficulty, issues with adherence, its effects on the rest of the training program the consequences of its limited ability for use.

Potential Benefit: Improved General Health

Although early studies suggested that HIIT might be more effective (at least relative to the time of the workout) for fat loss, the potential for HIIT to have more or less identical, or occasionally superior, effects on overall health has been a primary focus in research (4). In a general sense this is true with HIIT improving cardiovascular health, general health and other factors such as insulin sensitivity, usually with far shorter workouts than traditional aerobic work. There may be gender differences here with women not showing the same improvements in insulin sensitivity as men but this is probably a consequence of the fact that women start with higher insulin sensitivity than men and don't have as much room to improve (4a). Overall, this claim for HIIT is well supported although there are other factors to consider.

Potential Benefit: Increased Fat Loss

Perhaps one of the most long-standing claims for HIIT is that it generates superior fat loss compared to traditional aerobic work, especially in terms of the time required. That is, if both a 25 minute HIIT and 60 minute aerobic session generate the same fat loss, the HIIT is doing so with a shorter time commitment. At least some studies show this to be the case but there are few factors to take into account. The first is that, when diet is uncontrolled, neither aerobic exercise or HIIT is terribly effective in the first place with total fat losses for both being perhaps 2 lbs (1kg) fat lost over several months (5). Not only is this insignificant overall, it is only the case when the HIIT sessions are of a similar duration as the aerobic sessions in the first place. When the HIIT sessions are much shorter, continuous aerobic activity comes out slightly ahead in terms of fat loss although the effects are still small overall. Women do appear to lose more fat with HIIT than men although this is most likely due to starting with a higher BF% (6).

The general lack of effects is due to the diet not being controlled but demonstrates that, even if HIIT is as good as aerobic exercise for loss, both are relatively ineffective by themselves (again, HIIT can have many indirect benefits for fat loss when women are dieting). Much of this is probably due to increases in hunger or food intake and I'd note again that women seem to show more variability in this regard. If hunger is increased to a greater degree after HIIT than aerobic exercise, causing a woman to eat more, choosing the HIIT may do more harm than good. This is especially true given that HIIT tends to burn fewer calories during exercise than aerobic exercise.

This may seem confusing given the general claim that HIIT burns more total calories than aerobic work so I want to look at the actual math of it. Consider someone performing 5 intervals of 1 minute where they are burning 15 calories/minute during the work interval with 5 rest periods of 1 minute where they are burning 3 calories per minute. This yields an average calorie burn of 9 calories per minute (and this might be slightly higher or lower depending on the specific interval workout done) which is roughly the equivalent of what would be burned doing HISS at an RPE of 5.5. But since only 10 minutes of work is done, only 90 calories total will be burned plus the small amount burned during the warm-up and cool down and the total might be 120 calories with a small calorie burn after the workout is over. That same 120 calories could be burned with a 20 minute MISS workout burning 6 cal/min while a 60' MISS workout would burn 360 calories, far more.

Certainly if the number of intervals were doubled to 10, the calorie burn will increase to 180 plus a bit for warm-up and cool-down, for a total of perhaps 220 calories and the workout will now take 30 minutes. A 40 minute MISS workout (at 6 cal/min) would burn the same number of calories while only taking slightly more time (and being far less difficult). Finally, a 60 minute LISS workout burning 4 cal/minute burns 240 calories although it does take longer. In all cases, not only does the HIIT not provide an enormous time savings, but the LISS/MISS workouts will be much easier to complete. While many still focus on the supposed afterburn effect of HIIT, I'd reiterate that not only is the effect small overall but that women may generate an even smaller response than men. Regardless of the specific numbers, it's not only clear that HIIT is relatively inferior in terms of calorie burn but that it's only even equivalent in terms of fat loss when the workout duration is similar to aerobic exercise.

Potential Benefit: More Time Efficient

The final major claim for the superiority of HIIT is that the workouts are more time efficient than traditional continuous workouts. In a busy world where many people don't have time to exercise for extended periods, a workout which generates similar results in less time is a major benefit. And under at least some conditions, HIIT workouts can be fairly short. In some of the examples I gave above, a full workout may take only 20-25 minutes, half the time of the typical 45-60 minute aerobic workout. At the same time, it's also clear that HIIT workouts can become extremely long if a large number of longer intervals are being done. HIIT workouts are only equivalent in terms of the fat loss seen if they are of a similar duration to traditional aerobic work. So it's not always true that HIIT provides enormous time savings. By the time a HIIT workout is taking 40 minutes, there are minimal time savings compared to a 45-60 minute aerobic workout. And this comes along with the potential negatives of HIIT, discussed next.

Potential Negative: Difficulty

Perhaps the primary negative is that a properly done HIIT workout takes a great deal of effort (more recently, less intensive HIIT types of workouts have been researched to good effect). This means that the person must be willing to push themselves and work at a fairly high level. While this is rarely an issue with well trained or highly motivated athletes, it's questionable if the trainee seeking general fitness and health or who are just starting an exercise program will be capable of pushing themselves hard enough to make HIIT effective. A HIIT workout where the intervals are not sufficiently high-intensity will not come close to matching the benefits of a longer workout at a more moderate intensity. Related to this is the fact that only the most extreme aerobic workouts (i.e. HISS) come close to HIIT in terms of difficulty and this is important given that HIIT is often not much more time efficient than aerobic exercise to begin with. A 40 minute HIIT session is brutally difficult while a 45' MISS or 60' LISS session can be accomplished much more easily. With HIIT, ttrainee is working much harder for only a small potential benefit.

Potential Negative: Adherence

Related to this is a second potential negative of HIIT which has to do with exercise adherence. Done properly, HIIT is painful and, for many, unenjoyable. Even motivated athletes don't necessarily enjoy HIIT and do it only as a means to an end in terms of improving performance or fat loss. In the beginning stages of an exercise program, workouts that are found to be miserable or painful tend to be abandoned and HIIT can be both with many studies showing that adherence rates are lower for HIIT compared to moderate intensity aerobic activity (6). This isn't universal with some people preferring HIIT, often when the intervals are done at as slightly lower intensity, since the workout is shorter (7).

The adherence issue is especially prevalent if HIIT is attempted from the very beginning of a new exercise program or started too early. Lost by many HIIT advocates is that studies on the topic typically include several weeks of regular aerobic exercise before the HIIT is introduced. Often, a mixture of shorter and longer intervals is used which is combined with easier aerobic exercise. This gives new trainees a chance to develop fitness and work their way into the higher intensity work rather doing three HIIT sessions per week from day 1. In that vein, the combination of four aerobic sessions per week with 1 HIIT session (starting with fewer intervals which progressed over 12 weeks) provided superior benefits to only moderate activity while showing nearly 100% adherence (8). For most this is the better approach.

Potential Negative: Impact on Other Parts of the Workout

Adding to the above is an issue that I find is often forgotten or ignored which is that the inclusion of HIIT must be considered within the rest exercise program. Here I am talking about weight training which, like HIIT, represents another high-intensity stress to the body. Simply put, there is a limit to how much high-intensity work that can be done within a week's time before the person's ability to recover is overwhelmed. This can occur when the person is eating normally but becomes especially true under dieting conditions as the reduction in calorie intake further reduces the body's ability to recover. Most studies on this topic only compared HIIT to aerobic exercise or a mixture of the two with no other exercise being performed. Weight training was rarely included and subjects were usually not dieting. Yet when HIIT became popular, dieters tried to combine all three: HIIT, resistance training and dieting. For perspective, only the rarest athlete performs more than 2-3 truly high-intensity workouts per week. Yet someone performing 4 weight workouts per week who tries to add 2 (or more) HIIT sessions is now trying to perform 6 (or more). This would be a nearly impossible work load under the best of conditions but trying to do it while dieting rapidly leads to burnout or injury.

While overall physiological stress is an issue, there is also the factor that most forms of HIIT tend to involve the legs either exclusively or in addition to the upper body (i.e. elliptical, rowing machine) which overlaps enormously with any heavy lower body weight training that is being done. When a trainee is trying to gain muscle or strength in the legs, HIIT causes fatigue or hampers their weight training workouts. When dieting, the legs can become so fatigued that overtraining or injury occurs. This does interact with the nature of the weight training program itself. Someone training the legs once/week (which I do not recommend for women) might be able to add 2 HIIT sessions during the week as this would only amount to 3 total high-intensity workouts for the lower body. In contrast, someone training the legs intensely in the weight room 3 times per week who attempted to add another 2 HIIT sessions would now have 5 total high-intensity leg workouts per week and would be likely to overtrain or get injured.

Potential Negative: Limited Frequency of HIIT

The final potential negative of HIIT that I want to address is the fact that, due to its high intensity nature, HIIT must be limited in the number of times per week that it can be done (and this is even more true if other high-intensity work is being done). As I mentioned above, highly trained athletes rarely perform HIIT more than 2-3 times per week with 1-2 sessions being the maximum if other high-intensity work is being done. When a given goal requires that more aerobic work than this be done, this becomes limiting. In the case of general cardiovascular health, where a minimum of three sessions per week is required, HIIT cannot be the sole form of exercise. If only 1-2 of those sessions can be HIIT, than an additional 2 or 1 aerobic sessions would be needed. Women with PCOS often benefit from daily exercise due to its effect on insulin sensitivity. If HIIT is limited to 1-2 sessions, an additional 4-5 aerobic sessions are needed.

The same dynamic holds for dieters where some type of calorie burning activity to be done nearly daily. This may be by choice to create a deficit while allowing more food to be eaten or by necessity for the smaller extreme dieter who is trying to maintain a deficit in the face of metabolic slowdown. In either case, if the dieter is performing 6-7 non-weight training workouts per week, HIIT will be insufficient. At the very least more traditional aerobic work (LISS or perhaps the lower levels of MISS) would be required on the other days. In some cases, the addition of HIIT to a diet and heavy weight training program is simply untenable. In this case, HIIT must be eliminated entirely in favor of traditional aerobic exercise.

Summary

Before looking at guidelines, let me finish by saying that the above look at the potential benefits and negatives of HIIT isn't meant to say that HIIT should or should not necessarily be done. Whether seeking general health and fitness or for fat loss, it should be clear that HIIT is in no way required. It can certainly have benefits (i.e. the hormonal response, muscle glycogen depletion) under certain situations but that must be weighed against the potential for injury, burnout, excessive fatigue or quitting the exercise program. If HIIT is done, it must be introduced gradually and progressively while being limited in the total number of sessions that are done. Any additional conditioning work would then be done with more traditionally LISS/MISS types of aerobic exercise with the combination likely being superior than either by itself.

Guidelines for Cardiovascular/HIIT Exercise

Since I touched on them already above, I will only summarize guidelines for aerobic and HIIT training here. For aerobic exercise, a frequency of 3-6 times per week at an intensity ranging from an RPE of 3-6 and a duration of 20-60 minutes will be appropriate for most goals. The type of exercise is less important than the other components. For HIIT, a frequency 0-2 sessions per week at an intensity of 7 or higher on the RPE scale with intervals ranging from 15-90 seconds and a total workout time of 15-25 minutes would be appropriate. The type of exercise must be chosen for safety over everything else.

Jumping

I mentioned jumping as one type of exercise back in Chapter 4 both in terms of its use by athletes along with the benefits it can have on bone mineral density (BMD). While the use of jumping (often called plyometrics) by athletes is too involved to discuss meaningfully here, I do want to look at the topic in terms of the bone density issue and how it might be used or implemented towards this goal. Whether for general health to improve bone density or when dieting, to hopefully limit bone loss, jumping is one of the relatively safer ways for most women to put a proper stimulus on bone (both Olympic weight lifting and sprinting have this effect but both require enormous technical training). I will only address Intensity, Frequency and Time since, by definition, jumping is the Type of exercise being done.

Intensity

Unlike other forms of activity, there are few objective markers of intensity for jumping. In athletic practice, jumps are frequently classified based on such factors as their overall complexity or how much of a load they put on muscle or bones. An activity such as skipping rope or even hopping in place is fairly low intensity as it is simple and puts relatively lower stresses on the body. In contrast, jumping down off a box and either landing or jumping straight up again (called a depth landing or depth jump) not only requires good technique but puts an enormous load on the body overall and this is a very high intensity exercise. For the most part I am only including the above for completeness as most studies on the topic of jumping and bone density have used vertical jumps in place. This type of activity is done by bending the knees slightly before jumping as high as possible and then landing. This still requires proper technique, the knees must stay over the toes both when jumping and landing (and this is important as many women's knees will bow in during this type of movement, something I will discuss in more detail in Volume 2).

Frequency

As a high-intensity type of exercise, jumping should only be done with a limited frequency. Most athletes only perform it 2-3 times per week and there would be little benefit for a non-athlete to do more than this. It's best to space these workouts out throughout the week so three workouts might be done Monday/Wednesday/Friday or Tuesday/Thursday/Saturday. Two workouts could be spaced Monday/Thursday, Monday/Friday or some similar spacing based on convenience. In the sample templates I will put jumping exercise on any day where legs are trained in the weight room.

Time

For jumping exercises, the component of time has little to no meaning, a short jumping workout might take no more than 5 minutes while athletes might perform jumping exercises for much longer. Rather, it's most common to talk about jumping exercises in terms of the total number of jumps or foot contacts where 20 jumps and landings equals 20 foot contacts. How long that takes depends mostly on the rest interval taken between jumps. Some jumping exercises are done relatively continuously while others require a rest between jumps. Someone skipping rope might do 60 or more foot contacts in a minute while someone doing depth drops might do no more than 5 repetitions before taking a few minute break. Jumping can become extremely dangerous when it is done in a fatigued state and I mention this as there is a current trend of plyometrics classes where 40 or more minutes of relatively continuous work is being done. Not only is this excessive but potentially dangerous if and when form breaks down.

Guidelines for Jumping

The guidelines for jumping in terms of improving BMD are actually quite simple and are not as context specific as for the other types of exercise. While some research has used more than, typically 10-20 vertical jumps per workout with 30 seconds between repetitions have been used. Since each jump takes at most a few seconds, this entire workout might take 5-10 minutes or so to complete. Done with an appropriate frequency this is sufficient to have a positive impact on BMD. Because of its high skill component, jumping should be done near or at the beginning of a workout as jumping when the legs are not tired from either resistance training or hard aerobic activity increases injury risk. Let me note that jumping only impacts the bones of the leg meaningfully and there are others area of concern for women in terms of bone density. To adequately hit those, jumping must be combined with weight training.

Weight/Resistance Training Guidelines

As described in Chapter 4, weight training refers to any type of activity where the muscles work against a fairly high resistance for relatively short periods of time with the goal of making them stronger and/or larger (or preventing them from getting weaker and smaller in the case of dieting). Traditionally weight training is performed using free weights such as barbells, dumbbells or kettlebells or on specialized machines but technically anything that challenges the muscles sufficiently will be efective. Rubber tubing is popular for home exercise, cans or bottles could be filled with water or sand and many exercises can be done using body weight for resistance.

While resistance training is the single most important type of exercise that can or should be performed when dieting, it is also the most complex in terms of the concepts that surround it and the number of different parameters that can go into the setup of a routine or program. The full details of this will have to wait for Volume 2 and I will only provide an abbreviated set of guidelines here.

Basic Definitions

Since I can't assume that any given reader has a back ground in weight training, I want to start by defining some basic terms and concepts so that the next sections will make sense.

Muscle or Muscle Group: While weight training impacts on far more than just muscle (i.e. the nervous system, bones, ligaments, tendons, etc.) it's most common to describe weight training workouts in terms of the muscle or muscle groups (a group of overlapping muscles) being trained. So people will talk about training the chest (pectorals or pecs), quadriceps (quads), biceps, triceps, etc.

Exercise: This refers to the specific movements being done with weight training exercises training one or more muscles groups at a time. Weight training exercises are generally divided into compound and isolation exercises. Compound exercises generally work many several muscles or muscle groups at a time while isolation exercises put the majority of focus on a single muscle group. For example, the squat (a compound exercise) works the quadriceps, glutes, hamstrings, low back and other muscles while the leg extension (an isolation exercise) puts all of the focus only on the quadriceps.

Repetition/Rep: The single lifting and (usually) lowering of a weight is called a repetition or rep. I say usually as, in some sports, the weight is only lifted and then dropped but this is still called a repetition.

Set/Sets: A series of repetitions. Someone who lifts and lowers a weight 15 times has done one set of 15 reps. One or more sets of an exercise may be done with some amount of rest between them.

Repetition Maximum (RM): If a set of repetitions are taken to the point that no more reps can be done in good form, the weight being used is referred to as a repetition maximum or RM load. RM can apply to any repetition number so the weight that could only be lifted once in good form would be a 1RM and the weight that could only be lifted 10 times in good form would be a 10RM.

Rest Interval: The rest between sets is called the rest interval (RI) which can be listed in seconds (") or minutes ('). So an RI of 60" means that 60 seconds would be taken between sets. An RI of 90" (or 1'30") would mean that 90 seconds (1.5 minutes) would be taken.

Training Notation: So that the examples below will make sense and since there are other methods that exist, I want to show the training notation that I will be using. My notation will always be #Sets X #Reps/ RI. So 3 sets of 15 repetitions with 90 seconds rest would be written as 3X15/90" where 90 seconds is the rest between each set as well as before the next exercise. Often, training will be given with a range of numbers for any of the three components. A notation of 3-4X12-15/60-90" would indicate that 3 to 4 sets of 12 to 15 repetitions with a rest interval between 60 and 90 seconds between sets would be used.

Types of Workouts: The above components can be put together in a nearly unlimited number of ways in terms of exercise choices, sets, reps, rest periods, etc. to form individual workouts. Workouts can be divided into one of two types: whole- or full-body and muscle group workouts. A full-body workout is one where all of the major muscles groups are trained in the same single workout. In contrast, a muscle group workout is one in which only part of the body's muscle is trained. A muscle group workout might include a single muscle/muscle group, two to three total muscles groups or even the entire set of upper or lower body muscles depending on the specifics of the training program. I will discuss this more below.

Frequency

Frequency in weight training can be used to refer to one of two different concepts. The first is the total number of workouts per week. This might range from a minimum of 2 per week for a beginner up to 4-6 or more for a more advanced lifter (the occasional strength/power sport may have two workouts per day). The second concept is the number of times any given muscle group is trained within a week. In some cases, this may match the total number of training sessions per week and someone performing two full body workouts per week will be performing two total workouts and two workouts per muscle per week. In other cases, the total number of workouts and workouts per muscle group will not match. Someone who only trained their upper body twice a week and their lower body twice a week would be training four total times per week but each muscle group would only be trained twice per week.

Intensity

Weight training intensity can be represented in a number of different ways and I want to briefly look at them before suggesting the method that I prefer. Traditionally, the percentage of 1RM (the heaviest weight that can only be lifted once) has been used and recommendations might be to train at 75% or 85% or between 65 and 80% of 1RM for various goals. This approach is based on the average number of repetitions trainees can do with a given percentage of 1RM (i.e. 8 reps at 80%). As with the use of aerobic training percentages, there are several problems with this.

One is that the relationship between %age of 1RM and the repetitions done can vary depending on a number of factors including how well trained someone is (more well trained can usually do more reps) or their sport (endurance athletes typically do more reps at any given percentage than strength/power athletes). Importantly to this book, women often show a different relationship than men,. At intensities of 80% or higher, women and men typically can perform about the same number of repetitions at any given percentage but with lighter weights, women are able to do more. At 70% 1RM a woman might do 20 repetitions compared to a man's 15 and at 60% she may do 35 compared to his 20. Another problem is that using %age of 1RM means determining the 1RM somehow. Usually this means determining how much weight someone can lift only once but outside of strength/power athletes, most will not able to accurately or safely do this. There are equations to estimate 1RM from higher repetition sets but these are based on the average relationship between percentage of 1RM And repetitions to begin with and may not be accurate for women. So just as with aerobic/HIIT training, other methods of determining intensity are required.

One approach is to use the RM concept itself since repetitions per set tend to be related to the adaptations seen. A 15RM is, by definition, the heaviest weight that can be lifted only 15 times in good form while a 5RM is the heavier weight that can be lifted 5 times and this is true regardless of the percentage of 1RM it might or might not represent. While this is an improvement over percentage based methods, it requires that all sets be taken to the point of failure and this comes with it's own set of problems including injury or burnout over time. However, the RM concept can still be used by first determining the RM load and then training slightly below that level. If someone's 15RM in an exercise is 100 pounds, they could use 100 pounds and stop at 12 reps or do 15 reps at 80 pounds.

While some sports (notably powerlifting and Olympic lifting) still tend to base training on percentages, in most cases, the best solution to the above problems is the same as for aerobic training which is to use RPE along with another concept I will describe. Here I'll be discussing two slightly different but somewhat related RPE scales and hopefully this won't become too confusing. The first RPE scale is more of a global RPE scale to represent the overall difficulty of any given set (or perhaps workout). Given that weight training is a form of high-intensity training, anything much below a 6 RPE will be ineffective at stimulating any sorts of gains in strength, muscle or bone density. Beginners can often train at levels lower than this and make improvements and lower RPEs are appropriate for warm-up sets. But for the actual work sets, a 6-7 or higher RPE must be used. This is important to realize as many women shortchange themselves in the weight room by lifting loads far below their capabilities. In one study, for example, when women are allowed to self-select a lifting RPE, for example, they frequently choose values far below what is necessary to see any actual gains from their training (9).

The second approach to RPE is more specific to resistance training and effectively combined with the above. Here RPE is used to represent the number of repetitions in reserve (RIR) or how many repetitions below failure the weight is (10). The RPE/RIR chart appears below and it's important to understand that the RPE score and RIR are inversely related, which can be confusing. A 10 RPE would indicate that there are zero RIR. A 9.5 would indicate that there are zero RIR but the weight could be a bit heavier with a 9 indicating 1 RIR, etc. The chart is only shown to a 7RPE since sets that are done with more than 3 RIR typically are only really useful for warmup sets.

RPE	Description
10	Maximum (0 Reps in Reserve)
9.5	No RIR but could go heavier
9	1 Repetition in Reserve
8.5	1-2 Repetitions in Reserve
8	2 Repetitions in Reserve
7.5	2-3 Repetitions in Reserve
7	3 Repetitions in Reserve

Let me note that the above chart is irrespective of the number of goal repetitions. A woman doing sets of 15 repetitions should still be working at an RPE of 7 or higher according to the above chart. This means she should not be able to lift the weight more than 18 times or it is too light. A female powerlifter doing sets of 5 should only be able to do 8 or less repetitions with that weight (RIR of 3 or less). Similar to RIR is an approach called Estimated Reps to Failure or ERF. ERF represents the number of repetitions that could be done to failure if the set were continued to failure and is conceptually identical to the RIR without the reversed nature of the chart. An ERF of 3 would indicate that 3 more repetitions could be done before hitting failure and would be equivalent to an RPE of 7 with 3 reps in reserve. In general, the ERF approach can be very accurate although this depends slightly on the exercise in question (11).

Both the RPE/RIR and ERF approach are functionally identical in that they indicate how many more repetitions could be done to failure. As a general guideline, an RPE of 7+ (RIR of 3 or less) or ERF of 3 or less would is about the lowest that should be used for productive strength training and avoids the need to constantly go to failure. Certainly training to failure from time to time can be useful, if for no other reason than it will help people to get a feel for what an an RPE of 10 or 0 RIR/ERF can be. When a trainee is doing more than one set per exercise, is it normal for RPE to go up with each set with failure being approached or reached on the last set. Using one of the above approaches allows the intensity to be set appropriately for the first set of that exercise so that all sets can be completed.

Time/Volume

Similar to jumping, time has little meaning for weight training since the length of the workout has little to no relevance to the training outside of how long someone might practically have to exercise. This is due to the nature of weight training where only the time spent actually lifting is particularly important. Someone training with very short rest intervals might complete 15 sets in 30 minutes while someone training with long rest intervals might only complete 5 sets in that same amount of time. The workout duration is the same but the amount of actual lifting is not. At least conceptually simile to time for other types of exercise is the idea of weight training volume as a measure of the total amount of lifting that is actually done. As with intensity, volume can be expressed in different ways but I only want to look at two.

One approach, often used in research, is to look at the total number of sets done per workout or per muscle group or exercise. By this definition, someone doing 8 sets of exercises for the chest is doing more volume than someone doing 4 sets or 1 set. But this too can be misleading. Someone performing 8 sets of 1 repetition with very heavy weights may be doing much less total work than someone doing 4 sets of 10 repetitions. One is not necessarily better than the other with each being appropriate for a specific goal. Rather, just looking at the number of sets is not terribly informative. Better than total sets is to look at the total number of repetitions being done per exercise or per muscle group. Someone who performs 60 repetitions (i.e. 4 sets of 15 or 6 sets of 10) is doing double the volume of someone performing only 30 repetitions (i.e. 2 sets of 15 or 3 sets of 10).

Type

As the name suggests, weight training has traditionally been done with equipment such weight machines, barbells and dumbbells. Strictly speaking, anything that applies sufficient resistance to a muscle for an appropriate number of repetitions or time can generate the same types of results as weights themselves (hence the more general term resistance training). Bodyweight exercises such as squats and lunges, rubber tubing and others can all potentially be used. In recent years, less common activities such as swinging hammers, flipping tires and others have become popular as well.

Each type of resistance has its pros and cons but the primary limitation to most non-weights based training is that it can be difficult to apply progressive overload effectively. With tubing, it's often very difficult to make small changes in resistance and bodyweight exercises can only be modified so much to maintain a challenge to the muscles being trained. In contrast, when lifting weights, the amount of resistance both being used or added tends to be very well defined. Free weights are standardized in terms of plates and bars and even weight machines indicate the weight being used and can be progressed as someone's fitness improves. This makes applying progressive overload much easier comparatively speaking. This isn't to say that bodyweight or tubing exercises, both of which can be done at home, are useless or ineffective. Simply that as people improve, they can become limiting.

Guidelines for Weight Training

Although I discussed each above, I want to first summarize and present general guidelines for the frequency, intensity and volume of weight training. As with other types of exercise, a primary factor in what might be appropriate or optimal is the population being discussed. The beginner or someone seeking general fitness has different requirements than the serious trainee or competitive physique or performance athlete. With some slight modifications to make the recommendations more relevant to this book, I've summarized the current research (and practice) supported guidelines in the chart below (12-14). Intensity has been indicated in terms of RM load rather than percentage for reasons explained above with an RPE of 7 or higher being assumed and I described type of workout above (and will address it again below).

Population Group	Workout Frequency	Muscle Group Frequency	Intensity	Sets/Muscle	Total Reps Per Muscle Per Wkout.	Type of Workout
Beginner	2-3/Week	2-3X/week	20 RM	1-2	8-20	Whole body
General Health	2-3X/Week	2-3X/week	8-12RM	2-4	8-30	Whole body
Serious Trainee	3-4+/Week	2X/week	6-15RM	4-6	40-70	Split
Advanced Physique	3-6+/Week	2X/week	6-15RM	6-8 (10)	70-100?	Split

You can see that beginners only need a relatively small amount of training, 2-3 total workouts per week (and per muscle group) at a relatively low intensity (a weight that could be lifted 20 times even if it is lifted for less repetitions than this) and volume of training (1-2 total sets). This overlaps with general health training which has the same frequency, a higher intensity and allows for more total sets/rep per muscle group as desired. Recommendations change for the serious trainee and here more total workouts per week may be done although the frequency per muscle group is decreased. Finally is the advanced trainee (here I am focusing only on physique athletes) who may need to train the most frequently (although with the same lowered frequency per muscle group) using the largest potential number of sets and repetitions. The question mark after 100 indicates that little research has examined advanced trainees and most of the recommendations here are anecdotal or experiential. Certainly the advanced trainee is likely to need more total training than anyone else although, in my experience, most trainees do far more work than is necessary or optimal.

Types of Weight Training

While the different parameters of sets, reps, rest intervals, training intensity, exercise choice, etc. can technically be combined in nearly unlimited ways, in practice, there are only a handful of types of weight training which are defined based on certain combinations and the primary goal being sought. The four goals I will examine are increasing strength/power, increasing muscle size, metabolic/glycogen depletion work and finally maintenance training.

Although I won't discuss it further in this book, strength/power training generally consists of 4-8 sets of 5 or less repetitions with weights near the actual 1RM (although percentages are not ideal, 85% or higher would be typical) and RI's ranging from 2-5 minutes on average (Ol'er may take slightly less rest and other athletes may need more in some cases). For safety reasons this is always done with compound, and usually specific free weight exercises such as the squat, bench press, deadlift, or Olympic lifts as isolation exercises are inappropriate for this type of low repetition work. While this type of training is used predominantly by performance athletes, it is not unheard of for some beginning training programs to be based around sets of 5 (with much lighter weights) or for advanced physique athletes or dieters to use this type of loading.

General muscle growth, strength and bone density training can fall anywhere from 1-8 sets (depending on training status) of 6-15 repetitions (a rough range of 70-80% 1RM) using rest intervals of 1-2 minutes on average. This can be done with a mixture of compound and isolation work although it would be most common to use compound movements when lower repetitions (6-10) are being used and isolation movements when higher repetitions (10-15) are being done. This tends to be the range that the majority of trainees will fall into and I will call it hypertrophy (muscle growth) training going forwards.

Next is metabolic/glycogen depletion training, specifically aimed at those two goals. This starts to cross over with some of the non-traditional HIIT approaches I mentioned above. Here 2-4 sets of 15-20 repetitions using rest intervals of 45-60 seconds would be appropriate. While some have tried to do this with compound and/or complex movements such as squats or the Olympic lifts, I do not recommend this as the risk of injury increases as fatigue causes form to break down. Less compound movements (I.e. leg press) and isolation work tends to be a better choice here from a safety standpoint.

334

The above types of training are not discrete entities but lie on a continuum. Sets of 5 can generate muscle growth and certainly impact on bone density but have little impact on depleting muscle glycogen. Sets of 6-15 will increase strength and BMD and will deplete muscle glycogen to some degree. Sets of 15-20 can generate some growth, albeit somewhat inefficiently, have much smaller impacts on strength and bone but have the greatest metabolic effects.

Existing somewhat outside of the previous types of weight training is what I will call maintenance training. This is aimed at maintaining the current level of strength and will be discussed further when I talk about resistance training in the context of dieting in later chapters. Both research and practical experience has shown that fitness (of any sort) can be maintained with far less work than was necessary to build it in the first place. The question is then by how much it can be reduced and how it should be reducecd. Repeatedly, it has been found that training volume (number of sets/total reps) and frequency can be reduced by up to 2/3rds but only if intensity is maintained without any meaningful loss of fitness (15.16). Intensity is the key here with the same research showing that fitness will be lost if intensity is reduced even if the previous volumes and frequencies are maintained.

In the context of weight training, practically this means that 8 sets of 8-10 repetitions per muscle group twice weekly could reduce that to 2-3 sets of 8-10 done once weekly so long as the weight being lifted was unchanged. A strength power athlete who had been doing 5 sets of 5 repetitions could reduce this to 2-3 sets of 5 with the same weight or even 3 sets of 3 (a reduction in volume) with the same weight that was being lifted for 5 repetitions. In general, I recommend that most trainees perform 2-4 heavy sets per muscle group once or twice per week at most. As the general trainee or woman seeking health and fitness is usually doing a fairly small amount of training to begin with, there isn't much room to reduce training although someone who had been doing 4 sets per muscle group could easily reduce that to 1-2 heavy sets for maintenance. While this won't maintain fitness forever, it will do so for extended periods of time. This makes it useful for trainees who have a particularly busy time period where they can't maintain their previous training and many performance athletes will engage in this type of reduced training during their competition season to maintain strength while allowing for optimal recovery and performance.

I've summarized the guidelines for all four types of training below. As maintenance will be based on the previous training

Type	Sets	Reps	RI	Exercise Choice	Strength	Size	Bone	Glycogen
Strength	4-8	1-5	2-5'	Compound Complex	Highest	Medium	High	Low
Hypertrophy	1-8	6-15	60-120"	Compound Isolation	Medium	High	High	Medium
Depletion	2-4	15-20	45-60"	Isolation Machines	Low	Low	Low	High
Maintenance	Relative to training being previously done with volume/frequency reduced by up to 2/3rds with the goal of maintaining intensity (weight being lifted).							

Whole Body vs. Split Workouts

In the same way that the types of weight training can be subdivided, so can individual workouts/training programs. Here there are only two general categories which are whole or full-body routines and split routines. A full body routine is a type of training program where all of the major muscles/muscle groups of the body are trained in a single workout. This may include anywhere from 3-12 total exercises depending on the specific type of full-body workout being used. When fewer exercises are used, more sets per exercise are done and vice versa.

A split routine is a type of training program where only part of the body is trained in any given workout. Split routines can range from simple, dividing the body into two parts (i.e. upper and lower body) or the very complex, dividing it 3, 4 or more ways with only one to two muscle groups being trained in any given workout. A three way split might have a workout dedicated to chest/shoulders/triceps, one to back/biceps and one to legs and core for example. At the extremes, many will dedicate a single workout to one muscle group and train that muscle only once per week. As women generally recover more quickly between workouts than men, this is not optimal and I recommend a general frequency of twice per week per muscle group or once every five days. I've shown a few examples of how whole body or split routines might be set up/scheduled throughout the week in the chart below.

Type of Split	Monday	Tuesday	Wednesday	Thursday	Friday	Saturday	Sunday
Full Body	Full Body			Full Body			
Full Body	Full Body		Full Body		Full Body		
2-Way Split	Upper	Lower		Upper	Lower		
2-Way Split	Upper		Lower		Upper	Lower	
2-Way Split*	Upper		Lower		Upper		
	Lower		Upper		Lower		
3-Way Split*	CDT		BB		LC		
3-Way Split	CDT	BBi	LC	CDT	BBi	LC	
3-Way Split*	CDT	BBi	LC		CDT	BBi	
	LC	CDT	BBi		LC	CDT	

CDT = Chest, delts, triceps, Bbi = Back, biceps, LC = Legs and core

When a routine has two sets of notations, this is to indicate how the workouts might rotate across two weeks of training. I do want to address the splits with an asterisk after them. The first is a two-way split with only three workouts per week, so that each workout is done roughly every 5th day, matching my recommended frequency above. This is a good approach for women who can only train three times per week but want to use a basic split routine. It can also be good for older trainees who need more recovery between workouts. The first three-way split is an example of training each muscle group only once per week. As I mentioned above, I do not consider this optimal for most women. The final marked three-way split shows how three workouts can be spaced across only 5 workouts per week. Here, the workouts rotate on different days of the week and yield a training frequency of every 5th day.

Chapter 29: Sample Training Programs

Having looked at basic exercise guidelines in the previous chapter, I want to look at how those guidelines might be put together for different goals. Since training will be discussed in detail Volume 2, I will not address performance athletes and will only focus on the beginning exerciser, general dieter, trainee seeking general health and fitness, serious trainee and advanced trainee/dieter.

Beginning Exerciser

For someone just starting an exercise program, only the most minimal amounts of exercise are required. As I have discussed throughout this book, I cannot overemphasize the need for beginners to start slowly and build up gradually. This not only tends to improve adherence but also avoids the potential for women to excessively stress their bodies out in the initial stages.

For aerobic exercise, the first goal should be 20 minutes of continuous aerobic exercise done a minimum of three times per week at an RPE of 3-4 (challenging but not impossible). In situations where someone is very unfit, it may take several workouts or longer until even 20 minutes of continuous activity can be done. In this case, breaking the total amount of exercise time up into smaller blocks is just as effective and may be more manageable. Once 20 minutes three times per week has been achieved for several weeks, the duration of each workout can be increased to a maximum of 60 minutes, more workouts can be added or the intensity can be increased gradually as fitness improves. The choice of exercise is completely unimportant compared to that the frequency, intensity and time components are met and beginners should pick the exercise that they will do consistently.

True HIIT would be generally inappropriate at this level although trainees who intend to use it can start doing a pseudo-HIIT during their normal aerobic workouts after 4 weeks of consistent training. This could mean performing 30-60 seconds out of every five minute block of exercise at an RPE of 5-6 before returning to their normal 3-4. Every few workouts, the duration of the harder interval could be increased (to a maximum of 90 seconds), the frequency could be increased (i.e. 30-60 seconds hard every few minutes) or the RPE could be pushed up gradually. This not only prepares them for true HIIT down the road but will have benefits on improving fitness as well as making the training less boring.

Resistance training should be performed 2-3 times per week, using a full body routine. The focus should be on learning proper technique first with weight increases occurring second. While there are different philosophies about training beginners, I generally feel that staying in the 8-12 or 10-15 repetition range is most appropriate. It's heavy enough to have benefits (even lifting at 50% of maximum improves strength in beginners) but light enough to do properly and safely. Initially no more than 1 set per exercise should be done and this can be increased if desired to 2 sets after at least 4 weeks of consistent training. In the earliest stages of training, I would recommend an RPE of 7 or less such that at least 3 or more repetitions could be done in any given set. Over 4-8 weeks, this can increase until the trainee is working at an RPE of 7 or higher. The type of exercise (i.e. bodyweight vs. free weights vs. machines) is less important than the other parameters. If they are available, machines tend to be easier to learn initially with many free weight exercises being more complex and requiring coaching.

Other potential components of the exercise program can include jumping, stretching and balance exercises with the latter two being especially important for older trainees. As I described in the last chapter, jumping guidelines are fairly simple and studies have commonly used 20 vertical jumps several times per week with 30 seconds in between them. I would generally recommend waiting until several weeks of consistent aerobic/weight training has been done before introducing jumping. In the first week of jumping, no more than 5 jumps per session should be done, this can be increased by 5 jumps each week so that 20 jumps are being done after a month. It's critical that the jumping be done properly which means the knees must stay over the toes while the trainee crouches down and swings their arms up and jumps straight up. Upon landing, the balls of the feet should hit first and then the heels.

Stretching can be done for the major muscle groups with up to 60 seconds per stretch being performed (note that full range of motion weight training has a stretching effect in its own right). I'd reiterate that women are usually more flexible than men to begin with and, although they love stretching, it often isn't as necessary for them. Flexibility tends to be lost with age and stretching is arguably more valuable for the postmenopausal woman. Finally are balance exercises. This tends to be most important for the older woman as balance is often lost which can precipitate to falls and other issues. Weight training in general tends to improve balance itself and specific exercises may not be required if it is being done.

The above recommendations are summarized in the chart on the next page.

Exercise	Frequency/Week	Intensity	Time	Type
Aerobic	3+	RPE 3-4	20'+	Preferred
HIIT	0	N/A	N/A	N/A
Weights	2-3	RPE 7 or less to begin	1-2 sets per muscle group 8-15 repetitions per set	Full body workout, machines or free weights
Jumping	2-3	Maximum	10-20 vertical jumps	N/A

A typical training week might look as follows with Full indicating a full body weight workout.

Type	Mon	Tue	Wed	Thu	Fri	Sat	Sun
Jumping	Y	Off	Y	Off	Y	Off	Off
Weights	Full	Off	(Full)	Off	Full	Off	Off
Aerobic	Y	Off	Y	Off	Y	Off	Off

If only two weight training sessions are done, jumping could also be limited to that frequency. A third session could also be performed since the total workout only takes about 10 minutes and can be done at home. As well, if desired, aerobic training could be done on alternating days with weight training. This can have benefits with adherence but it may simply be more convenient to do it with the weight workouts.

I would consider someone a beginner for the first 8-12 weeks of consistent exercise at which point they will move to one of two categories: general fitness and health or general dieting. Based on the realities of the world, I would honestly expect most women to move into general dieting, which I will discuss next. If that is not the case and a woman is simply training for general health and fitness, she will move to that category which is based around a level of exercise that she should have reached if she progresses the amount and intensity of her activity as I described above.

General Dieting

As I have discussed throughout this book, it is ideal for exercise to be part of a proper approach to dieting and fat loss. I have also mentioned that, in the early stages, exercise has at best a small impact on either total weight or fat loss. Beginners simply cannot perform enough activity to increase the total weight loss significantly and calorie restriction will have a far greater effect.. This isn't to say that exercise is irrelevant and I've mentioned numerous benefits and reasons for it to be included throughout this book. As well, over weeks and months, as fitness improves and more/more intense activity can be done, exercise will start to play a larger role in the fat loss process. This means that the earlier that a proper exercise program is introduced, the sooner that fitness will improve and that exercise can start to have a larger impact.

For the most part, the exercise levels that have been reached by the end of the beginner exercise stage are more than sufficient when formal fat loss dieting starts but there are some places where one or two changes may be considered. Certainly continuing to increase the frequency, duration and/or intensity of aerobic exercise will burn proportionally more calories and, as this goes up over time, the need for calories to be restricted will go down. Working up to 45-60 minutes of aerobic activity 3 or more times per week at an RPE of 4-5 will start to have a significant impact on calorie expenditure and the inclusion of 1-2 HIIT sessions is also possible. This can be useful when someone doesn't have a lot of time to exercise on a given day along enhancing overall fat oxidation by depleting muscle glycogen. If the pseudo-HIIT I described above has not been performed, HIIT must be introduced gradually. The first workouts might include 2-3 total intervals of 15-30 seconds apiece but not done at maximal intensity. This would be increased over a number of weeks and I would reiterate that the choice of exercise for HIIT must be based around safety.

Two to three weight training sessions per week will still be more than sufficient here although more complex free weight exercises may be introduced if the trainee wishes and was not doing them as part of their beginner exercise program. A primary change to consider here would be to increase the number of repetitions per set of weight training exercises can be increased to 12-15 or even 15-20. So far as the RPE remains above 7, this will continue to build at least some muscle along with depleting muscle glycogen to enhance the use of fat for fuel. This will also deplete muscle glycogen more effectively, further enhancing the use of fat for fuel. Jumping, stretching and any balance exercises can remain unchanged. I have summarized the above information in the chart on the next page.

Exercise	Frequency/Week	Intensity	Time	Type
Aerobic	3+	RPE 3-5	45-60'	Preferred
HIIT	0-1	RPE 7+	10-15 second intervals to begin	Safe
Weights	2-3	RPE 7 or less to begin	1-4 sets per muscle group 12-15 (15-20) reps/set	Full body workout, machines or free weights
Jumping	2-3	Maximum	10-20 vertical jumps	N/A

A typical training week assuming three aerobic, one HIIT and three full-body weight workouts per week. As described above, more aerobic sessions could be done as desired.

Type	Mon	Tue	Wed	Thu	Fri	Sat	Sun
Jumping	Y	Off	Y	Off	Y	Off	Off
Weights	Full	Off	Full	Off	Full	Off	Off
Aerobic	Y	Off	Y	Off	Y	HIIT	Off

Jumping and weight training should always fall on the same day with the jumping being done first. While I have shown the aerobic sessions on the same days at the weight workouts, they can be moved to the off days (i.e. Tuesday/Thursday/Saturday). This means that some amount of activity would be done almost daily which may be beneficial from an adherence point of view (many are more attentive to their diet on days that they exercise) along with increasing overall energy expenditure. More aerobic sessions could be done as desired as well although it's important to work up gradually to that level.

General Health

For the most part, the exercise recommendations for a woman seeking general health and fitness is just an extension of the beginner exercise program. The total amounts that are recommended are a bit higher but for the most part, a woman who has progressed the beginner program properly will be at more or less the recommended amounts for developing optimal health and fitness (1).

In terms of aerobic training, the recommended amount is 150 or more total minutes of exercise per week which can come from a combination of moderate (RPE 3-4) and vigorous (RPE 5-6) exercise with the total duration spread across three or more total workouts. HIIT done 1-2 times per week may also be considered. Once again, HIIT isn't required but can provide an alternative to longer workouts along with adding some variety and improving fitness even further. Assuming the guidelines I gave above for doing pseudo-HIIT have been followed, true HIIT, starting with a small number of 15 second intervals can be done with gradual increases in the number of intervals or length of the interval. As with the general dieter, the primary criteria for choosing a HIIT activity must be safety above all.

The same general guidelines for resistance training hold with each muscle being trained 2-3 times per week for 2-4 total sets per muscle group. If a woman wants to perform the full 4 sets per muscle group, it may be best to move to a basic split routine so that the workout doesn't become excessively long. Even splitting the body into upper and lower body allows for more work to be done at each workout while limiting the duration. It also provides more flexibility in scheduling the weight workouts since they do not have to be done on alternate days of the week. This should be weighed against adherence and scheduling issues as training consistently three times per week but doing fewer sets is superior to attempting to do more training but constantly missing workouts. Maintaining a repetition count of 8-12 repetitions per set with an RPE of 7+ is still appropriate here with the focus being more on increasing the weight lifted than anything else. This will increase strength, build muscle mass and heavy loading is a key to improving bone density. Both higher and lower repetitions than this can be useful but a full discussion of this topic will have to wait for Volume 2 of this book. If coaching is available, and they aren't being done already, more complex free weight exercises can be introduced here as needed or desired.

Assuming the guidelines I gave for introducing jumping above were followed, 20 jumps per workout should be easily completed and this would be maintained. The same would hold for any stretching or balance type drills being done although I'd note again that proper weight training can often have similar if not superior effects on these components of fitness to begin with. These guidelines are summarized below.

Exercise	Frequency/Week	Intensity	Time	Type
Aerobic	3+	RPE 3-4 + 5-6	150' per week	Preferred
HIIT	0-2	RPE 7+	Longer intervals possible	Safe
Weight	2-4	RPE 7-10	2-4 sets per muscle group 8-15 repetitions per set	Full body workout, machines or free weights
Jumping	2-3	Maximum	20 vertical jumps	N/A

A typical training week, assuming 4 days/week of weights in a upper/lower split routine, 3 aerobic sessions and one HIIT session is shown below although the same 3/day per week weight training schedule from above can also be used.

Type	Mon	Tue	Wed	Thu	Fri	Sat	Sun
Jumping	Y	(Y)	Off	Y	(Y)	Off	Off
Weights	Lower	Upper	Off	Lower	Upper	Off	Off
Aerobic	Y	Y	Off	Y	HIIT	Off	Off

Any jumping would be done in conjunction with the lower body days twice/week although one to two additional sessions could be added. The HIIT workout is put at the end of the week prior to two days of rest over the weekend. For general health and fitness, there is no real need to do more training than shown above and this can be done for extended periods of time. So long as the overall training is progressive in terms of the intensity, fitness will continue to improve. That said, it's not uncommon for the goals of women training at this level to change over time. Even without explicit dieting, the higher levels of training being done often cause positive changes in body composition and woman may decide to explicitly diet, combining their training program with a calorically restricted diet as described in this book.

An equally common occurrence at this point is for women to become more serious in their training with a desire to push themselves further. This could be due to the changes in body composition or the feeling of improved fitness, especially strength. The latter is quite common with women who engage in a proper resistance training program that generates strength and muscular gains often wanting to see how much stronger than can get. This isn't universal and there's nothing wrong with that not being a goal but it's not uncommon. In any of these situations, the trainee would move into the serious trainee category, discussed next. I would recommend that at least 3-6 months of consistent training at the above level be done before any further increases occur.

Serious Trainee

By the time a woman reaches the level of serious trainee (once again defined as someone training at a fairly high level with no desire to compete) there tends to be somewhat more variability in the amount and types of training that are done. Unless she is focused solely on increasing strength or muscle size, it would be fairly uncommon for the serious trainee to be performing only weight training. Instead, it's far more common to see this level of trainee performing quite a bit (and often too much) aerobic and/or HIIT work. An hour or more of MISS level cardio might be done multiple times per week, combined with one or more HIIT sessions. The typical motivation here is a fear of fat gain but, not only does this far exceed what is necessary to accomplish this, the chronically excessive activity eventually takes it's toll.

This becomes even more true if this excessive level of aerobic work is then combined with equally excessive amounts of weight training. It is almost universally true that the serious trainee will be using a split routine, often training only 1-2 body parts per workout but this is usually done with far too many redundant exercises, too many sets and often an intensity that is far below what is optimal. Daily or near daily prolonged weight training workouts are often performed before or after aerobic work and it's not uncommon to see trainees in the gym for 2-3 hours most days of the week. Eventually, something will give. This may be physical in terms of injuries and it's common to see women (and men as well) pushing themselves through endless amounts of training with knee braces or other joint support due to chronic joint pain. There is also the physiological aspect of stress and burnout and this is exacerbated by the dietary restriction that may be present.

In terms of what might be a more ideal approach for the serious trainee, the amount of aerobic/HIIT training being done will depend somewhat on goals but it's likely that the serious trainee will want to do some. If the trainee has goals of making gradual increases in strength and muscle mass, this should be limited to perhaps 3-4 sessions per week with the intensity kept to MISS/LISS levels. HIIT sessions tend to harm recovery, especially for the legs and I don't recommend them under most circumstance. For the serious trainee concerned more with simply being extremely healthy and fit, this could be increased to 5 sessions per week although the majority of them should be no longer than 60 minutes (and perhaps shorter) at no higher than MISS intensity. One and possibly two HIIT sessions could be done. This is more than sufficient to avoid fat gain so long as even moderate dietary control is kept in place.

Moving to weight training, while some prefer to train 6 days/week, I generally feel that 4-5 workout per week is more than sufficient under most conditions so long as the workouts are done properly. A split routine would typically be used here and I'd reiterate that an average muscle group frequency of twice weekly or every 5 days with less total sets at each workout will be a better approach for most women in terms of strength or muscular gains. At the intermediate serious trainee level (perhaps 1-3 years of proper training), that would mean 6-8 sets or 40-70 total repetitions per muscle group at each workout. At the advanced serious trainee level, this could be increased to perhaps 8-10 sets and 80-100 total repetitions per muscle group at each workout. These numbers do not include warm-up sets and all work sets should be done at an RPE of 7 (3 RIR/ERF) or higher.

Multiple (2-3) exercises per muscle group would typically be done and this will most likely be a mixture of compound (and often free weight) and isolation movements. A mixture of repetition ranges including 6-8 up to 12-15 can be used with the lower repetitions being used on compound movements and higher repetitions on isolation movements. Assuming a split routine is being used, there are many potential approaches. Splitting the body into three different workouts would probably be the most appropriate given the number of sets that are being done and the goal training frequency. Jumping would be done before leg workouts for its benefits on bone density. I have summarized this below.

Exercise	Frequency/Week	Intensity	Time	Type
Aerobic	3-5	RPE 3-5	60' or less per workout	Preferred
HIIT	0-2	RPE 7+	Up to 90" intervals	Safe
Weights	4-5 (6 max) total	RPE 7-10	6-8 sets/40-70 reps (int) 8-10 sets/80-100 reps (adv) per muscle group per workout	Split routine 2-3 exercises per muscle group
Jumping	2-3	Maximum	20 vertical jumps	N/A

*Training each muscle group once every 5th day is sufficient may be required depending on the split routine used and total number of training days.

In the chart below, I've shown a training template for two different goals. The first is a serious trainee focusing primarily on increases in strength and muscle size while the second is one primarily concerned with high levels of health fitness and either gradual changes in or maintenance of body composition. In both cases, a three-way split routine consisting of Legs/Core (LC), chest/delts/triceps (CDT) and back/biceps (BBi) is being used with 5 total weight workouts per week. Since this will make the workouts rotate from week to week, I have shown two weeks of training for each and this gives a training frequency per muscle group of once every 5th day (i.e. Workout 1 is done on Mon and Fri the first week and again on Tue of the second week).

Goal	Type	Mon	Tue	Wed	Thu	Fri	Sat	Sun	Mon	Tue	Wed	Thu	Fri	Sat	Sun
Strength/Size	Jumping	Y				Y				Y			Y		
	Weights	LC	CDT	BI	Off	LC	CDT	Off	BBi	LC	CDT	Off	BBi	LC	Off
	Aerobic		Y	Y			Y		Y		Y		Y		
Body comp	Jumping	Y				Y				Y				Y	
	Weights	LC	CDT	BI	Off	LC	CDT	Off	BBi	LC	CDT	Off	BBi	LC	Off
	Aerobic	Y	Y	HIIT		Y	Y		HIIT	Y	Y		Y	Y	

The primary difference between the two situations is in the amount and type of aerobic training being done. For the trainee seeking strength and/or muscle mass gains, aerobic work is limited to only three days per week and is never done on the same day as the lower body training as this can impair growth in the legs. No HIIT is done in this case since it will interfere with strength and muscle gains. For the trainee seeking to maintain or gradually improve body composition, 5 total sessions are done as a mixture of aerobic and HIIT with the HIIT sessions always being done on a non-leg training day.

The Aggressive Diet

Before examining the extended Category 1 diet, I want to look briefly at how training should or should not be done when using an aggressive diet approach (1.5% per week target weight loss or 40-50%+ daily deficit). This information really applies to anyone using such an approach. This includes the general dieter, serious trainee, and physique athletes (I will address the aggressive diet for the physique athlete again in a later chapter). Aggressive diets are usually not appropriate for performance athletes as they are usually not able to reduce their training by the necessary degree (some strength/power athletes may be able to do this). On an aggressive diet, the first choice for exercise must always be resistance training. That, along with sufficient protein, will ensure that no LBM is lost and that the total weight loss is coming 100% from fat. This isn't quite as necessary for the beginner, especially in Category 2 or 3 but even here, strength and small muscle gains may be seen and there is no reason not to do at least some amount of resistance training so that a basic program will be in place once a more moderate diet is adopted.

That said, the amount of resistance training that should be done is very small. Without exception the maintenance recommendations I provided in the previous chapter should be used meaning that a maximum of 2-4 sets per muscle group per workout a maximum of 1-2 times per week should be done. I'd also recommend limiting the total number of training days to only 4 per week in which case a split routine of some sort would be used. Some dieters have reduced their training to only twice/week (regardless of their normal training approach) using a full body workout as well. Starting an aggressive diet with 1-2 depletion workouts (3-4 sets of 15-20 with 60" rest) to deplete glycogen can also be helpful.

There is little to nothing to discuss regarding HIIT as its use should not even be considered due to the severely decreased recovery that a dieter will have on an aggressive diet. In terms of aerobic exercise, an excessive amount will actually harm a dieter's results as it causes a more rapid decrease in metabolic rate. This runs counter to most dieter's beliefs and the single most common mistake on such diets is to perform too much aerobic exercise. For that reason, aerobic work should either be eliminated or reduce to no more than 3 days/week for 20-30 minutes at a low intensity. Any more is detrimental. For those who are performing it, I would suggest maintaining jumping at least two days per week. This is summarized below.

Exercise	Frequency/Week	Intensity	Time	Type
Aerobic	3 maximum	RPE 3-5	20-30'	Preferred
HIIT	N/A	N/A	N/A	N/A
Weight	2-4	RPE 7-10	2-4 sets Maintain weight on bar	Split routine 2-3 exercise/muscle
Jumping	2	Maximum	20 vertical jumps	N/A

Depending on how training is specifically implemented, a number of different schedules are possible for an aggressive diet and I've shown several options in the chart below. I will only focus on weight training as HIIT work is inappropriate and aerobic work should be severely limited.

	Mon	Tue	Wed	Thu	Fri	Sat	Sun
Option 1	D*	D*		U	L		
Option 2	U	L		U	L		
Option 3	CDT		LC		BBi		

* Only in week 1 of the diet, replace with heavy training in subsequent weeks

The first option includes two depletion workouts, which should only be done in the first week of the aggressive diet before being replaced with heavy work. Option 2 is what option 1 would look like after the first week but could be used by dieters not doing depletion work. Option 3 is a standard split routine.

342

The Category 1 Extended Diet

Next is Category 1 dieter and here I am focusing on the physique (bodybuilding, fitness, figure, bikini) competitor dieting to anywhere from 10-18% body fat depending on their sport's specific requirements. For decades this is an area that has been mostly governed by lore and tradition with most of the prevalent ideas coming from male bodybuilders who were using drugs of varying types. It's only recently that any sort of evidence or scientifically based strategies for contest preparation have been made. Perhaps the first paper on the topic was written by Helms et. al. and much of what I will write in this section comes from that paper (2). Arguably this paper, moreso than any other, has stimulated an increased amount of research on physique competitors with several excellent papers on females having been published recently (these are detailed in Chapter 34).

Aerobic Training

Looking first at aerobic training, it's been common for decades for physique competitors to perform a fairly large amount of it during their diet, albeit at very low intensities. One hour per day, usually in the morning before eating is common and more than this is often seen or recommended. I have discussed this issue repeatedly throughout this book and there are both pros and cons to performing this level of aerobic work. On the one hand, daily aerobic training can lessen the need to reduce food intake since more of the deficit will be coming from exercise. On the other hand, smaller women will not burn a significant number of calories during low-intensity activity. As well, introduced too quickly, done too intensely or done excessively, it can cause problems that I've discussed elsewhere in the book. So long as the intensity is kept under control and the amount of aerobic work being done is brought up gradually, these problems are lessened. As well, as I discussed in Chapter 27, for smaller females dieting to the lowest levels of body fat, food intake may reach a point where no further reductions can be realistically made. At this point, the amount of aerobic work being done will have to go up to compensate and frequently reach what most would consider excessive levels will be reached. So long as it is done progressively, there is little problem.

HIIT is has its own set of issues though I discussed most of them in the previous chapter and won't repeat them here. Certainly HIIT can have benefits in terms of hormonal response, glycogen depletion (and two of the Stubborn Fat Protocols in Appendix 1 use them) although weight training has similar overall effects. At the same time, adding HIIT to an extreme diet and a heavy weight training load can rapidly overwhelm a woman's recovery capacity and cause burn-out or injury. This is probably more true towards the end of the diet than at the beginning but it is always an issue. If HIIT is used at all, it should still be limited to no more than 2 sessions per week and many will not be able to sustain even that.

Moving to more specific recommendations, it is a rare woman who can diet to the lowest levels of body fat without some amount of aerobic (or HIIT) training. It isn't unheard of for men to do so but their larger body weights, higher calorie expenditures during weight workouts and lack of stubborn lower body fat makes this relatively more possible for them. For women, at least some will almost always be needed. How much is then the question and this is impossible to answer specifically. Some smaller women may need to do aerobic work daily (and often twice daily near the very end of their diet) while others may only need 3-4 total aerobic sessions (with or without HIIT) per week. In reference 2 cited above, it is recommended that dieters do as few total aerobic/HIIT sessions as are necessary to reach the dieting goal. Phrased differently, dieters should only perform daily LISS cardio because they need it to maintain fat loss rather than doing it that frequently because that is how physique competitors have always done it.

Resistance Training

Looking next at resistance training, a typical approach to contest dieting has been to use higher repetitions and shorter rest periods with the idea that this is a better fat burning stimulus and will improve muscular definition (often called "burning in the cuts"). There are many problems with this approach. First and foremost, definition and separation comes from the combination of sufficient muscular size and a low body fat level and no specific training can improve definition or muscular separation short of its impact on those two factors. Of even more importance is that removing the stimulus that built muscle in the first place (i.e. heavier weights and low-medium repetitions) by using lighter weights will cause muscle to be lost unless powerful drugs are being used (as they were when this approach was first developed). For a natural physique competitor, switching only to lighter weights and higher repetitions than were being used prior to the diet is disastrous (recall from Chapter 28 that lowering training intensity causes fitness loss) Which isn't to say that performing some of that this type of training may not be useful while dieting. It simply can't replace all of the normal heavy training that was being done. I'll come back to this below.

Phrased differently, the physique athlete should, to as great a degree as possible, maintain at least some of their normal heavy training, especially in terms of the weights being lifted. As this is the primary stimulus for muscle growth, it is also the primary stimulus to prevent muscle loss. Which isn't to say that dieters should expect their strength to remain unchanged throughout their diet. All lifters have good and bad days and it's common to lose some amount of strength, especially as the athletes approaches the lower limits of body fat. But the over-riding goal should be to maintain lifting poundages to as great a degree as possible. With the understanding of intensity/weight on bar being the key to avoiding muscle loss, the issue of frequency and volume (total sets or reps) needs to be considered.

In reference 2 cited above, the recommendation is made for contest dieters to maintain their previous training volumes and frequencies throughout the diet. So if 6-8 sets of 60-70 repetitions per muscle group were being done twice weekly, that should be maintained throughout the diet. The logic is that the amount of training that is optimal for building muscle will also be optimal for maintaining muscle during the diet. Essentially he argues that the previous weight training routine should be continued with the major changes coming from adjustment to the diet and any added aerobic/HIIT work. While these recommendations are certainly valid, there are other research supported approaches worth considering. I have traditionally recommended that dieters reduce their training proactively to the maintenance levels discussed in Chapter 28 fairly early in their diet. Training volume can always be increased during diet breaks as needed and there should be little fear of any real muscle loss with this reduced training approach is intensity is maintained. My logic here is that athletes dieting to the extreme tend to burn themselves out over time and become overtrained or injured when they try to maintain their training at pre-diet levels.

Both approaches have been shown to work both in research and the real world and I want to address both the pros and cons of each briefly. A benefit of maintaining the pre-diet training level is that it avoids the decrease in workout related energy expenditure that would occur if training volume is reduced. Noting that weight training workouts do not burn a large number of calories to begin with, there is no doubt that every bit of calorie expenditure from exercise helps at the extremes and may help dieters avoid the need to add excessive aerobic work to maintain their energy expenditures.

But this has to be balanced with the aforementioned risk of burnout and overtraining. I am in no way saying that either are inevitable but the training that a female trainee might have easily handled when she was eating at maintenance or above may become too much when her calories are reduced for extended periods. Reducing training volume and/or frequency while maintaining intensity basically avoids that issue completely. To that I'd add that reducing the total number of heavy sets per muscle group also allows metabolic weight training work to be added if desired . This would be impossible if the amount of heavy work were kept at pre-diet levels but can be done if it is reduced. With this approach, rather than performing the pre-diet 8 heavy sets per muscle group, only 2-3 heavy sets might be done followed by 3-4 higher repetitions sets done purely for metabolic and glycogen depletion purposes. This does seem to contradict the general idea of reducing the total training volume as the total number of repetitions being done may not change. In a sense this is true. However, the combination of fewer heavy sets followed by metabolic work is still a reduction in the total number of heavy sets and still fits into the overall paradigm of reducing the amount of truly heavy training to avoid burnout or overtraining.

The above two approaches are not mutually exclusive. Ignoring aggressive diets where training must be reduced immediately, dieters may find it relatively easy to maintain their pre-diet training volume and intensity earlier in the diet before fatigue sets in. This has the advantages I listed above in terms of maintaining energy expenditure. As the diet continues and lower levels of body fat are reached, this can become more problematic and the total training volume in the weight room may need to be reduced gradually. The focus should still be on maintaining intensity and weight on the bar but this is a situation where it is far better to do 4 heavier sets and stop rather than doing 6-8 sets with a lighter weight to maintain the pre-diet volume. This holds for individuals workouts: if the goal is 8 sets for a given muscle group and the lifter is exhausted after 6 sets, they should eliminate the final two sets and move on.

This is actually another reason that I tend to prefer reducing training volume at the start of a diet: motivated athletes and dieters are often a little bit too motivated. If the workout says to do 8 sets per muscle group for 3 muscle groups, they will push themselves through the entire workout no matter how exhausted they are or terrible they feel. In contrast, when they are only allowed to do 2-3 heavy sets (whether followed by depletion work or not), that's what they do before moving on. With few exceptions, when they are given the option to do more, the motivated training will always do more. In many cases, that will be too much. Simply, without a coach, most athletes tend to be somewhat bad at self-regulating themselves and I find that changing their training earlier helps to save them from themselves.

This raises the question of why my training recommendations often run counter to that of other coaches or even the recommendations made in reference 2 above. Generally the difference is whether or not the recommendations are being provided in written form or in person. Coaches who train hands-on, or even via online training, are able to adjust and modify their athletes training as needed based on that athletes responses. I will do the same when/if I am coaching someone individually but, more often, my recommendations are appearing in book or print form and I have no direct interaction with the person reading it. Having seen how most approach their diet in terms of training, I recommend reducing volume as much due to the science on the topic as to save the dieter from themselves. I am simply being proactive based on what I have seen dieters do over the years.

Regardless of the specific approach taken by a Category 1 dieter, it would be fairly standard for weight training to be performed 4-5 days per week and the training being done may be more or less identical to the pre-diet training routine or might be modified to include fewer heavy sets combined with more metabolic training. In both cases, at least some amount of heavy training must be maintained and this is the only absolutely mandatory aspect of training during dieting. Almost universally a split routine of some sort would be used at this level and dieting is one place where training a muscle group once per week may be viable for women since it falls within the maintenance recommendations I described above. While there is the occasional faddish interest in plyometrics for physique dieting, jumping has no real effect on fat loss. It is still valuable to perform (as always, prior to leg training) due to its benefits on bone density. This too can be lost and maintaining at least some impact stimulus will help to limit losses. Stretching and balance work has no direct impact on the Category 1 diet but may be done as desired.

One type of training that is only relevant to the extreme physique dieter is posing practice. Competitions have a series of mandatory poses along with a free pose routine where the athlete shows off their muscular development and this must be practiced to at least some degree. In general, some amount of posing practice, simply mastering the mandatory poses would begin as soon as the contest diet begins. After two to three months, most should have the mandatory poses relatively mastered leaving at least 3 months to choreograph and practice a posing routine. Posing practice should begin in front of a mirror and eventually be done without it. While seemingly simple, posing practice can be physically demanding and might realistically be done 1-4 times per week. Relatively new physique athletes will need more posing than more advanced but practice will be required regardless. This is summarized below:

Exercise	Frequency/Week	Intensity	Time	Type
Aerobic	As many as required	RPE 3-5	60' or less per workout	Preferred
HIIT	0-2	RPE 7+	Longer intervals possible	Safe
Weight	4-5 (6) total	RPE 7-10	Maintained Volume OR Reduced volume	Split routine 2-3 exercise/muscle
Jumping	2-3	Maximum	20 vertical jumps	N/A
Posing	1-4	N/A	Variable	N/A

In the chart below, I've shown two weeks of training based on a three way split of Legs/Core (LC), chest/delt/triceps (CDT) and back/biceps (BBi) and 5 total resistance training days per week. Aerobic work is performed 3 times per week with one HIIT session although this might be increased later in the diet as the body adapts metabolically.

Type	Mon	Tue	Wed	Thu	Fri	Sat	Sun	Mon	Tue	Wed	Thu	Fri	Sat	Sun
Jumping	Y				Y				Y				Y	
Weights	LC	CDT	BBi	Off	LC	CDT	Off	BBi	LC	CDT	Off	BBi	LC	
Aerobic	Y		HIIT		Y	Y		Y		HIIT		Y	Y	
Posing	Y		Y		Y			Y		Y		Y		

As with the serious trainee, you can see that the workouts rotate throughout each week with each workout being done every 5th day. There are three aerobic sessions per week with the HIIT sessions being done before the day off (the HIIT sessions could also go on Wednesday). This also ensures that it doesn't fall on a leg day. Posing is listed at 3X/week on training days but can be put anywhere during the week based on the competitor's preference or scheduling availability.

Muscle Gain

The final training goal I want to look at is that of explicit muscle gain and here primarily in terms of what a physique athlete might be doing between competitions to bring up weak points or increase their overall muscularity. Certainly performance athletes may also seek this goal, especially strength/power athletes but they are frequently working around their other training and I will save this for Volume 2.

Resistance training is by far and away the primary training that will be done when muscle gain is the goal and the guidelines I presented in the last chapter apply here with an average training frequency of twice/week or once every 5th day, a repetition range of 6-15 and and RPE of 7+ and roughly 40-70 repetitions per muscle per workout for intermediate up to 80-100 for advanced . A split routine would be used with 4-5 workout per week. The focus should be on gradual progression in weights being lifted along with a slight calorie surplus and proper around workout nutrition. This combination leads to growth.

Looking next at aerobic/HIIT work, there are a few issues I want to examine. It's not uncommon for physique athletes to maintain a large amount of aerobic and/or HIIT work during size gaining phases, usually in an attempt to limit fat gains (some coaches recommend an hour of morning cardio every day). At the same time, a great deal of research and practical experience shows that this tends to limit strength and muscular gains due to what is called the interference effect. As most aerobic exercise uses the legs, this tends to be most pronounced there but even upper body gains can be impaired. I discussed some of the reasons for this interference in Chapter 27 including fatigue that may limit weight room performance, differences in the adaptation 'signal' sent by different types of training, a general tendency to overtrain and the calorie burn that must be replaced. A large body of research supports this effect although, confusingly, some finds that aerobic (and possibly HIIT) can improve muscular gains (5). This tends to be most true in what are called Type I fibers (a type of muscle fiber geared towards endurance). But any positive effect here is predicated on the workout occurring 6-24 hours from the weight training workout for the same muscle groups along with the total volume being limited. Practically this means that no more than 2 lower body sessions per week might be combined with 2 and at most 3 aerobic sessions per week of which one might be HIIT. The intensity on the aerobic exercise must be kept at the LISS level with no more than a 3-4 RPE. Running has the largest negative impact on growth and should be avoided.

For issues primarily related to bone density, some amount of jumping should be done as part of the overall program . Since it is a high-intensity activity, it does have at least some potential to also impact positively on lower body muscle growth. As always it must be done prior to heavy weight training and only in limited amounts. I've summarized the recommendations for muscle growth below.

Exercise	Frequency/Week	Intensity	Time	Type
Aerobic	1-3	RPE 3-4	45' or less per workout	Non-impact
HIIT	0-1	RPE 7+	Longer intervals possible	Safe
Weights	4-5 (6 max) total 2 per muscle group*	RPE 7-10	6-8 sets/40-70 reps (int) 8-10 sets/80-100 reps (adv) per muscle group per workout	Split routine 2-3 exercise/muscle group
Jumping	2-3	Maximum	20 vertical jumps	N/A

In the chart below, I've shown a sample workout routine for a female trainee performing a three way split routine consisting of Legs/Core (LC), chest/delts/triceps (CDT) and back/biceps (BBi) across 6 workouts per week. Jumping is performed twice per week before the lower body training and the lifter will perform 3 LISS sessions of 45 minutes or less and one HIIT session (I'd reiterate that generally I think the inclusion of HIIT during a size gaining phase is a mistake but if it is being used it must be scheduled appropriately).. Note that all of the aerobic/HIIT sessions are done at least 24 hours away from lower body work to limit any possible interference effect. If even this is too much to adequately recover from (indicated by plateaus in strength gains or muscle growth), the HIIT workout would be eliminated with the aerobic sessions either being shortened or eliminated as needed to ensure progress.

Type	Mon	Tue	Wed	Thu	Fri	Sat	Sun	Mon	Tue	Wed	Thu	Fri	Sat	Sun
Jumping	Y				Y				Y				Y	
Weights	LC	CDT	BBI	LC	CDT	BBI	Off	LC	CDT	BBI	LC	CDT	BBI	Off
Aerobic		LISS	LISS		LISS	HIIT			LISS	LISS		LISS	HIIT	

Chapter 29: Hormonal Category Templates

Before presenting specific fat loss templates in the next chapters, I want to first summarize at least some of the information from the earlier parts of the book. Here I will be focusing on how changes during the menstrual cycle, or in response to the various hormonal modifiers impact on a woman's overall physiology (including fuel use, insulin sensitivity, metabolic rate and others) along with her choice of diet set up, specific supplements and/or potential changes in nutrient requirements.

For each hormonal situation, I will briefly describe it before looking at the change in physiology and recommendations that would be appropriate. To save space, I will assume that my general nutritional recommendations along with general use and sleep supplements, creatine or thermogenic compounds are appropriate in all situations and not list them specifically unless there is some particular exception to their use. If a given template lacks a specific category, no changes or modifications are necessary. Since it should almost exclusively apply to the Category 1 dieter approaching the lower levels of body fat percentage, I will provide a template for amenorrhea in a later chapter. Finally, since it applies to all of the templates (and honestly didn't fit anywhere else in the book), I will look at some of the potential differences that might exist for women who are not normally cycling at the end of the chapter.

The Normally Cycling Woman

As I described in detail in Chapter 2, the normally cycling woman is marked by cyclical changes in the hormones estrogen and progesterone on a roughly 28 day cycle (varying from 24-32 days) with specific changes in her overall physiology occurring due to those changes. Insulin sensitivity, fuel use, metabolic rate, hunger and others all vary with the primary differences being seen between the follicular and luteal phases with other smaller changes occurring within each phase. This has implications for the type of diet she will be setting up along with any changes that might occur in her nutrient or supplement recommendations. I've summarized these below.

Day	1 2 3 4 5 6 7	8 9 10 11 12 13 14	15 16 17 18 19 20 21	22 23 24 25 26 27 28
Phase	Early Follicular	Early Follicular	Early Luteal	Late Luteal
Note	Menses (~3-5 days)	Ovulation		PMS (~4-7 days)
Primary Hormone	Estrogen	Estrogen	Progesterone	Progesterone
Insulin Sensitivity	High	High	Lowered	Lowered
Fuel at Rest	Carbs	Carbs	Fat	Fat
Fat Storage	Lowered	Lowered	Increased	Increased
Metabolic Rate	Normal	Normal	Increased	Increased
Hunger	Lowered	Lowered	Increased	Increased
Blood Glucose	Stable	Stable	Unstable	Unstable
Water retention	Lowered	Increased	Lowered	Increased (highest)
Diet	Follicular Phase		Luteal Phase	
Dietary Changes		Reduce NA/Increase K*	Add Fruit, Chocolate	Add Fruit, Chocolate Reduce NA/Increase K*
Phase Specific Supps.	Aspirin/NSAID if needed		Luteal phase	Luteal Phase, Soy/Phyto. Aspirin/ NSAID

*Na is sodium and K is potassium. This is to help with water retention.

Looking at the specific recommendations, the normally cycling female will ideally set up both the follicular and luteal phase diets. Through both phases, primarily to ensure adequate nutrient intake and to protect her menstrual cycle, red meat or chicken, dairy foods and sufficient dietary fat should be consumed. During the late follicular phase, when water retention occurs, reducing sodium intake while increasing potassium can be beneficial. In the luteal phase, ensuring at least some fruit intake can help to maintain blood glucose and the allowance of a small amount chocolate may help with cravings. In the late luteal phase, when water retention is typically the worst, sodium can be reduced and potassium increased.

To address issues related to PMS, the normally cycling woman can add the luteal phase supplements during the second half of the cycle. Soy protein (25 g/day) or phytoestrogens (50 mg) could also be considered here as it may help to offset some of the problems that occur during this week. Aspirin or another NSAID can be used in the late luteal phase to control cramping and may still be useful during menstruation if cramping is still occurring.

PCOS/Hyperandrogenism: Introduction

Despite the relatively common occurrence of PCOS in women, the fact that it may represent many different combinations of primary symptoms makes it difficult to make more than general comments about it. For example, menstrual cycle irregularities such as oligomenorrhea (a cycle lasting 35-90 days) or amenorrhea are common but not universal. When oligomenorrhea is present, there is no way to predict what the PCOS woman's hormones will be on any given day. She will menstruate at some point and may experience PMS symptoms prior to this that would make the luteal phase supplements appropriate but it is impossible to know ahead of time when this may occur and can only be judged subjectively, adding the supplements when mood changes or other symptoms occur. Since none of that can be predicted in any meaningful fashion, I will present the cycle as if it were unchanging from week to week.

To this I'd add that elevated testosterone/androgens may not always be present. If they are, it is likely that certain physical characteristics such as oily skin, acne or increased body hair will be present.. A more male-like body fat pattern and increased muscle mass is also common. That said, insulin resistance is a hallmark of PCOS, especially if women are overweight or inactive and that category of PCOS women will be described as being in an androgen-like state. This is shown below.

PCOS/Hyperandrogenism: Obese and/or Inactive

Day	1 2 3 4 5 6 7 8 9 10 11 12 13 14 15 16 17 18 19 20 21 22 23 24 25 26 27 28
Effective Phase	Luteal
Hormone State	Androgen-Like
Fuel at Rest	Fat
Fat Storage	High?
Body Composition	Increased abdominal fat, Increased muscle mass (if hyperandrogeni)
Metabolic Rate	Normal
Diet	Luteal Phase/Very Low-Carbohydrate Diet (<80-100 g/day carbs)
Phase Specific Supps	PCOS supplements

Due to the insulin resistance, the luteal phase or even a very low-carbohydrate diet is appropriate here. The PCOS supplements can be used to improve either insulin sensitivity, metabolic health or fertility.

For those women who are leaner and/or regularly active, it will be more likely that insulin sensitivity will be improved (albeit not completely normalized) even if androgen levels are elevated. This will make it more similar to an estrogen like state in terms of diet set up and recommendations. The same overall comments will hold for the woman with subclinical hyperandrogenism. If she is overweight/inactive, she will be considered to be in an androgen-like state. If she is lean and active, an estrogen-like state.

PCOS/Hyperandrogenism: Lean and/or Active

Day	1 2 3 4 5 6 7 8 9 10 11 12 13 14 15 16 17 18 19 20 21 22 23 24 25 26 27 28
Effective Phase	Follicular
Hormone State	Estrogen-Like
Fuel at Rest	Carbs
Fat Storage	Normal?
Body Composition	Increased abdominal fat, Increased muscle mass (if hyperandrogenic)
Appetite/Hunger	Increased
Metabolic Rate	Normal
Diet	Follicular Phase
Phase Specific Supps	None

Due to improved insulin sensitivity, the follicular phase diet is appropriate here and there are no phase specific supplements to be considered.

Birth Control: Introduction

Of all of the hormonal modifiers, birth control is by far and away the most complex. Additionally, there is simply a lack of research in many cases, especially in terms of how the varying forms of birth control differ from one another in their physiological effects. For that reason, along with trying to keep things more simplified, I've grouped birth control based primarily on the progestin present. Specifically, first and second generation progestins will be considered as a single category since they tend to induce some degree of insulin resistance and a progesterone-like hormonal state. Progestin only BC will also be included here. Even here, any type of BC with a withdrawal week, even if first and second generation progestins are present allows for a rebound week that is more estrogen like.

Birth Control: First or Second Generation Progestin or Progestin Only

Day	1 2 3 4 5 6 7 8 9 10 11 12 13 14 15 16 17 18 19 20 21	22 23 24 25 26 27 28
Phase*	Effective Luteal	Effectively Early Follicular*
Hormone State	Progesterone-like	Estrogen
Fuel at Rest	Fat	Carbs
Fat Storage	Increased?	Normal?
Body Composition	Potentially Small Negative (LBM loss, fat gain)	N/A
Appetite/Hunger	Potentially Increased	Normal
Metabolic Rate	Potentially Increased	Normal
Diet	Luteal Phase	Follicular Phase
Dietary Changes	Increased B12, zinc, selenium, magnesium, Vitamin C requirements	None
Phase Specific Supps	Possibly Luteal Phase	None

*Women on progesterone only BC or without a withdrawal week should treat all 4 weeks as effectively luteal.

. The luteal phase supplements are only listed as a possibility as it is difficult to tell if they will be either necessary or beneficial in any specific case. If a woman is noticing PMS-like symptoms especially hunger or cravings, she may wish to at least test the luteal phase supplements to see if they offer any relief.

In contrast, third and fourth generation progestins do not seem to induce insulin resistance and I will consider them as an estrogen like state across the entire cycle of use regardless of the pattern of use. As the hormonal IUD only acts locally in terms of its hormonal effects and women using that should use the template for the normally cycling woman instead as the menstrual cycle will be intact.

Birth Control: Third or Fourth Generation Progestin

Day	1 2 3 4 5 6 7 8 9 10 11 12 13 14 15 16 17 18 19 20 21 22 23 24 25 26 27 28
Phase	Effectively Follicular
Hormone State	Estrogen-Like
Fuel at Rest	Carbs
Fat Storage	Normal?
Body Composition	None?
Appetite/Hunger	Unchanged
Metabolic Rate	Potentially Increased
Diet	Follicular Phase
Dietary Changes	Increased B12, zinc, selenium, magnesium, Vitamin C requirements

Readers may note several question marks in the templates above and that is simply due to there being little to no data available on those topics; what I put in the template is simply based on the underlying physiological state that is being created. Recall from Chapter 20 that BC may increase micronutrient requirements and making proper food choices is critical. There are no phase specific supplements.

Obesity

Although obesity (my Category 3) can technically occur alongside of any of the other hormonal modifiers (and is often seen hand in hand with PCOS specifically), it will tend to induce insulin resistance to enough of a degree that I will consider any situation where it is present as an effectively luteal phase/androgen-like state.

Day	1 2 3 4 5 6 7 8 9 10 11 12 13 14 15 16 17 18 19 20 21 22 23 24 25 26 27 28
Phase	Effectively Luteal
Hormone State	Androgen-Like
Fuel at Rest	Fat
Fat Storage	High
Body Composition	Increased body fat/lean body mass
Appetite/Hunger	Increased
Metabolic Rate	Normal
Diet	Luteal Phase/Very Low-Carbohydrate Diet (<80-100 g/day carbs)
Phase Specific Supps.	Possibly luteal phase

While not shown in the above template, I'd remind readers that research does find a number of nutrient deficiencies to be present in obesity; for this reason I might recommend the general use supplements more strongly in this population. While the menstrual cycle often becomes irregular in obesity, this is not universal. Category 3 women who are still normally cycling may benefit from the luteal phase supplements during the luteal phase of their cycle if they are experiencing PMS symptoms.

The Menopausal Transition: Introduction

Since they represent different stages of the menopausal transition, I will describe early peri-menopause, late peri-menopause, post-menopause without HRT and post-menopause with HRT together. As well, since it can be considered a type of surgical menopause, and utilizes (estrogen-only) HRT, I will include partial hysterectomy here. Since many of these hormonal situations are more similar than not and will have more or less identical descriptions, I will group them to save space and unnecessary repetition. Early peri-menopause, menopause with HRT and partial hysterectomy with HRT will all be considered an effectively follicular phase/estrogen-like state since insulin sensitivity will remain relatively high.

Early Peri-Menopause, Menopause w/HRT, Hysterectomy with HRT

Day	1 2 3 4 5 6 7 8 9 10 11 12 13 14 15 16 17 18 19 20 21 22 23 24 25 26 27 28
Phase	Effectively Follicular
Hormone State	Estrogen-Like
Fuel at Rest	Carbs
Fat Storage	Normal?
Body Composition	None outside of aging related changes
Appetite/Hunger	Unchanged
Metabolic Rate	Slow decrease with age
Diet	Follicular Phase
Dietary Changes	Decreased iron requirements (8 mg/day)

In contrast, late peri-menopause and menopause without HRT will be considered an effectively luteal phase/androgen-like state as insulin resistance typically develops due to decreased estrogen signaling

Late Peri-Menopause, Menopause w/o HRT

Day	1 2 3 4 5 6 7 8 9 10 11 12 13 14 15 16 17 18 19 20 21 22 23 24 25 26 27 28
Phase	Effectively Luteal
Hormone State	Androgen-Like
Fuel at Rest	Fat
Fat Storage	High
Body Composition	Increased body weight/body fat, shift in fat patterns, decreased muscle mass
Appetite/Hunger	Unchanged?
Metabolic Rate	Faster decrease with age
Diet	Luteal Phase/Very Low-Carbohydrate Diet (<80-100 g/day carbs)
Phase Specific Supps.	Menopause supplements, soy/phytoestrogens, Increased Calcium

Differences from the Normal Menstrual Cycle

While the majority of physiological factors that are specific to women and/or differ from men apply in any hormonal situation, there are several issues that only the normally cycling female will face that will not be an issue when a hormonal modifier is present. To avoid unnecessary repetition, I will only look at those places where differences do exist and readers may assume that any topic that is not listed here will be identical regardless of her hormonal situation. I will also only address each of those differences here rather than repeating them for every hormonal situation in the next chapters to save space.

Perhaps the largest difference is that tracking changes in body weight and body composition will generally be much easier for women without a menstrual cycle as hormone levels are more consistent overall. One exception to this might be triphasic BC (where the increasing levels of progestins may impact on water retention) or BC with a withdrawal week where the estrogen rebound occurs. Women will have to track over 1-2 monthly cycles to determine what their individual pattern is and this will indicate which weeks can or cannot be meaningfully compared (once the pattern is established, it should be relatively stable). If average weekly weight is changing weekly (triphasic) BC or staying stable for 3 weeks and then increasing (withdrawal), it will still be necessary to compare only like weeks (i.e. weeks 1-3 to each other and week 4 to week 4). Women with oligomenorrhea technically have hormones that are changing throughout their cycle but the variability and randomness here makes it impossible to predict or even meaningfully track changes. Just remember that any large scale changes within a week are water weight. Women who are not normally cycling may need to adjust their estimate of maintenance calories/Total Daily Energy Expenditure (TDEE) as discussed in Chapter 16 (strictly speaking, the normally cycling woman sees a small change from the follicular to luteal phase). The differences here do tend to be somewhat small and since TDEE is an estimate anyhow, some women may choose to ignore them completely and make adjustments based on real-world fat loss instead.

Chapter 30: The Category 2/3 Dieter

Since they share more commonalities than not, especially in terms of there being little worry of major hormonal or menstrual cycle dysfunction, I will be looking at both the Category 3 and Category 2 dieter in this chapter. For each, I will look briefly again at who a given category is likely to include (in terms of activity levels, etc.) along with some of the issues that I have discussed previously in this book before providing a sample diet and training template. For each template, I will choose a hormonal category and look at how training and diet would be integrated with it. For diet, this will include sample diet schedules for small, medium and large deficits (as appropriate) along with the frequency of diet breaks. To save needless repetition of essentially identical information, I will only provide only a single sample template for each Category, choosing one of the hormonal templates from the previous chapter. Women in other hormonal categories can simply apply the training and diet information to their own specific situation, keeping in mind any differences that I mentioned in the previous chapter. Finally, I will finish the chapter by looking at how to end the Category 2/3 dieter and move to long-term maintenance.

The Category 3 Dieter

While it is not impossible for the Category 3 female to be active or an athlete (i.e. a strength/power athlete such as a thrower, powerlifter or Olympic lifter), I will assume for the sake of this discussion that the dieter is inactive or minimally involved in formal exercise and use the beginner exercise program. So long as the guidelines for introducing exercise gradually are followed, a formal Pre-Diet Phase is probably not necessary (although it can always be implemented). Since the small deficit is likely to generate fat loss too slow to be effective, I have only shown the medium and large deficits below.

Day	1	2	3	4	5	6	7	8	9	10	11	12	13	14	15	16	17	18	19	20	21	22	23	24	25	26	27	28	
Effective Phase	Effectively Luteal																												
Hormone State	Androgen-like																												
Diet	Luteal Phase or Very Low-Carbohydrate Diet (<80-100 g/day carbs)																												
Supplements	Possibly Luteal, thermogenics (optional)																												
Day	1	2	3	4	5	6	7	8	9	10	11	12	13	14	15	16	17	18	19	20	21	22	23	24	25	26	27	28	Diet Break
Weights	T		(T)		T			T		(T)		T			T		(T)		T			T		(T)		T			
Aerobic		L		L		L			L		L		L			L		L		L			L		L		L		
Large Deficit	D	D	D		D	F	D	D	D	D	D	*	*	*	D	D	D		D	F	D	D	D	D	D	F	D	D	D	10-12 weeks
Med Deficit	D	D	D		D	F	D	D	D	D	D	*	*	*	D	D	D		D	F	D	D	D	D	D	F	D	D	D	12-16 weeks

T=Training, L = Low intensity aerobic exercise, D diet, F=free meal, ***=Maintenance (see below)

Looking at the training program, I've shown weight training to be performed at least two times per week with a third optional workout per week. Low intensity aerobic activity should be performed a minimum of three times per week. I have shown it on alternate days of the week from the weight workouts as this will have the largest impact on insulin sensitivity overall. As discussed previously, this may not be practical from a time or convenience standpoint. Women who find it easier to perform both weight training and aerobic training in the same workout should do that if it leads to more consistency overall.

For the large and medium deficits, I've shown the inclusion of one free meal per week along with the normal diet days. As I discussed in Chapter 20 on Flexible Eating Strategies, women who find that the free meal throws them off of their diet should eliminate it or at least wait until more consistent dietary habits have been established. For the Category 3 dieter on a large deficit, calories should be raised to maintenance for 2-3 days every 6 weeks of dieting (indicated by the ***). On a medium deficit, calories should be raised to maintenance for 2-3 days every 10 weeks of active dieting (indicated by the ***). As with free meals, dieters who find that this throws them off of their diet or makes returning to it difficult should forego the free meals and only implement the full diet breaks. These should occur every 10-12 weeks when a large deficit is being used or every 12-16 weeks if a moderate deficit is being used.

The Category 2 Dieter

As I discussed earlier in the book, the Category 2 dieter is likely to have the most variability in terms of the type of training that is or isn't being done. It could readily include inactive women, relative beginners, serious trainees and at least some types of athletes (either those with relatively moderate body fat requirements or those who have gained excess body fat for one reason or another). In the sample template, I will assume that the dieter is a serious trainee looking to lose fat/improve body composition who is using hormonal BC with a second generation progestin with a 21 day on/7 day off use pattern. She will be using a three-way split routine of Legs/Core (LC), Chest/Delts/Triceps (CDT), Back/Biceps (BBi) while performing 4 days per week of aerobic activity and one HIIT workout per week. Since all are possibilities for her diet, I will present dietary patterns for all three deficit sizes.

Day	1	2	3	4	5	6	7	8	9	10	11	12	13	14	15	16	17	18	19	20	21	22	23	24	25	26	27	28	
Eff. Phase	Effective Luteal																					Effectively Early Follicular							
Hormone State	Progesterone																					Estrogen							
Diet	Luteal Phase																					Follicular Phase							
Supplements	Possibly luteal phase supplements																					No specific supplements							
Day	1	2	3	4	5	6	7	8	9	10	11	12	13	14	15	16	17	18	19	20	21	22	23	24	25	26	27	28	Diet Break
Weights	LC	CDT	BBi		LC	CDT		BBi	LC	CDT		BBi	LC		LC	CDT	BBi		LC	CDT		BBi	LC	CDT		BBi	LC		
Aerobic	Y	Y	H		Y	Y		H	Y	Y		Y	Y		Y	Y	H		Y	Y		H	Y	Y		Y	Y		
Large Deficit	D	D	F	D	D	F	D	D	D	F	D	M2	M2	D	F	D	D	M1	M1	D	D	D	F	D	D	D	F	D	6-8 wks
Med. Deficit	D	D	D	D	D	F	D	D	D	D	D	D	F	D	D	D	D	D	D	F	D	D	D	D	D	M	M	D	8-12 wks
Small Deficit	D	D	D	D	D	F	D	D	D	D	D	D	F	D	D	D	D	D	M7	M7	D	D	D	D	D	D	F	D	12-14 wks

L = Low intensity aerobic exercise, H=HIIT, D=diet, F=free meal, M=Maintenance (see below)

As I showed in the last chapter, the serious trainee's workout rotates throughout each week with different workouts falling on different days. The aerobic and HIIT days change as well with a primary goal of keeping HIIT as far away from the leg workout as possible. For all deficit sizes, two free meals are shown during each week. I have shown them on Wednesday and Saturday as an example only and they can be placed as needed so long as they are not on back-to-back days. As with the Category 3 dieter, women who find that free meals do more harm than good in terms of their diet should eliminate them in favor of days at maintenance, possibly IIFYM and the full diet break. On any weeks when calories are brought to maintenance, one free meal should be eliminated.

Looking first at the large deficit diet, the general dieting week alternates full dieting days with days including a free meal. During a large deficit diet, the Category 2 woman should bring her calories to maintenance for 2 days every 3 weeks. The first time this occurs (M1) which would be in the third week of the diet (during this week, the maintenance days replace the Free Meal). The second time this occurs (M2) would be in the 6th week of the diet. I have placed the maintenance days to coincide with the last two workouts of the week but they can be placed anywhere in the week as desired. If a Full Diet Break was planned after 6 weeks (i.e. in week 7), these days would be eliminated. If the diet were being continued for 8 total weeks with a Full Diet Break in week 9, the second set of maintenance days should not be done.

For the medium deficit diet, the same basic dynamics are in place with each week consisting of 5 full dieting days with up to two free meals. Here calories only need to be raised to maintenance every four weeks and I have shown this in the template on Friday and Saturday of the fourth week to coincide with the two workouts. Once again, these days can be placed as desired during that week. A diet break should be taken every 8-12 weeks and the maintenance days in week 8 would be eliminated if the diet break will be starting in week 9. If the Category 2 dieter is planning to take a break at week 9, calories would be raised to maintenance at week 4 but not in week 8. The same would hold if she were taking a diet break at week 13 and she would raise calories to maintenance at week 4 and 8 but not in week 12.

Finally is the small deficit diet. Once again the weekly structure is the same with up to 2 free meals allowed. Calories only need to be raised to maintenance every 7 weeks in this diet which I have indicated by M7. A full diet break would be taken every 12-14 weeks which means that only one increase of calories to maintenance will ever be required during the active dieting phase. A second would only potentially occur in week 14 and since the diet break would be started, it would be eliminated anyhow.

Ending the Category 2/3 Diet

At some point, any fat loss diet will end. Whether for an inactive individual, exerciser, serious trainee or athlete, for the Category 2/3 dieter, this is most likely to be when the dieter has reached their original goal or simply needs to take an extended break from dieting (this may occur prior to another active dieting phase). In all cases, the goal is to maintain the weight/fat loss and avoid the weight and fat regain that is all too common when the diet is over. Regardless of the specifics, there are three issues I want to address. The first is how to adjust the diet and raise calorie levels. The second is how to adjust exercise. Third, and perhaps most importantly, are the strategies that have been found to best improve the chances for long-term success in weight maintenance after fat has been lost.

Adjusting Calorie Intake

The first step in ending a fat loss diet will be to return calories back to maintenance levels to bring the body back into energy balance. While technically activity could be decreased to eliminate the deficit, and this may occur in situations where it was increased to very high levels during a diet, I will focus only on increasing food intake to maintenance levels. This is important for several reasons. The first is that, by definition, if calories are not raised to maintenance, the person will still technically be dieting. The second is that by raising calories to maintenance, many of the metabolic adaptations that occurred will be reversed to some degree although they will never reverse completely. The adaptive component of resting metabolic rate may be cut in half and at least some research suggests that the reductions in Non-Exercise Activity Thermogenesis disappear when calories are higher. This potentially allows for even more food to be eaten without exceeding TDEE and causing fat gain.

Practically this means that calorie intake will need to be raised until it effectively matches the Total Daily Energy Expenditure (TDEE). This value will always be below the pre-diet level and should be based on the new current body weight. If a dieter started at 180 lbs and ended the diet at 160 lbs, they would be basing estimates of TDEE on that new 160 pound body weight. This must be further adjusted due to the other adaptations that occur in every component of TDEE. I generally recommend subtracting 10% from the estimate as a safety factor. So if a 160 lb female has an estimated TDEE of 16 cal/lb (as determined in Chapter 16) or 2560 calories per day, this would be reduced by 10% or roughly 250 calories per day, making the new estimated TDEE 2200 calories which should only act as a starting point.

With one exception, this is no different than the Full Diet Break I described in Chapter 21 although the goal is longer term maintenance rather than simply a break between active dieting blocks. That exception has to do with how quickly calories are raised when the diet is over. Unlike the Full Diet Break, where calories must be raised to maintenance within 2-3 days to get the benefits, food intake can be raised more slowly, over a span of a week or two when dieters are moving back to maintenance. This has two major benefits in this case.

The first is that small amounts of additional fat loss may occur even as hormone levels are improving due to the increased food intake (1). The second is that gradual increases in calorie intake reduce the risk of losing food control along with avoiding the type of rigid dietary thinking where someone is either on or off a diet. A gradual addition of foods to the baseline of a properly set up fat loss diet feels more like a transition from dieting to maintenance which can help with adherence. Slower increases in food intake can also help to avoid water retention, bloating and stomach upset which can cause mental stress. That said, I do not recommend taking longer than two weeks to reach the new estimated maintenance levels.

To do this, the dieter should determine how many calories will be need to be added to their diet which should be subdivided into smaller amounts which would be added every few days to the current diet. If a dieter needs to add 500 calories to their diet over the course of 2 weeks, they might add 100 calories every 2-3 days until the new calorie intake level has been reached. This only amounts to one serving of starchy carbohydrate, a piece of fruit or roughly 10 grams of fat (less than one tablespoon) over that time period. It's important to maintain the other components of the fat loss diet, especially sufficient protein intake during the return to maintenance and any increases in calorie intake should come from foods being added to the base of proper eating that has been established.

Adjusting Exercise

Exercise and activity levels are the next factor that may change when someone ends a diet although the specific recommendations are very situation specific. Ideally training should be a part of any fat loss approach for reasons I've discussed earlier in this book and I'll assume that it was being performed to at least some degree during the diet. How much and how that amount should be adjusted will depend heavily on which population is being discussed. Realistically the competition athlete will have been performing the most total activity although it the amount can vary considerably. Some will have increased activity levels during the diet to burn more calories while others may have decreased the amount they were doing to avoid overtraining when recovery was impaired. In both cases, training should be adjusted over 2-4 weeks towards relatively normal levels in terms of the amount, frequency and intensity of training that was being done prior to the dieting period. In the case of competition athletes, it is likely that the diet will end after the season is over in which case 1-2 or more weeks of relatively reduced training may be done to allow recovery from the previous season to dissipate. This can drastically reduce TDEE and it's important for those athletes to keep calorie intake in check to avoid excessive fat gain. As the next season begins, training will resume and progress towards more normal levels, increasing TDEE.

For the serious trainee, similar dynamics may hold although it's more common here for extra aerobic work to be added during a fat loss phase. If levels of aerobic activity were fairly high near the end of the diet this can be reduced fairly significantly with a minimum of 3 sessions per week of 30-45' being more than sufficient in most cases (realistically most females do far more than this). One of those sessions could conceivably be a High-Intensity Interval Training (HIIT) session but I'd recommend no more than that in general. Weight training 3-5 days per week would make up the rest of the training during the week.

Finally is the general dieter for whom exercise may not have played a significant role in the fat loss process due to the generally small amount that can typically be done. While this should have been progressively increased over the length of the diet, it is impossible to predict how much or how little any given women might be doing when her diet is over. At the very least, I would expect her to be performing 2 (and possibly 3) weight workouts per week and a minimum of 3 aerobic (and possibly one HIIT) session per week and, from this level, the amount of exercise can be increased as calories are increased. Quite in fact, this is likely where exercise will have its greatest role. Exercise helps to offset some of the metabolic adaptations to dieting which allows for more food to be eaten without creating a calorie surplus. When proper resistance training is coupled with a higher protein intake, a larger proportion of any weight gained will tend to be from muscle rather than fat. It does take a fairly large amount of exercise to have a real benefit here with 250 minutes per week or moderate to vigorous exercise being found to limit post-diet weight gain (2). This should include a mixture of resistance training, aerobic exercise and possibly HIIT.

Finally, in the situation where a dieter did not engage in any exercise during the diet itself, a program must be started when calories are being brought back to maintenance. The guidelines I have provided previously still hold and gradual increases in the frequency, intensity, time (or all three) should occur working towards the 250 minutes per week goal and mixture of exercise described above.

Long-Term Weight Maintenance: Introduction

While all dieters will need to adjust their calories and training at the end of a diet, only the serious recreational trainee and general dieter will have long-term maintenance of their new weight and BF%/body composition as a goal (athletes who dieted for a specific competition or competition season will almost always be regaining at least some fat afterwards). In a very real way, maintenance is a far more difficult process than fat loss itself with research consistently showing that a majority of dieters will regain some, if not all, of the weight and fat that they lost over the 1-3 years following the diet. In that sense, research examining the best way to lose weight or fat is not really examining the right question. Rather, the focus should be on improving long-term maintenance of those losses. This is actually an issue that is common to all behavioral changes: most can make changes in the short-term but long-term maintenance is difficult.

I want to make it clear that the commonly cited claim that only 5-10% of people successfully lose weight and keep it off is completely incorrect. It represents data from a few early studies of the most difficult cases, women and men who had done diet after diet without success and who are not representative of most dieters. Large numbers of people lose weight outside of research studies or even using a commercial program and the actual success rates for weight loss maintenance are 20-30% or higher depending on what criteria for long-term success is used. I mention this as I feel that the expectation of failure, driven by endless media stores that losing weight is impossible, mentally sets dieters up for failure from the outset. In expecting to fail, dieters ensure that they will.

There are of course many other reasons why diets fail so often and I want to examine some of them. Perhaps the largest contributor is in how dieters approach the goal of weight and fat loss in the first place. Frequently the process is conceptualized as a purely short-term change where diet and/or exercise will be changed briefly, weight will be lost and then, somehow, it will be maintained once they return to their previous eating and activity patterns. While this would be wonderful, it is not realistic and long-term maintenance of any changes in body composition can only occur if at least some of the changes that were made are also maintained.

Adding to this are the number of truly pathological dieting practices that are so commonly used. Whether it is through enormous calorie deficits along with staggering amounts of activity (neither of which can be maintained), poorly set up diets, a lack of exercise or absurd approaches that cannot possibly work, dieters do themselves more harm than good. The majority of this book has been aimed at addressing these issues and more in terms of dieting in the safest and most effective way to achieve optimal fat loss or changes in body composition, especially within the context of a woman's unique physiology. While this in no way guarantees success, it at least avoids the problems inherent to how dieting is typically approached.

Which brings me back to the fact that, while the percentage of total dieters succeeding is still fairly low at 30%, it's equally clear that a large number of people are successfully losing weight/fat and keeping it off. In general, they show many commonalities in their approach to the process and this helps to point to specific strategies that can be used to increase the chances of success for readers of this book. The first step to escape this trap is to realize that fat loss is a long-term process. First the fat must be lost and then that loss must be maintained in the long-term. This means that the behavior changes that were made to first lost the fat must be maintained, to one degree or another, in the long-term.

Strictly speaking, at least some behavior changes must be maintained forever and, while this may seem overwhelming, maintaining fat loss often becomes easier with time (3). This seems to contradict the fact that the biological adaptations to weight loss never dissipate completely and is probably due to eating and activity habits becoming more ingrained and automatic. But even this process takes time, far longer than most think (the idea that it takes only 3 weeks to establish a new habit is nonsense). Someone with 20+ years of certain eating and activity patterns cannot reverse those in a number of weeks, or even months. In this vein, longer diet interventions show better success than shorter and this is assuredly due to dietary habits becoming more well established.

I've mentioned other factors of relevance here, such as adopting more flexible eating attitudes and avoid the types of black and white thinking inherent to rigid eating attitudes. As I discussed in Chapter 15, many see themselves as either on or off a diet or see food as either diet foods of non-diet foods. Adopting flexible attitudes means realizing that essentially all foods can be incorporated both into a fat loss diet as well as maintenance. It's equally important to realize that individual days of eating are irrelevant in the big scheme and that a day of overeating can be compensated with small adjustments over the next few days is key. I suspect that Intermittent Calorie Restriction (ICR) approaches will have great utility. Not only do they automatically factor in more flexible eating patterns, they establish in the dieter's mind that dieting hard for several days is relatively easy. An ICR style dieter could easily introduce a day or two of "fasting" (25% of maintenance) if they felt that body weight was increasing or even include one proactively each week to ensure that any calorie surpluses during the week are pre-compensated for. Obviously this should not be used to justify excessive eating during the week.

I'd add that as common a reason for long-term failure has to do with a peculiarity of human behavior where we tend to focus on negatives more than positives. In the case of weight or fat loss, this may manifest by focusing on how far away the goal still is rather than on the progress that has already been made (it is the same logic by which a dieter will focus on a single day that they were not adherent to their diet rather than the weeks that they were). Of equal importance is that as soon as dieters regain some amounts of weight or fat, they often see their total efforts as having failed or been in vein. The amounts are almost irrelevant but a 2 lb fat regain will almost universally be seen as more negative than a 20 pound or more fat loss. Instead, it's better for the dieter to not only focus on what they have accomplished but to realize that they clearly know how to lose weight and fat to begin with since they already did it. Having done it previously, they can re-implement the changes they made previously to lose any regained weight.

There are many other reasons that dieters fail to maintain their losses in the long-term but, rather than attempting to detail them, I want to examine some of the habits and behavioral approaches that successful dieters have been found to use. Most of this information comes from a group called the National Weight Control Registry (NWCR), which represents a group of over 3000 dieters who have lost at least 30 pounds and maintained that loss for at least a year. Most in the NWCR are women and the average weight loss is over 60 pounds (ranging from 30 to 300 pounds) with a duration of long-term maintenance ranging from 1 to 66 years. Some members lost the weight rapidly, some lost it slowly and about half used some sort of specific diet program with the other half doing it on their own. While the majority of NWCR members used some form of carbohydrate based, low-fat diet there is a small number (about 10%) who report using low-carbohydrate diets and this number may increase over time.

Studies on the NWCR members have found a number of common habits suggesting that these are important for long-term weight maintenance and I want to look at some of the major ones (4). Nearly all members used a combination of diet and exercise to lose weight and 90% report performing daily activity equivalent to roughly an hour of brisk walking. Members report eating a reduced calorie, low-fat diet (again, increasing numbers have used low-carbohydrate diets) with the regular use of low- or no-calorie artificially sweetened beverages (once again countering the idea that these products make people gain weight). Most don't watch more than 10 hour per week of television (a time when many eat mindlessly while moving very little) but engage in NEAT type activities instead. Most NWCR members report eating breakfast which seems to contradict what I wrote about Intermittent Fasting (IF'ing) approaches but I suspect this is just a leftover habit based on the idea of breakfast being the most important meal of the day. NWCR dieters are often consistent in their eating patterns during the week and across weekends. Dieters who allow excessive flexibility on the weekends or holidays gain more weight than those who don't and, while this seems to contradict what I wrote about ICR and flexible dieting, I think this is an issue of semantics. It's one thing to adopt flexible attitudes about day-to-day food intake and another to fall into the trap of "It's a holiday and I can eat as much as I want."

Before looking at perhaps the most important habit that is seen in the NWCR group, I want to mention that there are other potential components to improving long-term weight maintenance, much of which is related to new technologies (5). Online communities can provide support and encouragement and feedback, sites exist to gamify exercise by allowing people to compete against others or earn badges for their accomplishments and various apps exist to track body composition or weight or send the person reminders to keep them focused on their diet. All of these and more that will be developed all provide support, accountability and followup which are critical to long-term success.

With that said, let me finish by discussing perhaps the single most important habit among the NWCR members which is consistently monitoring their body weight, often through daily weighing. This singular strategy, while simple, turns out to be a key component of successful weight loss maintenance (6). Not only does daily weighing remind and focus the individual on their goals, it acts as a form of immediate feedback. I'll mention again that daily variations must be ignored with a 7-day rolling average being far superior (the normally cycling woman must also take into account menstrual cycle related changes). Some new scales will actually keep the rolling average in memory and apps exist to to this. It has even been shown that people are less likely to weigh the day after they overeat and this would suggest that having to weigh the next morning might help to prevent overeating in the first place (7). Even with the knowledge that it's a purely temporary gain, nobody likes to see the number on the scale go up and anything that keeps the person focused on their eating and activity goals is good in the context of long-term weight maintenance. Essentially, an activity that may take no more than 15-30 seconds each morning can have a profound impact on the chance of long-term success. But even this raises an important question.

What is Weight Loss Maintenance?

To finish this chapter and topic, I want to address the question of what long-term maintenance actually is or should represent. Many tend to think of maintenance as the idea that body weight or BF% will be rigidly unchanging on a day-to-day or week-to-week basis and this represents yet another problem with how people approach the process of dieting and fat loss. Small fluctuations in body weight are normal to begin with due to changes in water weight, etc. and the measurement error in BF% may make that number move around slightly whether true fat gain is occurring or not. It would be a fairly rare individual who's eating and activity habits were so rigid (and if this occurred it would likely be in the Category 1 athletes in the first place) that there are truly zero change in weight or BF%. At the same time, a mistake that many dieter's make is to ignore actual changes when they are occurring, suddenly finding themselves back at their pre-diet level. Somewhere between those two extremes will be ideal and using a true weight gain cutoff of 3% over current body weight has been suggested as a definition of maintenance with action being taken if a true increase in body weight occurs beyond that level (4).

For a female who ended their diet at 160 pounds (72.7kg), 3% would be a 4.8 pound (2.1 kg) gain (this is calculated by multiplying weight by 0.03). If her actual weight by a 7-day rolling average reached 165 lbs, this would mean that she is backsliding and needs to take action. This could mean being stricter with her food intake or increasing her activity but something should be done. It might actually be better for women to use a smaller weight cutoff, in this case 2-3 lbs (~2%) as losing that much weight can be accomplished relatively rapidly for most women while larger losses start to become more difficult. This approach requires that regular monitoring be practiced, again supporting it's overall importance.

Given the relatively greater importance of body composition, it would be arguably better to use BF% to monitor change and a cutoff of 2-3% increase in BF% would be roughly equivalent to a 3% gain in body fat. The problem here is that most methods of measuring BF% have an inherent error of 3% or more which makes determining if this change has truly occurred much more difficult. Other methods could be used in this regard. Taking occasional tape measurements, at the waist and thigh for women, would give some indication of at regain and I mentioned in Chapter 6 that using a specific piece of clothing as an indicator may be the easiest of all. If it fits a certain way after the diet and starts to feel tighter (and menstrual cycle dynamics, if present, are accounted for), weight and body fat are likely being gained and the dieter will need to take action sooner rather than later. This alone will increase the chances of success enormously.

Chapter 32: The Category 1 Dieter and Amenorrhea

As I've discussed throughout this book, the Category 1 female faces the greatest number of issues for dieting. Women in all hormonal categories must deal with the issues of metabolic slowdown, hormonal disruption and slowed fat loss while the normally cycling female has the added issue of developing menstrual cycle dysfunction or amenorrhea. This can also occur for the PCOS or subclinically hyperandrogenic woman with oligomenorrhea. This is complicated further by the fact that Category 1 can span a fairly variable population of women. Certainly I would expect most women in this group to be athletes or serious trainees and even here they have the option of short aggressive diets which should be structured in one way and longer more extended diets, which should be structured and adjusted in another. As I have mentioned there is also a subgroup of inactive Category 1 women and I will discuss them first.

Inactive Category 1 Diet

As I have mentioned repeatedly in this book, the inactive Category 1 dieter is not only inactive, but often has a tendency to use problematic dieting practices (either unsustainable fad diets or those containing too little protein). This predisposes them towards muscle loss which brings with it a body fat rebound, often leaving them with a poorer body composition (or fat distribution) than they began with. Preventing this requires at least two changes. The first is to set up the fat loss diet properly, meaning according to the guidelines in this book. If absolutely no other guidelines are followed, women must consume enough protein on a day-do-day basis and this should be combined with at least some formal exercise, Resistance training should always be the first choice here and even two days per week will have a profound impact.

In an ideal world, women in this group would go through at least a 4 week Pre-Diet phase but, knowing full well that most will not want to wait that long to start their diet, I have presented a workable template below. I will be assuming that the woman in question is using a form of birth control with a third or fourth generation progestin that is being used on a 21-day on/7-day off pattern. This is combined with the beginner exercise program and I have shown diet schedules for small, medium and large deficits.

Day	1	2	3	4	5	6	7	8	9	10	11	12	13	14	15	16	17	18	19	20	21	22	23	24	25	26	27	28	
Effective Phase*	Follicular																												
Hormone State	Estrogen-like																												
Diet	Follicular																												
Supplements	No Phase Specific Supplements																												
Day	1	2	3	4	5	6	7	8	9	10	11	12	13	14	15	16	17	18	19	20	21	22	23	24	25	26	27	28	Diet Break
Weights	T	(T)		T			T		(T)	T			T		(T)	T			T			T		(T)	T				
Aerobic		L		L		L		L		L		L		L		L		L		L		L		L		L			
Large Deficit	D	D	D		D	M	D	D	D	D	M	D		D		D	M	D	D		D	M	D		D	D	D	D	2-4 weeks
Med. Deficit	D	D	D		D	F	D	D	D	D	D		D	M	M	D	D	D	D		D	F	D	D	D	D	M	M	6-8 weeks
Small Deficit	D	D	D		D	F	D	D	D	D	D		D	M2	M2	D	D	D	D		D	M1	M1	D	D	D	F	D	8-10 weeks

L = Low intensity aerobic exercise, D=diet, F=free meal, M=Maintenance (see below)

Weight training is shown as being done a minimum of two times per week with the possibility of an optional third workout indicated by (T). Aerobic activity would be done a minimum of three times per week although it could be done more frequently if desired and HIIT could be incorporated after 4 weeks of consistent aerobic work had been done. I've shown the aerobic work alternate with weight training days but they can be done on the same day if it fits the dieter's schedule better.

Looking first at the large/aggressive deficit, I'd reiterate that this should be a short-term approach only, with 2-4 weeks being a typical duration before a break is taken. Whether the diet is 2-4 weeks in length, readers can see that calories are raised to maintenance for one day roughly every 3-4 days. This is crucial to try to limit the adaptations to being below the critical Energy Availability (EA) threshold. They will still occur to some degree but this is manageable since the diet is meant to be short-term only. By the time any major problems start, the diet should be over. Moving to the medium deficit, the schedule allows for one free meal per week along with two days at maintenance every other week. I've placed these on Friday or Friday/Saturday to coincide with the weight training workout but this is not required. The medium deficit diet should last no longer than 6-8 weeks before a break is taken and the free meal or maintenance days in the last week of the diet should be eliminated. Finally is the small deficit diet. Here calories only need to be raised to maintenance for 2 days every 21 days which means during week 3 and 6 of an 8 week diet and weeks 3,6, and 9 of a 10 week diet (shown by M1 and M2). A free meal is allowed in other weeks and the diet break should occur at 8-10 weeks.

Aggressive Category 1 Diet for Athletes/Trainees

While it tends to be generally inappropriate for long-term dieting without major modifications (i.e. my own Ultimate Diet 2.0), I have mentioned a few times in the book that there may be times when an athletic Category 1 dieter may want or need to use a short, aggressive diet to reduce body fat quickly. This might be the strength/power athlete who finds that long diets harm their performance or an athlete who needs to offset the small gains in fat that often accompany off-season training. In occasional situations, the physique dieter who has fallen behind on their diet can consider 2 weeks of aggressive dieting to get back on schedule. As mentioned previously, this can cause more problems than it solves with women frequently not responding as well as men to this approach. If more than 2 weeks of aggressive dieting would be required to get back on schedule, a different competition should be chosen.

The main consideration for aggressive diets has to do with training. First and foremost, it must be accepted that few will make meaningful gains in any aspect of fitness during such a diet. The aim, rather, should be to prevent any loss of fitness and this can be easily accomplished with alterations in the current training program. This means moving to the maintenance training levels which I described in Chapter 28, reducing frequency and volume of training by 2/3rds while intensity is maintained. As I've noted, excessive aerobic work can harm results and should be limited to reasonable amounts of perhaps 20-30' of LISS only. HIIT should not be done under any circumstances.

For the template below, I will assume that the dieter is normally cycling and will actually show several different weight training schedules along with three diet schedules.

Day	1–7	8–14	15–21	22–28
Phase	Early Follicular	Late Follicular	Early Luteal	Late Luteal
Note	Menses (3-5 days)	Ovulation		PMS (4-7 days)
Hormone	Estrogen		Progesterone	
Diet	Follicular Phase		Luteal Phase	
Changes		Reduce NA/Increase K*	Add Fruit, Chocolate	Add Fruit, Chocolate; Reduce NA/IncreaseK*
Supps.	Aspirin/NSAID if needed		Luteal phase	Luteal Phase, Soy/Phyto. Aspirin/NSAID

Day	1	2	3	4	5	6	7	8	9	10	11	12	13	14	15	16	17	18	19	20	21	22	23	24	25	26	27	28
Weights 1	F		(F)		F			F		(F)		F			F		(F)		F			F		(F)		F		
Weights 2	U	L		U	L			U	L		U	L			U	L		U	L			U	L		U	L		
Weights 3	M	M		U	L			U	L		U	L			U	L		U	L			U	L		U	L		
Weights 4	Lc			CDT		BBi		Lc			CDT		BBi		Lc			CDT		BBi		Lc			CDT		BBi	
Diet 1	D	D	D	D	F	D	D	D	D	D	D	F	D	D	R	R	R	R	R	R	R	R	R	R	R	R	R	R
Diet 2	D	D	D	R	R	D	D	D	D	D	R	R	D	D	D	D	D	R	R	D	D	D	D	D	R	R	D	D
Diet 3	D	R	D	D	R	D	D	D	R	D	D	R	D	D	D	R	D	D	R	D	D	D	R	D	D	R	D	D

F=Full Body, U=Upper, L=Lower, M=Metabolic/Depletion, D=Diet, R =Refeed/Maintenance

Looking first at diet structure, Diet 1 represents a 2 week diet cycle. Here a free meal (if desired) can be used weekly but calories are not brought to maintenance until the break itself is taken in week 3. While there will be some negative hormonal adaptations due to being below the critical EA threshold, they will be small enough over only 2 weeks to not be of any real concern. As well, if training volume is lowered as recommended, there should be no real risk of glycogen depletion harming performance over this short of a time frame. The second diet schedule is based around a 4 week diet and here calories are raised to maintenance for 2 days every week. The third schedule is also a 4 week diet and has 2 days at maintenance per week spread out during the week.

Looking next at training, I've provided several possible approaches. The first is just two to three short full-body workouts spread throughout the week with perhaps 2-3 heavy sets per muscle group being done at each. For the short duration nature of the diet, this will be more than sufficient to maintain strength and muscle mass (any small amount lost will rapidly be regained when calories are raised again. The second is an upper/lower split for those who want to train slightly more frequently and could be used by some types of strength/power athletes or physique athletes with up to 4 total sets per muscle group being used. The third cycle is similar to the second but starts off the aggressive diet with two glycogen depletion (4 sets of 15-20 reps with a 60" rest interval per muscle group) workouts to enhance whole body fat oxidation. The final workout option is a legs/core, chest/delt/tris, back/biceps split with each trained once per week and again 4 total heavy sets per muscle group being done. This would be most appropriate for a physique competitor who wants to drop some fat before returning to attempting to gain muscle mass.

Extended Category 1 Dieter

Finally is the extended Category 1 diet template. Primarily here I am focusing on physique dieters although (though the principles apply to performance athletes) who is dieting to somewhere between 18% and 10-12% body fat. I have discussed the myriad issues that go into this type of diet throughout this book and rather than repeating them will only remind dieters that they must go through the process of estimating their dieting time, including a Pre-Diet phase as needed (generally the last month of their previous training block, etc). I'd reiterate that it is always better to err on the side of starting too early rather than too late, especially for new competitors who may not be familiar with their personal responses. A dieter who is ahead of schedule can always slow their fat loss to avoid hitting a peak too early while a dieter that has fallen behind must either pick a different contest or insert a potentially problematic aggressive diet.

In the template below, I will again use a normally cycling woman as it comes with all of the hormonal and metabolic problems I have discussed including the risk for menstrual cycle dysfunction and full-blown amenorrhea (which also exists for the oligomenorrheic woman). Women with any other hormonal modifier still face the same hormonal and metabolic adaptations and the template, with minor changes, would still apply. The template below will be slightly different than the previous ones in this book in several ways.

First, I will divide the template into three distinct phases based on target BF% ranges of 24-18%, 18-14% and 14-10%. I have also shown where various physique competitors might fall in those ranges. I will also not provide specific deficit schedules, assuming that dieters are using a larger weight loss goal earlier in the diet which decreases as the diet progresses. For each phase, I will show how the overall diet (in terms of the use of days at maintenance) change along with potential changes to training, primarily in terms of aerobic and HIIT frequency. A suggested frequency of diet breaks will also be shown for each phase.

Day	1	2	3	4	5	6	7	8	9	10	11	12	13	14	15	16	17	18	19	20	21	22	23	24	25	26	27	28	
Phase	Early Follicular							Late Follicular							Early Luteal							Late Luteal							
Note	Menses (3-5 days)							Ovulation														PMS (4-7 days)							
Hormone	Estrogen														Progesterone														
Diet	Follicular Phase														Luteal Phase														
Changes								Reduce NA/Increase K*							Add Fruit, Chocolate							Add Fruit, Chocolate Reduce NA/Increase K*							
Supps.	Aspirin/NSAID if needed														Luteal phase							Luteal Phase, Soy/Phyto. Aspirin/ NSAID							

Day	1	2	3	4	5	6	7	8	9	10	11	12	13	14	15	16	17	18	19	20	21	22	23	24	25	26	27	28	Break
1:24-18%	Bikini Competitors, Serious Trainee																												
Weights	LC	CDT	BBi		LC	CDT		BBi	LC	CDT		BBi	LC		LC	CDT	BBi		LC	CDT		BBi	LC	CDT	Of	BBi	LC		
Aerobic	L		L		L	L			L		L		L	L		L		L		L		L		L		L	L		
Diet	D	D	D	D	M	D		D	D	D	D	D	M	D	D	D	D	D	D	D	M	D	D	D	D	D	M	D	8-10 wks
2:18-14%	Figure (depending on requirements)																												
Weights	LC	CDT	BBi		LC	CDT		BBi	LC	CDT		BBi	LC		LC	CDT	BBi		LC	CDT		BBi	LC	CDT	Of	BBi	LC		
Aerobic	L	L		L	L	(H)		L	L		L	L	(H)		L	L		L	L	(H)		L	L		L	L	(H)		
Diet 1	D	D	M	D		M		D	D	M	D		M	D	D	D	M	D		M	D	D	D	M	D		M	D	
Diet 2	D	D	D	D	M	M		D	D	D	D	D	M	M	D	D	D	D	D	D	M	M	D	D	D	D	M	M	6-8 wks
3:14-10%	Bodybuilding, Physique																												
Weights	LC	CDT	BBi		LC	CDT		BBi	LC	CDT		BBi	LC		LC	CDT	BBi		LC	CDT		BBi	LC	CDT	Of	BBi	LC		
Aerobic	L	L		L	L	(H)	L	L	L		L	L	(H)	L	L	L		L	L	(H)	L	L	L		L	L	(H)	L	
Diet	D	M	D	D	M	M	D	D	M	D		D	M	M	D	M	D		D	M	M	D	D	M	D		D	M	M	D	6-8 wks

LC=Legs/Core, CDT=Chest,delts,triceps, BBi=back/biceps, L=LISS, H=HIIT, D=Diet, M=Maintenance

Looking at the template, I've indicated three primary changes which occur from the first to third phases. The first is that, if needed, the amount of aerobic work being done may be increased. The templates starts with 4 low-intensity days from 24-18% body fat, moves to 4 low intensity days with an optional HIIT session (which could be replaced with LISS) from 18-14% and this might increase further from 14-10% based on the dieter's needs (this might mean daily activity for smaller dieters). I'd reiterate the amount of aerobic/HIIT work is highly individual and that the goal should be to do as much as is needed to maintain fat loss but no more. If 3-4 days of low intensity aerobic work and/or one HIIT workout keeps fat loss at the appropriate rate, more should not be added simply for the sake of it. I'd mention that dieters who have reached the 18% body fat range may wish to consider the Stubborn Fat Protocols in Appendix 1.

The second change will be to the diet itself and there are two adjustments to be made, one of which is not shown in the template. This has to do with the goal weight loss which, in general, should be 1% per week in from 24-18% and 18-14% before dropping to 0.5% per week from 14-10% body fat. There are potential exceptions to this, a women who was only dieting to perhaps 18% might choose to use a 0.5% deficit for her entire diet since she has only a small amount of fat to lose.

The second change is in terms of how many days per week calories will need to be raised to maintenance to both maintain training intensity and help to offset metabolic and hormonal adaptations with the required number of days at maintenance going up as BF% goes down. I've reproduced the chart from Chapter 23 below showing how this would be implemented showing both the minimum and maximum number of days at maintenance that could be used.

BF%	Min. Days	Max. Days
24-18%	1	3
18-14%	2	3
14-10%	3	3

You can see that as the current/goal BF% range goes down, the number of maintenance days that are required, increasing from 1 to 2 to 3 days. As I discussed in Chapter 23, some trainees may prefer to use a larger number of days at maintenance from the outset of their diet and I'd refer readers back to page 258 for examples of how those days might be integrated with training in both cases. Finally are the diet breaks which I've shown becoming slightly more frequent as dieters move through each phase. As discussed in Chapter 21, the break can be implemented in one of two ways. The first is to space them evenly across the diet so a 24 week diet would have a break every 8 weeks. Alternately, a dieter might take 10 weeks before their first break, 8 before their second break and only 6 before their final break (and this might coincide with peak week to begin with).

Amenorrhea: Introduction

In an ideal world, the Category 1 dieter targeting the lower extremes of BF% would reach her goal without developing full-blown Functional Hypothalamic Amenorrhea (FHA). It is not unheard of and women are sometimes seen who reach 10-12% body fat who are still menstruating although they assuredly have one of the subclinical menstrual cycle disorders. Whether this is due to not chronically undereating/crossing the critical EA threshold, having less psychogenic stress or being more robust is unknown. Some women who avoid amenorrhea have a reproductive age over 14 but this is not universal. Regardless of the exceptions, the reality for most women is that it is less an issue of if amenorrhea will develop than when it will. Given that reality, I want to briefly re-examine the physiological effects that occur in amenorrhea before looking at how this practically impacts upon the set up of the diet or training program. Note that since amenorrhea generally developed at the ends of an extreme diet, many of the effects are a consequence of dieting in general and male dieters experience at least some of the same issues.

Hormonally, a number of changes occur including a drop in estrogen to ~33% of normal levels with progesterone dropping further and the normal cyclical changes of both also disappearing. The loss of estrogen signaling means that its appetite suppressing, anti-inflammatory and muscular remodeling effects are lost. There can also be negative cognitive changes. While the drop in estrogen should reduce insulin sensitivity, the opposite is true and insulin sensitivity improves. This causes a decrease in fatty acid mobilization from fat cells and a women's normally increased use of fat for fuel during aerobic exercise is lost (I mentioned in Chapter 12 that this can be reversed with a topical estrogen patch). This decrease in the use of fat for fuel may increase the use of protein for energy which can lead to muscle loss if the diet is not adjusted. As estrogen is part of what maintains breast tissue, an often underappreciated consequence of extreme dieting is that the breasts may shrink (some women report that they essentially collapse, often never returning to their previous size or shape).

While the loss of progesterone has some benefits (such as the loss of its direct fat storing effects), there will also be a loss of the normal small increase in metabolic rate in the second half of the cycle. Along with the changes in reproductive hormones, there will other changes such as decreased thyroid (T3), leptin, IGF-1 and other hormones with an increase in cortisol (a stress hormone). Resting metabolic rate may be decreased by up to 20% and this comes along with impaired immune system function, decreased recovery during exercise and adaptation to training, decreased muscular strength and increased injury risk.

I also mentioned that women's sleep patterns may be impaired and normal melatonin rhythms can be shifted to a place where they are high in the morning (causing fatigue) and low at night (making sleep difficult). Perhaps the largest negative consequence, and the one that is effectively "invisible" is the potential for the loss of bone mineral density (BMD). While this does occur slowly, the fact is that the longer amenorrhea is maintained, the worse the effects that are seen. Not only can this further increase injury risk (i.e. stress fractures), the bone loss is potentially permanent.

There are potentially a few small benefits to amenorrhea. One is that that any mood changes during the late luteal phase due to PMS/PMDD will typically be lost which, along with the loss of menstruation, which many women see as a positive. While mood and training performance are typically both negatively impaired during amenorrhea, they will at least be unchanging (many women find that their exercise performance can swing wildly throughout the month as I will discuss in detail in Volume 2). The loss of weekly water weight shifts will make tracking the diet marginally easier (though stress/cortisol related water retention can still cause problems). Weight class athletes also do not have to worry about a competition falling during a week when they might be retaining water. Please do not misread this as these small benefits ultimately pale to the enormous number of negatives that are occurring.

Amenorrhea in Women Not Actively Dieting

While FHA is often a consequence that must be accepted when dieting to the extremes, I want to briefly address a sub-population of women who may be experiencing amenorrhea who are not exercising or dieting to the extremes. Let me reiterate that there can can be many other causes of amenorrhea, including birth control along with endless medical reasons, and here I am assuming that these have been eliminated as possibilities and true FHA is present for one reason or another. Here I cannot overemphasize the need for a woman to do everything in her power to resume normal menstrual cycle functioning as rapidly as possible. Whether the amenorrhea is seen as a benefit or not, the long-term and potentially permanent damage to bone density that are occurring will have enormous consequences later in life.

This requires determining the actual cause of the FHA and there are several possible reasons why a woman who is not actively dieting might be amenorrheic. I already described a sub-population of women who, due to psychological stress (perfectionism, a need for external validation and others) can develop FHA in the absence of excessive exercise, a low EA or even fat loss. This is often accompanied by slight dietary changes such as a reduce calorie intake and very low fat intake (which is often reversed by therapy), psychological stress seems to be the primary cause and treatment should center around that. In least some cases, women with FHA who are not actively dieting will be exercising and often multiple hours per day in the gym are being done. This may be accompanied by a desire to maintain an unrealistic BF% in the long term and, at least in some women, this may be contributing to the problem. Even in the absence of fat loss, a woman may be near or below the critical EA threshold and training/diet should be examined.

Regardless of the cause, the goal of the non-dieting woman with amenorrhea should be to regain normal menstrual cycle function as soon as possible. Rather than address those issues here, I will refer women to the next chapter on ending the Category 1 diet as the recommendations are identical.

Amenorrhea in Category 1 Dieters

For those women who must accept amenorrhea as a possible consequence of the dieting and exercise required to reach their competition goals, I want to now discuss some changes to training, diet and supplements that should be considered or implemented once amenorrhea has developed.

Training Adjustments

There are two related issues that need to be taken into account in terms of how training may be adjusted when amenorrhea occurs. The first is the direct negative impact of amenorrhea itself on training as this will impair recovery both during and between workouts. The second is the general fatigue that occurs with the extended and intensive dieting and training that is required for women to reach the lower limits of female BF% to begin with. Addressing these would, in the most general sense, mean reducing the total amount of training that is being done, either within a given workout or in total during the week. However, given the requirements of dieting to the extremes, especially when there is a time frame, this is not always possible. Rather, it is more common for the amount of (primarily aerobic) exercise being done to increase to offset metabolic adaptations and maintain fat loss at the required rate. This will be most true for smaller females. What can be changed is the relative proportion of high- and low-intensity training.

This is probably impossible for most performance athletes as their training schedules tend to be fairly set but the physique competitor has much more flexibility in the types and amounts of training being done. As dieters following this book's recommendations should not be performing excessive amounts of HIIT or high-intensity aerobic activity, I am mainly focusing on weight training and the option of reducing the total amount of weight training being done (this is sometimes possible for strength/power athletes such as powerlifters or Olympic lifters as well). In my experience, when fatigue starts to accumulate,the ability to perform a large number of sets suffers more than strength per se (at the end of an extreme diet, strength is almost always lost). Training volume tends to contribute more to fatigue over time than intensity and, as I discussed in Chapter 28, reducing the total number of sets being done per workout, per exercise or per muscle group is often very beneficial to avoid complete burnout. Even in the face of extreme fatigue, most lifters can perform 2-4 heavy sets at or at least near their previous weights while 6-8 heavy sets would not be realistic without reducing the weight. Given the choice, fewer heavier sets will be superior.

At the extremes, dieters might reduce their resistance training to the level of maintenance training I have discussed previously. While lessening the potential to overtrain or burn out, this has the drawback that it will also reduce calorie expenditure although the difference may not be large. Dieters can compensate for this in one of two ways. The first is to replace eliminated heavy sets with lighter, depletion work. Six to eight heavy sets might realistically become 3 heavy sets followed by 3-4 sets of depletion work with a moderate weight. In some ways this might even be superior in that it both reduces the total amount of heavy work along with depleting muscle glycogen. Alternately, or in addition to that adjustment, additional low-intensity aerobic activity could be done afterwards to increase calorie expenditure.

As I discussed in Chapter 28, there are ways to implement the above concepts. The first is to proactively begin to reduce training slightly in the final phase of dieting (even if amenorrhea has not yet developed). The full reduction does not have to occur immediately but a dieter might drop 2 heavy sets per exercise or muscle group at the beginning of this phase to take into account the reduction in recovery. That might be replaced with 1 set of depletion work. Halfway through the phase, 2 more sets might be dropped as needed, also to be replaced with some higher repetition work. Athletes with concerns about reducing their volume may prefer to implement the above as needed rather than automatically. If a feeling of chronic exhaustion is starting to set in, the workout might be reduced in terms of the total number of heavy sets, for example. This can also be done during the workout where, if an athlete felt that they were excessively fatigued after 5 of 8 planned sets, they could just eliminate the last 3 sets for that day, either replacing them with depletion work, a few minutes of aerobic activity or ignoring them completely. On a day when they felt stronger, the full workout might be completed. This type of approach, referred to as autoregulation is far superior in the long run to trying to complete a workout in the face of exhaustion.

Finally is the issue of women's stubborn lower body fat where the combination of dieting in general and amenorrhea can make its loss very difficult. Some of this is moderated by the changes in the diet that I will describe below but the Stubborn Fat Protocols discussed in Appendix 1 can become more relevant here. I also feel that, limited research to the contrary, fasted cardio will be superior.

Diet Adjustments

The changes in a woman's physiology when she develops amenorrhea have implications for the way that her diet can or should change as she continues to lose fat. A large part of the changes here is primarily due to the decrease in energy expenditure that is occurring as she reaches the lower limits of female BF%. Recall that this is both due to her being lighter along with the adaptive component and this can become quite significant at the extremes. There are also the changes in how her body is using nutrients for fuel. Increasing insulin sensitivity means that more carbohydrates are being used and this comes along with more difficult fat mobilization and lower blood fatty acids. This adds up to more carbs and less fat being burned during the diet. There is also the increased use of protein for energy, which can put her at risk for muscle mass loss (remember that women are relatively more protected from this than men to begin with).

For the calculations below, I will continue to use the sample dieter who started at 150 lbs and 22% body fat with 117 lbs of LBM and assume that she is at 137 lbs and 14% body fat when amenorrhea develops. Realistically her calorie intake is likely to be in the 1400-1600 calorie range (or possibly lower) and I will assume she is eating 1500 calories for the sake of the calculations.

Adjusting Calorie Intake

Due to the drop in energy expenditure that is occurring, the Category 1 dieter's calorie levels must be adjusted to maintain the goal weekly fat loss. If it has not occurred already, the weekly weight loss goal should be reduced to a maximum of 0.5% per week. So long as the recommendations in this book have been followed, it's most likely that the diet would have been adjusted to this level before amenorrhea has developed in the first place. To maintain the same level of fat loss, the same weekly or bi-weekly adjustments in either calorie intake or activity (via LISS) that were discussed in Chapter 27 will need to be be made. Given the changes in RMR that occur with amenorrhea, it's conceivable that larger changes will need to be made at this point but, as always, actual weekly fat loss should be the determinant.

Adjusting Protein Intake

Although women are relatively more protected against the loss of LBM than men (at least partially due to carrying more body fat to begin with), the risk of LBM loss does increase as women reach the lower limits of BF%. Much of this is just related to carrying less body fat while the changes occurring in amenorrhea (i.e. the loss of estrogen signaling) contribute further. In addition to maintaining the intensity of weight training the second key to preventing LBM loss is potentially increasing protein intake from what may seem like already high levels. The maximum intake levels I gave in Chapter 19 are appropriate here and I've repeated them in the chart below for both endurance athletes along with those who perform weight training of any sort. The inactive column of the chart has been removed since no inactive individual should be trying to reach the lowest levels of BF% in the first place.

	Endurance	Weight Training
Normal Dieting	1.0 g/lb LBM (2.2 g/kg LBM)	1.1-1.2 g/lb LBM (2.4-2.6 g/kg LBM)
Maximum	1.2 g/lb LBM (2.65 g/kg LBM)	1.4-1.5 g/lb LBM (3.1-3.3 g/kg LBM)

While the highest levels recommended for weight training athletes may seem excessive several recent studies on physique competitors that I will discuss in Chapter 34 found that women were able to reach the lower limits of female BF% with essentially zero LBM loss while consuming this amount of protein (note that most were case studies with no control group). The sample dieting female at 117 lbs of LBM will consume the maximum intake of 1.5 g/lb LBM and her total grams and calories from protein appear below.

117 lbs LBM * 1.5 g/lb LBM protein = 175 grams protein per day
175 grams protein * 4 cal/g = 700 calories from protein

Her original diet contained 140 grams (560 calories) of protein per day so this represents an increase of 35 grams (140 calories) per day or roughly 9 extra grams per meal across 4 daily meals. The same recommendations in terms of protein sources, distribution, etc. will all still hold here. Twenty to thirty grams of protein should be consumed after (and possibly before) weight training workouts and an additional 20-30 grams at bedtime will help to stave off late-night hunger and muscle breakdown.

Adjusting Fat and Carbohydrate Intake: Introduction

Once calorie and protein intake has been set, the rest of the Category 1 diet will be made up of dietary fat and carbohydrate. While I discussed them separately in Chapter 19 during the initial diet set-up, I will address them together here since changes in one automatically mean that changes must occur in the other. Within any fixed calorie and protein intake, a decrease in fat intake will allow for an increase in carbohydrate intake and vice versa. I bring this up as there are two opposite approaches that may be potentially valid once the Category 1 female has developed amenorrhea. The first I will address is probably the more common approach and entails reducing dietary fat while increasing carbohydrates. While less common, the second entails reducing carbohydrates to low levels and increasing dietary fat and there are some potential benefits worth considering to this approach.

Option 1: Reduce Fat and Increase Carbohydrate

When I initially set up the diet, I set 25% dietary fat as a recommendation/requirement for the normally cycling woman as this keeps estrogen higher and should help to delay the onset of amenorrhea. Once amenorrhea has developed, estrogen has dropped and there is no menstrual cycle to protect, this is no longer important. Thus dietary fat can be reduced, an approach with both pros and cons. Perhaps the biggest benefit of reducing dietary fat is that it leaves slightly more room for carbohydrates. This will help to maintaining training intensity although the three maintenance days per week make this relatively less important. The cons to this approach is that very low fat intakes can limit food flexibility (i.e. some foods will be simply off limits) and may leave dieters chronically hungry. If this approach is used, dietary fat can be reduced from the minimum requirement of 25% to the minimum intake of 0.25 g/lb.

137 lbs * 0.25 g/lb = 35 grams fat
35 grams fat * 9 cal/g = 315 calories from fat

As the original diet contains 56 and 78 grams of fat during the follicular and luteal phases respectively, this represents a decrease of 21 (~200 calories) and 43 (~400 calories) grams of fat respectively which a considerable savings. As before, the total fat intake of 35 grams of fat should be divided relatively evenly across the day's meals although saving a bit more for evening may help to stave off hunger. The only requirement here is that the essential fatty acids (EFA's) be consumed. The rest of the day's fats can come from any source although there may not be room for much additional fat given that even the lowest fat foods may contain 1-2 grams already. With the reduction in dietary fat will come an increase in total carbohydrate intake and this is once again determined by the difference between the dieter's calorie intake and the calories from protein and fat. If she is consuming 1500 calories per day with protein providing 700 and dietary fat 315 calories per day, her carb intake is calculated as below.

Protein + Fat Calories = 700 + 315 = 1015 calories
1500 calories - 1015 calories = 485 calories from carbs
485 calories / 4 cal/gram = 121 grams carbohydrate per day

At her current bodyweight of 137 lbs, this is slightly below 1 g/lb (2.2 g/kg) but this is the consequence of her increased protein intake, being lighter and dieting to this level of extremes. While low in terms of her training, this is offset by the three maintenance days. So far as carbohydrate sources, the reality is that a majority of the daily carbohydrates are likely to coming from fibrous carbohydrates and vegetables and they may not be much room for starches as they often provide too many calories in fairly low volume of food. Including even a small amount of fruit would be valuable here as this can help to keep blood sugar more stable with starches being saved for the maintenance days to refill muscle glycogen.

The adjusted daily diet appears below:

Calories	1500 calories
Protein	175 g/day
Carbohydrate	121 g/day
Fat	35 g/day

These levels will have to be further adjusted as the diet continues and energy expenditure drops further. Since protein has to stay at fixed levels and she is already at the lower limits of fat intake, only carbohydrates can be further reduced, often below 100 grams, technically qualifying as a ketogenic diet (most studies use 50 g/day). While this is potentially problematic for reasons I have discussed, the three days at maintenance will offset this. I'll show how the maintenance days will be calculated below.

Option 2: Reduce Carbohydrate and Increase Fat Intake
In contrast to the above is the opposite approach of reducing carbohydrate intake to low levels and increasing dietary fat which also has its benefits and drawbacks. Probably the biggest potential benefit is that higher dietary fat intakes tend to keep at least some people fuller by slowing digestion (at the same time, less food is being eaten since fat is so calorically dense). At the end of an extreme diet when hunger can be uncontrollable, this can be significant and every little bit will help. Another potential benefit is that the reduced carbohydrate intake coupled with intense training will reduce muscle glycogen, enhancing fat burning in the body. A final potential benefit is that low-carbohydrate diets have a natural effect in inhibiting the alpha-2 receptors that make women's lower body fat more difficult to mobilize (1).

So far as negatives, I already mentioned one is that the high calorie density of fats can mean that there is less total food volume to eat per day. Food volume per se is a signal for fullness due to the stretching of the stomach and this is a trade-off against slower digestion rates (a high fibrous vegetable intake will also help to offset this with protein, fat and fiber giving the slowest digestion times of all). There are also the other drawbacks of very-low carbohydrate diets including mental fog, low energy, etc. This can potentially harm training ability, not only due to the general fatigue but reduced muscle glycogen. The latter is still much less of a problem if the 3 recommended days at maintenance are being incorporated in the diet. Sodium, potassium, and magnesium losses also increase which means more needs to be consumed. Ensuring sufficient amounts of each also helps to offset many of the fatigue issues.

If this approach is taken, carbohydrates would typically be reduced to 50 grams of even less. Technically anything under 100 grams per day is a ketogenic diet but as carbohydrates are already fairly low at this point, it will take a larger scale reduction to be particularly meaningful. There is no real benefit to going below 50 g/day and, assuming this intake, carbohydrates will make up 200 calories and dietary fat will be calculated as the remainder of the calories.

$$\text{Protein + Fat Calories} = 700 + 200 = 900 \text{ calories}$$
$$1500 \text{ calories} - 900 \text{ calories} = 600 \text{ calories from carbs}$$
$$600 \text{ calories} / 9 \text{ cal/g} = 67 \text{ grams fat per day}$$

While higher than the 35 grams of Option 1, the 67 grams of fat per day is still not enormous, falling between the original follicular and luteal phase intakes. This would allow just over 14 grams of fat per meal which can go a long ways towards increasing fullness and controlling appetite. Once again, some of that must come from the EFA's with the rest coming from other sources. As mentioned above, at 50 grams per day, most starchy carbohydrates will have to be eliminated but vegetables and perhaps a small amount of carbs before training can usually be worked in. In this approach is used, the daily diet will be:

Calories	1500 calories
Protein	175 g/day
Carbohydrate	50 g/day
Fat	67 g/day

Once again, these intake will eventually need to be adjusted and here, the adjustment will have to come from a reduction in dietary fat or an increase in aerobic activity.

Calculating Maintenance Days

Although it may occur earlier in the Category 1 diet (technically by the third phase from 14-10% body fat), by the time a dieter has become amenorrheic there should be three full maintenance days per week. As discussed in Chapter 23, this means that there will only be 4 diet days and that there should never be more than 2-3 days of active dieting before a maintenance days. On the maintenance days, both calories and carbohydrates will be raised and I want to show how to calculate how much they should increase. To do this, the weekly deficit should first be determined based on the weekly goal weight loss (which should be 0.5%) which is multiplied by 3,500 calories/pound and then divided by the number of diet days (which should be 4). I've shown this below for the sample dieter at 137 lbs.

$$137 \text{ lbs} * 0.005 = 0.68 \text{ lb/week target weight loss}$$
$$0.68 \text{ lb/week} * 3500 \text{ calories} = 2400 \text{ weekly calorie deficit}$$
$$2400 \text{ calories} / 4 \text{ diet days} = 600 \text{ calorie/day deficit on diet days}$$

Since 600 calories is her daily deficit on the diet days, she will need to add this back to her diet to reach maintenance. Ideally most if not all of this should come from carbohydrates which means that 150 grams (600 calories carbs / 4 cal/g = 150 grams) would be added. Assuming this is the case, I've shown her diet based on both Option 1 and Option 2 above.

	Option 1	Option 2
Calories	2100 calories	2100 calories
Protein	175 g/day	175 g/day
Carbohydrate	270 g/day	200 g/day
Fat	35 g/day	67 g/day

For option 1, dietary fat could be increased slightly by 10-20 grams (90-180 calories), requiring a 22-44 grams reduction in carbohydrate intake. This allows more food flexibility and may help to control hunger more effectively. For option 2, dietary fat could be reduced slightly, to perhaps 50 grams per day allowing 38 more grams of carbs to be eaten to help support training and I've shown these adjusted levels in the chart below.

	Option 1	Option 2
Calories	2100 calories	2100 calories
Protein	175 g/day	175 g/day
Carbohydrate	225 g/day	238 g/day
Fat	55 g/day	50 g/day

Which makes them effectively identical. In both cases, the majority of carbs should come from starchy sources although some simpler carbs may be included, allowing a treat to be included as desired.

Supplement Adjustments

The final adjustment that can occur when amenorrhea occurs will be to any dietary supplements that are being used. The general use supplements should always be taken, and will likely be even more important at this time as the lowered food intake will make it nearly impossible to obtain sufficient micronutrients no matter what food choices are made. As the luteal phase and any issues related to it or PMS has been lost, those supplements will no longer be needed . However, many of the same neurochemical changes in serotonin and dopamine occur with amenorrhea and both 5-HTP and vitex cagnus may benefit both mood and hunger and can be tested. Neither aspirin or sodium/potassium manipulation will be required due to the loss of the cycle.

Considering how common it is for sleep to become impaired at the end of a diet, the various sleep supplements are of potentially more importance at this time. The general sleep supplements and especially melatonin are all considerations. The latter is particularly important given the phase-shift in melatonin rhythms that can occur that I described in Chapter 12 where melatonin stays elevated in the morning while rising later at night. As I mentioned there, taking low dose (1 mg or less) melatonin 2 hours and again 1 hour prior to sleep can help to reset this. While not a supplement per se, this can be combined with the use of a light box providing 10,000 lux used for 30-60 minute upon awakening to reduce melatonin levels and improve mood and energy.

Given the lack of estrogen signaling, and the loss of its benefits, a final supplement worth considering would be soy protein or isolated phytoestrogens. While unnecessary for the normally cycling woman, here they will provide at least some estrogenic signaling. While this is unlikely to impact bone density, it may control hunger, maintain fat oxidation or protect the loss of breast tissue. A single serving of soy protein (20-25 grams) per day or 50-100 mg of isolated phytoestrogens would be an appropriate dose.

If they are not already being used, thermogenic compounds could be added. While their effect is small, even a 5% increase in energy expenditure might increase fat loss by 0.55-0.75 lbs/month. While small in an absolute sense this is significant for a small female dieter. The appetite blunting effect is an added benefit and taken before training, ephedrine/caffeine can improve training intensity. Let me note again that ephedrine is banned in many federations and cayenne, green tea or nicotine may be better choices if this is the case. Women struggling with lower body fat loss may also wish to consider yohimbine. I detailed it's use in Chapter 24 and will discuss it again within the context of the stubborn fat protocols in Appendix 1. Yohimbine is banned in many federations (or countries) and can cause anxiety.

Amenorrhea Hormonal Template

To summarize the information above, I've presented the same type of hormonal template that I provided for the other hormonal situations in Chapter 30. As before, I've left out the general use supplements and have only included any potential additions that might be made. Since I provided a training template above from 14-10% body fat, I will only list general training changes that might be made.

Day	1 2 3 4 5 6 7 8 9 10 11 12 13 14 15 16 17 18 19 20 21 22 23 24 25 26 27 28
Phase	None
Hormonal State	Low Estrogen, Low Progesterone
Diet	Increase protein, decrease fat (optional), carbohydrates are the difference
Supplements	5-HTP/Vitex, Melatonin, Soy Protein (20-25 g/day) OR Phytoestrogens (50-100 mg/day) Thermogenics, Yohimbine
Training	Reduced if possible, reduced high-intensity recommended Increased injury risk with high-skill/impact activities

While the above addresses the changes in amenorrhea, I want to reiterate that the long-term damaging effects mean that it must be reversed as rapidly as possibly when the diet is over.

Chapter 33: Ending the Category 1 Diet

The final issue I want to address in this book is how the woman dieting to anywhere from 16-18% to 10-12% body fat should end her diet. In the majority of cases, this will primarily involve physique and endurance athletes (some other performance sports may also require a very low BF%) with the major difference being when the diet is considered over and recovery should begin. In some cases, the dieter may only diet down for a single day or competition, in others they may need to remain lean for an extended competition period. This difference only impacts on when recovery should begin but has no effect on what should be done at that point. In this chapter I will examine a number of topics including what defines the end of the Category 1 diet, what should be done at that point and how to avoid an overshoot of body fat. First, let me re-examine the topic of realistically sustainable or optimal BF%.

Sustainable and Optimal BF% Levels

Once women have reached the lowest extremes of BF%, it is not uncommon for them to express the desire to remain at that level of leanness year-round or effectively forever. Ignoring the fact that this is both unrealistic and generally unsustainable, it is also potentially physically damaging in the long-term. Even if a woman at 12-13% is not amenorrheic, she is likely to have some form of menstrual cycle or other hormonal dysfunction. While not universal, this can cause bone density loss over time along with other hormonal or metabolic impairments. Performance athletes often find it difficult to improve any aspect of their fitness and performance and physique or strength/power athletes frequently find out the hard way that it is impossible to gain significant amounts of strength or muscle mass. The hormonal changes along with the amount of calorie restriction and training required to remain that lean make it nearly impossible, endurance athletes possibly excepted, to make progress. The condition of extreme or peak leanness is a temporary one and that normal physiological, hormonal and menstrual cycle function will not resume until both EA and BF% are at sufficient or optimal levels. But what BF% is optimal or sustainable?

Clearly some women are able to maintain a very low BF% for extended periods although there are frequently negative effects on health and physiology. It might be sustainable (in a sense) but is neither healthy nor optimal. For that reason, I will define a sustainable BF% as the lowest level that can be maintained for extended periods while allowing a woman's physiology to be mostly normal. Her hormones should be in a generally normal range (although they may still be slightly below pre-diet levels) and, unless she has a hormonal modifier that eliminates it, should have a menstrual cycle (luteal phase defect or anovulation may be present). Her EA should be well above the critical threshold of 13.6 cal/lb LBM (30 cal/kg LBM) although it may not reach the 20.5 cal/lb LBM (45 cal/kg LBM) EA that is considered sufficient. Her nutrient intake in terms of protein, carbohydrate and fats should also be in a proper range.

For most women, a BF% of roughly 18% (~21% by DEXA) will probably be in a roughly correct range to achieve this. There may be some variability here given the differences in women in terms of their robustness or reproductive age. Some may be able to sustain slightly lower levels (i.e. 16% and occasionally lower) while others need to be at 20% or higher to reach the above goals. While this may seem or feel "fat" for a woman who achieved 10%, it is extremely lean by most standards. If sufficient muscle mass is present most women will show good definition in their upper bodies, potentially the slightest hint of their abdominals and their hips and thighs will be lean although not excessively so.

Moving from sustainable BF% levels, I want to look at what might an optimal BF% might be. In the broadest sense, it would represent a situation where a woman's overall physiology is completely normal. Metabolic rate, hormone levels and, assuming no hormonal modifier, menstrual cycle function should be normal with no subclinical disorder present. A sufficient calorie intake, providing an optimal EA should be present along with optimal nutrient intake for all aspects of health. In a more specific sense, an optimal BF% for athletes would be one that allows for maximal gains in fitness or performance without being so high as to make reaching the competition goal excessively difficult when dieting is required again.

The specific BF% that the above will occur at is poorly researched and is likely to be sports specific. The nature of endurance training means that relatively lower BF% may be appropriate (as in a case study in Chapter 34) while any athlete seeking maximal gains in strength, power or muscle mass will likely need to be between 22-24% body fat (25-28% via DEXA) for optimal results. While higher than the 18-20% value above, this is still very lean and women with sufficient muscle mass will show some definition. While outside of the scope of this book, this BF%, or even slightly higher, would be near ideal for the woman wishing to both become pregnant and ensure the best outcome for her child.

The End of the Diet: Part 1

Having looked at both sustainable and optimal BF% levels, I want to start looking at when the diet ends and what should happen next. In the most general sense, the diet is over when the fat loss goal has been achieved. For the serious trainee, possibly bikini competitors and even some performance athletes this may be in the range of 16-18% body fat while physique competitors, some endurance and other athletes may drop to 10-12% body fat. Once that goal has been met, one of two situations will exist.

The first situation is that the fat loss goal will have been a purely temporary one. While unlikely to be in Category 1 or to be dieting to the extremes, this is common among the general dieter who may only be dieting for a wedding, anniversary or reunion. Traditionally, physique competitors have rarely done more than one show in a year and in this case, recovery should begin immediate after the competition has ended. At least some weight class athletes enter competitions rarely, only dieting down temporarily (and often manipulating water) before needing to enter recovery to begin their next training cycle.

The second situation is on where the new BF% level will need to be maintained for some extended period of time. For the serious trainee or general dieter who is only targeting a sustainable BF% level (i.e.18%), this would likely be for preference/appearance reasons and the goal will be to maintain the new BF% in the long-term. The modern physique athlete may also enter two (or occasionally more) competitions within a relatively short time span. In some cases, the first competition is being used to test peak-week strategies for the second or may be a qualifying event for a larger competition. In others it is simply a practical issue. Given the time (6 months) and effort required to diet down in the first place, it's logical to enter more than one contest before returning to a higher BF%. How this is ideally approached depends on many factors and the details are beyond the scope of this book.

For the competition athlete, most typically in the endurance sports, but occasionally in others such as sprinting, it is more common to diet down and maintain a very low BF% for the entire competition season, generally lasting 3-4 months. This can be somewhat problematic at the low extremes of BF% but performance athletes are generally doing such a large amount of training that a much larger food intake is possible. And while it is absolutely not healthy for an athlete to maintain this level of leanness for extended time periods, it is a necessary part of competitive sport.

Maintaining Current Body Fat Levels

Once the goal has moved from active fat loss to maintenance of the new BF% (for whatever reason), the dieter will need to adjust training and/or diet to bring themselves back into energy balance, with calorie intake equalling energy expenditure. If this is achieved, no change in BF% up or down should occur which is the definition of maintenance. The first step is to determine how many calories below maintenance the dieter current is. To do this, the dieter should first determine how large their current weekly deficit was before the end of the diet. This is done by multiplying the final week's fat loss by 3,500 calories and dividing by 7 to determine the daily calorie deficit. I've shown a sample calculation below for a dieter who has been losing 0.5 lbs in the last week of their diet prior to moving to maintenance.

0.5 lbs/week * 3500 calories = 1750 weekly calorie deficit
1750 calories/week / 7 days/week = 250 daily calorie deficit

In this case, achieving energy balance to stabilize BF% means either increasing calorie intake or decreasing exercise energy expenditure by 250 cal/day from their current levels. Whether this is best done by adjusting training or increasing calories depends on the situation. For the dieter who is on low calories and who is performing relatively less activity, it would probably be best to increase total calorie intake with a majority of those calories coming from carbohydrates (if dietary fat is extremely low it can be raised slightly as well). A 250 calorie increase would represent roughly 62 grams of carbohydrates per day.

In contrast, if activity levels were extremely high with a relatively higher calorie intake, reducing activity would be better. For a smaller female, 250 calories of low intensity aerobic activity represents about 45 minutes and this would represent a significant decrease in her activity levels. The performance athlete may not have this option unless they had added extra low-intensity work while dieting and here calories should be increased. I'd note that the calculated value may be slightly too low and dieters often show a gradual continued fat loss even after the adjustments have been made. This is due to the shift from dieting to relative maintenance reversing at least slightly some of the negative adaptations to dieting. The above should only be considered a starting point and dieters should re-adjust their diet or training based on real-world changes in BF% (which should be stable and relatively unchanging).

While women who finish their diet at 16-18% may be able to maintain level that in the long-term, any female dieter who's goal required that they attain/maintain a lower BF% than that will eventually move out of maintenance and truly end the diet, moving into recovery. At this point, they should treat themselves identically to the woman who's fat loss goals were only temporary in terms of what should be done.

The End of the Diet: Part 2

Whether the dietary goals were purely temporary or had to be maintained for some period of time, eventually the need to maintain that low BF% will be over and this will mark the true end of the extreme Category 1 diet. At this point there are two related goals. For the normally cycling woman or PCOS/hyperandrogenic women with oligomenorrhea, restoring their normal menstrual cycle function is of crucial importance. Even if she is not amenorrheic, it is almost assured that some degree of subclinical menstrual cycle dysfunction will be present (and recall from Chapter 12 that each step from normally cycling to amenorrheic is progressively worse both hormonally and physiologically).

For all women, restoring normal hormonal, metabolic and physiological function is equally important. Both are achieved through the same essential approach which is to raise EA (by adjusting training, diet or both) while regaining body weight and body fat (this will primarily occur as a consequence of adjusting diet and training). This will be true whether she intend to stabilize at 16-18% body fat for extended periods or increase to 20-24% body fat to optimize the ability to gain strength, muscle mass or improve performance during the off-season (again, endurance athletes may stay leaner than this).

Increasing EA

While there is far more to full recovery, the first step in restoring normal menstrual cycle dysfunction is to increase EA at least to and ideally above the critical threshold of 13.6 kcal/lb LBM (30 kcal/kg LBM) while making other changes to the diet described below. I have shown a sample calculation for a dieter with 120 lbs of LBM below.

Critical EA = 120 lbs LBM * 13.6 cal/lb LBM = 1632 calories/day

Recall from Chapter 12 that EA represents the number of calories available to the body after the energy expenditure from exercise has been accounted for. This means that the actual calorie intake will need to be adjusted from the above value depending on how much exercise is being done. In the chart below, I've shown the critical EA threshold for a female with 120 lbs of LBM along with the amount she would have to eat based on zero, 200, 400 or 600 calories per day of exercise below.

Critical EA	Exercise Expenditure	Total Calorie Intake
1632 calories/day	Zero calories	1632 calories/day
1632 calories/day	200 calories	1832 calories/day
1632 calories/day	400 calories	2032 calories/day
1632 calories/day	600 calories	2232 calories/day

Let me emphasize that the above should be considered the minimal EA rather than a specific target. EA can most certainly be higher but must not be lower at the end of a diet as no recovery will occur until the critical level is reached or exceeded and I will address the implications of this later in the chapter. Since EA represents the difference in total calorie intake and the calories burned during exercise, increasing EA above the critical threshold or higher can be accomplished by increasing calorie intake, decreasing activity levels or doing both at the same time. As usual, which is more appropriate depends on the specifics of the situation. The dieter who used a fairly moderate amount of activity with diet to reach 16-18% body fat will be better off increasing calorie intake since there is not much exercise to reduce. In contrast, the extreme dieter who increased activity significantly while reducing food intake may increase food intake while decreasing activity simultaneously. Since any change to the diet will depend on how much activity is altered, let me look at that first.

Adjusting Training: Part 1

Given the requirements of reaching the lower limits of BF% in general, it will be typical for most dieters to be doing a fairly large amount of exercise although the exact amount and type will depend on which group is being discussed. The physique athlete will generally be doing a combination of weight training, aerobic and/or HIIT training and there may be other components to the training such as posing being done. While physique competitors should attempt to do as little aerobic/HIIT work as is required to reach their goals, the reality is that smaller females will invariably be doing a fair amount to avoid reducing their calorie intake excessively (this may be offset if a large amount of weight training is maintained).

Other athletes will be doing various amounts of training based on the specific of their sport although most at the lower limits of BF% will typically be doing a fairly large total amount. Almost without exception, endurance athletes generally train the most, often 5-6 days per week with some days including two workouts (or one very long workout). This may be reduced during the competition season as the focus shifts towards intensity and peaking but the total amount is still generally high. Week may vary in terms of the amount done with significant reductions during weeks with important races but volume is almost always high. In many cases, extra low-intensity work may have been added to increase calorie expenditure.

With few exceptions, by the end of the diet/competition season, athletes tend to be both physically and psychologically exhausted. The physique athlete has spent months dieting down with strict calorie restriction along with large amounts of weight training and potentially aerobic work while the performance athlete may have been working relatively intensely for the better part of a year (their diet only makes up a small portion of that). Given this fact, with no exception I can think of, reducing or even eliminating much of the training that was being done should occur for at least some amount of time. Performance athletes do this as a matter of course, taking one or two weeks completely away from their sport once their final competition has ended (perhaps the only exception to this is the often exercise addicted endurance athlete). At most 3-4 very easy workouts might be done and it is not until the third or fourth week that any real training is reintroduced as the athlete begins their preparation for the next competition season.

While performance athletes have trained in the above fashion for decades, taking time off after their season is over, physique athletes are almost universally resistant to doing the same. Their lives (and some might say identity) tends to revolve around the gym and training and the idea of taking any time off, even after an exhausting 6+ month contest prep, is often psychologically distressing. To be sure, the amount of training that the typical physique dieter is doing during their diet is often much less than that of the performance athlete but it also tends to be of a higher intensity due to the focus on weight training. This reduced amount doesn't change the overall stress of severe calorie restriction, heavy training along with the psychogenic stress that is often present. Both the body and mind need a break after an extended and extreme diet but even the idea of performing several weeks of light training is met with resistance as athletes want to return to full intensity training immediately.

There is no doubt that successful athletes (and likely people who are successful in any field) usually have a single-minded focus about their sport and this is not a bad thing. However, it can become pathological, often leading athletes to engage in unhealthy and/or damaging behaviors. Athletes will continue to train through injury, sickness, extreme fatigue, etc. driving themselves into the depths of overtraining or, at the extreme, the adaptive hypocortisolism I discussed in Chapter 13. At the extremes, this represents exercise dependence which frequently borders on addiction. Perhaps surprisingly, there is no gender difference with exercise dependence being found in roughly 30-40% of athletes of both genders (1,2). For the exercise dependent athlete, the suggestion to reduce activity levels is likely to be met with resistance. Somewhat unsurprisingly, orthorexic attitudes and exercise addiction seem to be linked (2a).

In the performance athlete, the fear of losing fitness is always prevalent even if it is generally accepted that losing a small amount of fitness in the "off-season" will give them more potential to make progress in the long-term. For the physique athlete, the fear is of losing their hard-earned muscle mass or their perfect on-stage appearance tend to be the major factors at play. I will come back to the psychological need to stay extremely lean below but want to point out that the fear of muscle loss over short periods of not training is extremely overblown. Muscle is slowly gained but equally slowly lost and insignificant changes occur over a short time period with younger, but not older (65-75 years old) women losing less muscle and strength than men when they stop training (3,4). Taking a few days off from training has no impact.

I would note that while many, if not most, athlete are resistant to taking time off after their diet is over, some athletes go to the other extreme. Burnt out from months of dieting, and frequently poor dieting practices, they stop training for weeks of months while eating enormous amounts of food. They regain fat at an accelerated rate which causes negative physiological and psychological effects and women in the physique community often report a total loss of food control with extended periods of massive food intakes. In one study, female bodybuilders went from a calorie intake of 1500-1800 per day prior to their competition to over 3000 calories in the days immediately after the show, gaining 8.8 lbs (4kg), some of which was glycogen and water, within 3 weeks (5). Occasionally there are reports of women being unable to lose the fat gained again and this is attributed to "permanent metabolic damage" (as discussed in Chapter 9, this is not supported by research). Invariably this type of response following a competition is most prevalent in those women using the problematic dietary approaches I have discussed. They diet rigidly (often on only a handful of foods), combining excessive amounts of aerobic/HIIT work with early extreme calorie restriction and this is usually on a base of psychogenic or life stress. They never raise calories to maintenance or take breaks. Once the diet is over they rebound psychologically and physiologically.

Somewhere between the extremes of maintaining a large amount of training and doing none for extended periods will be the best approach. Small amounts of training help to reduce psychological stress and, for many, it improves food control but too much exercise will slow recovery after the diet. Athletes will often counter-argue that they can maintain their previous training load so long as they raise their calories sufficiently. While there is some truth to this, few are actually willing to raise their calories in this way to begin with and there is more to full recovery than just sufficient calorie intake an an adequate EA and training will have to be reduced to one degree or another. To what extent will depend on the specifics of the situation but I want to at least provide some general guidelines below.

Adjusting Training: Part 2

With very few exceptions, every athlete should take the day after their final competition completely off. Realistically performance athletes will have little to no choice in the matter due to the fatigue from the competition. Even if they could train, they probably won't want to. The physique athlete is likely to be equally fatigued due to their final peak week preparation, morning prejudging and evening posing routines. In an ideal world, perhaps 5-7 days would be taken completely off from training after the final competition and, as noted above, there will be no real loss in fitness, strength or muscle mass during that time period. In reality, I doubt that many athletes will be able to take a full week off from any training without some degree of psychological stress but I'd suggest that 2-3 days completely should be the goal and athletes who take even that amount of time off are invariably surprised by how much better they feel overall compared to before their competition. Brisk walking, light stretching or even a light yoga class could be useful here for further relaxation but nothing more intense should be considered.

For those athletes who simply cannot handle being that inactive for 3-7 days, some type of training that is different than their normal training should be done. For physique athletes this might mean working with kettlebells or doing exercises that are not part of their usual routine for at most 2-3 light sets. The high-intensity performance or mixed sport athlete can do something similar. Endurance athletes are often more limited in their activities but simply performing some activity that they don't typically do can be a good thing psychologically. Basically this can be a week to more or less play and get away from the training that is done for the better part of the rest of the year and this invariably leads to greater enthusiasm when normal training resumes. Depending on how much training was being done prior to the end of the diet, reducing or eliminating training may be sufficient to bring some athletes above the critical EA threshold without needing to adjust their diet (though this may still be required or beneficial).

What will occur after that initial 3-7 day period of relative rest will depend on the sport. The performance athlete often takes a second easy week (or performs some activity if the first week was taken completely off) or may start moving back into light training for their sport. This might mean three easy runs or bike rides for runners and cyclists or some easy drills for sprinters but this is best left to the athlete's coach and training program. I will simply caution here to avoid the urge to resume too much training too quickly when the goal should still be recovery. I would also suggest that endurance athletes initiate both resistance training and jumping during this time if that is not part of their normal training or was not done during the competition period. Most endurance activities have minimal benefit on bone density and the off-season/preparation phase is the only opportunity endurance athletes have to positive impact on this. Even if it will not have a major effect until menstrual cycle function has resumed, by introducing it earlier rather than later, the maximum benefits can be gained once the athlete has achieved physiological normalcy.

For the physique athlete and many strength/power athletes, the majority off training during the year is in the weight room although some prefer to keep in at least some amount of aerobic work in their training. For those physique athletes who want to maintain some some aerobic training during their recovery (and presumably into their next gaining phase), I would recommend a limit of 20-30' of low intensity (RPE 3-4) work a maximum of three times per week. More than this will not only impair overall recovery from the diet but will be detrimental to the goal of increasing muscle mass. Even if HIIT is going to be used in the off-season (I discussed how this might be done in Chapter 28), it should be eliminated for quite some time after the diet is over, probably until full physiologically recovery has occurred.

In terms of resistance training, after the first week of relatively light training/playing in the weight room has been completed, a gradual return towards the athlete's habitual training. In the initial stages, the amount done should always be fairly minimal and I would recommend perhaps three to four total weight workouts per week of no more than 45-60 minutes. A total of 2-4 sets per muscle group with less than maximal weights (an RPE of 6-7/repetitions in reserve of 3-4 or more) would a good place to start in the second and third week following the diet. Over the 4-6 weeks following the competition training volume and frequency can return towards normal levels but athletes should not expect to make any type of gains during this time. Until full recovery occurs, training at a maximal level is pointless.

In that vein I want to address the idea that there is an anabolic rebound that occurs following an extreme diet. Physique athletes often report that they muscles seems to grow rapidly as they come out of their diet and begin training again. This this occurs to some degree, it primarily represents the storage of glycogen and IMTG over the first week but this is not actual muscle gain (and no competitor ends up with more LBM than before their diet) . A recent study actually measured this, examining physique competitors 1 week before, 1 week after and again 4-6 weeks after their contest (6). In the first week, there was an increase in LBM but this represented glycogen and IMTG with essentially 100% fat being regained over the next 4-6 weeks (of some interest, metabolic rate was normalized after 4 weeks). Physiologically, the natural competitor's body is primed for fat storage after a diet and true muscle gain will be impossible until physiological normalcy is achieved. At best a physique competitor may end up with at their pre-diet LBM rapidly but actual gains will not occur until much later.

I would mention that athletes generally find that they have more energy and the ability to train more intensely as their calories go up and they start to recover. This is good in that it indicates that recovery is in fact occurring but bad in that some athletes may increase their training intensity (or volume) excessively. Not only is this unproductive in that few gains can be made but it can also limit recovery, requiring the athlete to raise calories even further to ensure that a sufficiently high EA is achieved to normal functioning

Adjusting the Diet: Introduction

Once the athlete has decided how to adjust their training, they will have a rough idea of how to adjust their diet to achieve and sustain a sufficient EA. Although they overlap, I will divide these into two phases with distinct goals and time frames. The first occurs immediately after the diet is over and revolves around ensuring that EA surpasses the critical threshold to begin the process of menstrual cycle, hormonal and physiological recovery. The second is more prolonged and involves regaining body fat to an optimal level. This might be a sustainable level such as 16-18% or to a higher level to complete recovery and allow the athlete to focus on improving their fitness. Just as with being resistant to adjusting training, it's common for dieters to show resistance to performing either phase at all, or in an optimal way. This is especially true in terms of regaining weight and body fat. I briefly want to look at why this is the case.

Primarily this revolves around appearance issues or, more accurately, the change in appearance that occurs when a very lean dieter is faced with the realities of regaining body fat. The physique sports by their very nature revolve around appearance and developing what is considered physical perfection (as defined by the sport). To either want to be involved in physique sports, or to be successful at it, means being somewhat body obsessed almost by definition as anyone who isn't simply can't reach the highest levels. Even in performance sports, with some exceptions (i.e. some throwing events, super heavy weight Olympic or powerlifters), there is almost always some focus on appearance. A great deal of this is not even sports related, women are and have always been exposed to more social pressure on their appearance. This is compounded in those sports emphasizing thinness for performance reasons, have an aesthetic component or require the female to wear form fitting or revealing clothing. At major events like the Olympics, it's not uncommon for sports commentators to explicitly focus on the female athlete's appearance, something they would never do to a male athlete. All of this adds up to athletes either having or developing a preoccupation with their body and appearance, sometimes even becoming more concerned with how they look than how they perform.

At the extremes this can manifest as body dysmorphia (technically Body Dysmorphic Disorder or BDD) where individuals may see a body in the mirror different from reality and have constant negative thoughts about their perceived physical imperfections. Perhaps surprisingly, women and men show roughly equal levels of BDD although there are gender differences in the parts of the body that each tends to be concerned with (7,8). Women, not surprisingly, are more likely to obsess about their skin, stomach, breasts, lower body and excessive facial hair while men were more concerned with their body build (height and muscularity), hair loss and genitals.

All of the above contribute to the frequent resistance to regain body fat but others compound it. One that is frequently unconsidered is that dieting to the lower limits of BF% (for both women and men) will forever skew the individual's idea of normal. Once a woman has reached 10-12% body fat with the staggering appearance changes that accompany it, she will tend to think that she is "fat" at even a relatively lean 18%. At a the recommended optimal (and healthy levels) of 22-24%, the formerly ripped athlete will both feel and look (to themselves) to be positively overweigh even if they are still leaner than the majority of people. Tangentially, this is a consideration that women considering a physique contest should seriously consider. Whatever good (i.e. proving that they can reach that level of development) might come out of it, the potential consequences afterwards may be severe. A woman may never see herself "normally" in the mirror again and, even in the case that a subclinical or overt eating disorder was not present to begin with, it's common for women to show some symptoms afterwards. True normalcy may never be fully achieved which is a high price to pay. I am in no way trying to dissuade readers of this book from pursuing this goal but only want to make them aware of the potentially enormous long-term consequences.

All of the above combines with the final factor which is the time involved going in both directions. From a reasonable BF%, reaching the extremes of leanness may take 6 months of meticulous, dedicated dieting and training. Yet that level of leanness and appearance can be lost seemingly overnight. The physique athlete will lose separation in their muscles simply by holding water from raising carbohydrates for several days and, in the same way that small amounts of fat loss have enormous appearance effects in very lean dieters, small amounts of fat gain have enormous negative effects. Even ignoring those short-term effects, the 6 months of strict dieting can be reversed in half that time or less. Watching their previously "perfect" physique disappear rapidly can make the entire effort seem wasted.

While I am in no way attempting to trivialize the realities of the above, the difficulty that the lean female may face in raising her calories or regaining body fat, I must re-emphasize the potentially permanent harm that women may do by not properly recovering after dieting to the low extremes. The menstrual cycle, if normally present but impaired, must be restored as rapidly as possible. Both normal hormone levels and normal physiological function must also be restored. Athletes will not be able to make significant improvements in any aspect of their fitness until this occurs and women, unlike men, face the potentially permanent loss of bone density that can occur if recovery does not happen. With that said, let me look at each phase of recovery in detail.

Adjusting the Diet: Phase 1

As stated above, the first phase of adjusting the diet occurs immediately after the end of the diet and the goal here is to begin the process of both menstrual cycle function and overall hormonal recovery. The primary requirement here is that calorie intake must be increased so that the critical EA threshold of 13.6 cal/lb LBM (30 cal/kg LBM) is met or surpassed since recovery cannot begin until that occurs. A secondary requirement is that dietary fat should be raised to a minimum of 0.44 g/lb (~1.0 g/kg) with at least 1/3rd of that from saturated fat as both are important for proper menstrual cycle function.

Strictly speaking, protein intake can be decreased as calorie intake is increasing as the highest levels recommended for the final phase of the diet were only necessary to prevent LBM loss. At the same time, protein is the most hunger blunting of all nutrients and keeping it relatively higher can help reduce the risk of excessive overeating due to runaway hunger that will be present when the diet is ended. I would suggest protein be lowered to no less than 1.2 g/lb LBM for physique or other strength/power athletes and 1.0 g/lb LBM For endurance athletes during this phase. I've shown these requirements below.

EA (minimum)	Protein Intake	Fat Intake
13.6 cal/lb LBM	1.0 g/lb (2.2 g/kg) endurance	0.44 g/lb
(30 cal/kg LBM)	1.2 g/lb (2.65 g/kg) all other	(~1.0 g/kg)

Once again, the EA represents a minimum, not a target and it can be taken higher. Focusing on physique or strength/power athletes, I've shown how the above numbers would calculate out for different body weights, assuming an ending BF% of 12%.

Wt (lb)	LBM (lb)	Minimum EA (cal)	Pro. (g)	Fat (g)	Sat. (g)
122	110	1496 + Exercise	110-132	54	18
133	120	1632 + Exercise	120-144	59	20
144	130	1768 + Exercise	130-156	63	21
155	140	1904 + Exercise	140-168	68	23

As shown in the chart, the minimum number of calories that will actually have to be eaten will be the critical EA threshold plus the number of calories being burned during exercise. Once the minimum daily calorie intake has been established, this will allow the number of carbohydrates that should be eaten to be determined. So assume the sample dieter who reached a weight of 130 lbs at 10% body fat and 117 lbs of LBM. She has reduced her training to only burn 300 calories per day (roughly an hour of weight training) and will be eating 1.2 g/lb LBM of protein while targeting 0.44 g/lb body weight from fat per day.

> 117 lbs LBM * 13.6 cal/lb LBM = 1591 calories + 300 exercise calories = 1891 calories
> 117 lbs LBM * 1.2 g/lb LBM = 140 g protein * 4 cal/g = 560 cal from protein
> 130 lbs * 0.44 g/lb = 54 grams fat * 9 cal/g = 486 calories from fat
> Calories from Carbs = 1891 calories - 560 cal - 486 cal = 845 calories
> 845 calories from carbs / 4 cal/g = 211 g carbs per day (1.6 g/lb or 3.65 g/kg)

So her diet to simply meet the critical EA threshold will be 1591 calories and, with 300 calories per day of exercise, she will need to eat a minimum of ~1900 calories per day (athletes may eat more than this but cannot eat less or recovery will not occur). This represents a calorie intake of 14.6 cal/lb (32 cal/kg) of total bodyweight (1891 calories / 130 lbs = 14.5 cal/lb) and this should be fairly close to her predicted maintenance after the diet. While 16 cal/lb might be a more normal value, I'd reiterate my suggestion to adjust this downwards by 10% as a safety valve. Reducing 16 cal/lb by 10% (1.6) yields 1.4 a nearly identical value. Of those 1900 calories, she will be eating 140 grams protein, 54 grams of fat (with ~18 grams from saturated fat) and 211 grams of carbohydrates per day. How much of a change this will represent from her current diet will depend on what she was eating at the end of the diet itself. Working from the adjusted diet I showed in the previous chapter on amenorrhea, I will assume that she ended her diet at roughly 1300 calories (10 cal/lb) with 175 g/day of protein, 35 g/day of dietary fat and 75 grams per day of carbohydrates on her diet days. I've shown how her diet would be adjusted during this phase below.

	End of Diet	Recovery	Change
Calories	1500 calories	1900	+400
Protein	175 g/day	140 g/day	-35 g/day
Carbohydrate	121 g/day	211 g/day	+90 g/day
Fat	35 g/day	54 g/day	+19 g/day

As shown, her calorie intake would increase by 400 with a reduction of 35 grams of protein and an increase of 20 grams of fat and 90 grams of carbohydrate per day. Once again this should represent a minimum target and more can be eaten (runaway hunger may make avoiding eating more impossible). Any further increases in calorie intake should come primarily from carbohydrate as this will have a larger impact on hormonal recovery than an increase in dietary fat.

How Long Should it Take to Raise Calories?
Now let me look at the issue of how long it should take to raise calories to the appropriate level. In the physique community, it is sometimes suggested that calories be raised very slowly over a 4-8 week span following a diet and three primary reasons have usually been given. The first is that raising calories, especially carbohydrates, more slowly can avoid some issues with stomach upset along with preventing major swings in water weight. While the former is a very real issue, I consider the second to be somewhat nonsensical. Certainly it can be psychologically demoralizing to see the scale jump by 5 pounds overnight after dieting for 6 months to lose 20 pounds but this is only water and food in the gut rather than body fat. To avoid mental stress, competitors should avoid the scale for the first week after a contest.

A very real argument can be made that raising calories too rapidly after a diet can cause the complete loss of food control. Given the changes that occur in hunger and appetite regulation while dieting to extremely low body fat levels, this is certainly a risk. For many, there is also somewhat of a psychological flip that switches when people end a diet as they go from a great deal of mental control over their food intake to seemingly none. In my experience, this usually shows up earlier in the diet, for example during days at maintenance or diet breaks. At the same time, the types of flexible approaches to eating recommended in this book, sufficient days at maintenance, diet breaks, IIFYM strategies tend to go a long way to preventing this problem. In my experience and that of other coaches, it is the extremely rigid 6 months of complete deprivation approaches to dieting that lead to the most extreme post-diet overeating. When a dieter has been able to fulfill their food cravings along with psychological and physiological needs during the diet, the need to binge on those foods after the diet is significantly reduced.

A third argument is one that I addressed earlier in the book and has to do with the incorrect idea that gradually raising calories can somehow increase metabolic rate without fat gain. Not only does this not generally occur with overfeeding from maintenance but it absolutely cannot occur during recovery from dieting. Hormones, and by extension, metabolism, does not and cannot recover to any significant degree if calorie intake is still below the critical EA threshold (recall that body fat sends a major signal to the brain in the form of leptin that is part of recovery). I'd remind readers of the study above where metabolic rate was at least normalized after 4 weeks but this was due to the fat gain that was occurring. Perhaps the final argument for or reason that dieters are often reluctant to raise calories quickly is to limit fat gain. While fat gain (in addition to the rapid water weight gain) is an issue, the reality is that dieters will have to regain body fat to either sustainable or optimal levels no matter what they do. Whether it occurs in 2 months or 6 months is irrelevant outside of potentially making it take longer to re-achieve hormonal normalcy. Dieters who take 4-8 weeks to even reach the critical EA threshold or start regaining body fat are doing nothing but delaying their recovery as they are, fundamentally, still dieting. Compared to the dieter who rapidly raises calories, the consequences can be severe and I will look at real world examples in the next chapter.

For all of the above reasons, I simply recommend that dieters take no more than 2 weeks to raise their calories and carbohydrates. The athlete is free to raise their calories faster than that, even doing so the day after their diet is over. But they should never take longer than 2 weeks to reach at least that level.

Fast vs. Slow Calorie Increases

With the understanding that the critical EA threshold must be crossed, let me look at the potential pros and cons of both fast and slow calorie increases. In the fast approach, the diet should be adjusted as described above over the 2-3 day span following the diet. If the athlete is taking those days completely off from training, it may take no more than adding a few hundred calories to the current diet to reach or cross the critical EA threshold. Calories will have to be increased further when activity is re-introduced and increased but this approach will start the recovery process essentially immediately (the peak week increase in calories will also help to start at least some of the recovery processes). The simplest way to approach the fast increase is to spend the 2-3 days following the contest performing a high carbohydrate, moderate protein, low/moderate fat refeed/days at maintenance. Given the hunger that is likely present, most dieters will cross the critical EA threshold without any real effort in this approach.

While a fast increase in calories is arguably the best approach, it does come with some drawbacks, most of which I described above. Stomach upset is not uncommon, especially if high-fiber carbohydrate are eaten, and body weight can go up significantly due to glycogen and water storage along with actually having food in the gut Appearance will also often suffer as there can be significant water retention at this point which will make the dieter look puffy and watery. As noted above, I would recommend avoiding both the scale and the mirror for a few days (water weight should be eliminated within a few days).

Perhaps the biggest problem with a fast approach is the potential for the total loss of food control with some stories of enormous food intakes in the day or two after a competition diet has ended. Even here, there isn't much to be concerned about. Only the most incredible binge can cause true fat gain to occur and, even so, body fat will have to be regained for full hormonal recovery in the first place so even this is a non-issue outside of psychological issues. Those dieters who find the idea of increasing calories rapidly over 1-3 days to be either psychologically or physiologically daunting may choose to increase calories over a maximum 2 week span following the end of their diet. At least some training will have been re-introduced at this point and many athletes find it less psychologically stressful to raise calories when they are doing at least some amount of training and giving those calories somewhere to "go". If this approach is being used, whatever calorie increase is needed (and activity must be factored in) can simply be divided out over that 1-2 week span with reasonable increases being made every few days.

The sample dieter has to increase her total calorie intake by 400 calories with the changes described above to protein, carbohydrate and dietary fat intake. If she decides to take a full week to raise her calories by this amount, that only amounts to 100 calories every 2 days. This is roughly one serving of starchy carbohydrates which could be added to any meal as desired. Over 2 weeks, the same 400 calorie increase only amounts to 50 calories every 2 days which is somewhat impractical to add to the diet. Rather, a 100 calorie increase every 4th day might work better. Alternately, raising calories by 200 at the end of the first week and again by 200 calories at the end of the second might be effective. If the athlete starts to increase the amount of exercise they are doing after those 2 weeks, calories will have to be increased further to remain above the critical EA threshold. Calorie increases will be higher if an EA threshold higher than the minimum is being targeted as well.

There is a compromise situation that may provide the best of both approaches. Given the often incredible hunger at the end of the diet, simply allowing an enormous calorie/carbohydrate intake over the first 1-3 days will cause an immediate improvement in hormonal status, energy levels and mood while allowing any leftover cravings to be addressed. In combination with a reduction in training, this will assuredly cause the athlete to cross the critical EA threshold as well. Following this 3 day span of increased food intake, more dietary control can be instituted for the remaining 2 weeks although calorie intake should never fall to take the dieter back below the critical EA threshold.

Adjusting the Diet: Phase 2

Once calories have been increased to or above the critical EA threshold over the first 2 weeks following the end of the diet, Phase 2 will begin. This phase is more extended and involves increasing body fat to either the sustainable (16-18%) or optimal (20-24%) levels I described earlier in the chapter. For the athlete seeking to improve fitness, strength, power or muscle mass, the faster that full recovery has occurred, the sooner productive training can resume and gains will be able to made.

How much body fat will need to be regained can be determined in one of two ways. If the athlete is simply returning to their pre-diet weight and BF%, they will need to regain the exact amount of actual fat that was lost. So in the case of this book's sample dieter who went from 150/22% body fat to 130/12% body fat she would need to regain 20 pounds of fat. If a female runner had gone from 135 lbs/18% body fat to 125 lbs/12% she would need to regain 10 lbs. If any LBM has been lost, it will need to be regained and this will change the values very slightly. Essentially, the athlete should aim to return to their pre-diet body weight and BF% and this will determine the total amount of weight and fat they need to regain.

In some cases, the athlete may wish to return to a slightly lower or higher BF% than they started at. Most commonly this will be the person who wants to attain the sustainable BF% level of 16-18% although the occasional dieter who started at 19-20% might want to return to 22% to better optimize their ability to make gains. The same equation I originally presented to determine the target weight for fat loss can be used here to determine how much fat will need to be regained to reach a specific BF%. Current LBM should be divided by 1 minus the goal BF% as a percentage and this will yield the ending bodyweight goal. I've shown the goal weight and required fat gain that the sample dieter at 130 lbs/117 lbs LBM would need to reach to achieve 18, 20 or 22% body fat below.

Goal Weight (18%) = 117 lbs/(1-0.18) = 117 lbs/0.82 = 143 lbs (13 lb fat gain)
Goal Weight (20%) = 117 lbs/(1-0.20) = 117 lbs/0.80 = 146 lbs (16 lb fat gain)
Goal Weight (22%) = 117 lbs/(1-0.22) = 117 lbs/0.78 = 150 lbs (20 lb fat gain)

The above calculation assumes 100% fat gain and if she gains LBM during this time, the total weight gain will be very slightly higher than calculated above.. How long it will take to achieve this weight gain will depend on how many calories are added back to the diet. Since there is no reason outside of avoiding psychological stress to use slow rates of weight gain, a weekly weight gain target of 1-1.5% can be used. For the sample dieter at 130 lbs this would represent a weekly gain of 1.3-2 lbs/week and the total fat gain would require 6-10, 8-12, and 10-15 weeks for the 13, 16 and 20 pound fat gains respectively. It's most likely that fat gain will be faster earlier in this phase due to the realities of post-diet hunger and metabolic rate suppression but it should slow as both return to normal and the dieter is coming closer to their goal weight and BF%. The 1.5% weekly weight gain may be used until the dieter is close to their goal before they move to 1% (alternately 1% could be used earlier in Phase 2 dropping to 0.5% gain when the goal is nearly achieved).

Determining the how much of a calorie surplus is required to gain at a given rate is more or less identical to determining the deficit and the value of 3,500 calories per pound can be used. In the early stages, where the body is primed for fat gain, this is likely to generate a true one pound fat gain but this may no longer be the case near the end of Phase 2. If the sample dieter was initially targeting a 1% gain of body weight, or 1.3 lbs, she would need 4,550 calories per week above her maintenance level (1.3 lbs * 3,500 calories/lb = 4550). Consumed across 7 days, this is a 650 calorie per day surplus which would yield a total calorie requirement of 2550 calories when added to her Phase 1 diet of ~1900 calories. Since protein is inefficiently used for gaining weight, the increase in calories should primarily come from carbohydrates and fat. For the sake of example, the sample dieter will increase her carbohydrates by 400 calories or 100 grams per day and her dietary fat for the other 250 calories or 27 grams per day. Her Phase 1 diet will change as follows.

	Phase 1	Phase 2	Change
Calories	1900	2550	+650
Protein	140 g/day	140 g/day	No Change
Carbohydrate	211 g/day	311 g/day	+100 g/day
Fat	54 g/day	71 g/day	+27 g/day

As her body weight increases, her energy expenditure will start to increase and this will necessitate a further increase in calories. Perhaps more importantly is that after the initial few weeks of light training, athletes will be starting to increase the amount and/or intensity of their training which will also increase their energy expenditure. Calories must continue to increase to compensate both to maintain the goal rate of fat gain along with ensuring that the athlete doesn't accidentally fall below the critical EA threshold (this should be of minimal concern unless activity increases rapidly over short time period). Regular body composition and bodyweight measurement should be used to ensure that she is gaining fat at a sufficient rate to reach full recovery within the 2-4 month goal depending on goal BF%.

Supplement Considerations

Finally, while most supplements will not be beneficial in terms of helping menstrual cycle recovery, there are two to consider. The first is some sort of liquid meal replacement drink (recall that studies on this provided a 360 calorie protein/carbohydrate drink) to increase total calorie intake This may have its greatest utility in the earliest stages of recover as liquids will not cause the stomach upset, bloating or potential weight gain that solid foods might. Liquids are often easier to consume and for those athletes having trouble eating enough during their recovery, this can be invaluable. Mind you, given that hunger is often absolutely staggering following a contest, eating too little is generally not an issue but this is a consideration. Another possibility would be the addition of acetyl-l-carnitine which, recall from Chapter 24 was shown in some women to help restore menstrual cycle function at a dose of 2 grams per day. A dose of 250 mg ALCAR and 500 mg L-carnitine also reduced cortisol and improved LH pulsatility. This cannot replace an increase in EA or the other changes described above but may be worthwhile.

Avoiding Body fat Overshoot

While it's clear that regaining body fat is a critical aspect of restoring normal physiological function at the end of an extreme diet, athletes must avoid overshooting their previous BF% and ending up with more fat than they began. The only exception to this is if their pre-diet BF% was too low to begin with (i.e. the dieter who started their diet at 15% should target a higher BF% when the diet is over). Rather the goal should be to reach either the sustainable 16-18% or optimal 22-24% body fat levels but no higher. More specifically, the athlete should ideally reach an ideal/their pre-diet body composition level in terms of both the amount of fat and LBM that they are carrying. As I discussed earlier in the book but want to address again, it is actually the LBM component that is of critical importance here. Because while body fat clearly plays a major role in the adaptations that occur to dieting, LBM plays a separate independent role in driving hunger. Until it has been regained, hunger will remain high and fat will continue to be gained.

Perhaps the clearest demonstration of this effect was the Minnesota Semi-Starvation study that I detailed in Chapter 9. Briefly, lean men were placed on 50% of maintenance calories for 6 months and lost 25% of their total weight before being placed on a recovery diet. During recovery, the men not only regained all of the fat that they had lost initially but ended up significantly fatter than they had started. In fact, it wasn't until they had regained all of the LBM that they had lost that their metabolic rate recovered completely and their appetite normalized itself. At least part of this is due to the relationship between LBM and metabolic rate itself but it's now known that LBM is sending it's own signal of hunger to the brain with low or lowered levels of LBM stimulating overeating in an attempt to rebuild itself (9).

This has several practical implications. The first is that excessive LBM loss on a diet will tend to lower metabolic rate and stimulate hunger more than would otherwise occur. Limiting or eliminating LBM loss on a diet is critical to its overall success. Here women have a slight advantage over men in that they tend to lose less LBM than men in the first place so long as they set up their diet and training appropriately. By extension, if LBM is lost during a diet, it must be regained during the recovery period as hunger and metabolic rate will not return to normal until this occurs. A delay in LBM recovery following a diet has the potential to cause a body fat overshoot and the gain of more fat than the athlete started with.

The solution to both issues, avoiding LBM loss while dieting and ensuring it is regained afterwards, is actually the same and relatively simple: proper resistance training must be combined with a sufficient dietary protein intake. If the diet and training is set up appropriately in the first place, LBM loss should be minimal approaching zero (this will be clearly demonstrated in the next chapter). The protein recommendations in this book are more than sufficient for both dieting and the recovery period and I've already mentioned that resistance training should be part of the training done by all athletes during recovery from their diet. I provided guidelines in Chapter 28 and by the time the athlete is in a position to regain LBM, their training levels should be approaching the levels I described.

Physique athletes will be performing weight training as a matter of course but I'll reiterate the importance for other athletes to include it at this time both to ensure recovery of any lost LBM and to stimulate improvements in bone density. Ultimately, so long as an athlete in Phase 2 ensures that any lost LBM is regained while she is regaining fat, there is no reason to expect her body fat levels to overshoot their original levels.   By the time she reaches an optimal BF%, her physiology including her hunger and metabolic rate will be normalized and there will be no biological drive to continue overeating.

When to Stop Gaining Fat?

At some point, the dieter will have finished Phase 2, having reached either their pre-diet or some optimal target body fat or body composition goal. Depending on how controlled or not calorie intake was, this should take somewhere between 2-4 months (if it takes much longer than this, the athlete was not eating enough).   At this point, hormonal status should be normalized although it may take longer for menstrual cycle function to resume completely. At this point, the diet will need to be adjusted one further time, moving back to the set up I originally described in this book. The normally cycling female will need to set up a follicular and luteal phase diet and women with other hormonal modifiers will set up the appropriate diet for their situation.

I would recommend that calories be initially set at maintenance levels at this point and kept there for roughly 2 weeks before any other changes are made. This is just a final stabilization phase and may necessitate a slight decrease in calorie intake from the previous week if fat is still being gained. How much of a decrease will depend on what the final weekly rate of fat gain was. If it had dropped to one half pound per week, for example, that would indicate that the weekly surplus was only 1750 calories or roughly 250 per day. Calories would be decreased by this much during the stabilization phase (training could technically be increased but that would represent a fairly large increase). After those two weeks, the athlete will be completely prepared to begin working on improvements to their muscle mass, strength/power or other components of fitness. Training should have returned to more or less normal levels by this point and, combined with the slight surpluses described before, they can start improving for their next season. I've summarized the overall schedule for the post-diet recovery below.

	Phase 1	Phase 2	Stabilization	Gaining
	First 2 weeks	2-4 Months	Two weeks	Remainder of Year
Goal	Begin Recovery	Increase BF%	Stabilize weight and BF%	Improve fitness
Calories	Move to 13.6 cal/lb+ Fast or Slow	500+ cal above the current level	Adjust calories to maintenance	Combine proper training with a slight calorie surplus
Training	Off/Light Different/Fun	Gradual build up for 4 weeks	Maintain training volume and intensity	

At the risk of beating a dead horse, let me re-iterate the absolute need for the above to occur as rapidly as is realistically possible. Not only can normal training and gains be made until it does, a woman may be doing actual physical (potentially permanent) damage to herself if it does not occur. Any psychological or mental resistance must be overcome to ensure that recovery proceeds properly.

Chapter 34: Studies of Dieting in Elite Athletes

To wrap up this book, I want to finish by examining the (admittedly) limited research that has been done on elite athletes dieting to the extremes. I will be looking at the studies in question in some detail, primarily to show how the athletes did (or did not) follow the approach that I have described in the preceding two chapters. In all but one, the approach taken was effectively identical to what I have recommended in this book with the expected results occurring. The one exception demonstrates not only the traditional dieting approach but shows concretely how damaging it can actually be.

Case Study of Fat Loss in a Cyclist

I want to start with a recent case study of an elite female cyclist who was attempting to lose body fat, regain lean body mass (LBM) and regain fitness following a viral infection (1). She engaged in a 10 week plan where she was instructed to reduce her energy availability (EA) from the current level of 18.6 cal/lb LBM (41 cal/kg LBM) to between 13.6-18 cal/lb LBM (30-40 cal/kg LBM) and she averaged an EA of 15.9 cal/lb LBM (35 cal/kg LBM). Her calories dropped from 3135 calories/day (24 cal/lb) to 2742 cal/day (22.6 cal/lb) or a roughly 400 calorie/day deficit. While these are very high values, I've noted that this is common for endurance athletes due to the high amount of total training that they do. For perspective, by week 8 of the intervention, she was performing 2 5-hour rides per week in addition to her other training.

Before the intervention she was consuming 143 grams of protein per day, 481 grams of carbohydrate per day and 71 grams of fat and this was altered to 155 grams of protein, 382 grams of carbs and 66 grams of fat per day. The increased protein intake came from increased dairy protein twice/day along with an increase in her portions of meat proteins and amounts to 1.6 g/lb LBM (above even my maximum recommendations). She performed weight training three times per week along with multiple fasted morning bike rides lasting 30 minutes. During rides longer than 2 hours she consumed 60 g/hour of carbs and ensured 20 grams of high quality protein after both her weight workouts and long rides to improve recovery. Over the 10 weeks her BF% dropped from ~23% to 19.5% with a total fat loss of 7.6 lbs (3.47 kg) or .76 lbs (0.34 kg) per week for weekly weight loss of 0.58%. She regained just under 2 lbs (0.8 kg) of LBM and achieved her previous power outputs. EA was raised to adequate levels following the diet.

With minor variation (i.e. slightly higher protein than my recommendations which is really not a problem), the above matches with every recommendation in this book. The athlete created a moderate deficit for a controlled period of time with the combination of a reduction in total carbohydrate and fat, a gradually increasing training volume and the addition of short low-intensity workouts done fasted in the morning. Longer workouts were supported with adequate carbohydrate to ensure optimal performance and protein was consumed following training to ensure recovery. This allowed her to reduce her BF% while regaining LBM and performance before returning to an EA sufficient to support her training.

Case Study of an Olympic Runner

The second case study I want to examine was performed on an Olympic level female distance runner (2). Lasting an incredible 9 years, from the time she was 27 to 35 years old with numerous measurements made including body composition, DEXA and others The athlete ran the 1500m event, a race predicated both on aerobic and anaerobic capacities and involving a variety of training. Recognizing that it is impossible to maintain peak competition body composition year round, she would alternate between her competition and off-season. During the off-season, her primary training period, she allowed her body weight and body fat to increase by 2-4% which put her at ~12-13% body fat, allowing an adequate EA to sustain training. Prior to competing, she engaged in a 6-8 week diet during which she would reduce her calories by 300 cal/day to generate a fat loss of about 4 lbs (2 kg) or roughly 0.5 lbs/week (~0.4% current body weight). This allowed her to achieve her peak BF% of 10% prior to the competition season.

During her diet, her protein intake was maintained at 1-1.2 g/lb LBM (2.2-2.7 g/kg LBM). Her snacking and carbohydrate intake were also reduced on her easier training days to facilitate a calorie reduction. During her dieting phase she maintained heavy weight training and repeated DEXA scans showed a higher than average bone mineral density (BMD). She missed 2.8 menstrual cycles per year (which I suspect occurred during the competition season) and never became fully amenorrheic. She made the world championships 7 times and was the finalist in 3 while only sustaining 2 injuries in that time. She was within 1% of her best 11 times and this occurred in 5 of the 9 seasons and her ability to remain injury free was likely a huge contributor to this. While very gradual, she gained LBM in her lower body over the course of her career, assuredly during her off-season when her calorie intake was higher.

Once again, with very minor variations, the athlete in question's approach mirrored what I have recommended in this book.   In the most general sense, she made no attempt to maintain the lowest limits of BF%, allowing weight and fat regain during her off-season. This allowed for hormonal recovery to occur and gave her the ability to eat sufficient calories and maintain an adequate EA to train more effectively. While she maintained a lower BF% in the off-season than I would tend to think is ideal in most cases, her lack of menstrual cycle dysfunction or BMD suggests that this was not problematic. This could be due to her being able to maintain an adequate EA during this time period of due to her higher reproductive age and I'd reiterate that women will vary in what a sustainable BF% is likely to be. During her diet, she used a slow rate of fat loss consistent with the rates recommended in this book and her protein intake of up to 1.2 g/lb LBM is identical to my recommendations in Chapter 19 for endurance athletes. Combined with weight training, this allowed her to maintain LBM while reducing her BF% to goal levels.

Research on the Extreme Physique Dieter

Finally let me look at a number of studies that have been done on physique dieters in recent years. While there are a limited number of studies (most of them on single individuals) examining them in the aggregate helps to show what successful real world physique competitors are doing and whether it matches up with the recommendations that I have made in this book. For each, I will present in some detail what was reported as having been done in terms of diet or training along with any other relevant measures. Primarily I will be focusing on factors such as EA, menstrual cycle function (both dysfunction and recovery), fat loss and LBM. When other data is available, I will present it as well and in most cases I will compare or contrast it to recommendations made earlier in this book.

The first study I want to discuss followed 30 female physique competitors dieting for a contest during both their dieting and recovery phases for their competition (3). The primary goal was to monitor their hormonal status and the 27 competitors (17 bikini, 9 body fitness and 1 fitness competitor; the study was from Scandinavia which uses different division names) who completed the study were compared to 23 non-dieting women. I'd note that 19 of the 27 were using birth control although the type was not indicated. The women were an average of 27 years old with the average diet period being 20 weeks and the average recovery period being 17.5 weeks. Hormonal status, body composition (by three methods) and strength were measured at three time points: start of the diet, immediately post-contest and after the recovery period.

During the diet, all of the women performed weight training using some form of split routine, training 4-5 times per week with workouts lasting 40-90 minutes. Either HIIT exclusively or a mix of HIIT and aerobic training was performed an average of 5 times per week.   During the recovery period resistance training was maintained while aerobic training was decreased to 2 times per week. During the diet, the women consumed an average of 1800 calories per day. Their protein intake was 187 grams per day which was 1.4 g/lb (3.0 g/kg), identical to my recommendation earlier in this book. Their carbohydrate intake was 127 grams per day, nearly identical to the 121 grams per day I calculated in diet Option 1 in Chapter 32. Their fat intake of 52 g/day is slightly higher than the value from Chapter 32 due to the women eating more calories. If the women utilized any sort of refeed or eating at maintenance days during the diet, it was not indicated in the paper and I can only assume that it was not done. During the recovery period, calorie intake increased to 2200 calories per day with carbohydrates being increased to 190 grams/day.

The women's body fat percentage dropped from 23-24% to roughly 12% although the specific numbers depended on the measurement method being used. It's interesting to note that the use of birth control by a majority of the women seemed to cause no problem in reaching their competition goals. There was either no or a small loss of LBM (depending on the method of measurement) as well and this occurred with a small loss of bone density. Body weight, BF%, LBM and bone density all recovered to their pre-diet levels during the recovery period.   The women's hormones changed as expected with leptin, testosterone, T3 and estrogen decreasing.   Leptin and estrogen returned to normal while testosterone and T3 remained slightly lower than before the diet during the recovery period. Three of the 27 women were amenorrheic before the diet with an additional 10 having menstrual irregularities. During the diet itself, more women developed menstrual irregularities or became amenorrheic although specific numbers were not provided. Following recovery, 7 of the women remained amenorrheic. In all cases, the frequency of menstrual cycle dysfunction was much higher in the dieting group than in the controls which is not surprising.

Overall this study, in a fairly large number of competitors supports what I have written in this book. The women combined a high protein intake with resistance training and reasonable amount of aerobic/HIIT exercise while starting their diet relatively early and this allowed them to reach competition shape with no loss of LBM. Following the contest, their BF% and bodyweight returned to normal with the combination of increased calorie intake and reduced aerobic work and there was essentially a normalization of their hormonal status. While many women showed some form of menstrual cycle dysfunction, it was not universal although the fact that 7 of the women had not regained menstrual cycle function after recovery is concerning. The recovery period of 17.5 weeks is just over 4 months which is admittedly on the shorter side and a longer post-study duration might have shown full recovery.

The next study was a case study which followed a single drug-free figure competitor over 32 weeks of contest dieting (4). The dieter was 29 years old and divided her diet into two phases of 22 and 10 weeks respectively. She performed a high-frequency and high-volume of weight training through both phases along with what appears to be exclusively HIIT exercise. Over the 32 weeks she lost 16 lbs (7.2 kg), representing a loss of roughly 0.5% of her bodyweight per week, with her BF% decreasing from 23.5% to 11.3%. She gained a small amount of LBM during the diet and her bone mineral density was unchanged. Most of the changes occurred in the final 24 weeks of her diet making her actual dieting time 6 months. Her starting calorie intake was 2400 calories, yielding an EA was roughly 19 cal/lb LBM (42 cal/kg LBM), near sufficient levels. This decreased over the duration of the diet to nearly 1200 calories at the end. Looking at the final 10 weeks of her diet, her protein intake was 1.3-1.6 g/lb (2.8-3.5 g/kg), again consistent with my recommendations. Following the contest, she experienced a "rapid regain of body fat" to her pre-contest level suggesting that her calorie intake was raised rapidly (they were not reported)

Of some importance, the dieter did not become amenorrheic until 1 month before her contest and regained her cycle within one month after the contest. She did show two more months of a shortened cycle, indicating luteal phase defect, and cramping before complete normalization occurred by month 4. This means that her approach, starting at a reasonable BF% and EA while using an extended dieting time led to a complete loss of menstrual cycle of only 2 months with 2 more months of slight dysfunction.

In the most recent study on the topic, a single female physique competitors was followed over 6 months of contest dieting (5). During that time her BF% dropped from 30% to 15.5% while losing 22 lbs (10.1 kg) of body fat, an average weekly loss of 0.6%. While her starting BF% contradicts my comments about women above 24% being unable to realistically achieve contest shape, I suspect this is a methodological issue in terms of how BF% was measured. Note that her 15% drop in BF% is essentially identical to the 14% a woman would lose going from 24% to 10%. She began her diet at 2550 calories/day (17 cal/lb) and this dropped to 1500 per day (12 cal/lb) by the end of the diet. Her protein intake was set at 150 g/day or roughly 1.5 g/b LBM (3.3 g/kg), consistent with my recommendations. She was also consuming 70 grams of carbohydrate per day with 70 grams of dietary fat nearly identical to my Option 2 diet presented in Chapter 32 On her single refeed day she consumed 125 grams of protein, 300 grams of carbohydrate and 25 grams of fat, also nearly identical to the Option 1 I presented for maintenance days.

Her training program was not detailed but can be assumed to have included both resistance training and some amount of aerobic and/or HIIT work and she demonstrated no loss of LBM during her diet. While it was not calculated in the study, my own rough estimates suggest that she dropped below the critical EA threshold in roughly month 3 or 4 of her diet and she showed a lengthened menstrual cycle into months 5 and 6 with no further menstrual cycle disruption. She was not tracked following her diet but I would assume that the minor changes to her menstrual cycle resolved themselves when her diet was over.

The final study I want to examine is another case study of a single dieter followed over a 20 week competition diet and 20 week recovery period (6). While the dieter did in fact reach her competition goals, as I'll show, her diet represents a perfect example of how not to approach an extreme diet. The study followed a 26 year old woman competing in figure competition who had her body composition along with her diet and exercise status measured at a number of time points during her diet and recovery. During her diet, she performed weight training 4-5 days per week with HIIT 1-2 days/week and aerobic work 1 day/week. She used a carb cycling approach with 2 high carb (180-230 g/day) days, 3 moderate carb (150-180 g/day) days and 2 low carb (100-150 g/day) days per week. These were synchronized with her training. Her protein intake was 150 g/day which represented 1.2-1.4 g/lb (2.7-3.0 g/kg) with a fat intake of roughly 40 g/day. This is all consistent with my dietary and training suggestions.

Over 20 weeks of dieting, she lost roughly 11 lbs (5 kg) with no measured LBM loss. Her BF% via DEXA showed a drop from 15.1% to 8.6% although this is an underestimate given that the lower limit for women is closer to 10%. I would consider a drop from 17% to 10% to be more accurate and will use those values below. But this is where the problems start. Due to being too lean at the outset, the dieter was already starting with an EA of 14.5 cal/lb LBM (32 cal/kg LBM) and dropped below the critical threshold immediately upon starting her diet. She began to show menstrual cycle irregularity within one month of dieting and became amenorrheic after only 11 weeks of dieting.

This would be bad enough in its own right but her approach to post workout recovery was equally problematic. Due to a fear of regaining body fat, she used a very slow increase in calories over the next 10 weeks and only achieved her pre-diet BF% after 20 weeks at which point her EA was still only 16 cal/lb LBM (35 cal/kg), still near the critical EA threshold and below what is considered adequate. Most likely due to this, the dieter did not resume menstrual cycle function for 71 weeks or nearly 18 months following the end of her contest. Bone mineral density was unfortunately not measured but can be assumed to have been lost during this time. Essentially the dieter started too lean while eating too little, dropped below the critical EA threshold immediately, lost her menstrual cycle earlier than necessary and, by raising calories far too slowly (which only delayed her eventual return to her previous BF% level) delayed normalization of her menstrual cycle for a year and a half.

I have summarized key information from the four studies described above in the chart below.

	Hulmi (2017)	Petrizzo (2017)	Rohrig (2017)	Halliday (2016)
Type of Study	27 Subjects	Case study	Case study	Case study
Age	27 years old	29 years old	24	26-27 years old
Birth control	19 of 27 dieters	Not indicated	No	No
Diet Duration	20 weeks	24 weeks	24 weeks	20 weeks
Resistance training	4-5 days per week	4-5 days/week	Yes (not described)	4-5 days/week
Aerobic work	~5 times/week Mix aerobic/HIIT	4 days/week	Not described	1 aerobic and 1-2 HIIT/week
Calorie Intake	1800 calories/day	2300 to 1300 over 22 wks.	2550 to 1500 over 24 wks.	1800 to 1500 over 10 wks.
Protein Intake	1.4 g/lb (3.0 g/kg)	1.3-1.5 g/lb (2.8-3.5 g/kg)	1.5 g/lb (3.3 g/kg)	1.4 g/lb (3.0 g/kg)
Carbohydrate Intake	127 g/day	Below 100 g/day at end of diet	Below 70 g/day at end of diet	Carb cycling
Fat Intake	52 g/day	20-40 g/day at end of diet	70 g/day at end of diet	40 g/day
BF% Change	23-24% -> 12%	24.3->11%	30%->15%	15->8.6% (adjusted 18->11%)
LBM Loss	None	Slight decrease	None	None
Bone Mineral Density	Small loss (regained after diet)	None	Not measured	Not measured
Rate Weight Loss	0.85 lb/wk (0.4 kg/wk)	0.55 lb/week (0.25 kg/wk)	0.0.9 lb/week (0.42 kg/wk)	0.65 /lb/week (0.3 kg/wk)
Pre-Diet EA	Not Determined	~19 cal/lb LBM (42 cal/kg LBM)	Not determined	14.5 cal/lb LBM (32 cal/kg LBM)
EA During Diet	Not Determined	Below threshold at week 10	Not Determined	Immediately below threshold
Menstrual Cycle	44% developed dysfunction	Lost after 5 months of dieting	Lengthened at 5-6 months	Lost 1 month into diet
Post-Diet				
Calorie increase	Not indicated	Rapid increase in calories	Not indicated	10 weeks to increase calories
Regain BF%	17.5 weeks to pre-diet BF%	Rapid increase in BF%	Not indicated	20 weeks to pre-diet BF%
Menstrual Cycle	7 remained amenorrheic at 17.5 wks	1 month to return	Not indicated	71 weeks to return

Despite the limited nature of and methodological differences in the studies, a general pattern starts to emerge. Clearly the combination of resistance training along with aerobic work, high protein (and relatively moderated carbohydrate and fat intakes) allows for the Category 1 dieter to reach the lower limits of female BF% with essentially zero lean body mass loss and this goes against the common idea that LBM must be lost on a diet (this assertion is much more true for men who are targeting 4-5% boyfat). This is especially true when combined with sufficiently long dieting periods and relatively slow rates of weekly weight and fat losses (the studies all fall between 0.5-0.6% of current weight per week or so).

Perhaps the biggest difference in the studies is in terms of the rate of menstrual dysfunction during the diet along with its recovery. The limited number of study participants makes drawing strong conclusions here but the Hulmi study clearly found a fairly large proportion (nearly half) who showed some degree of dysfunction, some of which were not reversed nearly 4 months after the diet (again recall from Chapter 12 that shorter studies often show less menstrual cycle recovery compared to longer and 4 months may simply have been insufficient to see full recovery. It is the case studies which present the starkest contrast. In the first, amenorrhea was avoided until one month before the end of the diet due the dieter starting at a higher BF%, an adequate calorie intake and not crossing the critical EA threshold until later in the diet.

Combined with a rapid increase in calories and BF%, this allowed the dieter to regain her cycle within one month and completely normal menstrual cycle function within 3 months. In the second, a similar pattern was seen where only minor menstrual cycle dysfunction was seen and amenorrhea did not occur as the dieter did not cross the critical EA threshold until relatively late in the diet. This is in direct contrast to the final case study where an early loss of cycle occurred due to the dieter starting too lean with a low EA which caused her to immediately drop below the critical EA threshold. A slow increase in calories and regain of body fat following the contest prevented menstrual cycle record for nearly 1.5 years potentially and likely causing bone density loss (unfortunately not measured)

Again, while limited, the above studies certainly support the recommendations I have made in this book in at least a broad sense. The combination of high protein intakes, resistance training, relatively slow rates of fat loss, etc. cause significant amounts of fat loss with essentially no LBM loss. More importantly, menstrual cycle dysfunction or outright amenorrhea may be avoided or at least delayed with proper dieting practices. By that I mean starting at a sufficient BF% with an adequate calorie intake and approaching or crossing the critical EA threshold as late in the diet as possible. Combined with a rapid increase in calories to increase weight and BF% (which ultimately has to be regained regardless of the rate), menstrual cycle and hormonal/physiological recovery can occur as rapidly as possible.

Appendix 1: The Stubborn Fat Protocols

I mentioned earlier in this book that women's lower body (hip/thigh) fat is not only one place she differs substantially from men but is far more resistant to loss. It's more likely to store fat after a meal (especially in the luteal/progesterone dominant phase) and releases stored fat to less of a degree. Years ago, in a book called <u>The Stubborn Fat Solution</u>), I addressed this in detail, covering the endless physiology of what makes stubborn fat stubborn and offering solutions. Some were based on diet (I mentioned in this book that low-carbohydrate diets can make lower body fat easier to mobilize), some on supplements (I mentioned yohimbine in this book) and then I presented four distinct cardio based protocols ranging from low-intensity (which can be done daily) to very high-intensity (which should be limited to one or two days per week). These protocols are only for the Category 1 dieter and the two high-intensity protocols are only for the dieter already involved in a training program. After much thought, I have decided to reproduce the protocols in this book since I want it to be a singular resource on the topic. Readers who want to read more about stubborn fat than they ever wanted to know can find everything in **The Stubborn Fat Solution**.

A Quick Warning

I've found out the hard way that if I put the warnings on stuff at the end of a chapter people often "forget" to read them and that's why I'm presenting them here first. It is not an over-exaggeration to say that individuals trying to strip off that last bit of fat can become a bit obsessed. Put a little less gently, most of them lose their freaking mind towards the end of the diet (or, frankly, even the beginning). It's easy enough to overtrain on a diet, most people in my experience train too hard too often without taking a break. They destroy themselves and, as often as not, they still don't get to where they want to be. Even if they do reach their goals, they blow up after the diet is done due to fatigue and exhaustion. Neither is good.

Now, a problem with modern dieting is that, for reasons ranging from reasonable to completely wrong, old school steady state cardio has gotten a bad rap. Never mind that four decades of bodybuilders got contest lean with nothing but low-intensity cardio, many have been convinced that steady state is either worthless (or in some cases actively detrimental) to fat loss. As I've repeatedly discussed, more is not better, but reasonable amounts are not only helpful but in many cases required.

The fact is, right or wrong, most people who are trying to eliminate the last bit of stubborn fat (whether for a contest or another goal) do some type of training nearly daily when they are contest dieting with many training more than once daily. So long as it is worked up to progressively, this would be completely fine so long as the intensity were kept in check. Unfortunately, this is frequently not the case. If someone has been convinced that low-intensity work is useless, and they want to do metabolic work every day, where exactly does that leave them? It leaves them trying to handle a training load that no human being could survive even at maintenance calories while much less while dieting to a low BF%. Depressingly, this is being recommended by some contest prep coaches and dieters are getting destroyed.

I'm bringing this up here because two of the advanced stubborn fat protocols (SFP 1.0 and 2.0) are very intense and dieters who lose sight of the above can cause themselves real problems. Those protocols simply cannot be done daily or even every other day under most circumstances. At best, the SFP1.0/2.0 can be done twice weekly with the very occasional trainee surviving three times per week. I mentioned repeatedly throughout this book to limit HIIT to twice weekly under most conditions and both protocols are HIIT based. Women are absolutely unique compared to men but almost nobody is unique enough to handle that amount of truly high-intensity work. The logical extension of this being that the protocols can and should be mixed. The interval protocols may be done 1-2X weekly with the other protocols making up the remainder of training.

The Phantom Tingle

When performing the stubborn fat protocols, and this seems to be more prevalent following a a day at maintenance or higher calories, some people report sort of an itchiness or tingle in their lower body. It's not universal but it's common enough for me to describe. It doesn't necessarily mean anything in terms of fat loss per se (actual fat loss is the only true metric of fat loss but remember how water retention and such can mask it) but it seems to be associated with drops in hip and thigh skinfolds over time. Often the fat in this area will get a little bit squishy or dimpled visually (and it feels different, softer than the typical very hard hip and thigh fat) and this usually comes before a whoosh and visible fat loss. I suspect that the tingle is due to increased blood flow and an absence of the tingle should not be taken as a lack of effectiveness or fat loss in the area. And with that let me present the protocols themselves.

Protocol 1: LISS with a Low-Carbohydrate Diet

As I stated, very low-carbohydrate diets (below 100 g/day) have a naturally fat mobilizing effect on the lower body fat but not all dieters are happy with them. They can make a lot of women depressed although this is highly variable and can be dealt with slightly with 5-HTP. Category 1 dieters with PCOS/hyperandrogenism often benefit from low-carbohydrate diets and the already moderated carb luteal phase diet can be adjusted by bringing carbs down further and increasing dietary fat. Very active dieters find that their training performance suffers due to glycogen depletion and they eventually have to insert a day at maintenance (this should be done as a matter of course). This approach can be useful for female dieters who can't use, won't use or simply can't get yohimbine (it's banned in some countries).

Protocol 2: LISS with Yohimbine

For females who can't or won't follow a low-carbohydrate diet, adding oral yohimbine (0.2 mg/kg or 0.09 mg/lb) and caffeine (200 mg) an hour before fasted low-intensity cardio will have the same effect. As always start with a half-dose for the first few days and then bring it up to assess your personal response. Remember that yohimbine builds up in the system (working better over time) but can cause water retention which can mask fat loss. It must be dropped at least a week out from a competition to allow water loss to occur. While yohimbine would ideally be used before morning fasted cardio this is not always possible. If a dieter is doing cardio after their weight workout, it should be taken an hour before the cardio will start. If they must do cardio after having eaten, it should be done 3-4 hours after that meal. Recall that yohimbine is banned in many federations and causes anxiety in some women so it it not for everyone.

Protocol 3: The Original Stubborn Fat 1.0 Protocol

The original Stubborn Fat Protocol (SFP 1.0) was developed over a decade ago based on what I knew about the topic at the time and many readers may have seen it reproduced (usually without credit to me) in various places. Most of the physiology underlying it was discussed earlier in this book but the basic idea is to use a short HIIT (using longer intervals) to generate a hormonal response that has a profound fat mobilizing effect and overcomes the normal resistance to mobilization of stubborn fat. At the time I was focused on the adrenaline and noradrenaline response although atrial natriuretic peptide (ANP), which I discussed earlier in the book, is likely to be highly involved in this as well.

For reasons discussed in more detail in my original book, while high intensity exercise mobilizes fatty acids within the fat cells, they are often trapped in there to some degree, being released only after about 5 minutes. This explains the short break after the HIIT session. Once those fatty acids have been released into the bloodstream, they must be burned off with some amount of LISS so that they are not re-esterified within either the lower body fat cells or elsewhere.

> 1. Ideally this should be done first thing in the morning but it can be done after weights or at least 3-4 hours after a meal
> 2. Take 200 mg of caffeine an hour before. If you drink coffee, take it black.
> 3. Do a 5-10' easy warmup (RPE 3-4)
> 4. 10 total minutes of interval training. 10X1' on/1' off would be appropriate at an RPE of 7.
> 5. Rest completely for 5 minutes. Get a drink of water, change machines if you want.
> 6. Perform 20-40 minutes of LISS (RPE 3-4)

Let me reiterate that the above protocol is intense and should not even be considered more than once or twice weekly, especially on a background of intense weight training. It can actually be used by endurance athletes who are approaching extreme levels of leanness as well as it can act as a quality workout. Other types of female athletes who need to achieve extreme levels of leanness may be able to use it as written or modify it slightly based on the specifics of their sport. As I described in Chapter 28, the choice of activity for the HIIT should be based on safety above all. Cycling, rowing, elliptical machines or perhaps a Stair Stepper are far superior to attempting to run intervals for all but trained runners or sprinters. As well, there is at least some indication that more calories (and potentially fat) will be burned by performing the LISS on a different machine than a person typically uses. So a trainee might do their warm-up and HIIT on a bicycle before taking a 5' break and then walking briskly on a treadmill or using the EFX to perform their LISS.

Protocol 4: The Stubborn Fat Protocol 2.0

Deriving from the first protocol, the Stubborn Fat Protocol 2.0 (SFP 2.0) was developed solely for **The Stubborn Fat Solution**. The basic idea behind the protocol is similar to the first in that it uses a HIIT workout to mobilize fatty acids, a short break so that they can be released into the bloodstream and then LISS to oxidize those fatty acids. This is then followed by another short HIIT session with the goal of generating at least a small post-workout calorie burn to burn off whatever fatty acids remain in the bloodstream (preventing their re-storage). Readers may note that the initial HIIT session is based around shorter intervals, this is to generate a maximal hormonal response in terms of adrenaline/noradrenaline and ANP without causing the same "trapping" effect of the fatty acids within the fat cell. The post-LISS HIIT work is longer to generate more metabolic stress to generate the largest post-exercise calorie burn possible. It will also deplete muscle glycogen to further increase fatty acid oxidation.

1. Ideally this should be done first thing in the morning but it can be done after weights or at least 3-4 hours after a meal
2. Take 200 mg of caffeine an hour before. If you drink coffee, take it black.
3. Do a 5-10' easy warmup (RPE 3-4)
4. 5 total minutes of interval training. 5X15-20" second intervals with 40-45 second rest at an RPE of 7-8.
5. Rest completely for 5 minutes. Get a drink of water, change machines if you want.
6. Perform 20-40 minutes of LISS (RPE 3-4)
7. Do another 5-10 minutes of longer intervals. 5-10X1' on/1' off maximum.
8. Perform 3-5 minutes for cool-down.

Compared to the SFP 1.0, SFP 2.0 is an extreme step up in difficulty. Even those dieters who are able to include the SFP 1.0 may find the above too demanding in which case it should be eliminated in favor of the SFP 1.0 and the two LISS only protocols. The same comments above in terms of the HIIT and LISS hold here. The choice of exercise machine for both HIIT segments should be based around safety with only trained runners or sprinters even considering that as an activity. All other trainees should stay with the bike, rower, elliptical, etc. A different machine can be done for the LISS portion if desired and the trainee should move back to a safe mode of exercise for the second round of HIIT.

References

Chapter 1: Introduction to Women's Physiology
1. "Gender Differences in Metabolism." Edited by Mark Tarnopolsky. (1999) CRC Press: Boca Raton, FL.
2. Robertson C1 et. al. should weight loss and maintenance programmes be designed differently for men? A systematic review of long-term randomised controlled trials presenting data for men and women: The ROMEO project. Obes Res Clin Pract. (2016) 10(1):70-84.
3. "Women, Sports and Performance, A Physiological Perspective, 2nd Edition" Edited by Wells, CL. 1991, Champaign, Ill. Human Kinetics.
4. Charniga, A. "A De-Masculinzation of Strength" 2012: Michigan: Sportnivny Press
5. Anderson LA et. al.The effects of androgens and estrogens on preadipocyte proliferation in human adipose tissue: influence of gender and site. J Clin Endocrinol Metab. (2001) 86(10):5045-51.
6. Mazzeo SE1, Bulik CM. Environmental and genetic risk factors for eating disorders: what the clinician needs to know. Child Adolesc Psychiatr Clin N Am. (2009) 18(1):67-82.
8. Strother, E et. al. Eating Disorders in Men: Underdiagnosed, Undertreated, and Misunderstood. Eat Disord. (2012) 20(5): 346–355
9. Coelho GM et. al. Prevention of eating disorders in female athletes. J Sports Med. (2014) 5:105–113.
10. Keating C. Sex differences precipitating anorexia nervosa in females: the estrogen paradox and a novel framework for targeting sex-specific neurocircuits and behavior.Curr Top Behav Neurosci. (2011) 8:189-20
11. Hönekopp J et al. Second to fourth digit length ratio (2D:4D) and adult sex hormone levels: new data and a meta-analytic review. Psychoneuroendocrinology. (2007) 32(4):313-21.
12. Fink B et. al. Second to fourth digit ratio, body mass index, waist-to-hip ratio, and waist-to-chest ratio: their relationships in heterosexual men and women. Ann Hum Biol. (2003) 30(6):728-38.
13. Hampson E et. al. On the relation between 2D:4D and sex-dimorphic personality traits. Arch Sex Behav. (2008) 37(1):133-44.
14. Moffit DM1, Swanik CB. The association between athleticism, prenatal testosterone, and finger length. J Strength Cond Res. (2011) 25(4):1085-8.
15. Bookstein, FL. et. al. Second to fourth digit ratio and face shape. Proc Biol Sci. (2005) 272(1576): 1995–2001.
16. Meindl K. et. al.Second-to-fourth digit ratio and facial shape in boys: the lower the digit ratio, the more robust the face. Proc Biol Sci. (2012) 279(1737): 2457–2463.
17. DeLecce TL et al. Sociosexual orientation and 2D:4D ratios in women: Relationship to men's desirability ratings as a long-term pair bond. Arch Sex Behav. (2014) 43(2):319-27.
18. Discussed briefly at http://sheltongstevens.blogspot.com/2014/04/a-look-behind-gold-of-chinese.html
19. Valla, J and Stephen Ceci. Can Sex Differences in Science Be Tied to the Long Reach of Prenatal Hormones? Brain Organization Theory, Digit Ratio (2D/4D), and Sex Differences in Preferences and Cognition Perspect Psychol Sci. (2011) 6(2): 134–136.
20. Alexander GM. Associations among gender-linked toy preferences, spatial ability, and digit ratio: evidence from eye-tracking analysis. Arch Sex Behav. (2006) 35(6):699-709.
21. Hines M et. al.Testosterone during pregnancy and gender role behavior of preschool children: a longitudinal, population study. Child Dev. (2002) 73(6):1678-87.
22. Honk, J et. al. P Testosterone administration impairs cognitive empathy in women depending on second-to-fourth digit ratio. Proc Natl Acad Sci U S A. (2011) 108(8): 3448–3452.
23. Benderlioglu Z an RJ Nelson. Digit length ratios predict reactive aggression in women, but not in men. Horm Behav. (2004) 46(5):558-64.
24. Klump KL et. al.Sex Differences in Binge Eating: Gonadal Hormone Effects Across Development.Annu Rev Clin Psychol. (2017) 13:183-207
25. Wrublevsky EP. Individual approach to women's training in speed and power track and field events. New Studies in Athletics. (2004) 4:17-26

Chapter 2: The Normal Menstrual Cycle
1. Ryu A, Kim TH. Premenstrual syndrome: A mini review. Maturitas. (2015) 82(4):436-40
1a. Bernardi, Mariagiulia et al. "Dysmenorrhea and Related Disorders." F1000Research 6 (2017): 1645. PMC. Web. 2 Oct. 2017.
2. Stevens J. Obesity, fat patterning and cardiovascular risk. Adv Exp Med Biol. (1995) 369:21-7.
3. Baghaei F et. al. The lean woman. Obes Res. 2(002) 10(2):115-21.
4. Gems D. Evolution of sexually dimorphic longevity in humans. Aging. (2014) 6(2):84-91
5. Escobar-Morreale HF et .al. The striking similarities in the metabolic associations of female androgen excess and male androgen deficiency. Hum Reprod. (2014) 29(10):2083-91.
6. Sherwin BB. Estrogen and cognitive functioning in women. Endocr Rev. (2003) 24(2):133-51.
7. Pedersen SB et. al. Estrogen controls lipolysis by up-regulating alpha2A-adrenergic receptors directly in human adipose tissue through the estrogen receptor alpha. Implications for the female fat distribution. J Clin Endocrinol Metab. (2004) 89(4):1869-78.

8. Gavin KM et. al. Estradiol effects on subcutaneous adipose tissue lipolysis in premenopausal women are adipose tissue depot specific and treatment dependent. Am J Physiol Endocrinol Metab. (2013) 304(11):E1167-74

9. Avram MM.Cellulite: a review of its physiology and treatment. J Cosmet Laser Ther. (2004) 6(4):181-5.

9a. Price TM et. al. Estrogen regulation of adipose tissue lipoprotein lipase--possible mechanism of body fat distribution. Am J Obstet Gynecol. (1998) 178(1 Pt 1):101-7.

10. Lundsgaard AM AND B Kiens. Gender Differences in Skeletal Muscle Substrate Metabolism – Molecular Mechanisms and Insulin Sensitivity Front Endocrinol (Lausanne). (2014) 5: 195

11. O'Sullivan AJ. Does oestrogen allow women to store fat more efficiently? A biological advantage for fertility and gestation. Obes Rev. (2009) 10(2):168-77.

12. Brown LM1, Clegg DJ.Central effects of estradiol in the regulation of food intake, body weight, and adiposity. J Steroid Biochem Mol Biol. (2010) 122(1-3):65-73.

13. Gao Q and TL Horvath. Cross-talk between estrogen and leptin signaling in the hypothalamus. Am J Physiol Endocrinol Metab. (2008) 294(5):E817-26.

14. L Davidsen et. al. Impact of the menstrual cycle on determinants of energy balance: a putative role in weight loss attempts. International Journal of Obesity (2007) 31: 887-890

15. Tiidus PM. Estrogen and gender effects on muscle damage, inflammation, and oxidative stress. Can J Appl Physiol. (2000) 25(4):274-87.

16. Hansen M1, Kjaer M. Influence of sex and estrogen on musculotendinous protein turnover at rest and after exercise. Exerc Sport Sci Rev. (2014) 42(4):183-92.

16a. Hallam J et. al. Gender-related Differences in Food Craving and Obesity. Yale J Biol Med. (2016) 89(2):161-73.

16b. Arnoni-Bauer Y et. al. Is It Me or My Hormones? Neuroendocrine Activation Profiles to Visual Food Stimuli Across the Menstrual Cycle. J Clin Endocrinol Metab. (2017) 102(9):3406-3414.

17. Hirschberg AL et. al. Sex hormones, appetite and eating behaviour in women. Maturitas.(2012) 71(3):248-56.

17a. Rebuffe-Scrive M et. al. Effect of local application of progesterone on human adipose tissue lipoprotein lipase. Horm Metab Res. (1983) 15(11):566.

18. Saleh J. Acylation stimulating protein: a female lipogenic factor? Obes Rev. (2011) 12(6):440-8.

19. Colagiuri S1, Brand Miller J. The 'carnivore connection'--evolutionary aspects of insulin resistance. Eur J Clin Nutr. (2002) 56: (Suppl 1):S30-5.

20. Parry BL et. al.Increased sensitivity to light-induced melatonin suppression in premenstrual dysphoric disorder. Chronobiol Int. (2010) 27(7):1438-53.

21. Biggs WS1, Demuth RH. Premenstrual syndrome and premenstrual dysphoric disorder.Am Fam Physician. (2011) 84(8):918-24.

21a. Hahn PM et. al.Menopausal-like hot flashes reported in women of reproductive age. Fertil Steril. (1998) 70(5):913-8.

21b. Amanda Daley.The role of exercise in the treatment of menstrual disorders: the evidence. Br J Gen Pract. (2009) 59: 241–242.

22. Oladosu FA et. al. NSAID resistance in dysmenorrhea: epidemiology, causes, and treatment. Am J Obstet Gynecol. (2017) Sep 6.

23. Lombardi A et. al. Regulation of skeletal muscle mitochondrial activity by thyroid hormones: focus on the "old" triiodothyronine and the "emerging" 3,5-diiodothyronine. Front Physiol. (2015) 21;6:237.

24. Santin AP and TW Furlanetto. Role of Estrogen in Thyroid Function and Growth Regulation. J Thyroid Res. (2011) 2011: 875125.

25. Biondi B and L Wartofsky. Combination treatment with T4 and T3: toward personalized replacement therapy in hypothyroidism? J Clin Endocrinol Metab. (2012) 97(7):2256-71.

26. Park HK an RS Ahima. Physiology of leptin: energy homeostasis, neuroendocrine function and metabolism. Metabolism. (2015) 64(1):24-34.

Chapter 3: Hormonal Modifiers

1. Badawy A and A Elnashar. Treatment options for polycystic ovary syndrome Int J Womens Health. (2011) 3: 25–35.

1a. Ovesen P et. al. Normal basal and insulin-stimulated fuel metabolism in lean women with the polycystic ovary syndrome. J Clin Endocrinol Metab. (1993) 77(6):1636-40.

1b. Goyal M and AS Dawood. Debates Regarding Lean Patients with Polycystic Ovary Syndrome: A Narrative Review J Hum Reprod Sci. (2017) 10(3): 154–161.

1c. Kowalczyk K et. al. Thyroid disorders in polycystic ovary syndrome. Eur Rev Med Pharmacol Sci. (2017) 21(2):346-360.

2. Harrison CL et. al. The impact of intensified exercise training on insulin resistance and fitness in overweight and obese women with and without polycystic ovary syndrome. Clin Endocrinol (Oxf). (2012) 76(3):351-7

2a. Awdishu S et. al. Oligomenorrhoea in exercising women: a polycystic ovarian syndrome phenotype or distinct entity? Sports Med. (2009) 39(12):1055-69.

3. Rickenlund A et. al. Hyperandrogenicity is an alternative mechanism underlying oligomenorrhea or amenorrhea in female athletes and may improve physical performance. Fertil Steril. (2003) 79(4):947-55.

4. Hagmar M et. al. Hyperandrogenism may explain reproductive dysfunction in olympic athletes. Med Sci Sports Exerc. (2009) 41(6):1241-8.

5. Collins DC. Sex hormone receptor binding, progestin selectivity, and the new oral contraceptives. Am J Obstet Gynecol. (1994) 170(5 Pt 2):1508-13.

6. Y. Zimmerman et. al. The effect of combined oral contraception on testosterone levels in healthy women: a systematic review and meta-analysis Hum Reprod Update. (2014) 20(1): 76–105.

6a. Caruso S et al. Improvement of Low Sexual Desire Due to Antiandrogenic Combined Oral Contraceptives After Switching to an Oral Contraceptive Containing 17β-Estradiol. J Womens Health (Larchmt). (2017) Mar 21. [Epub ahead of print]

7. Lopez LM et. al. Steroidal contraceptives: effect on carbohydrate metabolism in women without diabetes mellitus. Cochrane Database Syst Rev. (2014) 30;4:CD006133.

8. Gallo MF et. al. Combination contraceptives: effects on weight. Cochrane Database Syst Rev. (2014) 29;1:CD003987.

9. Uras R et. al. Evidence that in healthy young women, a six-cycle treatment with oral contraceptive containing 30 mcg of ethinylestradiol plus 2 mg of chlormadinone acetate reduces fat mass. Contraception. (2009) 79(2):117-21.

10. Lopez LM et. al. Progestin-only contraceptives: effects on weight. Cochrane Database Syst Rev. (2016) Aug 28;8:CD008815.

11. Berenson, AB and Mahbubur Rahman. Changes in weight, total fat, percent body fat, and central-to-peripheral fat ratio associated with injectable and oral contraceptive use. Am J Obstet Gynecol. (2009) 200(3): 329.e1–329

12. Steward RG et. al.The impact of short-term depot-medroxyprogesterone acetate treatment on resting metabolic rate. Contraception. (2016) 93(4):317-322

12a. Basu T et. al. The Effect of Depo Medroxyprogesterone Acetate (DMPA) on Cerebral Food Motivation Centers: A Pilot Study using Functional Magnetic Resonance Imaging. Contraception. (2016) 94(4):321-7

12b. Diffey B et. al.The effect of oral contraceptive agents on the basal metabolic rate of young women.Br J Nutr. (1997)77(6):853-62.

12c. Dal'Ava N et. al. Body weight and composition in users of levonorgestrel-releasing intrauterine system. Contraception. (2012) 86(4):350-3.

12d. Santos deNazare et. al. Changes in Body Composition in Women using Long-acting Reversible Contraception. Contraception. (2016) 95(4):382-389.

12e. Rosenberg M.Weight change with oral contraceptive use and during the menstrual cycle. Results of daily measurements. Contraception. 1998 58(6):345-9.

12f. Zevidah V et. al. Weight Change at 12 Months in Users of Three Progestin-Only Contraceptive Methods. Contraception. (2013) 88(4): 503–508.

12g. Grimes DA1, Schulz KF. Nonspecific side effects of oral contraceptives: nocebo or noise? Contraception. (2011) 83(1):5-9.1

13. Griffin L et. al. Postpartum Weight Loss in Overweight and Obese Women Using the Etonogestrel Subdermal Implant: a Pilot Study. Contraception. (2017) 95(6):564-570

13a. Liu SL and CM Lebrun. Effect of oral contraceptives and hormone replacement therapy on bone mineral density in premenopausal and perimenopausal women: a systematic review Br J Sports Med. (2006) 40(1): 11–24.

13b. Lopez LM et. al. Steroidal contraceptives and bone fractures in women: evidence from observational studies.Cochrane Database Syst Rev. 2015 Jul 21;(7):CD009849.

14. Diamanti-Kandarakis E, HA Kandarakis. Obesity and gonadal function of women.Pediatr Endocrinol Rev.(2004) Suppl 3:465-70.

15.Baker LJ and PM O'Brien. Premenstrual syndrome (PMS): a peri-menopausal perspective. Maturitas. (2012) 72:121-5.

16. S Chakravarti et.al. Hormonal profiles after the menopause. British Medical Journal (1976) 2: 784-786.

17. Burger H1. The menopausal transition--endocrinology.J Sex Med. (2008) 5(10):2266-73.

18. Markopoulos MC et. al. Hyperandrogenism after menopause. European Journal of Endocrinology (2015) 172: R79–R91.

19. Poehlman ET. Menopause, energy expenditure, and body composition. Acta Obstet Gynecol Scand. (2002) 81(7):603-11.

20. Simkin-Silverman LR and RR Wing. Weight gain during menopause. Is it inevitable or can it be prevented? Postgrad Med. (2000) 108(3):47-50, 53-6.

20a. Norman RJ et. al. Oestrogen and progestogen hormone replacement therapy for peri-menopausal and post-menopausal women: weight and body fat distribution. Cochrane Database Syst Rev. (2000) 2: CD001018.

21. Verkooijen HM et. al.The incidence of breast cancer and changes in the use of hormone replacement therapy: a review of the evidence. Maturitas. (2009) 64(2):80-5.

22. Gurney EP et. al. The Women's Health Initiative trial and related studies: 10 years later: a clinician's view. J Steroid Biochem Mol Biol. (2014) 142:4-11.

23. Hodis HN and WJ Mack. Hormone replacement therapy and the association with coronary heart disease and overall mortality: clinical application of the timing hypothesis. J Steroid Biochem Mol Biol. (2014) 142:68-75

24. Sood R et. al. Prescribing menopausal hormone therapy: an evidence-based approach Int J Womens Health. (2014) 6: 47–57.

25. Wild RA1, Manson JE2. Insights from the Women's Health Initiative: individualizing risk assessment for hormone therapy decisions. Semin Reprod Med. (2014) 32(6):433-7.

26. Palacios S1.Advances in hormone replacement therapy: making the menopause manageable. BMC Womens Health. (2008) 8:22.

27. Genant HK et. al.Low-dose esterified estrogen therapy: effects on bone, plasma estradiol concentrations, endometrium, and lipid levels. Estratab/Osteoporosis Study Group. Arch Intern Med. (1997) Dec 157(22):2609-15.

28. North American Menopause Society. The role of testosterone therapy in postmenopausal women: position statement of The North American Menopause Society. Menopause. (2005) 12(5):496-511

29. Maia H et,al.Testosterone replacement therapy in the climacteric: benefits beyond sexuality.Gynecol Endocrinol. (2009) 25:12-20.

30. Goodman MP. Are all estrogens created equal? A review of oral vs. transdermal therapy. J Womens Health (Larchmt). (2012) (2):161-9.

31. Ho KK. Metabolic effects of oestrogens: impact of the route of administration. Ann Endocrinol (Paris). (2003) 64(2):170-7.

32. Irahara M etl al. Associations of estrogen and testosterone with insulin resistance in pre- and postmenopausal women with and without hormone therapy. Int J Endocrinol Metab. (2013) 11(2):65-70.

33. Fineberg SE. Glycaemic control and hormone replacement therapy: implications of the Postmenopausal Estrogen/Progestogen Intervention (PEPI) study. Drugs Aging. (2000) 17(6):453-61.

34. Haney AF an RA Wild.Options for hormone therapy in women who have had a hysterectomy.Menopause (2007) 14(3 Pt 2):592-7.

35. Files JA. et. al. Bioidentical Hormone Therapy Mayo Clin Proc. (2011) 86(7): 673–680.

36. Holtorf K. The bioidentical hormone debate: are bioidentical hormones (estradiol, estriol, and progesterone) safer or more efficacious than commonly used synthetic versions in hormone replacement. Postgrad Med.(2009) 121:73-85.

37. L'hermite M et. al.Could transdermal estradiol + progesterone be a safer postmenopausal HRT? A review. Maturitas. (2008) 60(3-4):185-201.

38. Schmidt JW et. al. Hormone replacement therapy in menopausal women: Past problems and future possibilities. Gynecol Endocrinol. (2006) 22(10):564-77.

39. L'Hermite M. Bioidentical menopausal hormone therapy: registered hormones (non-oral estradiol ± progesterone) are optimal. Climacteric. (2017) 16:1-8.

40. Grandi G et. al. Estradiol in hormonal contraception: real evolution or just same old wine in a new bottle? Eur J Contracept Reprod Health Care. (2017) 22(4):245-246.

Chapter 5: What is Body Composition?

1. Sidossis L, Kajimura S. Brown and beige fat in humans: thermogenic adipocytes that control energy and glucose homeostasis. J Clin Invest. (2015) 125(2):478-86.

2. Galic S et. al. Adipose tissue as an endocrine organ Mol Cell Endocrinol. (2010) 316(2):129-39.

3. Hassan M et. al.Adipose tissue: friend or foe? Nat Rev Cardiol. (2012) 9(12):689-702.

4. Hamdy O et. al.Metabolic obesity: the paradox between visceral and subcutaneous fat. Curr Diabetes Rev. (2006) 2(4):367-73.

5. Kreitzman SN et. al. Glycogen storage: illusions of easy weight loss, excessive weight regain, and distortions in estimates of body composition. Am J Clin Nutr (1992) 56: 292S-293S.

6. Ross R1, Bradshaw AJ. The future of obesity reduction: beyond weight loss.Nat Rev Endocrinol.(2009) 5(6):319-25.

Chapter 6: Measuring and Tracking Body Composition

1. Prado CM et. al.Body composition phenotypes and obesity paradox. Curr Opin Clin Nutr Metab Care. (2015) 18(6):535-51.

2. Deurenberg, P et. al. Body mass index as a measure of body fatness: age- and sex-specific prediction formulas. Br J Nutr. (1991) 65(2):105-14.

3. Ball S et. al. Comparison of anthropometry to dual energy X-ray absorptiometry: a new prediction equation for women. Res Q Exerc Sport. (2004) Sep;75(3):248-58.

4. Steinberg DM et. al. Weighing every day matters: daily weighing improves weight loss and adoption of weight control behaviors. J Acad Nutr Diet. (2015) 115(4):511-8.

5. Levistky, DA et. al. Monitoring weight daily blocks the freshman weight gain: a model for combating the epidemic of obesity. Int J Obes (Lond). (2006) 30(6):1003-10.

6. Butryn ML et. al. Consistent self-monitoring of weight: a key component of successful weight loss maintenance. Obesity (Silver Spring). (2007) 15(12):3091-6.

7. Stevens J et. al. The definition of weight maintenance. Int J Obes (Lond). (2006) 30(3):391-9.

8. Benn Y et. al. What is the psychological impact of self-weighing? A meta-analysis Health Psychol Rev. (2016) 10(2): 187–203.

9. Stachoń AJ. Menstrual Changes in Body Composition of Female Athletes. Coll Antropol. (2016) 40(2):111-22.

Chapter 7: Altering Body Composition

1. McClave SA, Snider HL. Dissecting the energy needs of the body. Curr Opin Clin Nutr Metab Care. (2001) 4(2):143-7.

1a. Lemmer JT et. al.Effect of strength training on resting metabolic rate and physical activity: age and gender comparisons. Med Sci Sports Exerc. (2001) 33(4):532-41.

1b. Cullinen K1, Caldwell M. Weight training increases fat-free mass and strength in untrained young women. J Am Diet Assoc. (1998) 98(4):414-8.

2. Marks BL and JM Rippe.The importance of fat free mass maintenance in weight loss programmes.Sports Med. (1996) 22(5):273-81.

3. Dulloo AG et. al. How dieting makes the lean fatter: from a perspective of body composition autoregulation through adipostats and proteinstats awaiting discovery. Obes Rev. (2015) 16 Suppl 1:25-35

4. Phillips SM. A brief review of critical processes in exercise-induced muscular hypertrophy Sports Med. (2014) Suppl 1:S71-7.

4a. Häkkinen K et. al. Neuromuscular adaptations and serum hormones in women during short-term intensive strength training. Eur J Appl Physiol Occup Physiol. (1992) 64(2):106-11.

5. Tchoukalova YD et. al. Regional differences in cellular mechanisms of adipose tissue gain with overfeeding. Proc Natl Acad Sci USA. (2010) 107(42):18226-31.

6. Shah M and A. Garg. High-fat and high-carbohydrate diets and energy balance. Diabetes Care. (1996) 19(10):1142-52.

7. Hellerstein MK. De novo lipogenesis in humans: metabolic and regulatory aspects. Eur J Clin Nutr. (1999) 53 (Suppl 1):S53-65.

8. Shadid S et. al. Direct free fatty acid uptake into human adipocytes in vivo: relation to body fat distribution. Diabetes.(2007) 56(5):1369-75.

9. Jensen MD. Cytokine regulation of lipolysis in humans? J Clin Endocrinol Metab. (2003) 88:3003-4.

10. Langin D et al.Millennium fat-cell lipolysis reveals unsuspected novel tracks. Horm Metab Res. (2000) 32(11-12):443-52.

11. Frayn KN and F Karpe. Regulation of human subcutaneous adipose tissue blood flow. Int J Obes (Lond). (2014) 38(8):1019-26.

12. White UA and YD Tchoukalova. Sex dimorphism and depot differences in adipose tissue function. Biochim Biophys Acta. (2014) 1842(3): 377–392.

13. Rebuffé-Scrive M, et. al. Metabolism of mammary, abdominal, and femoral adipocytes in women before and after menopause. Metabolism. (1986) 35(9):792-7.

Chapter 8: Energy Balance

1. Weyer C et. al.Determinants of energy expenditure and fuel utilization in man: effects of body composition, age, sex, ethnicity and glucose tolerance in 916 subjects. Int J Obes Relat Metab Disord. (1999) 23(7):715-22.

2. Levine JA. Non-exercise activity thermogenesis (NEAT).Best Pract Res Clin Endocrinol Metab. (2002) 16(4):679-702.

3. Donahoo WT et. al. Variability in energy expenditure and its components. Curr Opin Clin Nutr Metab Care. (2004) 7(6):599-605.

4. Garland T Jr et. al.The biological control of voluntary exercise, spontaneous physical activity and daily energy expenditure in relation to obesity:human and rodent perspectives. J Exp Biol. (2011) 214:206-29.

5. Thomas DM et. al. Can a weight loss of one pound a week be achieved with a 3500-kcal deficit? Commentary on a commonly accepted rule.Int J Obes (Lond). (2013) 37(12):1611-3.

6. Heymsfield SB et. al. Energy content of weight loss: kinetic features during voluntary caloric restriction. Metabolism. (2012) 61(7):937-43.

7. Dhurandhar EJ et. al. Predicting adult weight change in the real world: a systematic review and meta-analysis accounting for compensatory changes in energy intake or expenditure. Int J Obes (Lond) (2015) 39(8):1181-7.

8. Trexler ET et. al. Metabolic adaptation to weight loss: implications for the athlete. J Int Soc Sports Nutr. (2014) 27;11(1):7.

Chapter 9: Metabolic Adaptation

1. Maclean PS et al.Biology's response to dieting: the impetus for weight regain. Am J Physiol Regul Integr Comp Physiol. (2011) 301(3):R581-600.

2.Melanson EL et. al.Resistance to exercise-induced weight loss: compensatory behavioral adaptations Med Sci Sports Exerc. (2013) 45(8): 1600–1609.

3. Shetty PS. Adaptation to low energy intakes: the responses and limits to low intakes in infants, children and adults. Eur J Clin Nutr. (1999) 53 (Suppl 1):S14-33.

4. Tremblay A et. al. Adaptive thermogenesis can make a difference in the ability of obese individuals to lose body weight. Int J Obes (Lond). (2013) 37(6):759-64.

5. Rosenbaum M and Leibel RL.Adaptive thermogenesis in humans.Int J Obes (Lond).(2010) 34 (Suppl 1) :S47-55.

6.. Redman LM et. al. Metabolic and behavioral compensations in response to caloric restriction: implications for the maintenance of weight loss. (2009) PLos One 4: e4377

7. Tremblay A et. al.Adaptive thermogenesis can make a difference in the ability of obese individuals to lose body weight. Int J Obes (Lond). (2013) 37(6):759-64

8. Dulloo AG et. al. Autoregulation of body composition during weight recovery in human: the Minnesota Experiment revisited. Int J Obes Relat Metab Disord. (1996) 20(5):393-405.

9. Lutter M, Nestler EJ. Homeostatic and hedonic signals interact in the regulation of food intake. J Nutr. (2009) 139(3):629-32.

10. Volkow ND et. al. Obesity and addiction: neurobiological overlaps. Obes Rev. (2013) 14(1):2-18.

11. Stice E et. al. Relation of obesity to consummatory and anticipatory food reward. Physiol Behav. (2009) 97(5):551-60.

12. Huda M et. al. Gut peptides and the regulation of appetite. Obes Rev. (2006) 7(2):163-82.

13. Dulloo AG et. al. Poststarvation hyperphagia and body fat overshooting in humans: a role for feedback signals from lean and fat tissues. Am J Clin Nutr. (1997) 65(3):717-23.

14. King NA et. al. Exercise, appetite and weight management: understanding the compensatory responses in eating behaviour and how they contribute to variability in exercise-induced weight loss. Br J Sports Med. (2012) 46(5):315-22.

15. Finlayson G et. ao. Low fat loss response after medium-term supervised exercise in obese is associated with exercise-induced increase in food reward. J Obes. (2011) pii: 615624.

16. Hazell TJ et. al. Effects of exercise intensity on plasma concentrations of appetite-regulating hormones: Potential mechanisms. Appetite. (2016) 98: 80–88

17. Rossow, LM. Natural bodybuilding competition preparation and recovery: a 12-month case study. Int J Sports Physiol Perform. (2013) 8(5):582-92

18. Müller MJ et. al.Metabolic adaptation to caloric restriction and subsequent refeeding: the Minnesota Starvation Experiment revisited. Am J Clin Nutr. (2015) 102(4):807-19

19. Johannsen DL et. al. Metabolic slowing with massive weight loss despite preservation of fat-free mass. J Clin Endocrinol Metab. (2012) 97(7):2489-96.

20. Weigle DS et. al.Weight loss leads to a marked decrease in nonresting energy expenditure in ambulatory human subjects. Metabolism. (1988) 37(10):930-6.

21. Rosenbaum M et. al. Effects of experimental weight perturbation on skeletal muscle work efficiency in human subjects. Am J Physiol Regul Integr Comp Physiol. (2003) 285(1):R183-92.

21a. Weigle DA and JD Brunzell. Assessment of energy expenditure in ambulatory reduced-obese subjects by the techniques of weight stabilization and exogenous weight replacement. Int J Obes. (1990) 14 (Suppl 1):69-77.

22. Martin CK et. al.Effect of calorie restriction on the free-living physical activity levels of nonobese humans: results of three randomized trials. J Appl Physiol (1985). (2011) 110(4):956-63.

23. Weyer C et. al.Energy metabolism after 2 y of energy restriction: the biosphere 2 experiment.Am J Clin Nutr. (2000) 72(4):946-53.

24. Reinhardt M et. al. A Human Thrifty Phenotype Associated With Less Weight Loss During Caloric Restriction. Diabetes.(2015) 64(8):2859-67

25. Pontzer H. Constrained Total Energy Expenditure and the Evolutionary Biology of Energy Balance.
 Exerc Sport Sci Rev. (2015) 43(3):110-6.

26. Donnelly JE et. al. Effects of a 16-month randomized controlled exercise trial on body weight and composition in young, overweight men and women: the Midwest Exercise Trial. Arch Intern Med. (2003) 163(11):1343-50

27. Bayon V et. al. Sleep debt and obesity. Ann Med. (2014) 46(5):264-72.27.

28. Teske JA et. al. Neuropeptidergic mediators of spontaneous physical activity and non-exercise activity thermogenesis. Neuroendocrinology. (2008) 87(2):71-90.

29. Hall KD. Body fat and fat-free mass inter-relationships: Forbes's theory revisited. Br J Nutr. (2007) 97(6):1059-63.

30. Rosenbaum M et. al. Long-term persistence of adaptive thermogenesis in subjects who have maintained a reduced body weight. Am J Clin Nutr. (2008) 88(4):906-12.

31. Astrup A et. al.Meta-analysis of resting metabolic rate in formerly obese subjects. Am J Clin Nutr. (1999) 69(6):1117-22.

32. Swift DL et. al.The role of exercise and physical activity in weight loss and maintenance. Prog Cardiovasc Dis (2014) 56(4):441-7.

33. Harris AM et. al. Weekly changes in basal metabolic rate with eight weeks of overfeeding. Obesity (Silver Spring). (2006) 14(4):690-5.31.

34. Tremblay A et. al.Overfeeding and energy expenditure in humans.Am J Clin Nutr.(1992) 56(5):857-62.

35. Levine JA et. al. Role of nonexercise activity thermogenesis in resistance to fat gain in humans. Science. (1999) 283(5399):212-4.

36. Wijers SL et. al. Individual thermogenic responses to mild cold and overfeeding are closely related. J Clin Endocrinol Metab. (2007) 92(11):4299-305.

37. Weyer C et. al. Changes in energy metabolism in response to 48 h of overfeeding and fasting in Caucasians and Pima Indians. Int J Obes Relat Metab Disord. (2001) 25(5):593-600.

38. Byrne NM et. al.Influence of distribution of lean body mass on resting metabolic rate after weight loss and weight regain: comparison of responses in white and black women. Am J Clin Nutr. (2003) 77(6):1368-73.

39. van Dale D1, Saris WH. Repetitive weight loss and weight regain: effects on weight reduction, resting metabolic rate, and lipolytic activity before and after exercise and/or diet treatment. Am J Clin Nutr. (1989) 49(3):409-16.

40. Steen SN et. al. Metabolic effects of repeated weight loss and regain in adolescent wrestlers. JAMA. (1988) 260(1):47-50.

41. Polito A et. al. Basal metabolic rate in anorexia nervosa: relation to body composition and leptin concentrations.

Am J Clin Nutr. (2000) 71(6):1495-502.

42. Knuth ND et. al. Metabolic adaptation following massive weight loss is related to the degree of energy imbalance and changes in circulating leptin. Obesity (Silver Spring). (2014) 22(12):2563-9.

43. Rosenbaum M et.al. Low-dose leptin reverses skeletal muscle, autonomic, and neuroendocrine adaptations to maintenance of reduced weight.. J Clin Invest. (2005) 115(12):3579-86.

44. Ravussin Y et. al. A missing link in body weight homeostasis: the catabolic signal of the overfed state.Cell Metab. (2014) 20(4):565-72

45. Schwartz MW et. al. Is the energy homeostasis system inherently biased toward weight gain? Diabetes. (2003) 52(2):232-8.

Chapter 10: Women, Fat Gain and Fat Loss: Part 1

1. Palmer B and DJ CLegg.The sexual dimorphism of obesity. Mol Cell Endocrinol. (2015). 15:113-9.

2. Santosa S and MD Jensen. The Sexual Dimorphism of Lipid Kinetics in Humans. Front Endocrinol (Lausanne). (2015); 6: 103.

3. Blaak E1. Gender differences in fat metabolism. Curr Opin Clin Nutr Metab Care. (2001) 4(6):499-502.

4. Comitato R et. al.Sex hormones and macronutrient metabolism. Crit Rev Food Sci Nutr (2015) 55:227-241.

5. Lovejoy JC et al. Obes Rev. Sex differences in obesity and the regulation of energy homeostasis. (2009) 10(2):154-67.

6. Mauvais-Jarvis F.Sex differences in metabolic homeostasis, diabetes, and obesity. Biol Sex Differ. (2015) 6:14.

7. Karastergiou K et. al. Sex differences in human adipose tissues – the biology of pear shape. Biol Sex Differ. (2012) 3: 13.

8. Power ML1, Schulkin J. Sex differences in fat storage, fat metabolism, and the health risks from obesity: possible evolutionary origins. Br J Nutr. (2008) 99(5):931-40.

9. Geer EB and Wei Shen. Gender Differences in Insulin Resistance, Body Composition, and Energy Balance Gend Med. (2009) 6(Suppl 1): 60–75.

9a. Katch VL et. al. Contribution of breast volume and weight to body fat distribution in females. Am J Phys Anthropol. (1980) 53(1):93-100.

9b. Jannsen I et. al. Skeletal muscle mass and distribution in 468 men and women aged 18–88 yr. J of Applied Physiology (1985) (2000) 89(1): 81-88.

9b. Poehlman ET. Menopause, energy expenditure, and body composition. Acta Obstet Gynecol Scand. (2002) 81(7):603-11.

10. Asarian L1, Geary N.Sex differences in the physiology of eating.   Am J Physiol Regul Integr Comp Physiol. (2013) 305(11):R1215-67.

11. Drewnowski A1 et. al. Food preferences in human obesity: carbohydrates versus fats.Appetite. (1992) 18(3):207-21.

12. Paul DR et. al. Effects of the interaction of sex and food intake on the relation between energy expenditure and body composition. Am J Clin Nutr. (2004) 79(3):385-9.

12a. Brennan IM et. al.Effects of the phases of the menstrual cycle on gastric emptying, glycemia, plasma GLP-1 and insulin, and energy intake in healthy lean women. Am J Physiol Gastrointest Liver Physiol. (2009) 297(3):G602-10.

13. Bryant EJ et. al. Disinhibition: its effects on appetite and weight regulation. Obes Rev. (2008) 9:409-19.

14. Neumark-Sztainer D et. al.Weight control behaviors among adult men and women: cause for concern? Obes Res. (1999)7:179-88.

15. Hirschberg AL et. al. Impaired cholecystokinin secretion and disturbed appetite regulation in women with polycystic ovary syndrome. Gynecol Endocrinol. (2004) 19(2):79-87.

15a. Jeanes YM et. al. Binge eating behaviours and food cravings in women with Polycystic Ovary Syndrome. Appetite. (2016) [Epub ahead of print]

15b. Lee I et. al. Increased risk of disordered eating in polycystic ovary syndrome. Fertil Steril. (2017) S0015-0282(16)63086-8.

16. Cunningham JJ.Body composition and resting metabolic rate: the myth of feminine metabolism. Am J Clin Nutr. (1982) 36(4):721-6.

16a. Gougeon R et. al. Increase in the thermic effect of food in women by adrenergic amines extracted from citrus aurantium. Obes Res. (2005) 13(7):1187-94.

16b. Tai MM et. al. Thermic effect of food during each phase of the menstrual cycle. Am J Clin Nutr. (1997) 66(5):1110-5.

17. Rosenfeld CS. Sex-dependent differences in voluntary physical activity. J Neurosci Res. (2017) 95(1-2):279-290.

17a. Jonason PK et. al. An evolutionary psychology perspective on sex differences in exercise behaviors and motivations. J Soc Psychol. (2007) 147(1):5-14.

18. von Loeffelholz C. The Role of Non-exercise Activity Thermogenesis in Human Obesity. [Updated 2014 Jun 5]. In: De Groot LJ, Beck-Peccoz P, Chrousos G, et al., editors. Endotext [Internet]. South Dartmouth (MA): MDText.com, Inc.; 2000-. Available: http://www.ncbi.nlm.nih.gov/books/NBK279077/

18a. Segal KR and Dunaif A. Resting metabolic rate and postprandial thermogenesis in polycystic ovarian syndrome. Int J Obes. (1990) 14(7):559-67.

18b.Broskey NT et. al. Assessing energy requirements in women with polycystic ovary syndrome: a comparison against doubly-labeled water. J Clin Endocrinol Metab. (2017) 102(6):1951-1959

19.Geisler C et. al.Gender-Specific Associations in Age-Related Changes in Resting Energy Expenditure (REE) and MRI Measured Body Composition in Healthy Caucasians. J Gerontol A Biol Sci Med Sci. (2015) 20. pii: glv211.

20. St-Onge MP and Gallagher D. Body composition changes with aging: the cause or the result of alterations in metabolic rate and macronutrient oxidation? Nutrition. (2010) 26(2):152-5.

21. Tipton KD et. al. Gender differences in protein metabolism. Curr Opin Clin Nutr Metab Care. (2001) ;4(6):493-8.

21a. Miller BF et. al.No effect of menstrual cycle on myofibrillar and connective tissue protein synthesis in contracting skeletal muscle. Am J Physiol Endocrinol Metab. (2006) 290(1):E163-E168.

22. Center for Substance Abuse Treatment. Substance Abuse Treatment: Addressing the Specific Needs of Women. Rockville (MD): Substance Abuse and Mental Health Services Administration (US); 2009. (Treatment Improvement Protocol (TIP) Series, No. 51.) Chapter 3: Physiological Effects of Alcohol, Drugs, and Tobacco on Women.

23. Sayon-Orea C et. al.Alcohol consumption and body weight: a systematic review. Nutr Rev. (2011) 69(8):419-31.

24. Votruba SB1, Jensen MD. Sex-specific differences in leg fat uptake are revealed with a high-fat meal. Am J Physiol Endocrinol Metab. (2006) 291(5):E1115-23.

25. Votruba SB1, Jensen MD. Short-term regional meal fat storage in nonobese humans is not a predictor of long-term regional fat gain. Am J Physiol Endocrinol Metab. (2012)15;302(9):E1078-83.

26. Nielsen S et. al. Energy expenditure, sex, and endogenous fuel availability in humans. J Clin Invest. (2003) 111(7):981-8

27. Koutsari C et. al. Nonoxidative free fatty acid disposal is greater in young women than men. J Clin Endocrinol Metab. (2011) 96(2):541-7.

28. Roepstorff C et. al.Gender differences in substrate utilization during submaximal exercise in endurance-trained subjects Am J Physiol Endocrinol Metab. (2002) 282(2):E435-47.

29. Steffensen, CH et. al. Myocellular triacylglycerol breakdown in females but not in males during exercise American Journal of Physiology - Endocrinology and Metabolism(2002) Vol. 282: E634-E642

30. Koutsari, C. et. al.Storage Rates of Circulating Free Fatty Acid Into Adipose Tissue During Eating or Walking in Humans Diabetes. (2012) 61(2): 329–338.

31. Paoli A et. al.Exercising fasting or fed to enhance fat loss? Influence of food intake on respiratory ratio and excess postexercise oxygen consumption after a bout of endurance training. Int J Sport Nutr Exerc Metab. (2011) 21(1):48-54.

32. Henderson GC1, Alderman BL.Determinants of resting lipid oxidation in response to a prior bout of endurance exercise. J Appl Physiol (1985). (2014) 116(1):95-103.

33. Henderson GC et. al. Lipolysis and fatty acid metabolism in men and women during the postexercise recovery period J Physiol. (2007) 584(Pt 3): 963–981.

33a. Towsend LK et. al. Mode of exercise and sex are not important for oxygen consumption during and in recovery from sprint interval training. Appl Physiol Nutr Metab. (2014) 39(12):1388-94.

34. Matsuo T et. al. Effects of the menstrual cycle on excess postexercise oxygen consumption in healthy young women. Metabolism. (1999) 48(3):275-7.

35. Lamont LS et. al.Fat-free mass and gender influences the rapid-phase excess postexercise oxygen consumption. Appl Physiol Nutr Metab. (2010) 35(1):23-6.

36. Wahrenberg H et. al. Divergent effects of weight reduction and oral anticonception treatment on adrenergic lipolysis regulation in obese women with the polycystic ovary syndrome. J Clin Endocrinol Metab. (1999) 84(6):2182-7.

37. Moro C et. al. Aerobic exercise training improves atrial natriuretic peptide and catecholamine-mediated lipolysis in obese women with polycystic ovary syndrome. J Clin Endocrinol Metab. (2009) 94(7):2579-86.

38. Jacobs KA et. al.Fatty acid reesterification but not oxidation is increased by oral contraceptive use in women. J Appl Physiol (1985). (2005) 98(5):1720-31.

39. Goodpaster BH et. al. Effects of obesity on substrate utilization during exercise. Obes Res. (2002) 10(7):575-84.

40. Isacco L et. al. Influence of hormonal status on substrate utilization at rest and during exercise in the female population. Sports Med. (2012) 42(4):327-42.

41. Millward DJ et. al.Sex differences in the composition of weight gain and loss in overweight and obese adults. Br J Nutr. (2014) 111(5):933-43.

42. Pietrobelli A et. al. Sexual dimorphism in the energy content of weight change. Int J Obes Relat Metab Disord. (2002) 26(10):1339-48.

43. Singh, P. et. al.Effects of weight gain and weight loss on regional fat distribution Am J Clin Nutr. (2012) 96(2): 229–233.

44. Nindl BC et. al. Regional body composition changes in women after 6 months of periodized physical training.J Appl Physiol (1985). (2000) 88(6):22

45. Bosy-Westphal A et. al. Effect of weight loss and regain on adipose tissue distribution, composition of lean mass and resting energy expenditure in young overweight and obese adults. Int J Obes (Lond). (2013) 37(10):1371-7

46. van der Kooy K et. al. Effect of a weight cycle on visceral fat accumulation. Am J Clin Nutr. (1993) 58(6):853-7.

Chapter 11: Women, Fat Gain and Fat Loss: Part 2

1. Williams, RL et. al. Effectiveness of weight loss interventions – is there a difference between men and women: a systematic review Obes Rev. (2015) 16(2): 171–186.

2. Franz MJ. Effectiveness of weight loss and maintenance interventions in women. Curr Diab Rep. (2004) 4(5):387-93.

3. Soltani S et. al.The effects of weight loss approaches on bone mineral density in adults: a systematic review and meta-analysis of randomized controlled trials. Osteoporos Int. (2016) 27(9):2655-2671

3a. Miller T et. al. Resistance Training Combined With Diet Decreases Body Fat While Preserving Lean Mass Independent of Resting Metabolic Rate: A Randomized Trial. Int J Sport Nutr Exerc Metab. (2017) 5:1-24.

4. Zurlo F et. al.Spontaneous physical activity and obesity: cross-sectional and longitudinal studies in Pima Indians. Am J Physiol. (1992) 263(2 Pt 1):E296-300.

5. Meijer GA et. al. The effect of a 5-month endurance-training programme on physical activity: evidence for a sex-difference in the metabolic response to exercise.Eur J Appl Physiol Occup Physiol. (1991) 62(1):11-7.

5a. Burrup R et. al. Strength training and body composition in middle-age women. (2017) J Sports Med Phys Fitness. 2017 Feb 8. doi: 10.23736/S0022-4707.17.06706-8. [Epub ahead of print]

6. Donnelly JE1, Smith BK. Is exercise effective for weight loss with ad libitum diet? Energy balance, compensation, and gender differences. Exerc Sport Sci Rev. (2005) 33(4):169-74.

7. Després JP et. al. Effects of exercise-training and detraining on fat cell lipolysis in men and women. Eur J Appl Physiol Occup Physiol. (1984) 53(1):25-30.

8. Melanson EL et. al.Resistance to exercise-induced weight loss: compensatory behavioral adaptations Med Sci Sports Exerc. (2013) 45(8): 1600–1609.

8a. Jackson M et. al. Exercise training and weight loss, not always a happy marriage: single blind exercise trials in females with diverse BMI. Appl Physiol Nutr Metab. (2017) Nov 2. doi: 10.1139/apnm-2017-0577. [Epub ahead of print]

9. Manthou E et. al.Behavioral compensatory adjustments to exercise training in overweight women. Med Sci Sports Exerc. (2010) 42(6):1121-8.

10. Donnelly JE et. al. Effects of a 16-month randomized controlled exercise trial on body weight and composition in young, overweight men and women: the Midwest Exercise Trial. Arch Intern Med. (2003) 163(11):1343-50.

11. Thomas DM et. al.Why do individuals not lose more weight from an exercise intervention at a defined dose? An energy balance analysis Obes Rev. (2012) 13(10): 835–847.

12. Westerterp KR et. al.Long-term effect of physical activity on energy balance and body composition. Br J Nutr. (1992)68(1):21-30.

13. Caudwell P. Exercise and weight loss: no sex differences in body weight response to exercise. Exerc Sport Sci Rev. (2014) 42(3):92-101.

14. Ballor DL1, Keesey RE.A meta-analysis of the factors affecting exercise-induced changes in body mass, fat mass and fat-free mass in males and females. Int J Obes. (1991) 15(11):717-26

15. Donnelly, JE et. al.Aerobic exercise alone results in clinically significant weight loss for men and women: Midwest Exercise Trial-2 Obesity (Silver Spring). (2013) 21(3): E219–E228.

16. Caudwell P et. al.No sex difference in body fat in response to supervised and measured exercise. Med Sci Sports Exerc. (2013) 45(2):351-8.

17. Melanson EL et. al.Effect of exercise intensity on 24-h energy expenditure and nutrient oxidation. J Appl Physiol (1985). (2002) 92(3):1045-52.

18. van Aggel-Leijssen DP et. al. The effect of low-intensity exercise training on fat metabolism of obese women. Obes Res. (2001) 9(2):86-96.

19. Krotkiewski M, Björntorp P.Muscle tissue in obesity with different distribution of adipose tissue. Effects of physical training. Int J Obes. (1986). 10(4):331-41.

20. Després JP et. al.Physical training and changes in regional adipose tissue distribution. Acta Med Scand Suppl. (1988) 723:205-12.

21. Andersson B et. al. The effects of exercise, training on body composition and metabolism in men and women. Int J Obes. (1991) Jan;15(1):75-81.

22. Woo R, Pi-Sunyer FX. Effect of increased physical activity on voluntary intake in lean women. Metabolism. (1985) 34(9):836-41.

23. Woo R et. al. Voluntary food intake during prolonged exercise in obese women. Am J Clin Nutr. (1982) 36(3):478-84.

23a. Durrant ML et. al. Effect of exercise on energy intake and eating patterns in lean and obese humans. Physiol Behav. (1982) 29(3):449-54.

24. Bilski J, Telegaoʹw A, Zahradnik-Bilska J, Dembicski A, Warzecha Z. Effects of exercise on appetite and food intake regulation. Medicina Sportiva. (2009). 13(2):82Y94.

25. Hagobian TA1, Braun B. Physical activity and hormonal regulation of appetite: sex differences and weight control. Exerc Sport Sci Rev. (2010) 38(1):25-30.

26. Howe SM et. al.Exercise-Trained Men and Women: Role of Exercise and Diet on Appetite and Energy Intake Nutrients. (2014) 6(11): 4935–4960.

27. Howe SM et. al. Nutrients. No Effect of Exercise Intensity on Appetite in Highly-Trained Endurance Women. (2016) 18;8(4).

28. Shi H Sexual differences in the control of energy homeostasis. Front Endocrinologist (2009) 30(3):396-404.

29. Woods SC et. al. Gender differences in the control of energy homeostasis. Exp Biol Med (Maywood). (2003)

228(10):1175-80.

30. Cortright RN, Koves TR.Sex differences in substrate metabolism and energy homeostasis.Can J Appl Physiol. (2000) 25:288-311.

31. Benedict C et. al.Differential sensitivity of men and women to anorexigenic and memory-improving effects of intranasal insulin. J Clin Endocrinol Metab. (2008)93(4):1339-44.

32. Kennedy A et. al.The metabolic significance of leptin in humans: gender-based differences in relationship to adiposity, insulin sensitivity, and energy expenditure. J Clin Endocrinol Metab. (1997) 82(4):1293-300.

33. Weigle DS et. al.Effect of fasting, refeeding, and dietary fat restriction on plasma leptin levels. J Clin Endocrinol Metab. (1997) 82(2):561-5.

34. Nicklas BJ et. al. Gender differences in the response of plasma leptin concentrations to weight loss in obese older individuals. Obes Res. (1997) 5(1):62-8.

35. Hickey MS et. al. Gender-dependent effects of exercise training on serum leptin levels in humans. Am J Physiol. (1997) 272(4 Pt 1):E562-6.

36. Hagobian TA1, Braun B. Physical activity and hormonal regulation of appetite: sex differences and weight control. Exerc Sport Sci Rev. (2010) 38(1):25-30.

37. Frank A. The role of hypothalamic estrogen receptors in metabolic regulation. Front Neuroendocrinol. (2014) 35(4):550-7.

38. Williams NI et. al. Estrogen and progesterone exposure is reduced in response to energy deficiency in women aged 25-40 years. Hum Reprod. (2010) 25(9):2328-39.

39. Hoyenga KB, Hoyenga KT Gender and energy balance: sex differences in adaptations for feast and famine. Physiol Behav. (1982) 28(3):545-63.

40. Fessler DM. No time to eat: an adaptationist account of periovulatory behavioral changes. Q Rev Biol. (2003) 78(1):3-21.

41. Roney JR and ZL Simmons. Ovarian hormone fluctuations predict within-cycle shifts in women's food intake. Horm Behav. (2017) 90:8-14.

41. Danel D1, Pawlowski B. Attractiveness of men's faces in relation to women's phase of menstrual cycle. Coll Antropol. (2006) 30(2):285-9.

42. Gueguen N. The receptivity of women to courtship solicitation across the menstrual cycle: a field experiment. Biol Psychol. (2009) 80(3):321-4.

43. Provost MP et. al. Differences in Gait Across the Menstrual Cycle and Their Attractiveness to Men. Archives of Sexual Behavior. (2008) 37(4): 598-604.

44 Russell VM. et. al. The association between discontinuing hormonal contraceptives and wives' marital satisfaction depends on husbands' facial attractiveness. Proc Natl Acad Sci U S A. (2014) 111(48):17081-6.

45. Strassmann BI.The evolution of endometrial cycles and menstruation.Q Rev Biol.(1996)71(2):181-220.

46. Barber, N. The evolutionary psychology of physical attractiveness: Sexual selection and human morphology. Ethology Sociobiology (1995) 16(5): 395-424.

Chapter 12: Menstrual Cycle Dysfunction

1. De Souza MJ1, Williams NI. Physiological aspects and clinical sequelae of energy deficiency and hypoestrogenism in exercising women Hum Reprod Update. (2004) 10(5):433-48.

2. De Souza MJ et. al. High prevalence of subtle and severe menstrual disturbances in exercising women: confirmation using daily hormone measures. Hum Reprod. (2010) 25(2):491-503.

3. Frisch RE.The right weight: body fat, menarche and fertility. Proc Nutr Soc. (1994) 53(1):113-29.

4. Beckie TM. A systematic review of allostatic load, health, and health disparities. Biol Res Nurs. (2012) 14(4):311-46.

5.Ellison, P. Human Ovarian Function and Reproductive Ecology: New Hypotheses. American Anthropologist. (1990) 92: 933-952.

6. Warren MP1, Perlroth NE. The effects of intense exercise on the female reproductive system. J Endocrinol. (2001) 170(1):3-11.

7. Boyden TW et. al.Impaired gonadotropin responses to gonadotropin-releasing hormone stimulation in endurance-trained women. Fertil Steril. (1984) 41(3):359-63.

8. Bonen A. Recreational exercise does not impair menstrual cycles: a prospective study. Int J Sports Med. (1992) 13(2):110-20.

9. Rogol AD et. al.Durability of the reproductive axis in eumenorrheic women during 1 yr of endurance training. J Appl Physiol (1985). (1992) 72(4):1571-80.

10. Bullen BA et. al. Endurance training effects on plasma hormonal responsiveness and sex hormone excretion.J Appl Physiol Respir Environ Exerc Physiol. (1984) 56(6):1453-63.

11. Williams NI. Effects of short-term strenuous endurance exercise upon corpus luteum function. Med Sci Sports Exerc. (1999) 31(7):949-58.

12. Roupas ND and NA Georgopoulos. Menstrual function in sports. Hormones (Athens) (2011)10:104-16.

13. Schweiger U et. al. Diet-induced menstrual irregularities: effects of age and weight loss. Fertil Steril. (1987) 48(5):746-51.

14. Lager C and PT Ellison. Effect of moderate weight loss on ovarian function assessed by salivary progesterone

measurements. American Journal of Human Biology (1990) 2: 303-312.

14a. Wade GN et. al. Control of fertility by metabolic cues. Am J Physiol. (1996) 270(1 Pt 1):E1-19.

15. Loucks AB. Energy availability, not body fatness, regulates reproductive function in women. Exerc Sport Sci Rev. (2003) 31(3):144-8.

16. Pirke KM et. al. Dieting causes menstrual irregularities in normal weight young women through impairment of episodic luteinizing hormone secretion. Fertil Steril. (1989) 51(2):263-8.

17. Loucks AB et. al. Low energy availability, not stress of exercise, alters LH pulsatility in exercising women. J Appl Physiol (1985). (1998) 84(1):37-46.

18. Williams NI et. al. Strenuous exercise with caloric restriction: effect on luteinizing hormone secretion. Med Sci Sports Exerc. (1995) 27(10):1390-8.

19. Loucks AB and JR Thuma. Luteinizing hormone pulsatility is disrupted at a threshold of energy availability in regularly menstruating women. J Clin Endocrinol Metab. (2003) 88(1):297-311.

20. Ihle R1, and AB Loucks. Dose-response relationships between energy availability and bone turnover in young exercising women. J Bone Miner Res. (2004) 19(8):1231-40.

21. Reed JL. et. al.Energy availability discriminates clinical menstrual status in exercising women . J Int Soc Sports Nutr.(2015) 12:11.2

21a, Leiberman JL, De Souza MJ, Williams NI. Luteal phase defects induced by ex- ercise and diet are associated with low energy availability. Med Sci Sports Exerc 2013;45(S5):520–1

22. Lieberman JL et. al.Menstrual Disruption with Exercise is not Linked to an Energy Availability Threshold. Med Sci Sports Exerc. (2017) Oct 10. doi: 10.1249/MSS.0000000000001451. [Epub ahead of print]

22a. Tenforde AS et. al. Parallels with the Female Athlete Triad in Male Athletes. Sports Med. 2016 Feb;46(2):171-82.

22b. Koehler K et at.al.Low energy availability in exercising men is associated with reduced leptin and insulin but not with changes in other metabolic hormones. J Sports Sci. (2016) 6:1-9. [Epub ahead of print]

22c. Papageorgiou M et. al. Effects of reduced energy availability on bone metabolism in women and men. Bone. (2017) 105:191-199.

22d. Fagerberg P. Negative Consequences of Low Energy Availability in Natural Male Bodybuilding: A Review. Int J Sport Nutr Exerc Metab. (2017) 22:1-31.

23. Chou SH, Mantzoros C. 20 years of leptin: role of leptin in human reproductive disorders. J Endocrinol. (2014) 223(1):T49-62.

24. Thong FS1, McLean C, Graham TE. Plasma leptin in female athletes: relationship with body fat, reproductive, nutritional, and endocrine factors. J Appl Physiol (1985). (2000) 88(6):2037-44.

25. Köpp W et. al. Low leptin levels predict amenorrhea in underweight and eating disordered females. Mol Psychiatry. (1997) 2(4):335-40.

26. Chou SH et. al. Leptin is an effective treatment for hypothalamic amenorrhea. Proc Natl Acad Sci U S A. (2011) 108(16):6585-90

27. Alvero RJ et. al. Effects of fasting on neuroendocrine function and follicle development in lean women. Clin Endocrinol Metab. (1998) 83(1):76-80

28. Schweiger U et. al. Caloric intake, stress, and menstrual function in athletes. Fertil Steril. (1988) 49(3):447-50.

29. Laughlin GA et. al. Nutritional and endocrine-metabolic aberrations in women with functional hypothalamic amenorrhea. J Clin Endocrinol Metab. (1998) 83(1):25-32.

30. Vescovi JD et. al.Cognitive dietary restraint: impact on bone, menstrual and metabolic status in young women. Physiol Behav. (2008) 95(1-2):48-55.

30a. Giles DE and SL Berga. Cognitive and psychiatric correlates of functional hypothalamic amenorrhea: a controlled comparison. Fertil Steril. (1993) 60(3):486-92.

31. Meczekalski B et. al.Functional hypothalamic amenorrhea: current view on neuroendocrine aberrations. Gynecol Endocrinol. (2008) 24(1):4-11.

32. Berga SL and T Louck. Use of cognitive behavior therapy for functional hypothalamic amenorrhea Ann N Y Acad Sci. (2006) 1092:114-29.

32a. Berga SL et. al.Recovery of ovarian activity in women with functional hypothalamic amenorrhea who were treated with cognitive behavior therapy. Fertil Steril. 2003 Oct;80(4):976-81.

32b. Michopoulos V et. al. Neuroendocrine recovery initiated by cognitive behavioral therapy in women with functional hypothalamic amenorrhea: a randomized, controlled trial. Fertil Steril. (2013) 99(7):2084-91

33. Dorgan JF et. al. Relation of energy, fat, and fiber intakes to plasma concentrations of estrogens and androgens in premenopausal women. Am J Clin Nutr. (1996) 64(1):25-31.

34. Wu AH, Pike MC, Stram DO. Meta-analysis: dietary fat intake, serum estrogen levels, and the risk of breast cancer. J Natl Cancer Inst. (1999) 91:529–34.

35. Jones DY. Influence of dietary fat on self-reported menstrual symptoms. Physiol Behav. (1987) 40(4):483-7.

36. Boyd NF et. al. Effects at two years of a low-fat, high-carbohydrate diet on radiologic features of the breast: results from a randomized trial. Canadian Diet and Breast Cancer Prevention Study Group. J Natl Cancer Inst. (1997) 89(7):488-96.

37. Remer T et. al.Short-term impact of a lactovegetarian diet on adrenocortical activity and adrenal androgens. J Clin Endocrinol Metab. (1998) 83(6):2132-7.

38. Barr SI. Vegetarianism and menstrual cycle disturbances: is there an association? Am J Clin Nutr. (1999) 70(3

Suppl):549S-54S.

39. Andrews MA et. al.Dietary factors and luteal phase deficiency in healthy eumenorrheic women.Hum Reprod. (2015)30:1942-51.

40. Kaiserauer S et. alNutritional, physiological, and menstrual status of distance runners.Med Sci Sports Exerc. (1989) 21(2):120-5.

41. Mavropoulos JC et. al. The effects of a low-carbohydrate, ketogenic diet on the polycystic ovary syndrome: A pilot study . Nutr Metab (Lond). (2005) 2:35.

42. Tolino A et. al. Evaluation of ovarian functionality after a dietary treatment in obese women with polycystic ovary syndrome. Eur J Obstet Gynecol Reprod Biol. (2005) 119(1):87-93.

43. Sirven J et. al. The ketogenic diet for intractable epilepsy in adults: preliminary results. Epilepsia. (1999) 40(12):1721-6.

44. Loucks AB et. al. Energy availability in athletes. J Sports Sci. (2011) 29 (Suppl 1):S7-15.

44a. Reed JL et. al. Exercising women with menstrual disturbances consume low energy dense foods and beverages. Appl Physiol Nutr Metab. (2011) 36(3):382-94.

45. Beals KA1, Manore MM. The prevalence and consequences of subclinical eating disorders in female athletes. Int J Sport Nutr. (1994) 4(2):175-95.

45a. Caronia LM et. al. A genetic basis for functional hypothalamic amenorrhea. N Engl J Med. (2011) 364(3):215-25.

46. Loucks AB. The response of luteinizing hormone pulsatility to 5 days of low energy availability disappears by 14 years of gynecological age. J Clin Endocrinol Metab. (2006) 91(8):3158-64.

47. Kurzer MS, Calloway DH. Effects of energy deprivation on sex hormone patterns in healthy menstruating women. Am J Physiol. (1986) 251(4 Pt 1):E483-8.

48. Williams NI et. al. Magnitude of daily energy deficit predicts frequency but not severity of menstrual disturbances associated with exercise and caloric restriction. Am J Physiol Endocrinol Metab. (2015) 308(1):E29-39.

49. Ruby BC et. al. Effects of estradiol on substrate turnover during exercise in amenorrheic females. Med Sci Sports Exerc. (1997) 29(9):1160-9.

49a. Sanders KM et. al. Heightened Cortisol Response to Exercise Challenge in Women with Functional Hypothalamic Amenorrhea. Am J Obstet Gynecol. 2017 Nov 20. pii: S0002-9378(17)32346-3.

50. Myerson M et. al. Resting metabolic rate and energy balance in amenorrheic and eumenorrheic runners. Med Sci Sports Exerc. (1991) 23(1):15-22.

51. Graham TE et. al. Thermal and metabolic responses to cold by men and by eumenorrheic and amenorrheic women. J Appl Physiol (1985). (1989) 67(1):282-90.

52. De Souza MJ1, Metzger DA. Reproductive dysfunction in amenorrheic athletes and anorexic patients: a review. Med Sci Sports Exerc. (1991) 23(9):995-1007.

53. Danilenko KV et. al. Diurnal and seasonal variations of melatonin and serotonin in women with seasonal affective disorder. Arctic Med Res. (1994) 53(3):137-45.

54. Alfred J. Lewy, MD, PhD et. al. The phase shift hypothesis for the circadian component of winter depression Dialogues Clin Neurosci. (2007) 9(3): 291–300.

55. Brzezinski A et. al. The circadian rhythm of plasma melatonin during the normal menstrual cycle and in amenorrheic women. J Clin Endocrinol Metab. (1988) 66(5):891-5.

56. Kadva A et. al. Elevated nocturnal melatonin is a consequence of gonadotropin-releasing hormone deficiency in women with hypothalamic amenorrhea. J Clin Endocrinol Metab. (1998) 83(10):3653-62.

57. Lloyd T et. al. Women athletes with menstrual irregularity have increased musculoskeletal injuries. Med Sci Sports Exerc. (1986) 18(4):374-9.

58. Keen AD, Drinkwater BL.Irreversible bone loss in former amenorrheic athletes. Osteoporos Int. (1997) 7(4):311-5.

59. Fredericson M1 and K Kent K. Normalization of bone density in a previously amenorrheic runner with osteoporosis. Med Sci Sports Exerc. (2005) 37(9):1481-6.

60. Zanker CL et. al. Annual changes of bone density over 12 years in an amenorrheic athlete. Med Sci Sports Exerc. (2004) 36(1):137-42.

61. Ducher G et. al. Obstacles in the optimization of bone health outcomes in the female athlete triad. Sports Med. (2011)41(7):587-607.

62.De Souza MJ etl al.Severity of energy-related menstrual disturbances increases in proportion to indices of energy conservation in exercising women. Fertil Steril. (2007) 88(4):971-5.

63. De Souza MJ. Menstrual disturbances in athletes: a focus on luteal phase defects. Med Sci Sports Exerc. (2003) 35(9):1553-63.

64. Manore MM et. al. The female athlete triad: components, nutrition issues, and health consequences. J Sports Sci. (2007) 25 (Suppl 1):S61-71.

65. Mallinson RJ and MJ DeSouza. Current perspectives on the etiology and manifestation of the "silent" component of the Female Athlete Triad Current perspectives on the etiology and manifestation of the "silent" component of the Int J Womens Health. (2014); 6: 451–467.

66. Mountjoy M et. al. The IOC consensus statement: beyond the Female Athlete Triad--Relative Energy Deficiency in Sport (RED-S). Br J Sports Med. (2014) 48(7):491-7.

67. De Souza MJ et. al.Misunderstanding the female athlete triad: refuting the IOC consensus statement on Relative Energy Deficiency in Sport (RED-S). Br J Sports Med. (2014) 48(20):1461-5.

68. Mountjoy M et. al. Authors' 2015 additions to the IOC consensus statement: Relative Energy Deficiency in Sport (RED-S). Br J Sports Med. (2015) 49(7):417-20.

69. Sara Márquez and Olga Molinero Energy availability, menstrual dysfunction and bone health in sports; an overview of the female athlete triad Nutr Hosp. (2013) 28(4):1010-1017.

70. Kopp-Woodroffe SA et. al. Energy and nutrient status of amenorrheic athletes participating in a diet and exercise training intervention program. Int J Sport Nutr. (1999) 9(1):70-88.

71. Arends JC et. al.Restoration of menses with nonpharmacologic therapy in college athletes with menstrual disturbances: a 5-year retrospective study. Int J Sport Nutr Exerc Metab. (2012) 22(2):98-108.

72.Dueck CA et. al.Treatment of athletic amenorrhea with a diet and training intervention program. Int J Sport Nutr. (1996) 6(1):24-40.

73. Lagowska K et. al. Effects of dietary intervention in young female athletes with menstrual disorders J Int Soc Sports Nutr. (2014); 11: 21.

74. Cialdella-Kam L et. al.Dietary intervention restored menses in female athletes with exercise-associated menstrual dysfunction with limited impact on bone and muscle health. Nutrients. (2014) 6(8):3018-39.

75. Allaway HC et. al. The physiology of functional hypothalamic amenorrhea associated with energy deficiency in exercising women and in women with anorexia nervosa. Horm Mol Biol Clin Investig. (2016) 25(2):91-119. doi: 10.1515/hmbci-2015-0053.

76. Mallinson RJ et. al. A case report of recovery of menstrual function following a nutritional intervention in two exercising women with amenorrhea of varying duration. J Int Soc Sports Nutr. (2013); 10: 34.

77. Kyriakidis M et. al. Functional hypothalamic amenorrhoea: leptin treatment, dietary intervention and counselling as alternatives to traditional practice - systematic review. Eur J Obstet Gynecol Reprod Biol. (2016) 198:131-137.

Chapter 13: Stress

1. McEwen BS.Physiology and neurobiology of stress and adaptation: central role of the brain. Physiol Rev. (2007) 87(3):873-904.

2. Lee MJ et. al.Deconstructing the roles of glucocorticoids in adipose tissue biology and the development of central obesity. Biochim Biophys Acta. (2014) 1842(3):473-81.

3. Nieuwenhuizen AG and F. Rutters. The hypothalamic-pituitary-adrenal-axis in the regulation of energy balance. Physiol Behav. (2008) 94(2):169-77.

4. Ulrich-Lai YM. Self-medication with sucrose. Curr Opin Behav Sci. (2016) 9:78-83.

4a. Kajantie E1, Phillips DI. The effects of sex and hormonal status on the physiological response to acute psychosocial stress. Psychoneuroendocrinology. (2006) 31(2):151-78.

5. Kudielka BM1, Kirschbaum C. Sex differences in HPA axis responses to stress: a review. Biol Psychol. (2005) 69(1):113-32.

6. Jaillon S et. al. Sexual Dimorphism in Innate Immunity. Clin Rev Allergy Immunol. (2017) Sep 30. doi: 10.1007/s12016-017-8648-x. [Epub ahead of print]

7. Fernández-Guasti A et. al. Sex, stress, and mood disorders: at the intersection of adrenal and gonadal hormones. Horm Metab Res. (2012) 44(8):607-18.

8. Goel N et. al.Sex differences in the HPA axis. Compr Physiol. (2014) 4(3):1121-55.

9. Taylor SE et. al. Biobehavioral responses to stress in females: tend-and-befriend, not fight-or-flight. Psychol Rev. (2000) 107(3):411-29.

10. Kudielka BM et al.Why do we respond so differently? Reviewing determinants of human salivary cortisol responses to challenge. Psychoneuroendocrinology. (2009) 34(1):2-18.

11. Kirschbaum C et. al. Short-term estradiol treatment enhances pituitary-adrenal axis and sympathetic responses to psychosocial stress in healthy young men. J Clin Endocrinol Metab. (1996) 81(10):3639-43.

12. Altemus M et. al. Increased vasopressin and adrenocorticotropin responses to stress in the midluteal phase of the menstrual cycle. J Clin Endocrinol Metab. (2001) 86(6):2525-30.

13. Kirschbaum C et. al.Impact of gender, menstrual cycle phase, and oral contraceptives on the activity of the hypothalamus-pituitary-adrenal axis. Psychosom Med. (1999) 61(2):154-62.

14. Meczekalski B et. al. Hypothalamic amenorrhea with normal body weight: ACTH, allopregnanolone and cortisol responses to corticotropin-releasing hormone test. Eur J Endocrinol. (2000) 142(3):280-5.

15. Rodin A et. al. Hyperandrogenism in polycystic ovary syndrome. Evidence of dysregulation of 11 beta-hydroxysteroid dehydrogenase. N Engl J Med. (1994) 17;330(7):460-5.

16. Pasquali R. The hypothalamic–pituitary–adrenal axis and sex hormones in chronic stress and obesity: pathophysiological and clinical aspects. Ann N Y Acad Sci. (2012) 1264(1): 20–35.

17. Otte C et. al.A meta-analysis of cortisol response to challenge in human aging: importance of gender. Psychoneuroendocrinology. (2005) 30(1):80-91.

18. Edwards KM and PJ Mills. Effects of estrogen versus estrogen and progesterone on cortisol and interleukin-6 Maturitas. (2008) 61(4): 330–333.

19. Traustadóttir T et al. The HPA axis response to stress in women: effects of aging and fitness. Psychoneuroendocrinology. (2005) 30(4):392-402. Epub 2005 Jan 11.

20. Carpenter T et. al. Sex differences in early-life programming of the hypothalamic-pituitary-adrenal axis in humans suggest increased vulnerability in females: a systematic review. J Dev Orig Health Dis. (2017) 8(2):244-255.

21. Farrell PA, Garthwaite TL, Gustafson AB. Plasma adrenocorticotropin and cortisol responses to submaximal and exhaustive exercise. J Appl Physiol Respirat Environ Exercise Physiol. (1983) 55:1441.

22. Deuster PA et. al.High intensity exercise promotes escape of adrenocorticotropin and cortisol from suppression by dexamethasone: sexually dimorphic responses. J Clin Endocrinol Metab. (1998) 83(9):3332-8.

23. Redman LM, Loucks AB. Menstrual disorders in athletes. Sports Med. (2005) 35(9):747-55.

24. Bobbert T et. al. Adaptation of the hypothalamic-pituitary hormones during intensive endurance training. Clin Endocrinol (Oxf). (2005) 63(5):530-6.

25. Fichter MM, Pirke KM. Effect of experimental and pathological weight loss upon the hypothalamo-pituitary-adrenal axis. Psycho- neuroendocrinology. (1986) 11:295.

26. Tomiyama AJ et. al. Low calorie dieting increases cortisol. Psychosom Med. (2010) 72(4):357-64.

27. Lemmens SG et. al. Influence of Consumption of a High-Protein vs. High-Carbohydrate Meal on the Physiological Cortisol and Psychological Mood Response in Men and Women PLoS One. (2011) 6(2): e16826.

28. Vicennati V et. al.Comment: response of the hypothalamic-pituitary-adrenocortical axis to high-protein/fat and high-carbohydrate meals in women with different obesity phenotypes. J Clin Endocrinol Metab. (2002) 87(8):3984-8.

29. Lovallo WR et. al.Caffeine Stimulation of Cortisol Secretion Across the Waking Hours in Relation to Caffeine Intake Levels Psychosom Med. (2005) 67(5): 734–739.

30. Lovallo, WR. Cortisol responses to mental stress, exercise, and meals following caffeine intake in men and women. Pharmacol Biochem Behav. (2006) 83(3): 441–447.

31. Stults-Kolehmainen MA1, Bartholomew JB. Psychological stress impairs short-term muscular recovery from resistance exercise. Med Sci Sports Exerc. (2012) 44(11):2220-7.

32. Bartholomew JB et. al. Strength gains after resistance training: the effect of stressful, negative life events. J Strength Cond Res. (2008) 22(4):1215-21.

33. Rutters F et. al. Hyperactivity of the HPA axis is related to dietary restraint in normal weight women.Physiol Behav. (2009) 16;96(2):315-9.

34. McLean JA et. al.Cognitive dietary restraint is associated with higher urinary cortisol excretion in healthy premenopausal women. Am J Clin Nutr. (2001) 73(1):7-12.

35. Schweiger U et. al. Everyday eating behavior and menstrual function in young women. Fertil Steril. (1992) 57(4):771-5.

36. Guest NS1, Barr SI. Cognitive dietary restraint is associated with stress fractures in women runners. Int J Sport Nutr Exerc Metab. (2005) 15(2):147-59.

37. McLean JA et. al. Dietary restraint, exercise, and bone density in young women: are they related? Med Sci Sports Exerc. (2001) 33(8):1292-6.s

38. Newman E et. al. Daily hassles and eating behaviour: the role of cortisol reactivity status. Psychoneuroendocrinology. (2007) 32(2):125-32. Epub 2007 Jan 2.

39. Niemeier HM et. al. Internal disinhibition predicts weight regain following weight loss and weight loss maintenance. Obesity (Silver Spring). (2007) 15(10):2485-94.

40. Berga SL. Stress and reproduction: a tale of false dichotomy? Endocrinology. (2008) 149(3):867-8.

41. Loucks, AB. Is Stress Measured in Joules? Military Psychology (2009) 21: S101-S107

42. Pauli SA1, Berga SL. Athletic amenorrhea: energy deficit or psychogenic challenge? Ann N Y Acad Sci. (2010) 1205:33-8.

43. Stewart TM et. al. Rigid vs. flexible dieting: association with eating disorder symptoms in nonobese women. Appetite. (2002) 38(1):39-44.

44. Oberle CD et. al. Orthorexia nervosa: Assessment and correlates with gender, BMI, and personality. Appetite. (2016) Jan 1;108:303-310. doi: 10.1016/j.appet.2016.10.021. Epub 2016 Oct 15.

44a. Pascoe MC et. al. Yoga, mindfulness-based stress reduction and stress-related physiological measures: A meta-analysis. Psychoneuroendocrinology. (2017) 30;86:152-168.

45. Melamed S et. al.Burnout and risk of cardiovascular disease: evidence, possible causal paths, and promising research directions. Psychol Bull. (2006) 132(3):327-53.

46. Heim C et. al.The potential role of hypocortisolism in the pathophysiology of stress-related bodily disorders. Psychoneuroendocrinology. (2000) 25(1):1-35.

47. Angeli A. et al. The overtraining syndrome in athletes: a stress-related disorder. J Endocrinol Invest. (2004) 27(6):603-12.

48. KA Brooks and JG Carter. Overtraining, Exercise, and Adrenal Insufficiency J Nov Physiother. (2013) 3(125): 11717.

49. Cadegiani FA and CE Kater. Adrenal fatigue does not exist: a systematic review. BMC Endocr Disord. (2016); 16(1): 48.

50. Fries E et. al. A new view on hypocortisolism. Psychoneuroendocrinology. (2005) 30(10):1010-6.

51. Raison CL and AH Miller. When not enough is too much: the role of insufficient glucocorticoid signaling in the pathophysiology of stress-related disorders. Am J Psychiatry. (2003) 160(9):1554-65.

52. Allolio B1 et. al. DHEA: why, when, and how much--DHEA replacement in adrenal insufficiency. Ann Endocrinol (Paris). (2007) 68(4):268-73.

Chapter 14: Fixing the Problems

1. Wu BN and AJ O'Sullivan. Sex differences in energy metabolism need to be considered with lifestyle modifications in humans. J Nutr Metab. (2011) 2011:391809.

2. Garthe I et. al. Effect of nutritional intervention on body composition and performance in elite athletes. Eur J Sport Sci. (2013) 13(3):295-303.

3. Wilkin TJ et. al. Maximum calorie (sub-threshold) dieting of the obese and its hormonal response. Acta Endocrinol (Copenh). (1983) 103(2):184-7.

4. Garthe I et. al. Effect of two different weight-loss rates on body composition and strength and power-related performance in elite athletes. Int J Sport Nutr Exerc Metab. (2011) 21(2):97-104.

5. Garthe I et. al. Long-term effect of weight loss on body composition and performance in elite athletes. Int J Sport Nutr Exerc Metab. (2011) 21(5):426-35.

6. Kevin D. Hall. Body Fat and Fat-Free Mass Interrelationships Forbes's Theory Revisited. Br J Nutr. (2007) 97(6): 1059–1063.

7. Thomas DM et. al. Effect of dietary adherence on the body weight plateau: a mathematical model incorporating intermittent compliance with energy intake prescription. Am J Clin Nutr. (2014) 100 :787-95

8. A. Astrup and S. Rossner. Lessons from obesity management: Greater initial weight loss improves long-term maintenance. Obes Rev (2000) 1: 17-19.

9. Johnstone AM. Fasting - the ultimate diet? Obes Rev. (2007) 8(3):211-22.

10. Wisse BE et. al.Effect of prolonged moderate and severe energy restriction and refeeding on plasma leptin concentrations in obese women. Am J Clin Nutr. (1999) 70(3):321-30.

11. Friedl KE et. al. Endocrine markers of semistarvation in healthy lean men in a multistressor environment. J Appl Physiol (1985). (2000) 88(5):1820-30.

12. Loucks AB and M Verdun. Slow restoration of LH pulsatility by refeeding in energetically disrupted women. Am J Physiol. (1998) 275(4 Pt 2):R1218-26.

13. Olson BR et. al. Short-term fasting affects luteinizing hormone secretory dynamics but not reproductive function in normal-weight sedentary women. J Clin Endocrinol Metab. (1995) 80(4):1187-93.

14. Schrauwen P et. a. Fat balance in obese subjects: role of glycogen stores. Am J Physiol. (1998) 274(6 Pt 1):E1027-33.

15. Schrauwen P et. al.Role of glycogen-lowering exercise in the change of fat oxidation in response to a high-fat diet. Am J Physiol. (1997) 273(3 Pt 1):E623-9.

16. Paoli A. Exercising fasting or fed to enhance fat loss? Influence of food intake on respiratory ratio and excess postexercise oxygen consumption after a bout of endurance training. Int J Sport Nutr Exerc Metab. (2011) 21(1):48-54.

17. Schoenfeld BJ et. al. Body composition changes associated with fasted versus non-fasted aerobic exercise. Journal of the International Society of Sports Nutrition (2014) 11:54

18. Liljedahl ME et. al. Different responses of skeletal muscle following sprint training in men and women. European Journal of Applied Physiology and Occupational Physiology. (1996) 74(4): 375-383

19. Szallar SE et. al. Regulators of human white adipose browning: evidence for sympathetic control and sexual dimorphic responses to sprint interval training. PLoS One. (2014) 9(6):e90696.

20. Esbjörnsson M et. al. Greater growth hormone and insulin response in women than in men during repeated bouts of sprint exercise. Acta Physiol (Oxf). (2009) 197(2):107-15.

21. Brooks S et. al. The hormonal responses to repetitive brief maximal exercise in humans. Eur J Appl Physiol Occup Physiol. (1990) 60(2):144-8.

21a. Trapp EG et. al. The effects of high-intensity intermittent exercise training on fat loss and fasting insulin levels of young women. Int J Obes (Lond). (2008) 32(4):684-91.

22. Esbjörnsson-Liljedahl M. et. al.Metabolic response in type I and type II muscle fibers during a 30-s cycle sprint in men and women. J Appl Physiol (1985). (1999) 87(4):1326-32.

23. Billaut F and D Bishop. Muscle fatigue in males and females during multiple-sprint exercise. Sports Med. (2009) 39(4):257-78.

24. Essén-Gustavsson B and PA Tesch. Glycogen and triglyceride utilization in relation to muscle metabolic characteristics in men performing heavy-resistance exercise. Eur J Appl Physiol Occup Physiol. (1990) 61(1-2):5-10.

25. Koopman et. al. Intramyocellular lipid and glycogen content are reduced following resistance exercise in untrained healthy males. Eur J Appl Physiol. (2006) 96(5):525-34.

26 Bell DG, Jacobs I. Muscle fiber-specific glycogen utilization in strength-trained males and females. Med Sci Sports Exerc. (1989) 21(6):649-54

27. Binzen CA et. al. Postexercise oxygen consumption and substrate use after resistance exercise in women. Med Sci Sports Exerc. (2001) 33(6):932-8.

28. Osterberg KL and Melby, CL. Effect of acute resistance exercise on postexercise oxygen consumption and resting metabolic rate in young women. Int J Sport Nutr Exerc Metab. (2000) 10(1):71-81.

29. Staron RS et. al. Strength and skeletal muscle adaptations in heavy-resistance-trained women after detraining and retraining. J Appl Physiol (1985). (1991) 70(2):631-40.

30. Labayen I et. al. Basal and postprandial substrate oxidation rates in obese women receiving two test meals with different protein content.Clin Nutr. (2004)23(4):571-8.

31. Trexler ET et. al.Dietary macronutrient distribution influences post-exercise substrate utilization in women: a cross-

sectional evaluation of metabolic flexibility. J Sports Med Phys Fitness. (2016) March 9. doi: 10.23736/S0022-4707.16.06284-8

Chapter 15: Introduction to Dieting

1. Mata J et. al. When weight management lasts. Lower perceived rule complexity increases adherence. Appetite. (2010) 54(1):37-43.
2. Loria-Kohen V et. al. Evaluation of the usefulness of a low-calorie diet with or without bread in the treatment of overweight/obesity. Clin Nutr. (2012) Aug;31(4):455-61.
3. Westenhoefer J. Dietary restraint and disinhibition: is restraint a homogeneous construct? Appetite. (1991) 16(1):45-55.
5. Polivy J1 and P Herman.Is the body the self? Women and body image. Coll Antropol. (2007) 31(1):63-7.
5. Smith CF et. al. Flexible vs. Rigid dieting strategies: relationship with adverse behavioral outcomes. Appetite. (1999)32(3):295-305.
6, Westenhoefer J et. al. Cognitive and weight-related correlates of flexible and rigid restrained eating behaviour. Eat Behav. (2013) 14(1):69-72.
7. Stewart TM et. al.Rigid vs. flexible dieting: association with eating disorder symptoms in nonobese women. Appetite. (2002) 38(1):39-44.
8.Westenhoefer J et. al.Validation of the flexible and rigid control dimensions of dietary restraint. Int J Eat Disord. (1999) 26(1):53-64.
9. Westenhoefer J et. al.Behavioural correlates of successful weight reduction over 3 y. Results from the Lean Habits Study. Int J Obes Relat Metab Disord. (2004) 28(2):334-5.
10. Hill AJ. The psychology of food craving. Proc Nutr Soc. (2007) 66(2):277-85.
11. Wing RR and RW Jeffrey. Prescribed 'Breaks' as a means to disrupt weight control efforts. Obes Res (2003) 11:287-291.
12. Vale, RC et. al. The benefits of behaving badly on occasion: Successful regulation by planned hedonic deviations. Journal of Consumer Psychology (2016) 26:17–28
13. Davidsen L et. al. Impact of the menstrual cycle on determinants of energy balance: a putative role in weight loss attempts. Int J Obes (Lond). (2007) (12):1777-85.

Chapter 16: Determining Maintenance Calories

1. Black AE et. al.Human energy expenditure in affluent societies: an analysis of 574 doubly-labelled water measurements. Eur J Clin Nutr. (1996) 50(2):72-92.
2. Ismail MN et. al.Energy expenditure studies to predict requirements of selected national athletes. Malays J Nutr. (1997) 3(1):71-81.
3. van Erp-Baart AM et. al.Nationwide survey on nutritional habits in elite athletes. Part I. Energy, carbohydrate, protein, and fat intake. Int J Sports Med. (1989) 10 (Suppl) 1:S3-10.
4. Rodriquez NR et. al.American College of Sports Medicine position stand. Nutrition and athletic performance. Med Sci Sports Exerc. (2009) 41(3):709-31.

Chapter 17: Adjusting Daily Calories

1. Garthe I et. al. Effect of nutritional intervention on body composition and performance in elite athletes. Eur J Sport Sci. (2013) 13(3):295-303.
2. Hilton LK and AB Loucks. Low energy availability, not exercise stress, suppresses the diurnal rhythm of leptin in healthy young women. Am J Physiol Endocrinol Metab. (2000) 278(1):E43-9.
3. Blundell JE et. al. Appetite control and energy balance: impact of exercise. Obes Rev. (2015) 16 (Suppl 1):67-76.
4.Hopkins M et. al. Individual variability in compensatory eating following acute exercise in overweight and obese women. Br J Sports Med. (2014) 48(20):1472-6.
5. Stiegler P and A Cunliffe. The role of diet and exercise for the maintenance of fat-free mass and resting metabolic rate during weight loss. Sports Med. (2006) 36(3):239-62.
6. Verheggen RJ et. al.A systematic review and meta-analysis on the effects of exercise training versus hypocaloric diet: distinct effects on body weight and visceral adipose tissue. Obes Rev. (2016) 17(8):664-90.
7. Ismail I et. al.A systematic review and meta-analysis of the effect of aerobic vs. resistance exercise training on visceral fat. Obes Rev. (2012) 13(1):68-91.
8. Abe T et. al.Relationship between training frequency and subcutaneous and visceral fat in women. Med Sci Sports Exerc. (1997) 29(12):1549-53.
9. Sanal E et. al. Effects of aerobic or combined aerobic resistance exercise on body composition in overweight and obese adults: gender differences. A randomized intervention study. Eur J Phys Rehabil Med .(2013) 49(1):1-11
10. Miller T et. al. Resistance Training Combined With Diet Decreases Body Fat While Preserving Lean Mass Independent of Resting Metabolic Rate: A Randomized Trial. Int J Sport Nutr Exerc Metab. (2017) 5:1-24.
11. Jakicic JM. The effect of physical activity on body weight. Obesity (Silver Spring). (2009) 17 (Suppl 3):S34-8
12. Donnelly JE et. al. The role of exercise for weight loss and maintenance. Best Pract Res Clin Gastroenterol. (2004) 18(6):1009-29.
13. Wu T et. al. Long-term effectiveness of diet-plus-exercise interventions vs. diet-only interventions for weight loss:

a meta-analysis. Obes Rev. (2009) 10(3):313-23.

14. Krupa S et. al. Low or Moderate Dietary Energy Restriction for Long-term Weight Loss: What Works Best? Obesity (Silver Spring). Obesity (Silver Spring). (2009) 17(11): 2019–2024.

Chapter 18: Goal Setting

1. Healy ML et. al. Endocrine profiles in 693 elite athletes in the postcompetition setting. Clin Endocrinol (Oxf) (2014) 81(2):294-305.

2. Rynkiewicz M et. al. Body composition of male and female elite Polish sumo wrestlers in different weight category. J Combat Sports Martial Arts (2013) 2(2): 153-157

3. Johnson GO et. al.A physiological comparison of female body builders and power lifters. J Sports Med Phys Fitness. (1990) 30(4):361-4.

4. van der Ploeg GE et. al. Body composition changes in female bodybuilders during preparation for competition. Eur J Clin Nutr. (2001) 55(4):268-77.

5. Alway SE et. al. Contrasts in muscle and myofibers of elite male and female bodybuilders. J Appl Physiol (1985). (1989). 67(1):24-31.

6. Abe T et. al. Gender differences in FFM accumulation and architectural characteristics of muscle. Med Sci Sports Exerc. (1998) 30(7):1066-70.

7. Wamsteker EW et. al.Unrealistic weight-loss goals among obese patients are associated with age and causal attributions. J Am Diet Assoc. (2009) 109(11):1903-8.

8. Foster GD et. al.What is a reasonable weight loss? Patients' expectations and evaluations of obesity treatment outcomes. J Consult Clin Psychol. (1997) 65(1):79-85.

10. Dutton GR Weight loss goals of patients in a health maintenance organization. Eat Behav. (2010) 11(2):74-8.

11. Linde JA et. al.Are unrealistic weight loss goals associated with outcomes for overweight women? Obes Res. (2004) 12(3):569-76.

12..Reale R et. al.Acute Weight Loss Strategies for Combat Sports and Applications to Olympic Success. Int J Sports Physiol Perform. (2016) 24:1-30.

13. Fogelholm M et. al.Effects of bodyweight reduction on sports performance. Sports Med. (1994) 18(4):249-67.

14. Sundgot-Borgen J and I Garthe. Elite athletes in aesthetic and Olympic weight-class sports and the challenge of body weight and body compositions. J Sports Sci. (2011) 29 (Suppl 1):S101-14

Chapter 19: Calculating Nutrient Requirements

1. Marino M et.al.Nutrition and human health from a sex-gender perspective. Mol Aspects Med. (2011) 32(1):1-70.

2. Phillips SM et al. Protein "requirements" beyond the RDA: implications for optimizing health. Appl Physiol Nutr Metab. (2016) 9:1-8.

3. Paddon-Jones D. and H. Leidy. Dietary protein and muscle in older persons Curr Opin Clin Nutr Metab Care. (2014) 17(1): 5–11.

3a. Phillips SM1, Van Loon LJ. Dietary protein for athletes: from requirements to optimum adaptation. J Sports Sci. (2011) 29 (Suppl 1):S29-38.

4. Simpson SJ, Raubenheimer D. Obesity: the protein leverage hypothesis. Obes Rev. (2005);6(2):133-42.

5. Helms ER et. al.A systematic review of dietary protein during caloric restriction in resistance trained lean athletes: a case for higher intakes. Int J Sport Nutr Exerc Metab. (2014) 24(2):127-38.

6. Martens EA1, Westerterp-Plantenga MS. Protein diets, body weight loss and weight maintenance. Curr Opin Clin Nutr Metab Care. (2014) 17(1):75-9.

7. Layman DK et. al.Dietary protein and exercise have additive effects on body composition during weight loss in adult women. J Nutr. (2005) 135(8):1903-10.

8. Antonio J et. al. A high protein diet (3.4 g/kg/d) combined with a heavy resistance training program improves body composition in healthy trained men and women--a follow-up investigation. J Int Soc Sports Nutr. 2015 Oct 20;12:39.

9. Martin WF et. al. Dietary protein intake and renal function. Nutr Metab (2005) 2: 25.

10. Poortmans JR and Dellalieux O. Do regular high protein diets have potential health risks on kidney function in athletes? Int J Sport Nutr Exerc Metab. (2000) 10(1):28-38

11. Bonjour JP. Dietary protein: an essential nutrient for bone health. J Am Coll Nutr. (2005) 24(6 Suppl):526S-36S.

12. Elmadfa I, Freisling H. Fat intake, diet variety and health promotion. Forum Nutr. (2005) (57):1-10.

13. Wyness L.The role of red meat in the diet: nutrition and health benefits. Proc Nutr Soc. 2015 Dec 8:1-6.

14. Biesalski HK. Meat and cancer: meat as a component of a healthy diet. Eur J Clin Nutr. (2002) 56 Suppl 1:S2-11.

15. Tarnopolsky M.Protein requirements for endurance athletes Nutrition. 2004 Jul-Aug;20(7-8):662-8.

16. Houltham SD and DS Rowlands. A snapshot of nitrogen balance in endurance-trained women. Appl Physiol Nutr Metab. (2014) 39(2):219-25.

17. Volek JS et. al. Nutritional aspects of women strength athletes. Br J Sports Med. (2006) 40(9):742-8.

18. Tobias DK et. al. Effect of low-fat diet interventions versus other diet interventions on long-term weight change in adults: a systematic review and meta-analysis. Lancet Diabetes Endocrinol. (2015) 3(12):968-79.

19. Fleming JA, Kris-Etherton PM. Macronutrient Content of the Diet: What Do We Know About Energy Balance and Weight Maintenance? Curr Obes Rep. (2016) 5(2):208-13

20. McDevitt RM et. al. Macronutrient disposal during controlled overfeeding with glucose, fructose,

sucrose, or fat in lean and obese women. Am J Clin Nutr. (2000) 72(2):369-77.

21. Venkatraman JT et. al. Dietary fats and immune status in athletes: clinical implications. Med Sci Sports Exerc. (2000) 32(7 Suppl):S389-95.

22. Gerlach KE et. al. Fat intake and injury in female runners. J Int Soc Sports Nutr. (2008) 5:1.

23. Horvath PJ et. al.The effects of varying dietary fat on the nutrient intake in male and female runners. J Am Coll Nutr. (2000) 19(1):42-51.

24. Riccardi G1, Rivellese AA. Dietary treatment of the metabolic syndrome--the optimal diet. Br J Nutr. (2000) 83 (Suppl 1):S143-8.

25. Moran LJ et. al. Dietary composition in the treatment of polycystic ovary syndrome: a systematic review to inform evidence-based guidelines. J Acad Nutr Diet. (2013) 113(4):520-45.

26. Slater G and SM Phillips. Nutrition guidelines for strength sports: sprinting, weightlifting, throwing events, and bodybuilding. J Sports Sci. (2011) 29 (Suppl 1):S67-77.

27. Stellingwerff T et. al. Nutrition for power sports: middle-distance running, track cycling, rowing, canoeing/kayaking, and swimming. J Sports Sci. (2011); 29 (Suppl 1):S79-89.

28. Holway FE and LL Spriet. Sport-specific nutrition: practical strategies for team sports. J Sports Sci.(2011) 29 (Suppl 1):S115-25.

29. Sundgot-Borgen J and I Garthe. Elite athletes in aesthetic and Olympic weight-class sports and the challenge of body weight and body compositions. J Sports Sci. (2011) 29 (Suppl 1):S101-14.

30. Paoli A. Ketogenic diet for obesity: friend or foe? Int J Environ Res Public Health. (2014)11:2092-107.

30a. Esposity, T et. al. Effects of low-carbohydrate diet therapy in overweight subjects with autoimmune thyroiditis: possible synergism with ChREBP Drug Des Devel Ther. (2016) 10: 2939–2946.

31. Gesta S et. al. In vitro and in vivo impairment of alpha2-adrenergic receptor-dependent antilipolysis by fatty acids in human adipose tissue. Horm Metab Res. (2001) 33(12):701- 7.

32. Burke LM Sports Med. Re-Examining High-Fat Diets for Sports Performance: Did We Call the 'Nail in the Coffin' Too Soon? (2015) 45 (Suppl 1):S33-49.

38. Geiker NR et. al. A weight-loss program adapted to the menstrual cycle increases weight loss in healthy, overweight, premenopausal women: a 6-mo randomized controlled trial. Am J Clin Nutr (2016) 104(1):15-20

Chapter 20: Nutrient Sources, Electrolytes, Fluids and Diet Products

1. McClung JP et. al. Female athletes: a population at risk of vitamin and mineral deficiencies affecting health and performance. J Trace Elem Med Biol. (2014) 28(4):388-92.

2. Manore MM. Dietary recommendations and athletic menstrual dysfunction. Sports Med. (2002) 32(14):887-901.

2a. Rossi A et. al.Fibromyalgia and nutrition: what news? Clin Exp Rheumatol. (2015) 33(1 Suppl 88):S117-25.

2b. Murray-Kolb LE.Iron status and neuropsychological consequences in women of reproductive age: what do we know and where are we headed? J Nutr. (2011) 141(4):747S-755S.

2c. Petkus DL et, ak, The Unexplored Crossroads of the Female Athlete Triad and Iron Deficiency: A Narrative Review. Sports Med. (2017) Mar 13. doi: 10.1007/s40279-017-0706-2.

3. Hess SY. The impact of common micronutrient deficiencies on iodine and thyroid metabolism: the evidence from human studies. Best Pract Res Clin Endocrinol Metab. (2010) 24(1):117-32.

4. Weaver CM. The role of nutrition on optimizing peak bone mass. Asia Pac J Clin Nutr. (2008);17 (Suppl 1):135-7.

5. von Hurst PR and K. Vitamin D and skeletal muscle function in athletes. Curr Opin Clin Nutr Metab Care. (2014) 17(6):539-45.

5a. Nair R and A. Maseeh. Vitamin D: The "sunshine" vitamin. J Pharmacol Pharmacother. (2012) 3(2): 118–126.

6. Lanham-New SA.Importance of calcium, vitamin D and vitamin K for osteoporosis prevention and treatment. Proc Nutr Soc. (2008) 67(2):163-76.

7. García OP Impact of micronutrient deficiencies on obesity. Nutr Rev. (2009) 67(10):559-72.

7a. Palmery M et. al.Oral contraceptives and changes in nutritional requirements. Eur Rev Med Pharmacol Sci. (2013) 17(13):1804-13

8. Ganapathy S and SL Volpe. Zinc, exercise, and thyroid hormone function. Crit Rev Food Sci Nutr. (1999) 39(4):369-90.

9. Beard J1, Tobin B. Iron status and exercise. Am J Clin Nutr. (2000) 72(2 Suppl):594S-7S.

9a. Kretsch MJ et. al.Cognitive function, iron status, and hemoglobin concentration in obese dieting women. Eur J Clin Nutr. (1998) 52(7):512-8.

10. Barr SI, Rideout CA.Nutritional considerations for vegetarian athletes. Nutrition.(2004) 20:696-703.

10a. 6. Coad J1, Conlon C. Iron deficiency in women: assessment, causes and consequences. Curr Opin Clin Nutr Metab Care. (2011) 14(6):625-34.

10b. Elmadfa I, Freisling H. Fat intake, diet variety and health promotion. Forum Nutr. (2005) (57):1-10.

11. Biesalski HK.Meat and cancer: meat as a component of a healthy diet. Eur J Clin Nutr. (2002) 56 Suppl 1:S2-11.

12. Lyle RM et. al. Iron status in exercising women: the effect of oral iron therapy vs increased consumption of muscle foods. Am J Clin Nutr. (1992) 56(6):1049-55.

13. Miranda, JM et. al.Egg and Egg-Derived Foods: Effects on Human Health and Use as Functional Foods Nutrients. (2015) 7(1): 706–729.

14. Melnik BC1, Schmitz G. Role of insulin, insulin-like growth factor-1, hyperglycaemic food and milk consumption

in the pathogenesis of acne vulgaris. Exp Dermatol. (2009) 18(10):833-41.

15. Dougkas A et. al.Associations between dairy consumption and body weight: a review of the evidence and underlying mechanisms. Nutr Res Rev. (2011) 24(1):72-95

16. Josse AR et. al.Increased consumption of dairy foods and protein during diet- and exercise-induced weight loss promotes fat mass loss and lean mass gain in overweight and obese premenopausal women. J Nutr. (2011) 141(9):1626-34.

16a. Josse AR and SM Phillips. Impact of milk consumption and resistance training on body composition of female athletes. Med Sport Sci. (2012);59:94-103.

17. McGregorcor RA and SD Poppitt. Milk protein for improved metabolic health: a review of the evidence. Nutr Metab (Lond). (2013) 10: 46.

17a. Panahi S and A Tremblay. The Potential Role of Yogurt in Weight Management and Prevention of Type 2 Diabetes. J Am Coll Nutr. 35(8):717-731.

18. Calder PC1, Yaqoob P.Omega-3 polyunsaturated fatty acids and human health outcomes. Biofactors. (2009) 35(3):266-72.

19. Simopoulos AP.Omega-3 fatty acids in inflammation and autoimmune diseases. J Am Coll Nutr. (2002) 21(6):495-505.

20. Navarini L et. al. Polyunsaturated fatty acids: any role in rheumatoid arthritis? Lipids Health Dis. 2017 Oct 10;16(1):197.

20a. Wilson PB and LA Madrigal. Associations among Omega-3 Fatty Acid Status, Anxiety, and Mental Toughness in Female Collegiate Athletes. J Am Coll Nutr. (2017) Sep 14:1-6.

20b. Buckley JD1, Howe PR. Anti-obesity effects of long-chain omega-3 polyunsaturated fatty acids. Obes Rev. (2009) 10(6):648-59

21. Visioli F et. al. Dietary intake of fish vs. formulations leads to higher plasma concentrations of n-3 fatty acids. Lipids. (2003) 38(4):415-8.

21a. Plourde M, Cunnane SC. Extremely limited synthesis of long chain polyunsaturates in adults: implications for their dietary essentiality and use as supplements. Appl Physiol Nutr Metab. (2007) Aug;32(4):619-34.

21b. Giltay EJ et. al.Docosahexaenoic acid concentrations are higher in women than in men because of estrogenic effects. Am J Clin Nutr. (2004) 80(5):1167-74.

22. Grundy SM What is the desirable ratio of saturated, polyunsaturated, and monounsaturated fatty acids in the diet? Am J Clin Nutr. (1997) 66(4 Suppl):988S-990S.

23. White JS. Straight talk about high-fructose corn syrup: what it is and what it ain't. Am J Clin Nutr. (2008) 88(6):1716S-1721S.

24. Wolf A et. al. A short history of beverages and how our body treats them.Obes Rev.(2008) 9(2):151-64.

25. Choo VL and Sievenpiper JL. The ecologic validity of fructose feeding trials: supraphysiological feeding of fructose in human trials requires careful consideration when drawing conclusions on cardiometabolic risk. Front Nutr. (2015) 6;2:12

26. World Health Organization . Guideline: Sugars Intake for Adults and Children. World Health Organization; Geneva, Switzerland: (2015). pp. 1–49.

27. Biesiekierski JR et. al. Nutr Clin Pract. Characterization of Adults With a Self-Diagnosis of Nonceliac Gluten Sensitivity. (2014) 16;29(4):504-509.

27a. Vici G et. al. Gluten free diet and nutrient deficiencies: A review. Clin Nutr. (2016) 5(6):1236-1241

28. Higdon JV et. al. Cruciferous Vegetables and Human Cancer Risk: Epidemiologic Evidence and Mechanistic Basis. Pharmacol Res. (2007) 55(3): 224–236.

29. Tan J et. al.The role of short-chain fatty acids in health and disease. Adv Immunol. (2014);121:91-119.

30. Cordain L et. al. Origins and evolution of the Western diet: health implications for the 21st century. Am J Clin Nutr. (2005) 81(2):341-54.

31. Brownley KA et. Dietary sodium restriction alters postprandial ghrelin: implications for race differences in obesity. al. Ethn Dis. (2006) 16(4):844-51.

32. Thys-Jacobs S et. al. Calcium carbonate and the premenstrual syndrome: effects on premenstrual and menstrual symptoms. Premenstrual Syndrome Study Group. Am J Obstet Gynecol. (1998) 179(2):444-52.

33. Popkin BM et. al. Water, hydration, and health. Nutr Rev. (2010) 68(8):439-58.

34. Daniels MC1, Popkin BM. Impact of water intake on energy intake and weight status: a systematic review. Nutr Rev. (2010) 68(9):505-21.

34a. Thornton SN. Increased Hydration Can Be Associated with Weight Loss. Front Nutr. (2016) 3: 18.

35. Zhang Ye et. al.Caffeine and diuresis during rest and exercise: A meta-analysis. J Sci Med Sport. (2015) 18(5):569-74.

36. DiMeglio DP and RD Mattes. Liquid versus solid carbohydrate: effects on food intake and body weight. Int J Obes Relat Metab Disord. (2000) 24(6):794-800.

37. Rogers PJ et. al.Does low-energy sweetener consumption affect energy intake and body weight? A systematic review, including meta-analyses, of the evidence from human and animal studies. Int J Obes (Lond). (2016) 40(3):381-94

38 Phelan, S et. al.Use of artificial sweeteners and fat-modified foods in weight loss maintainers and always normal weight individuals Int J Obes (Lond). (2009) 33(10): 1183–1190.

39. Peters, JC et. al. The effects of water and non- nutritive sweetened beverages on weight loss and weight maintenance: A randomized clinical trial Obesity (Silver Spring). (2016) 24(2): 297–304.

40. Greenberg JA et. al. Coffee, diabetes, and weight control. Am J Clin Nutr. (2006) 84(4):682-93.

41. Patwardhan RV et. al. Impaired elimination of caffeine by oral contraceptive steroids. J Lab Clin Med. (1980) 95(4):603-8.

41a. Heaney RP. Effects of caffeine on bone and the calcium economy. Food Chem Toxicol. (2002) 40(9):1263-70.

42. Ilich JZ1, Kerstetter JE. Nutrition in bone health revisited: a story beyond calcium. J Am Coll Nutr. (2000) 19(6):715-37.

43. Hetherington MM1, Boyland E. Short-term effects of chewing gum on snack intake and appetite. Appetite. (2007) 48(3):397-401.

44. Shikany JM et. al. Randomized controlled trial of chewing gum for weight loss. Obesity (Silver Spring). (2012) 20(3):547-52.

45. Heymsfield SB et. al.Weight management using a meal replacement strategy: meta and pooling analysis from six studies. Int J Obes Relat Metab Disord. (2003) 27(5):537-49.

Chapter 21: Flexible Eating Strategies

1. Byrne, NM et. al. Intermittent energy restriction improves weight loss efficiency in obese men: the MATADOR study. Int J Obes (2017). [Epub befpre print]

1a. Westerterp-Plantenga MS et. al. High protein intake sustains weight maintenance after body weight loss in humans. Int J Obes Relat Metab Disord. (2004) 28(1):57-64.

2. Swift DL et. al. The role of exercise and physical activity in weight loss and maintenance. Prog Cardiovasc Dis. (2014) 56(4):441-7.

3. Acheson KJ et. al. Glycogen storage capacity and de novo lipogenesis during massive carbohydrate overfeeding in man. Am J Clin Nutr. (1988) 48(2):240-7.

4. Le DS et. al. Less activation in the left dorsolateral prefrontal cortex in the reanalysis of the response to a meal in obese than in lean women and its association with successful weight loss. Am J Clin Nutr. (2007) 86(3):573-9.

5. Paul J. Kenny. Reward Mechanisms in Obesity: New Insights and Future DirectionsNeuron. (2011) 69(4): 664–679.

6. Hebebrand J et. al."Eating addiction", rather than "food addiction", better captures addictive-like eating behavior. Neurosci Biobehav Rev. (2014) 47:295-306.

7. Gorczyca AM et. al. Changes in macronutrient, micronutrient, and food group intakes throughout the menstrual cycle in healthy, premenopausal women. Eur J Nutr. (2015) 55(3):1181-8

8. Michener W1, Rozin P. Pharmacological versus sensory factors in the satiation of chocolate craving. Physiol Behav. (1994). 56(3):419-22.

9. Bruinsma K and Taren DL. Chocolate: food or drug? J Am Diet Assoc. (1999) 99(10):1249-56.

10. Martin FP et. al. Metabolic effects of dark chocolate consumption on energy, gut microbiota, and stress-related metabolism in free-living subjects. J Proteome Res.(2009) 8(12):5568-79.

Chapter 22: Around Workout Nutrition

1. Denison, HJ et. al.Prevention and optimal management of sarcopenia: a review of combined exercise and nutrition interventions to improve muscle outcomes in older people.Clin Interv Aging (2015)10:859-69.

2. Goulet ED. Effect of exercise-induced dehydration on endurance performance: evaluating the impact of exercise protocols on outcomes using a meta-analytic procedure. Br J Sports Med. (2013) 47(11):679-86.

3. Cotter JD et. al. Are we being drowned in hydration advice? Thirsty for more? Extrem Physiol Med. (2014) 3: 18.

4. Mayer EA et. al. Sex-based differences in gastrointestinal pain. Eur J Pain. (2004) 8(5):451-63.

5. de Oliveira EP et. al.Gastrointestinal complaints during exercise: prevalence, etiology, and nutritional recommendations. Sports Med. (2014) 44 (Suppl 1):S79-85.

5a. Haakonssen, EC et. al. The Effects of a Calcium-Rich Pre-Exercise Meal on Biomarkers of Calcium Homeostasis in Competitive Female Cyclists: A Randomised Crossover Trial. PLoS One. (2015) 10(5): e0123302.

6. Tipton KD et. al. Timing of amino acid-carbohydrate ingestion alters anabolic response of muscle to resistance exercise. Am J Physiol Endocrinol Metab. (2001) 281(2):E197-206.

7. Sims ST et. al. Preexercise sodium loading aids fluid balance and endurance for women exercising in the heat. J Appl Physiol (1985). (2007) 103(2):534-41.

8. Currell K and AE Jeukendrup. Superior endurance performance with ingestion of multiple transportable carbohydrates. Med Sci Sports Exerc. (2008) 40(2):275-81.

9. de Ataide e Silva T et. al. Can carbohydrate mouth rinse improve performance during exercise? A systematic review. Nutrients. (2013) 6(1):1-10.

10. Campbell SE et. al. Glucose kinetics and exercise performance during phases of the menstrual cycle: effect of glucose ingestion. Am J Physiol Endocrinol Metab. (2001) 281(4):E817-25.

10a. Hashimoto H et. al. Menstrual cycle phase and carbohydrate ingestion alter immune response following endurance exercise and high intensity time trial performance test under hot conditions. J Int Soc Sports Nutr. (2014) 11:39.

11. Van Loon, LJC. Is There a Need for Protein Ingestion During Exercise? Sports Med. (2014); 44(Suppl 1):105–111.

12. Kaciuba-Uscilko H and R Grucza. Gender differences in thermoregulation. Curr Opin Clin Nutr Metab Care. (2001) 4(6):533-6.

13. Marsh SA and DG Jenkins. Physiological responses to the menstrual cycle: implications for the development of heat illness in female athletes. Sports Med. (2002) 32(10):601-14.

13a. Hashimoto H et. al. The effect of the menstrual cycle and water consumption on physiological responses during prolonged exercise at moderate intensity in hot conditions. J Sports Med Phys Fitness. (2016) 56(9):951-60.

13b. Mee JA et. al. A comparison of males and females' temporal patterning to short- and long-term heat acclimation. Scand J Med Sci Sports. (2015) 25 (Suppl) 1:250-8.

14. Rosner MH, Kirven J. Exercise-associated hyponatremia. Clin J Am Soc Nephrol. (2007) 2:151-61.

15. Hausswirth C1, Le Meur Y. Physiological and nutritional aspects of post-exercise recovery: specific recommendations for female athletes. Sports Med. (2011) 41(10):861-82.

16. Witard OC et. al. Protein Considerations for Optimising Skeletal Muscle Mass in Healthy Young and Older Adults. Nutrients. (2016) 23;8(4):181

17. Kerksick CM et. al. International Society Sports Nutrition Position Stand: Nutrient Timing. JISSN (2017) 14:33

18. Areta JL Reduced resting skeletal muscle protein synthesis is rescued by resistance exercise and protein ingestion following short-term energy deficit. Am J Physiol Endocrinol Metab. (2014) 306(8):E989-97.

19. van Vliet S et. al. The Skeletal Muscle Anabolic Response to Plant- versus Animal-Based Protein Consumption. J Nutr. (2015) 145(9):1981-91.

20. Devries MC1, Phillips SM. Supplemental protein in support of muscle mass and health: advantage whey. J Food Sci. (2015) 80 (Suppl 1):A8-A15.

21. Babault N et. al. Pea proteins oral supplementation promotes muscle thickness gains during resistance training: a double-blind, randomized, Placebo-controlled clinical trial vs. Whey protein. J Int Soc Sports Nutr. (2015) 12(1):3.

22. Jentjens R and A Jeukendrup. Determinants of post-exercise glycogen synthesis during short-term recovery. Sports Med. (2003) 33(2):117-44.

23. Betts JA, Williams C. Short-term recovery from prolonged exercise: exploring the potential for protein ingestion to accentuate the benefits of carbohydrate supplements. Sports Med. (2010) 40(11):941-59.

24. Roy BD. Milk: the new sports drink? A Review J Int Soc Sports Nutr. (2008) 5: 15.

25. Desbrow B et. al. Comparing the rehydration potential of different milk-based drinks to a carbohydrate-electrolyte beverage. Appl Physiol Nutr Metab. (2014) 39(12):1366-72.

26. Saunders MJ. Carbohydrate-protein intake and recovery from endurance exercise: is chocolate milk the answer? Curr Sports Med Rep. (2011) 10(4):203-10.

27. Pritchett K1, Pritchett R. Chocolate milk: a post-exercise recovery beverage for endurance sports. Med Sport Sci. (2012) 59:127-34.

28. Hartman JW et. al. Consumption of fat-free fluid milk after resistance exercise promotes greater lean mass accretion than does consumption of soy or carbohydrate in young, novice, male weightlifters. Am J Clin Nutr. (2007) 86(2):373-81.

28a. Josse AR et. al. Body composition and strength changes in women with milk and resistance exercise. Med Sci Sports Exerc. (2010) 42(6):1122-30.

29. Jakeman JR et. al. Lower limb compression garment improves recovery from exercise-induced muscle damage in young, active females. Eur J Appl Physiol. (2010) 109(6):1137-44

30. Schoenfeld BJ et. al. Body composition changes associated with fasted versus non-fasted aerobic exercise. J Int Soc Sports Nutr. (2014) 11: 54.

31. Hawley JA et. al. Ramping up the signal: promoting endurance training adaptation in skeletal muscle by nutritional manipulation. Clin Exp Pharmacol Physiol. (2014) 41(8):608-13.

31a. Stannard SR et. al. Adaptations to skeletal muscle with endurance exercise training in the acutely fed versus overnight-fasted state. J Sci Med Sport. (2010) 13(4):465-9.

32. Deldicque L et. al. Increased p70s6k phosphorylation during intake of a protein-carbohydrate drink following resistance exercise in the fasted state. Eur J Appl Physiol. (2010) 108(4):791-800.

Chapter 23: Meal Frequency and Patterning

1. Quatela A et. al. The Energy Content and Composition of Meals Consumed after an Overnight Fast and Their Effects on Diet Induced Thermogenesis: A Systematic Review, Meta-Analyses and Meta-Regressions. Nutrients. (2016) O8(11). pii: E670.

1a. Kinabo JL and JV Durnin Effect of meal frequency on the thermic effect of food in women. Eur J Clin Nutr. (1990) 44(5):389-95.

2. Zauner C et. al. Resting energy expenditure in short-term starvation is increased as a result of an increase in serum norepinephrine. Am J Clin Nutr. (2000) 71(6):1511-5.

2a. Schoenfeld BJ et. al. Effects of meal frequency on weight loss and body composition: a meta-analysis Nutrition Reviews (2015) Vol. 73(2):69–82

3. Ohkawara K. Effects of increased meal frequency on fat oxidation and perceived hunger. Obesity (Silver Spring). (2013)21(2):336-43

4. Papakonstantinou E et. al. Effect of meal frequency on glucose and insulin levels in women with polycystic ovary syndrome: a randomised trial. Eur J Clin Nutr. (2016) 70(5):588-94

5. Moore DR et. al. Daytime pattern of post-exercise protein intake affects whole-body protein turnover in resistance-trained males. Nutr Metab (Lond). (2012) 16;9(1):91.

6. Trommelen J and LJ van Loon. Pre-Sleep Protein Ingestion to Improve the Skeletal Muscle Adaptive Response to Exercise Training. Nutrients. (2016) 8(12). pii: E763.

7. Jakubowicz D et. al.Effects of caloric intake timing on insulin resistance and hyperandrogenism in lean women with polycystic ovary syndrome. Clin Sci (Lond). (2013) 125(9):423-32.

8. Kinsey AW and MJ Ormsbee. The Health Impact of Nighttime Eating: Old and New Perspectives. Nutrients. (2015) Apr; 7(4): 2648–2662.

9. Arnal MA et. al. Protein pulse feeding improves protein retention in elderly women. Am J Clin Nutr. (1999) 69(6):1202-8.

10. Levitsky DA and CR Pacanowski. Effect of skipping breakfast on subsequent energy intake. Physiol Behav (2013) 2: 119:9-16.

11. Thomas EA et. al. Usual breakfast eating habits affect response to breakfast skipping in overweight women. Obesity (Silver Spring). (2015) 23(4):750-9.

12. Rothschild J et. al. Time-restricted feeding and risk of metabolic disease: a review of human and animal studies. Nutr Rev. (2014) 72(5):308-18.

13. Shephard RJ. The impact of Ramadan observance upon athletic performance. Nutrients. (2012) 4(6):491-505.

14. Tinsley GM et. al.Time-restricted feeding in young men performing resistance training: A randomized controlled trial. Eur J Sport Sci. (2016) 17(2):200-207

15. Moro T et. al.Effects of eight weeks of time-restricted feeding (16/8) on basal metabolism, maximal strength, body composition, inflammation, and cardiovascular risk factors in resistance-trained males. J Transl Med. (2016) 14(1):290.

15a. Harvie M and A Howell. Potential Benefits and Harms of Intermittent Energy Restriction and Intermittent Fasting Amongst Obese, Overweight and Normal Weight Subjects-A Narrative Review of Human and Animal Evidence. Behav Sci (Basel). (2017) 7(1).

16. Varady KA Intermittent versus daily calorie restriction: which diet regimen is more effective for weight loss? Obes Rev. (2011) 12(7):e593-601.

17. Davoodi SH et. al. Calorie Shifting Diet Versus Calorie Restriction Diet: A Comparative Clinical Trial Study Int J Prev Med. (2014) 5(4): 447–456.

18. Harvie, MN et. al. The effects of intermittent or continuous energy restriction on weight loss and metabolic disease risk markers: a randomised trial in young overweight women. Int J Obes (Lond). (2011) 35(5): 714–727.

19. Tinsley, GM et. al. Intermittent fasting programs and their effects on body composition: implications for weight-restricted sports. Strength & Conditioning Journal (2015) 37: 60-71.

20. http://paleoforwomen.com/shattering-the-myth-of-fasting-for-women-a-review-of-female-specific-responses-to-fasting-in-the-literature/Trommelen

21. http://andersnedergaard.dk/en/kropblog/intermittent-fasting-for-women/

22. Yavangi, M et. al.Does Ramadan fasting has any effects on menstrual cycles? Iran J Reprod Med. (2013) Feb; 11(2): 145–150.

23. Nair PM and PG Khawale. Role of therapeutic fasting in women's health: An overview. J Midlife Health. (2016) 7(2):61-4.

24. Hoddy KK et. al. Safety of alternate day fasting and effect on disordered eating behaviors. Nutr J. (2015) 14: 44.

25. Laessle RG et. al. Biological and psychological correlates of intermittent dieting behavior in young women. A model for bulimia nervosa. Physiol Behav. (1996) 60(1):1-5.

Chapter 24: Supplements

1. Chiou WB et. al. Ironic effects of dietary supplementation: illusory invulnerability created by taking dietary supplements licenses health-risk behaviors. Psychol Sci. (2011) 22(8):1081-6.

2. Chang YY and WB Chiou. Taking weight-loss supplements may elicit liberation from dietary control. A laboratory experiment. Appetite. (2014) 72:8-12.

2a. Kleiner SM et. al. Nutritional status of nationally ranked elite bodybuilders. Int J Sport Nutr. (1994) ;4(1):54-69.

2b. Ismaeel, A et. al. A Comparison of the Nutrient Intakes of Macronutrient-based Dieting and Strict Dieting Bodybuilders. Int J Sports Nutr Exerc Metab (2017) [Epub ahead of print]

3. García OP et. al. Impact of micronutrient deficiencies on obesity. Nutr Rev.(2009) 67(10):559-72.

4. Major GC Multivitamin and dietary supplements, body weight and appetite: results from a cross-sectional and a randomised double-blind placebo-controlled study. Br J Nutr. (2008) 99(5):1157-67.

4a. Major GC et. al. Multivitamin and dietary supplements, body weight and appetite: results from a cross-sectional and a randomised double-blind placebo-controlled study. Br J Nutr. (2008) 99(5):1157-67.

5. Omotayo O et. al. Modulation of Gut Microbiota in the Management of Metabolic Disorders: The Prospects and Challenges Int J Mol Sci. (2014) 15(3): 4158–4188.

5a. Conterno L et. al. Obesity and the gut microbiota: does up-regulating colonic fermentation protect against obesity and metabolic disease? Genes Nutr. (2011) 6(3): 241–260.

5b. Haro C et. al. Intestinal Microbiota Is Influenced by Gender and Body Mass Index. PLoS One. (2016) 26;11(5):e0154090.

6. De-Regil, L-M et. al. Iron Supplementation Benefits Physical Performance in Women of Reproductive Age: A Systematic Review and Meta-Analysis. J Nutr (2014) 144(6): 906-914.

7. Alaunyte I et. al. Iron and the female athlete: a review of dietary treatment methods for improving iron status and exercise performance. J Int Soc Sports Nutr. (2015) 6;12:38.

8. Tremblay A and JA Gilbert. Human obesity: is insufficient calcium/dairy intake part of the problem? J Am Coll Nutr. (2011) 30(5 Suppl 1):449S-53S.

8a. Mason C et. al. trial. Vitamin D3 supplementation during weight loss: a double-blind randomized controlled trial1,2,3 Am J Clin Nutr. (2014) 99(5): 1015–1025.

9. LeBlanc ES et. al. Vitamin D levels and menopause-related symptoms. Menopause. (2014) 21:1197-203

9a. Iolascon G et. al. Can vitamin D deficiency influence muscle performance in post-menopausal women? A multicenter retrospective study. Eur J Phys Rehabil Med. (2017) Jul 10. doi: 10.23736/S1973-9087.17.04533-6. [Epub ahead of print]

10. Buggio L et. al.Vitamin D and benign gynaecological diseases: A critical analysis of the current evidence. Gynecol Endocrinol. (2016) 32(4):259-63.

10a. Cannell JJ Athletic performance and vitamin D. Med Sci Sports Exerc. (2009) 41(5):1102-10.

10b. Bourre JM et al. Dietary omega-3 fatty acids for women. Biomed Pharmacother. (2007) 61(2-3):105-12.

11. Filho, EAR et. al.Essential fatty acids for premenstrual syndrome and their effect on prolactin and total cholesterol levels: a randomized, double blind, placebo-controlled study Reprod Health. (2011) Jan 17;8:2

11a. Noreen EE et. al.Effects of supplemental fish oil on resting metabolic rate, body composition, and salivary cortisol in healthy adults J Int Soc Sports Nutr. 2010; 7: 31. Published online (2010) Oct 8.

12. Sampalis F et. al.Evaluation of the effects of Neptune Krill Oil on the management of premenstrual syndrome and dysmenorrhea. Altern Med Rev. (2003) 8(2):171-9.

13. Zofková I et. al. Trace elements and bone health. Clin Chem Lab Med .(2013) Aug;51(8):1555-61

14. Maxwell C1, Volpe SL. Effect of zinc supplementation on thyroid hormone function. A case study of two college females. Ann Nutr Metab. (2007) 51(2):188-94.

15. Radziwoń-Zaleska M et.al. Antidepressant activity of zinc and magnesium in view of the current hypotheses of antidepressant action. Pharmacol Rep. (2008) 60(5):588-9.

15a. Parazzini F et. al. Magnesium in the gynecological practice: a literature review. Magnes Res. (2017) 30(1):1-7.

16. Phillips SM. The science of muscle hypertrophy: making dietary protein count. Proc Nutr Soc. (2011) 70(1):100-3.

17. Patisaul HB and W. Jeferson. The pros and cons of phytoestrogens. Front Neuroendocrinol. (2010) 31(4): 400–419.

18. Patisaul HB. Endocrine disruption by dietary phyto-oestrogens: impact on dimorphic sexual systems and behaviours. Proc Nutr Soc. (2017) 76(2):130-144

19. Hooper L. et. al. Effects of soy protein and isoflavones on circulating hormone concentrations in pre- and post-menopausal women: a systematic review and meta-analysis Hum Reprod Update. (2009) 15(4): 423–440.

20. Bryant M et. al. Effect of consumption of soy isoflavones on behavioural, somatic and affective symptoms in women with premenstrual syndrome. Br J Nutr. (2005)93(5):731-9.

201. Sunita P and SP Pattanayak. Phytoestrogens in postmenopausal indications: A theoretical perspective Pharmacogn Rev. (2011) 5(9): 41–47.

22. Messina M, Redmond G. Effects of soy protein and soybean isoflavones on thyroid function in healthy adults and hypothyroid patients: a review of the relevant literature. Thyroid. (2006) 16:249-58.

22a. Marritt RJ and BH Jenks. Safety of Soy-Based Infant Formulas Containing Isoflavones: The Clinical Evidence. J. Nutr. (2004) 134 (5): 1220S-1224S

22b. Vandenplas Y et. al. Safety of soya-based infant formulas in children. Br J Nutr. (2014) 28;111(8):1340-60

23. Mesiano S et. al.Phytoestrogens alter adrenocortical function: genistein and daidzein suppress glucocorticoid and stimulate androgen production by cultured adrenal cortical cells. J Clin Endocrinol Metab. (1999) 84(7):2443-8.

24. Velasquez MT. Role of Dietary Soy Protein in Obesity. Int J Med Sci. (2007) 4(2): 72–82.

24a. Wang S et. al. Anti-obesity molecular mechanism of soy isoflavones: weaving the way to new therapeutic routes. Food Funct. (2017) 8(11):3831-3846

25. Jamilian M amd Z Asemi. The Effects of Soy Isoflavones on Metabolic Status of Patients With Polycystic Ovary Syndrome. J Clin Endocrinol Metab. (2016) 101(9):3386-94

26. Dante G and Facchinetti F.Herbal treatments for alleviating premenstrual symptoms: a systematic review J Psychosom Obstet Gynaecol. (2011) 32(1):42-51

27. van Die MD et. al. Vitex agnus-castus extracts for female reproductive disorders: a systematic review of clinical trials. Planta Med. (2013) 79(7):562-75.

28. Marjoribanks J et. al. Nonsteroidal anti-inflammatory drugs for dysmenorrhoea. Cochrane Database Syst Rev. (2015) Jul 30;(7):CD001751.

28a. Lewy AJ et. al. The circadian basis of winter depression. Proc Natl Acad Sci U S A. (2006) 103(19): 7414–7419.

29. Genazzani AD et al. Acetyl-L-carnitine (ALC) administration positively affects reproductive axis in hypogonadotropic women with functional hypothalamic amenorrhea. J Endocrinol Invest. (2011) 34(4):287-91.

30. Genazzani AD et. al.Acetyl-l-carnitine as possible drug in the treatment of hypothalamic amenorrhea. Acta Obstet Gynecol Scand. (1991) 70(6):487-92.

30a. Genazzani AD et. al. Modulatory effects of l-carnitine plus l-acetyl-carnitine on neuroendocrine control of hypothalamic functions in functional hypothalamic amenorrhea (FHA). Gynecol Endocrinol. (2017) 33(12):963-967

31. Nadjarzadeh A. et. al.The effect of omega-3 supplementation on androgen profile and menstrual status in women with polycystic ovary syndrome: A randomized clinical trial Iran J Reprod Med. (2013) 11(8): 665–672.

32. Foroozanfard F et al. Effects of zinc supplementation on markers of insulin resistance and lipid profiles in women with polycystic ovary syndrome: a randomized, double-blind, placebo-controlled trial. Exp Clin Endocrinol Diabetes. (2015) 123(4):215-20.

32a. Ebrahimi A et. al. The Effects of Magnesium and Zinc Co-Supplementation on Biomarkers of Inflammation and Oxidative Stress, and Gene Expression Related to Inflammation in Polycystic Ovary Biol Trace Elem Res. (2017) Nov 10. doi: 10.1007/s12011-017-1198-5. [Epub ahead of print}

32b. Jafari-Sfidvajani A et. al. The effect of vitamin D supplementation in combination with low-calorie diet on anthropometric indices and androgen hormones in women with polycystic ovary syndrome: a double-blind, randomized, placebo-controlled trial. J Endocrinol Invest. (2017) Nov 6. doi: 10.1007/s40618-017-0785-9. [Epub ahead of print]

33. Wehr E et. al. Association of hypovitaminosis D with metabolic disturbances in polycystic ovary syndrome Eur J Endocrinol. (2009) 161(4):575-82.

33a. Foroozanfard F et. al. Effect of Two Different Doses of Vitamin D Supplementation on Metabolic Profiles of Insulin-Resistant Patients with Polycystic Ovary Syndrome: A Randomized, Double-Blind, Placebo-Controlled Trial. Horm Metab Res. (2017) Jul 5. doi: 10.1055/s-0043-112346. [Epub ahead of print]

34. Tagliaferri V et. al. Melatonin Treatment May Be Able to Restore Menstrual Cyclicity in Women With PCOS: A Pilot Study. Reprod Sci. (2017) Jan 1 doi: 10.1177/1933719117711262. [Epub ahead of print]

35.. Masharani U et. al.Effects of Controlled-Release Alpha Lipoic Acid In Lean, Nondiabetic Patients with Polycystic Ovary Syndrome J Diabetes Sci Technol. (2010) 4(2): 359–364

36. Fulghesu AM et. al. N-acetyl-cysteine treatment improves insulin sensitivity in women with polycystic ovary syndrome.Fertil Steril. (2002) 77(6):1128-35.

37. Javanmanesh F et. al. Gynecol Endocrinol.A comparison between the effects of metformin and N-acetyl cysteine (NAC) on some metabolic and endocrine characteristics of women with polycystic ovary syndrome. Gynecol Endocrinol (2015) 32(4):285-9

38. Kort DH1, Lobo RA1. Preliminary evidence that cinnamon improves menstrual cyclicity in women with polycystic ovary syndrome: a randomized controlled trial. Am J Obstet Gynecol. (2014) 211(5):487.e1-6.

39. Sedigheh Amooee et al. Metformin versus chromium picolinate in clomiphene citrate-resistant patients with PCOs: A double-blind randomized clinical trial Iran J Reprod Med. (2013) 11(8): 611–618.

40. Morgante G et. al. Polycystic ovary syndrome (PCOS) and hyperandrogenism: the role of a new natural association. Minerva Ginecol. (2015) 67(5):457-63.

40a. Samimi M et. al.The effects of coenzyme Q10 supplementation on glucose metabolism and lipid profiles in women with polycystic ovary syndrome: a randomized, double-blind, placebo-controlled trial. Clin Endocrinol (Oxf). (2016) 86(4):560-566

41. Bevilacqua A and M Bizzarri. Physiological role and clinical utility of inositols in polycystic ovary syndrome. Best Pract Res Clin Obstet Gynaecol. (2016) 37:129-139.

42. Unfer V et. al. Effects of myo-inositol in women with PCOS: a systematic review of randomized controlled trials. Gynecol Endocrinol. (2012) 28(7):509-15.

43. Sacchinelli A et. al. The Efficacy of Inositol and N-Acetyl Cysteine Administration (Ovaric HP) in Improving the Ovarian Function in Infertile Women with PCOS with or without Insulin Resistance. Obstet Gynecol Int. (2014) 2014:141020.

44. Pizzo A1, Laganà AS, Barbaro L. Comparison between effects of myo-inositol and D-chiro-inositol on ovarian function and metabolic factors in women with PCOS. Gynecol Endocrinol. (2014) 30(3):205-8.

45. Schindler AE1.Climacteric symptoms and hormones. Gynecol Endocrinol. (2006) Mar;22(3):151-4.

45a. Maevsky EI et. al. A succinate-based composition reverses menopausal symptoms without sex hormone replacement therapy. Adv Gerontol. (2008) 21(2):298-305.

45b. Burchakov DI et. al. Treatment of climacteric symptoms with an ammonium succinate-based dietary supplement: a randomized, double-blind, placebo-controlled trial. Gynecol Endocrinol. (2016) 32(sup2):64-68.

46. Geller SE1, Studee L. Contemporary alternatives to plant estrogens for menopause. Maturitas. (2006) 55 (Suppl 1):S3-13.

47. Toffol E et. al. Melatonin in perimenopausal and postmenopausal women: associations with mood, sleep, climacteric symptoms, and quality of life. Menopause. (2014) 21(5):493-500.

48. Amstrup AK et. al. Reduced fat mass and increased lean mass in response to one year of melatonin treatment in postmenopausal women: A randomized placebo controlled trial.Clin Endocrinol (Oxf). (2015) 84(3):342-7.

49. Walecka-Kapica E et. al.The effect of melatonin supplementation on the quality of sleep and weight status in postmenopausal women. Prz Menopauzalny. (2014) 13(6):334-8.

50. Parandavar N et. al.The Effect of Melatonin on Climacteric Symptoms in Menopausal Women; A Double-Blind, Randomized Controlled, Clinical Trial Iran J Public Health. (2014) 43(10): 1405–1416.

52. Kotlarczyk MP et. al. Melatonin osteoporosis prevention study (MOPS): a randomized, double-blind, placebo-controlled study examining the effects of melatonin on bone health and quality of life in perimenopausal women. J Pineal Res. (2012) 52(4):414-26.

52a. D'Anna R et. al. Myo-inositol and melatonin in the menopausal transition. Gynecol Endocrinol. (2016) 33(4):279-282

53.Labrie F.DHEA,important source of sex steroids in men and even more in women. Prog Brain Res.(2010)182:97-148.

54. Diepvens K. Obesity and thermogenesis related to the consumption of caffeine, ephedrine, capsaicin, and green tea. Am J Physiol Regul Integr Comp Physiol. (2007) 292(1):R77-85.

55. Greenberg JA et. al. Coffee, diabetes, and weight control. Am J Clin Nutr. (2006) 84(4):682-93.

55a. Harpaz E. et. al. The effect of caffeine on energy balance. J Basic Clin Physiol Pharmacol. (2016) 28(1):1-10.

55b. Davoodi, SH et. al. Caffeine Treatment Prevented from Weight Regain after Calorie Shifting Diet Induced Weight Loss. Iran J Pharm Res. (2014) 13(2): 707–718.

56. Abernethy DR, Todd EL. Impairment of caffeine clearance by chronic use of low-dose oestrogen-containing oral contraceptives. Eur J Clin Pharmacol. (1985) 28(4):425-8.

57. Shekelle PG et. al.Efficacy and safety of ephedra and ephedrine for weight loss and athletic performance: a meta-analysis. JAMA. (2003) 289(12):1537-45.

58. Astrup A Enhanced thermogenic responsiveness during chronic ephedrine treatment in man. Am J Clin Nutr. (1985) 42(1):83-94.

59. Lafontan M et. al.Alpha-2 adrenoceptors in lipolysis: alpha 2 antagonists and lipid-mobilizing strategies.Am J Clin Nutr.(1992)55(1 Suppl):219S-227S.

60. Graham TE Caffeine and exercise: metabolism, endurance and performance. Sports Med. (2001) 31(11):785-807.

61. Ganio MS et. al. Effect of caffeine on sport-specific endurance performance: a systematic review. J Strength Cond Res. (2009) 23(1):315-24.

62. Brooks et al. Caffeine Supplementation as an Ergogenic Aid for Muscular Strength and Endurance: A Recommendation for Coaches and Athletes. J Athl Enhanc (2016) 5:4

63. Goldstein E et. al.Caffeine enhances upper body strength in resistance-trained women. J Int Soc Sports Nutr. (2010) May 14;7:18.

64. Magkos F and SA Kavouras. Caffeine and ephedrine: physiological, metabolic and performance-enhancing effects. Sports Med. (2004) 34(13):871-89.

65. Tarnopolsky MA.Gender differences in metabolism; nutrition and supplements.J Sci Med Sport.(2000) 3:287-98.

66. Mihic S et. al. Acute creatine loading increases fat-free mass, but does not affect blood pressure, plasma creatinine, or CK activity in men and women. Med Sci Sports Exerc. (2000) 32(2):291-6.

67.Bemben MG and HS Lamont. Creatine supplementation and exercise performance: recent findings. Sports Med. (2005) 35(2):107-25.

68. Ellery SJ et. al. Creatine for women: a review of the relationship between creatine and the reproductive cycle and female-specific benefits of creatine therapy. Amino Acids. (2016) 48(8):1807-17

69. Candow DG et. al. Creatine supplementation and aging musculoskeletal health. Endocrine. (2014) 45(3):354-61.

70. Roitman S et. al.Creatine monohydrate in resistant depression: a preliminary study. Bipolar Disord. (2007) 9(7):754-8.

71. Saunders B et. al. β-alanine supplementation to improve exercise capacity and performance: a systematic review and meta-analysis. Br J Sports Med. (2016) 51:658-669.

72. Bennink HJ et. al. Maintaining physiological testosterone levels by adding dehydroepiandrosterone to combined oral contraceptives: I. Endocrine effects. Contraception. (2016) 96(5):322-329

Chapter 25: Estimating Dieting Times

1. Hall KD et. al. Quantification of the effect of energy imbalance on bodyweight. Lancet. (2011) 378(9793):826-37.

2. Koehler K et. al. Less-than-expected weight loss in normal-weight women undergoing caloric restriction and exercise is accompanied by preservation of fat-free mass and metabolic adaptations. Eur J Clin Nutr. (2016) 71(3):365-371

Chapter 26: Identifying and Breaking Plateaus

1. Schoeller DA et. al. Effect of dietary adherence on the body weight plateau: a mathematical model incorporating intermittent compliance with energy intake prescription. Am J Clin Nutr. (2014) 100(3):787-95.

2. Macdiarmid J and J Blundell. Assessing dietary intake: Who, what and why of under-reporting. Nutr Res Rev. (1998) 11(2):231-53.

3. de Castro JM. Weekly rhythms of spontaneous nutrient intake and meal pattern of humans. Physiol Behav. (1991) 50(4):729-38.

4. Gaillard RC et. al. Cytokines, leptin, and the hypothalamo-pituitary-adrenal axis. Ann N Y Acad Sci. (2000) 917:647-57.

5. Laaksonen DE Changes in abdominal subcutaneous fat water content with rapid weight loss and long-term weight maintenance in abdominally obese men and women. Int J Obes Relat Metab Disord. (2003) 27(6):677-83.

Chapter 27: Adjusting for Metabolic Adaptation

1. Byrne NM et. al. Does metabolic compensation explain the majority of less-than-expected weight loss in obese adults during a short-term severe diet and exercise intervention? Int J Obes (Lond). (2012) 36:1472-8.

2. Johannsen, DL et. al.Metabolic Slowing with Massive Weight Loss despite Preservation of Fat-Free Mass J Clin Endocrinol Metab. (2012) 97(7): 2489–2496.

3. Leibel RL et. al. Changes in energy expenditure resulting from altered body weight. N Engl J Med. (1995) 332(10):621-8.

4. Redman LM et. al. Metabolic and behavioral compensations in response to caloric restriction: implications for the maintenance of weight loss. PLoS One. (2009) 4(2):e4377.

5. Martin CK et. al. Effect of calorie restriction on the free-living physical activity levels of nonobese humans: results of three randomized trials. J Appl Physiol (1985) .(2011) 110(4):956-63

6. Halliday TM et. al.Dietary Intake, Body Composition, and Menstrual Cycle Changes during Competition Preparation and Recovery in a Drug-Free Figure Competitor: A Case Study. Nutrients. (2016) 20 8(11).

7. Price K et. al. Validation of the Fitbit One, Garmin Vivofit and Jawbone UP activity tracker in estimation of energy expenditure during treadmill walking and running. J Med Eng Technol. (2016) 5:1-8.

8.El-Amrawy F et. al. Are Currently Available Wearable Devices for Activity Tracking and Heart Rate Monitoring Accurate, Precise, and Medically Beneficial? Healthc Inform Res. (2015) 21(4): 315–320.

Chapter 28: Training Guidelines

1. Gulati M et. al. Heart rate response to exercise stress testing in asymptomatic women: the st. James women take heart project. Circulation. (2010) 122(2):130-7.

2. Mann T et. al. Methods of prescribing relative exercise intensity: physiological and practical considerations.Sports Med. (2013) 43(7):613-25.

3. Ekkekakis P et. al.The pleasure and displeasure people feel when they exercise at different intensities: decennial update and progress towards a tripartite rationale for exercise intensity prescription. Sports Med. (2011) 41(8):641-71.

4. Gibala MJ et. al. Physiological adaptations to low-volume, high-intensity interval training in health and disease J Physiol. (2012) 590(Pt 5): 1077–1084.

5. Keating SE et. al. A systematic review and meta-analysis of interval training versus moderate-intensity continuous training on body adiposity. Obes Rev. (2017) 8(8):943-964

6. Astorino TA et. al. Effect of periodized high intensity interval training (HIIT) on body composition and attitudes towards hunger in active men and women. Sports Med Phys Fitness. (2017) Jun 21. doi: 10.23736/S0022-4707.17.07297-8. [Epub ahead of print]

6. De Feo. Is high-intensity exercise better than moderate-intensity exercise for weight loss? Nutr Metab Cardiovasc Dis. (2013) 23(11):1037-42.

7. Thum JS et. al. High-Intensity Interval Training Elicits Higher Enjoyment than Moderate Intensity Continuous Exercise PLoS One. (2017) 12(1): e0166299.

8. Roxburgh BH et. al. Is Moderate Intensity Exercise Training Combined with High Intensity Interval Training More Effective at Improving Cardiorespiratory Fitness than Moderate Intensity Exercise Training Alone? J Sports Sci Med. (2014) 13(3): 702–707.

9. Cotter JA et. al. Ratings of Perceived Exertion During Acute Resistance Exercise Performed at Imposed and Self-Selected Loads in Recreationally Trained Women. J Strength Cond Res. (2017). 1(8):2313-2318

10. Helms ER et. al. Application of the Repetitions in Reserve-Based Rating of Perceived Exertion Scale for Resistance Training Strength Cond J. (2016) 38(4): 42–49.

11. Hackett DA et. al. Accuracy in Estimating Repetitions to Failure During Resistance Exercise. Journal of Strength & Conditioning Research. (2017) 31(8): 2162-2168.

12. Rhea MR et. al. A meta-analysis to determine the dose response for strength development. Med Sci Sports Exerc. (2003) 35(3):456-64.

13. Peterson MD et. al.Applications of the dose-response for muscular strength development: a review of meta-analytic efficacy and reliability for designing training prescription. J Strength Cond Res. (2005) 19(4):950-8.

14. Wernbom M et. al.The influence of frequency, intensity, volume and mode of strength training on whole muscle cross-sectional area in humans. Sports Med. (2007) 37(3):225-64.

15. Mujika I. Intense training: the key to optimal performance before and during the taper. Scand J Med Sci Sports. (2010) 20 (Suppl 2):24-31.

16. Bosquet L et. al. Effects of tapering on performance: a meta-analysis. Med Sci Sports Exerc. (2007) 39(8):1358-65.

Chapter 29: Sample Training Programs

1. Garber CE et. al. American College of Sports Medicine position stand. Quantity and quality of exercise for developing and maintaining cardiorespiratory, musculoskeletal, and neuromotor fitness in apparently healthy adults: guidance for prescribing exercise. Med Sci Sports Exerc. (2011) 43(7):1334-59.

2. Helms, E et. al. Evidence-based recommendations for natural bodybuilding contest preparation: nutrition and supplementation. Journal of the International Society of Sports Nutrition (2014) 11:20

3. Mujika I. Intense training: the key to optimal performance before and during the taper. Scand J Med Sci Sports. (2010) 20 (Suppl 2):24-31.

4. Bosquet L et. al. Effects of tapering on performance: a meta-analysis. Med Sci Sports Exerc. (2007) 39(8):1358-65.

5. Murach KA and JR Bagley. Skeletal Muscle Hypertrophy with Concurrent Exercise Training: Contrary Evidence for an Interference Effect. Sports Med. (2016) 46(8):1029-39

Chapter 31: The Category 2/3 Dieter

1. Wisse BE et. al. Effect of prolonged moderate and severe energy restriction and refeeding on plasma leptin concentrations in obese women. Am J Clin Nutr. (1999) 70(3):321-30.

2. Donnelly JE et. al. American College of Sports Medicine Position Stand. Appropriate physical activity intervention strategies for weight loss and prevention of weight regain for adults. Med Sci Sports Exerc. (2009) 41(2):459-71.
3. Jeffery RW Long-term maintenance of weight loss: current status. Health Psychol. (2000) 19(1 Suppl):5-16.
4. Hill JO et. al.The National Weight Control Registry: is it useful in helping deal with our obesity epidemic? J Nutr Educ Behav. (2005) 37(4):206-10.
5. Khaylis A et. al. A review of efficacious technology-based weight-loss interventions: five key components. Telemed J E Health. (2010) 16(9):931-8.
6. Butryn ML et. al. Consistent self-monitoring of weight: a key component of successful weight loss maintenance. Obesity (Silver Spring). (2007) 15(12):3091-6.
7. Tanenbaum ML et. al. Overeat today, skip the scale tomorrow: An examination of caloric intake predicting nonadherence to daily self-weighing. Obesity (Silver Spring). (2016) 24(11):2341-2343.
8. Stevens J et. al. The definition of weight maintenance. Int J Obes (Lond). (2006) 30(3):391-9.

Chapter 32: The Category 1 Dieter and Amenorrhea
1. Gesta S et. al. In vitro and in vivo impairment of alpha2-adrenergic receptor-dependent antilipolysis by fatty acids in human adipose tissue. Horm Metab Res. (2001) 33(12):701- 7.

Chapter 33: Ending the Category 1 Diet
1. Modolo V et. al. Negative addiction to exercise: are there differences between genders? Clinics (Sao Paulo). (2011) 66(2): 255–260.
2.Furst DM and K Germone. Negative addiction in male and female runners and exercisers. Percept Mot Skills. (1993) 77(1):192-4.
3. Ivey FM et. al. Effects of strength training and detraining on muscle quality: age and gender comparisons. J Gerontol A Biol Sci Med Sci. (2000) 55(3):B152-7; discussion B158-9.
2a. Oberle CD et. al. Orthorexic eating behaviors related to exercise addiction and internal motivations in a sample of university students. Eat Weight Disord. 2017 Dec 20. doi: 10.1007/s40519-017-0470-1. [Epub ahead of print]
4. Fozard JL et. al.Effects of age, gender, and myostatin genotype on the hypertrophic response to heavy resistance strength training. J Gerontol A Biol Sci Med Sci. (2000) 55(11):M641-8.
5. Walberg-Rankin J et. al. Diet and weight changes of female bodybuilders before and after competition. Int J Sport Nutr. (1993) 3(1):87-102.
6. Trexler ET et. al. Physiological Changes Following Competition in Male and Female Physique Athletes: A Pilot Study. Int J Sport Nutr Exerc Metab. (2017) 27(5):458-466.
7. Phillips KA and Diaz. Gender differences in body dysmorphic disorder. J Nerv Ment Dis. (1997) 185(9):570-7.
8. Phillips, KA et. al. Gender similarities and differences in 200 individuals with body dysmorphic disorder.Compr Psychiatry. (2006) 47(2): 77–87.
9. Dulloo AG. Collateral fattening: When a deficit in lean body mass drives overeating. Obesity (Silver Spring). (2017) 25(2):277-279.

Chapter 34: Studies of Dieting in Elite Athletes
1. Haakonssen EC et. al.Increased lean mass with reduced fat mass in an elite female cyclist returning to competition: case study. Int J Sports Physiol Perform. (2013) 8(6):699-701.
2. Stellingwerff T. Case-Study: Body Composition Periodization in an Olympic-Level Female Middle-Distance Runner Over a 9-Year Career. Int J Sport Nutr Exerc Metab. (2017) 15:1-19.
3. Hulmi JJ et. al. The Effects of Intensive Weight Reduction on Body Composition and Serum Hormones in Female Fitness Competitors. Front Physiol (2017) Jan 10. doi: 10.3389/fphys.2016.00689 [Epub before print]
4. Petrizzo J et. al. Case Study: The Effect of 32 Weeks of Figure-Contest Preparation on a Self-Proclaimed Drug-free Female's Lean Body and Bone Mass. Int J Sport Nutr Exerc Metab. (2017) 2:1-21.
5. Rohrig BJ et. al.Psychophysiological Tracking of a Female Physique Competitor through Competition Preparation.Int J Exerc Sci.(2017) 10(2):301-311.
6. Halliday TM et. al. Dietary Intake, Body Composition, and Menstrual Cycle Changes during Competition Preparation and Recovery in a Drug-Free Figure Competitor: A Case Study. Nutrients. (2016) 8(11). pii: E740.